Diseases of the Liver and Biliary Tract

Diseases of the Liver and Biliary Tract

EDITOR

Gary Gitnick, *M.D.*
Professor of Medicine
University of California, Los Angeles
Los Angeles, California

ASSOCIATE EDITORS

Douglas R. LaBrecque, *M.D.*
Professor of Medicine
Director of Liver Service
University of Iowa
Chief of Gastroenterology/Hepatology
VA Medical Center
Iowa City, Iowa

Frank G. Moody, *M.D.*
Denton A. Cooley Professor and Chairman
Department of Surgery
University of Texas Medical School
Houston, Texas

With 193 illustrations

Mosby Year Book

St. Louis Baltimore Boston Chicago London Philadelphia Sydney Toronto

Mosby Year Book

Dedicated to Publishing Excellence

Sponsoring Editors: Sandy Reinhardt and Stephanie Manning
Assistant Editor: Jane Petrash
Project Manager: Mark Spann
Production Editor: Christine M. Ripperda
Book Designer: Susan Lane

Printed in the United States of America

Mosby-Year Book, Inc.
11830 Westline Industrial Drive
St. Louis, Missouri 63146

Library of Congress Cataloging-in-Publication Data

Diseases of the liver and biliary tract / [edited by] Gary Gitnick, Douglas R. LaBrecque, Frank G. Moody.
p. cm.
Includes bibliographical references and index.
ISBN 0-8016-6075-0
1. Liver—Diseases. 2. Biliary tract—Diseases. I. Gitnick Gary II. LaBrecque, Douglas R. III. Moody, Frank G.
[DNLM: 1. Biliary Tract Diseases—physiopathology. 2. Liver Diseases—physiopathology. WI 700 D6115]
RC845.D56 1991
616.3′62—dc20
DNLM/DLC 91-18453
for Library of Congress CIP

C/MV/MV 9 8 7 6 5 4 3 2 1

Contributors

Bruce R. Bacon, *MD*
Professor of Internal Medicine
Director
Division of Gastroenterology and Hepatology
St. Louis University School of Medicine
St. Louis, Missouri

Alfred L. Baker, *MD*
Professor of Medicine
Director
Liver Study Unit
Department of Medicine
University of Chicago
Chicago, Illinois

Willliam F. Balistreri, *MD*
Dorothy M.M. Kersten Professor of Pediatrics
Director
Division of Pediatric Gastroenterology and Nutrition
University of Cincinnati Medical Center and Children's Hospital Medical Center
Cincinnati, Ohio

Neville Basman, *MD*
Fellow
Hepatology and Gastroenterology
Department of Medicine
University of Chicago
Chicago, Illinois

Michael Gerber, *MD*
Professor
Department of Pathology
Tulane University School of Medicine
New Orleans, Louisiana

C.N. Ghent, *MD, FRCP(C)*
Associate Professor
Department of Medicine
University of Western Ontario
London, Ontario
Canada

Charles F. Gholson, *MD*
Assistant Professor of Medicine
Department of Medicine and Gastroenterology
St. Louis University School of Medicine
St. Louis, Missouri

Patricia Greenwel, *MS*
Graduate Student
Department of Pathology
Albert Einstein College of Medicine of Yeshiva University
Bronx, New York

David A. Gremse, *MD*
Assistant Professor of Pediatrics
Director
Division of Pediatric Gastroenterology and Nutrition
University of South Alabama Medical Center
Mobile, Alabama

J. Michael Henderson, *MD*
Professor of Surgery
Department of Surgery
Emory University School of Medicine
Atlanta, Georgia

Frederick Johlin, *MD*
Assistant Professor
Department of Internal Medicine
University of Iowa
Iowa City, Iowa

Albert L. Jones, *MD*
Associate Chief of Staff for Research and Development
Professor of Medicine and Anatomy
University of California, San Francisco
San Francisco, California

Gary A. Levy, *MD*
Professor of Medicine
Director
Division of Gastroenterology
University of Toronto
Toronto
Canada

Kenneth L. Mattox, *MD*
Professor of Surgery
Baylor College of Medicine
Houston, Texas

S. Chris Pappas, *MD*
Assistant Professor
Department of Medicine
University of Toronto
Toronto
Canada

Robert P. Perrillo, *MD*
Professor of Medicine
Washington University School of Medicine
Chief of Gastroenterology
Veterans Administration Medical Center
St. Louis, Missouri

Fredric Regenstein, *MD*
Clinical Assistant Professor of Medicine
Gastroenterology Division
Tulane University School of Medicine
New Orleans, Louisiana

Robert J. Richardson, *MD*
Assistant Professor
Department of Surgery
Baylor College of Medicine
Houston, Texas

Charles Edwin Riggs, Jr., *MD*
Associate Professor of Internal Medicine
Department of Internal Medicine
College of Medicine
University of Iowa
Iowa City, Iowa

Marcos Rojkind, *MD*
Professor of Medicine and Pathology
Albert Einstein College of Medicine of Yeshiva University
Bronx, New York

Jerry L. Rosenblum, *MD*
Assistant Professor of Pediatrics
Washington University School of Medicine
St. Louis, Missouri

Robert J. Rothbaum, *MD*
Assistant Professor of Pediatrics
Division of Pediatric Gastroenterology and Nutrition
Washington University School of Medicine
St. Louis, Missouri

Byers W. Shaw, Jr., *MD*
Shackleford-Marischal Professor of Surgery
Department of Surgery
University of Nebraska Medical Center
Omaha, Nebraska

Stephen B. Sinclair, *MD*
Research Fellow
Division of Gastroenterology
University of Toronto
Toronto
Canada

Carlo H. Tamburro, *MD, MPH*
Professor of Medicine
Professor of Pharmacology and Toxicology
Chief
Division of Occupational Toxicology
University of Louisville School of Medicine
Louisville, Kentucky

Swan N. Thung, *MD*
Professor of Pathology
Department of Pathology
Mount Sinai School of Medicine
New York, New York

Cheree Trent-Mills, *MD*
Instructor of Medicine
Department of Internal Medicine and Gastroenterology
Washington University School of Medicine
St. Louis, Missouri

Michele Woodley, *MD*
Gastroenterology Fellow
Washington University School of Medicine
St. Louis, Missouri

Rowen Zetterman, *MD*
Professor of Internal Medicine
Department of Internal Medicine
University of Nebraska Medical Center
Omaha, Nebraska

This book is dedicated to my wife, **Cherna,**
who has consistently put up with my frequent absences,
and to my children, **Neil, Kim, Jill,** *and* **Tracy,**
from whom I took the time to develop this and other texts.
It is also dedicated to my brother, **Jerry,** *his wife,* **Saranne,**
their children, **Andrea** *and* **Nan Marie,**
and to my mother, **Ann,** *who made it all possible.*

Preface

In our own clinical practice of hepatology and in our teaching of students and house staff, the associate editors of this text and I saw a need for yet another textbook of liver disease. Although many comprehensive and excellent books are available, few of our students and colleagues were able to devote the time to reading these encyclopedic texts. Thus we perceived the need for a practical, clinically oriented text that was comprehensive and yet concise. To accomplish this seemingly impossible task, we chose to concentrate on facts and avoid the exposition of opinions or unproven concepts. Thus, although we cover pathophysiology throughout the book, we concentrate on only those areas that have been firmly established. The text is oriented to the needs of the clinician. However, it does provide an authoritative discussion of pathophysiology of each of the disease processes discussed and an understanding of liver function. The laboratory and clinical manifestations of liver disease are discussed, and diagnostic and treatment strategies are documented. In many areas, controversies persist regarding the appropriateness of diagnostic procedures and the applications of therapies. These controversies are discussed frankly, and the reader is allowed to make his or her own determinations. It is our hope that this text will serve to stimulate readers to expand their knowledge of the increasing spectrum of diseases of the liver. I am indebted to my associate editors, Douglas R. LaBrecque, M.D., and Frank G. Moody, M.D., for their exceptional efforts in developing a text that is streamlined to the needs of the clinician. I am also indebted to Susan Dashe, who diligently worked to bring together this text in a timely and efficient manner.

Gary Gitnick

Contents

SECTION FOUR **Disorders**

Diseases of the Liver and Biliary Tract

SECTION ONE

Basic Concepts

1 Introduction

Gary Gitnick

The design of the liver enables this complex organ to respond to unique functional demands. Comprising approximately 2.5% of total body weight, the liver metabolizes amino acids, carbohydrates, lipids, and vitamins. It also filters foreign substances and handles the products of heme metabolism. Intestinal substrates are taken up and stored, metabolized, and distributed to bile and to blood. Transformation in bile of drugs, toxins, and endogenous metabolites is another one of the liver's major functions. The liver distributes various substances, many of which are metabolites, to a variety of organs. Immune complexes enter the liver from the lymphatic system and from the spleen, and endotoxins enter from the intestine (where they are produced by bacterial flora). The sinusoidal lining cells of the liver are potent sources of phagocytosis and endocytosis. Finally, the liver participates in the regulation of blood volume and blood flow.

The organization of the vascular elements and parenchymal cells of the liver is specifically designed to interact with the digestive tract and other organ systems. This interaction is demonstrated by the liver's handling of amino acids, carbohydrates, lipids, vitamins, and a variety of pollutants that enter the body during ingestion of water or food. The uptake of substrates from the intestine and their subsequent storage, metabolism, and distribution by blood and bile are essential functions of the liver. The transformation of drugs, pollutants, and metabolites by complex biochemical mechanisms is an equally important function. These are simply examples of the many metabolic functions of the liver, all of which are affected by regulatory factors. The liver is an effective source of phagocytosis of materials, such as bacteria. It possesses certain unique features and functions.

The liver harbors exocrine and metabolic functions in the same cell. It has a double blood supply from the hepatic arterial and the portal systems. It also has a unique enterohepatic circulation, in which biliary solutes are reabsorbed in the intestine and then recirculated. The unique arrangement of cells facilitates the exchange between blood and liver cells. Vast biochemical activities between liver cells and the membranes of other cells regulate specific functions of the liver.

Disease states produce varying demands on the liver and may actually alter its structure. The process of tissue repair, involving regeneration of liver cells or formation of nodules, is well documented. Cirrhosis is characterized not only by these features but also by abnormal communication between the afferent and efferent blood supply. Cholestasis alters the relationship between the parasinusoidal spaces and the canaliculi, thereby altering bile flow. Thus structural and functional interrelationships exist in health and in disease. These interrelationships help to develop the important physiologic and biologic alterations that occur in both the normal and the diseased liver. These alterations are explained in greater depth in the chapters that follow.

This fascinating and complex organ is subject to a great variety of disease states. This text integrates a background in hepatic structure and function with an understanding of disease pathophysiology, diagnosis, and treatment. Advances in our understanding of liver disease have irrevocably changed previously held concepts. Among these advances has been the discovery of viruses associated with many forms of hepatitis. Viruses were initially implicated as causes of hepatitis A and hepatitis B and have now been documented as causes of hepatitis C, hepatitis D, and hepatitis E. It is likely that one or more additional hepatitis viruses also exists. We have witnessed the development of hepatitis vaccines and observed the relationship between chronic viral hepatitis and the development of chronic hepatitis and the subsequent development of cirrhosis and hepatocellular carcinoma. We have also found that interferon can improve symptoms and biochemical test results.

Primary sclerosing cholangitis has increased in incidence; fortunately there are new tools for its management, including ursodeoxycholic acid. Using new serologic assays, we can detect primary biliary cirrhosis at an earlier stage than before. New approaches to treatment include ursodeoxycholic acid, cyclosporine, and other, more controversial, approaches. We have seen the rapid development of hepatobiliary imaging and the usefulness of endoscopic diagnostic techniques, including endoscopic ultrasound. We have also extended endoscopy into the treatment arena with endoscopic sphincterotomy and extraction of common duct stones. Biliary monometry has assumed an important new role. We have new methods of lithotripsy and medical dissolution of gallstones. All of these advancements have provided new insights and new challenges.

In the case of ascites, new diuretics are more effective. Medical treatment of pyogenic liver abscesses has become possible, and hepatic transplantation has virtually revolutionized our approach to treatment of severe liver disease. Many other advances will be described in the chapters that follow.

These remarkable accomplishments in science and technology are outweighed by the continuing necessity to promote effective doctor-patient relationships. Advances only help patients who feel comfortable enough with their physicians to comply with treatment. The symptoms of the physical disease are only a small part of what patients with chronic diseases suffer. Nowhere in medicine is it more important for a physician to be both understanding and compassionate than in management of chronic liver disease. Most of our patients have diseases that last throughout their lives, which are likely to be shortened as a result of their disease; therefore effective treatment is based largely on the ability of the physician to communicate in an intelligent and compassionate manner. Too often physicians' adherence to scientific objectivity precludes their ability to treat patients who require not only science but also compassion. Regrettably, compassion cannot be taught by a book, only by example. The following text may enhance physicians' basic skills in diagnosis and treatment. It is hoped that the reader will complement these skills not only with the love of medicine but also with a sincere and dedicated attempt to treat the whole patient and not just the liver.

2 Morphology of the Liver

Albert L. Jones *and* ***Douglas R. LaBrecque***

GENERAL ORGANIZATIONAL STRUCTURE

The liver is the largest gland in the mammalian body. In the human neonate it accounts for one twentieth of the body weight, and in the adult it accounts for one fiftieth of the body weight. The most prominent cell in the liver is the hepatocyte, which accounts for 80% of the liver's volume. The liver of a 70 kg man reportedly contains 250 billion hepatocytes. The cells range from 20μm to 30 μm in diameter. They are polyhedral and are arranged in plates interspersed between vascular channels or sinusoids (Figure 2-1). Centrally located between adjacent hepa-

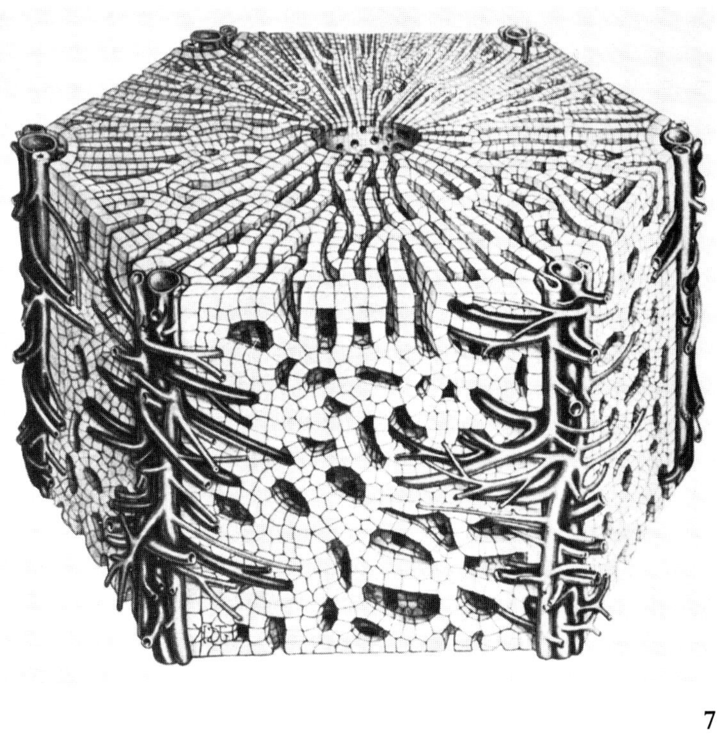

Figure 2-1
Diagram of the classic liver lobule. The central vein (terminal hepatic venule) lies in the center of the figure surrounded by anastomosing cords of block-shaped hepatocytes. Around the periphery of the lobule are six "triads" (portal areas), evenly spaced. Each triad consists of branches of the portal vein, hepatic artery, and bile duct.

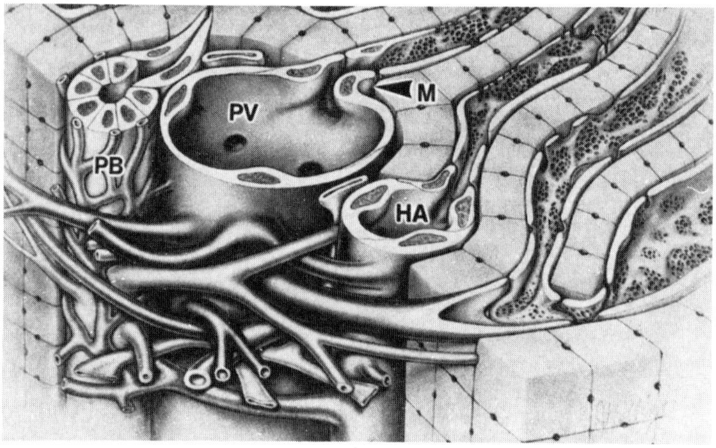

Figure 2-2
Schematic view of the liver portal area shown in greater detail than in Figure 2-1. This view shows the relationship of the branches of the portal vein, *PV,* hepatic artery, *HA,* and bile duct, *BD. PB,* peribiliary plexus; *M,* space of Mall. The blood in the PB comes entirely from the HA.

tocytes are the biliary channels, or bile canaliculi. To accomplish their diversity of functions, hepatocytes contain almost every organelle found in the animal kingdom. The liver also has an unusual dual blood supply. Two major vessels supply blood to the liver (Figure 2-2). One is the portal vein, which carries 75% of the blood into the liver from the alimentary tract, including the pancreas. This blood is rich in nutrients. The other major vessel is the hepatic artery, which supplies 25% of the blood. Blood from the hepatic artery contains the majority of oxygen that the liver needs for survival. Tributaries from the hepatic artery surround the entire triad of the liver (portal vein, hepatic artery, and bile ducts). In fact, when the supply of blood from the hepatic artery is compromised, these structures are in jeopardy (Figure 2-2). Bile ducts accompany the hepatic artery and portal vein and are composed of epithelium designed to be noncorroding and to deliver biliary products from the liver to the common bile duct and eventually to the small intestine.

CONNECTIVE TISSUE AND LIVER LOBES

The liver is divided into a left and right half by a fold of peritoneal tissue called the falciform ligament. The falciform ligament connects the liver to the diaphragm and to the anterior abdominal wall (Figure 2-3). Although anatomically it divides the right and left sides of the liver, physiologically it is not the falciform ligament that divides the liver into different planes but rather an imaginary plane that passes through the gallbladder and inferior vena cava. This imaginary plane marks the division, or branch point, of the portal vein, hepatic artery, and bile duct and divides the liver at the hilum into the right and left physiologic halves (Figure 2-4). The liver is further subdivided into four lobes, supplied with blood by the right and left branches of the portal vein and hepatic artery proper (Figure 2-4). Bile from these lobes drains into the right and left hepatic ducts, which accompany the vascular supply. Because each subdivision of the liver contains the same triad (portal vein, hepatic artery, and bile ducts), it is

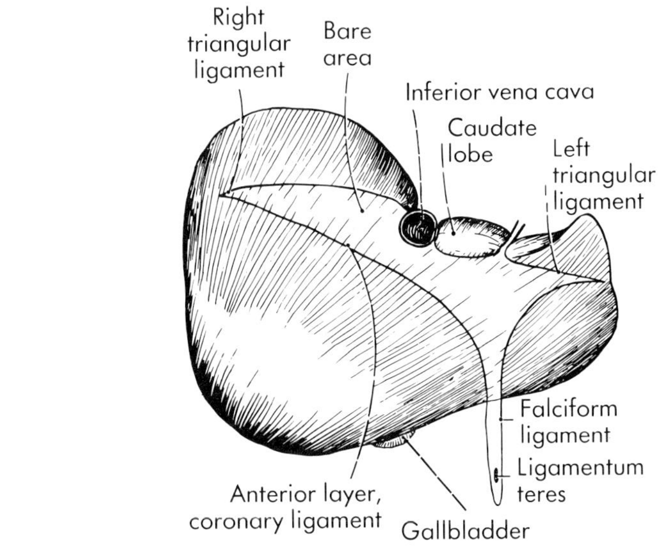

Figure 2-3
The diaphragmatic surface of the liver showing the relationships of the hepatic ligaments. (From Woodurne AM: Essentials of human anatomy, ed 8, London, 1965, Oxford University Press, p. 442).

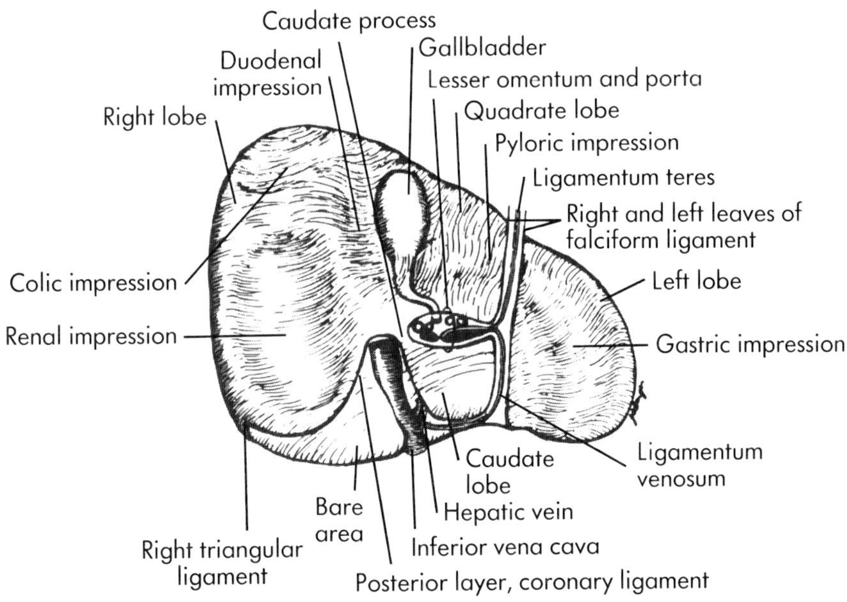

Figure 2-4
Diagram of the visceral surface of the liver. Notice the H pattern made up of the gallbladder, inferior vena cava, lesser omentum and porta, ligamentum teres, and ligamentum venosum. (From Woodburne AM: Essentials of human anatomy, ed 8, London, 1965, Oxford University Press, p. 442).

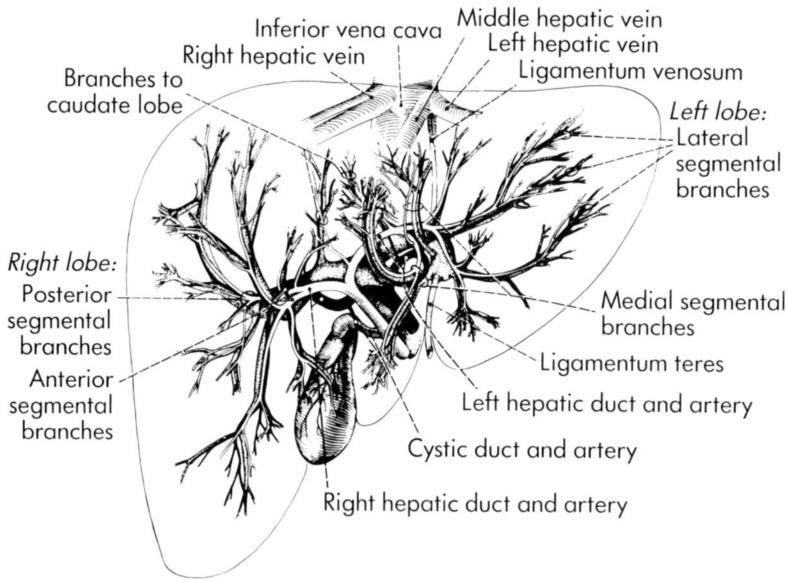

Figure 2-5
Composite drawing illustrating the usual pattern of branching of the bile ducts (white), the hepatic artery (black), and the portal vein (stripped). (From Woodburne AM: Essentials of human anatomy, ed 8, London, 1965, Oxford University Press, p. 442.)

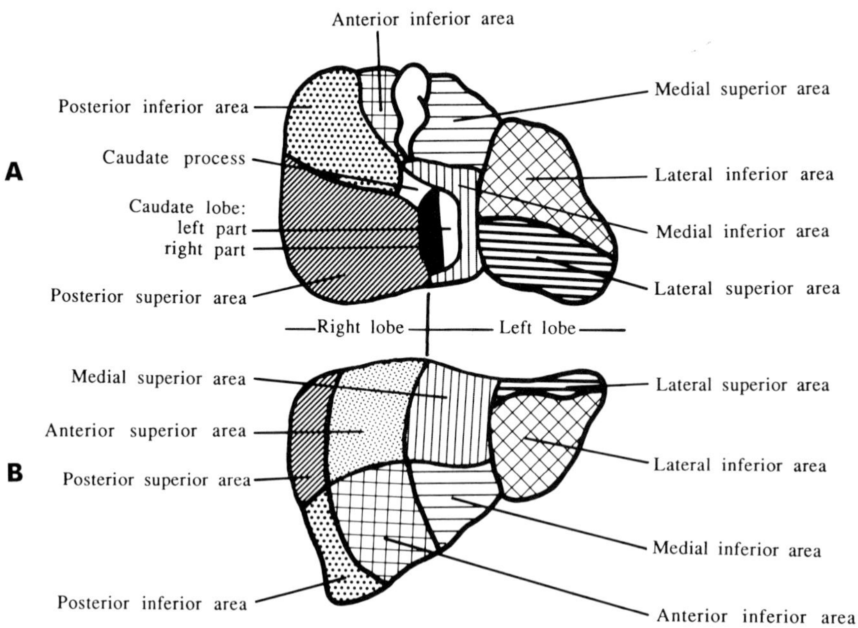

Figure 2-6
The segmentation of the liver, based on the principal divisions of the HA and ducts. **A,** the visceral surface. **B,** the diaphragmatic surface.

possible to subdivide the liver even further into subsections (Figure 2-5). Some surgeons feel that this subdivision is of critical importance, particularly when dissecting small lesions in these areas (Figure 2-6). The functional unit of the liver consists of the portal vein, hepatic artery, and bile duct. The area in which these structures enter (or leave, in the case of the bile duct) the liver is referred to as the porta hepatis.

LIGAMENTS

The ligaments of the liver actually represent a folding of peritoneum so that two layers are compressed against each other and comprise a small amount of connective tissue. The falciform ligament in the adult (ligamentum teres) was in the fetus the umbilical vein from the placenta. When they reach the liver, these two fused layers of peritoneum spread across its surface. Where the liver is pressed against the diaphragm, there is a bare area of the liver not covered by the peritoneum that is referred to as the "bare area" (Figure 2-3). The divergence of the two layers of peritoneum form other ligaments, referred to as the "triangular ligaments." The entire external surface of the liver is covered by a thin connective tissue capsule (Glisson's capsule). It lies just beneath the layer of flat peritoneal mesothelial cells, but it is also continuous with all of the connective tissue within the portal areas and sinusoids of the liver. In general, it is made up of type I and type III collagen.

LIVER LOBULATION

The circulation patterns of the liver lobule produce lobular gradients in the distribution of nutrients, biologically active molecules, and oxygen that are characterized by heterogeneities in cell structure and function. Without an appreciation of the differences in function along the lobule, it is difficult to understand the varying patterns of hepatic dysfunction due to liver injury. Three models of liver lobulation have been described, but most hepatologists have settled on a combination of two models. The classical description of the liver lobule emphasizes the central vein at the center of the lobule and the portal triads at the periphery of the lobule (Figure 2-1). In the Rappaport liver acinus model, parenchymal cells are grouped into concentric zones surrounding the terminal afferent vessels. In either concept, cells referred to as "zone 1" cells are nearest the blood inflow to the lobules, and cells referred to as "zone 3" are near the outflow. Zone 1 cells are the first to receive blood and in general the last to undergo necrosis and the first to regenerate after injury or partial hepatectomy. Cells in zones 2 and 3 receive blood with lower concentrations of nutrients and oxygen and are less resistant to injury. Zone 3 cells also contain the largest quantities of drug-metabolizing enzymes, which convert many harmless compounds, such as carbon tetrachloride and acetaminophen, into hepatotoxins. Zone 1 cells are the first to regenerate following certain forms of liver injury, perhaps because they are continuously sequestering all of the circulating epidermal growth factor (EGF), a promotor of DNA synthesis, and may have preprogramed cells to regenerate lost portions of liver. An appreciation of the cell biology of liver heterogeneity is also essential to the understanding of the pharmacokinetics of drugs and to the development of appropriate liver function tests

Table 2-1

Periportal zone	Perivenous zone
Oxidative energy metabolism	
Fatty acid oxidation	
Citrate cycle	
Respiratory chain	
Glucose release	Glucose uptake
Gluconeogenesis	Glycolysis
Glycogen synthesis from lactate	Glycogen synthesis from glucose
Glycogen degradation to glucose	Glycogen degradation to lactate
Amino acid utilization	
Amino acid conversion to glucose	
Amino acid degradation	
Ureagenesis from amino acid nitrogen	
Cholesterol synthesis	Ketogenesis
NH_3 detoxification	
Urea formation	Glutamine formation
	Biotransformation
	Monooxygenation
	Mercapturic acid formation
	Glucuronidation
Oxidation protection	
GSH peroxidation	
Bile formation	
Cholic acid excretion	
Bilirubin excretion	

From Jungermann K. In Diabetes Metab Rev 3:269-293, 1987.

(Table 2-1). For example, the aminopyrene breath test takes advantage of zone 3 drug metabolism and would be more sensitive to evaluate zone 3 damage than serum bile acids, which are taken up largely by zone 1 cells.

THE BILIARY TREE

The smallest branches of the biliary tree are the bile canaliculi, which actually represent specialized regions of the liver parenchymal cells (hepatocytes, Figure 2-7). Bile proceeds down the bile canaliculi, moving from zone 3 to zone 1 and into the perilobular or interlobular portal triads (Figure 2-1). The canalicular bile enters these small terminal bile ductules or "canals of Hering," which consist of a few fusiform cells held together by junctional complexes. Some light and electron microscope autoradiographic evidence suggests that these cells are multipotential and are the cells that become "oval" cells

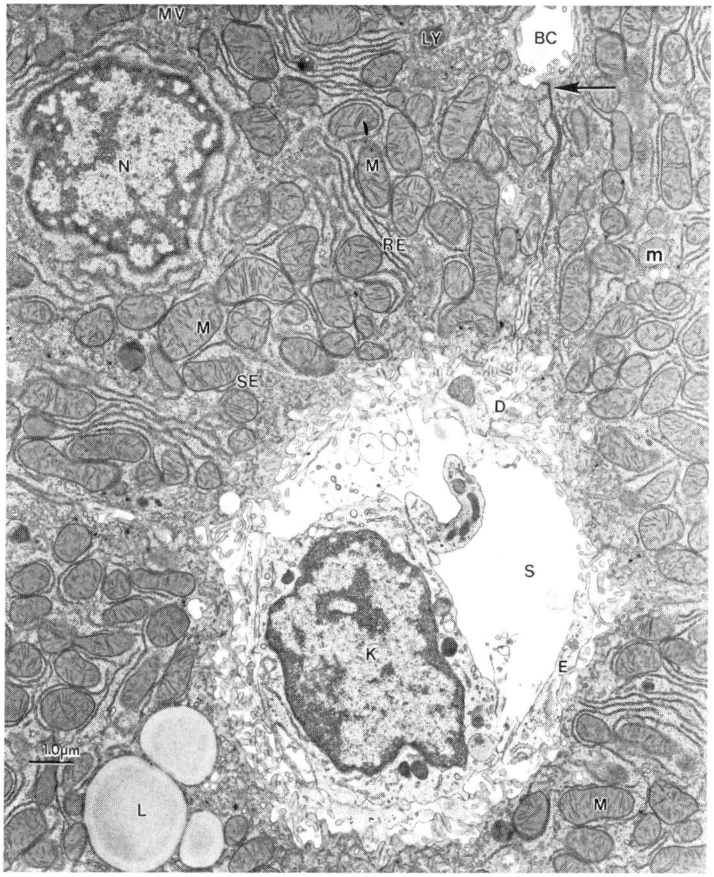

Figure 2-7
Electron micrograph showing portions of four rat liver parenchymal cells surrounding a sinusoid. *K,* Kupffer cell; *E,* endothelial cell; *M,* mitochondria; *D,* space of Disse; *m,* microbody; *L,* lipid; *BC,* bile canaliculus; *LY,* lysosome; *RE,* rough-surfaced endoplasmic reticulum; *SE,* smooth-surfaced endoplasmic reticulum; *N,* nucleus of parenchymal cell; *MV,* multivesicular body; and *S,* sinusoid.

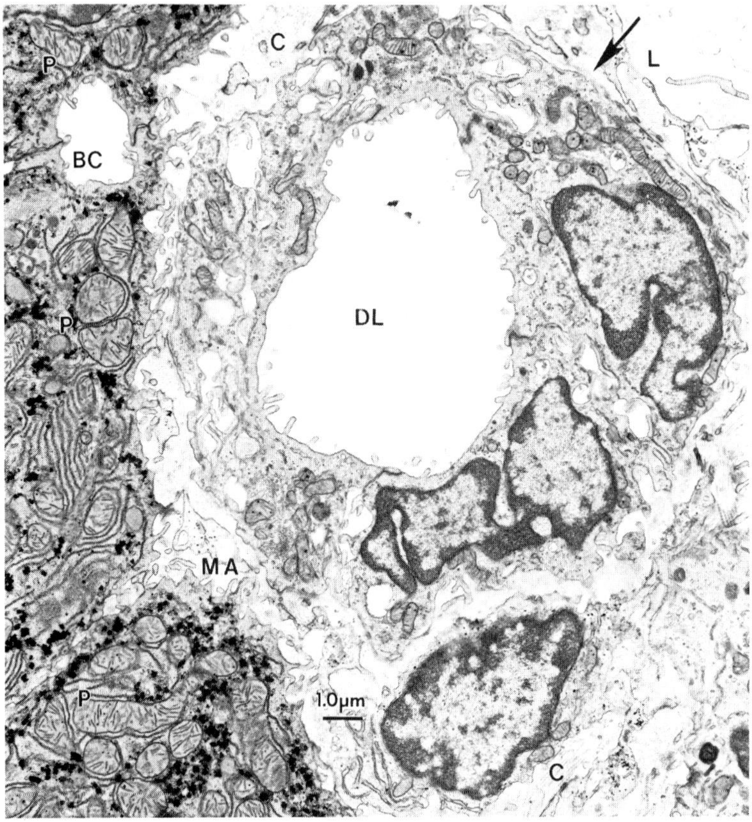

Figure 2-8
An electron micrograph of a small perilobular bile ductule close to liver parenchymal cells, *P*. A small canal of Hering epithelial cells (not shown) will conduct bile in the bile canaliculus, *BC* into the ductular lumen, *DL*. A thin basement membrane surrounds the bile ductule (arrow). *L*, lymphatic lumen; *MA*, space of Mall; *C*, collagen.

or liver-stem cells after fulminant hepatic injury. The appearance of oval cells may be an important positive sign in liver recovery. They may also be the cells that proliferate during cholestasis to form multiple bile ductules. From the terminal ductules bile enters larger ducts, the cuboidal epithelial cells of which are enriched in transport vesicles and undoubtedly are involved in modifying biliary components (Figure 2-8).

SINUSOIDS AND LYMPHATICS

The sinusoids form a rich intralobular vascular network converging toward the central vein (Figures 2-1, 2-2, 2-7). They differ from typical capillaries in that their walls are lined by two distinct cell types (endothelial cells and Kupffer cells) and their lumina are larger and variable in caliber (Figure 2-7). 2.8% of nonhepatocytes consist of endothelial cells, as do 2.1% of

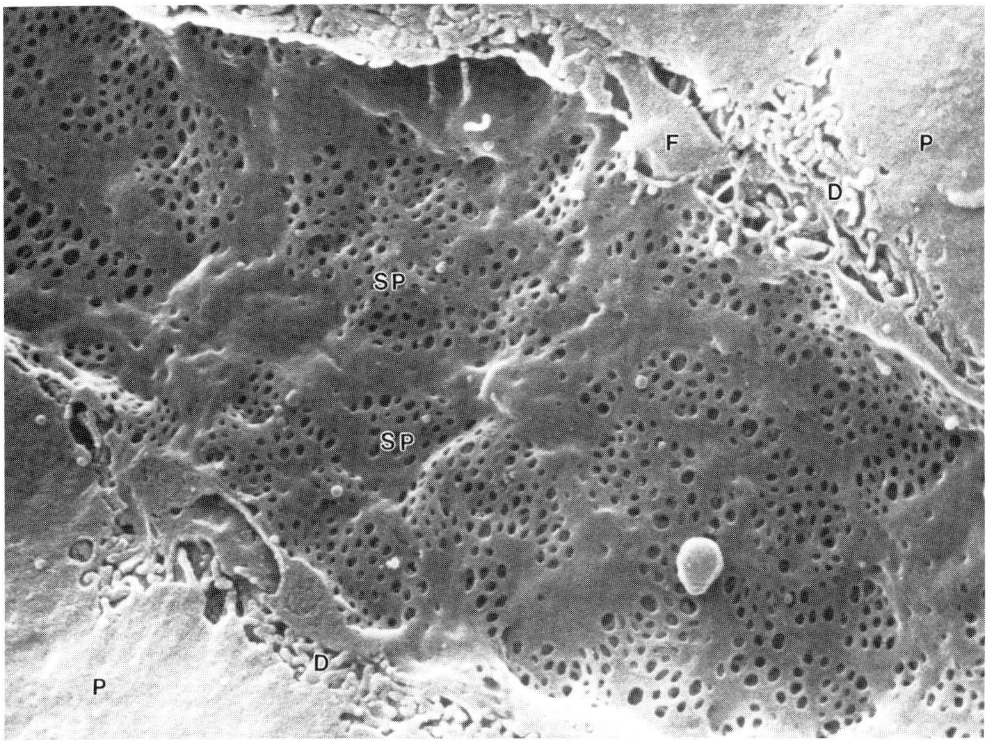

Figure 2-9
A high-power scanning electron micrograph depicting the sieve plates, *SP,* which are separated from each other by the "arms" of endothelial cells. The fenestrae vary in size but are about 1000Å in diameter. *D,* space of Disse; *F,* fat-storage cell; *P,* parenchymal cell with microvilli. (From Wisse E et al: The liver sieve: considerations concerning the structure and function of endothelial fenestrae, the sinusoidal wall and the space of Disse, Hepatology 5:683-692, 1985.)

Kupffer cells. The endothelial lining of the sinusoid is unique in that it does not have a typical basement membrane and its endothelial cells have fenestrae without diaphragms (except in ruminants, Figure 2-7). Therefore in most mammals there are no discernible barriers for exchange of materials between the blood and hepatocytes (Figure 2-9). However, this architecture allows for a forced sieving of material within the space of Disse. Soft, fast-moving structures such as blood cells promote the flow of fluid or macromolecules into and out of the space of Disse (Figure 2-10). Of course, this flow not only aids the liver in rapidly responding to changes in the internal milieu but also makes it more susceptible to toxic agents. Kupffer cells are the largest group of fixed macrophages (Figures 2-7 and 2-11). Kupffer cells endocytose bacteria, endotoxins, and effete erythrocytes from the blood and play a role in iron metabolism. In iron-storage diseases large quantities of iron accumulate in Kupffer cells in the form of ferritin and hemosiderin and in parenchy-

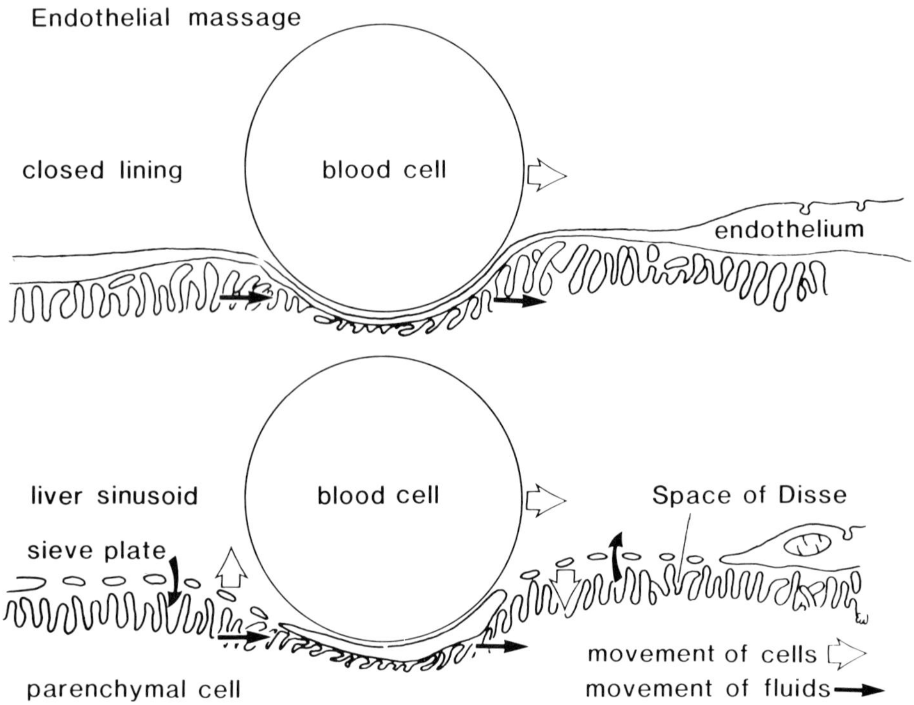

Figure 2-10
Diagram of the concept of endothelial massage. One of the effects of compression of the space of Disse by moving white blood cells is displacement of fluids within this space in a downstream direction. When fenestrae are encountered, fluid flows out of the space. When white blood cells move past, the microvilli and the endothelial lining return to precompression position. As a result, fresh plasma is sucked into the Disse's space. In in vivo microscopy preparations of rat liver, it has been seen that white blood cells can retard the flow rate in sinusoids without interrupting blood flow. This retardation reportedly represents an optimal situation for endothelial massage.

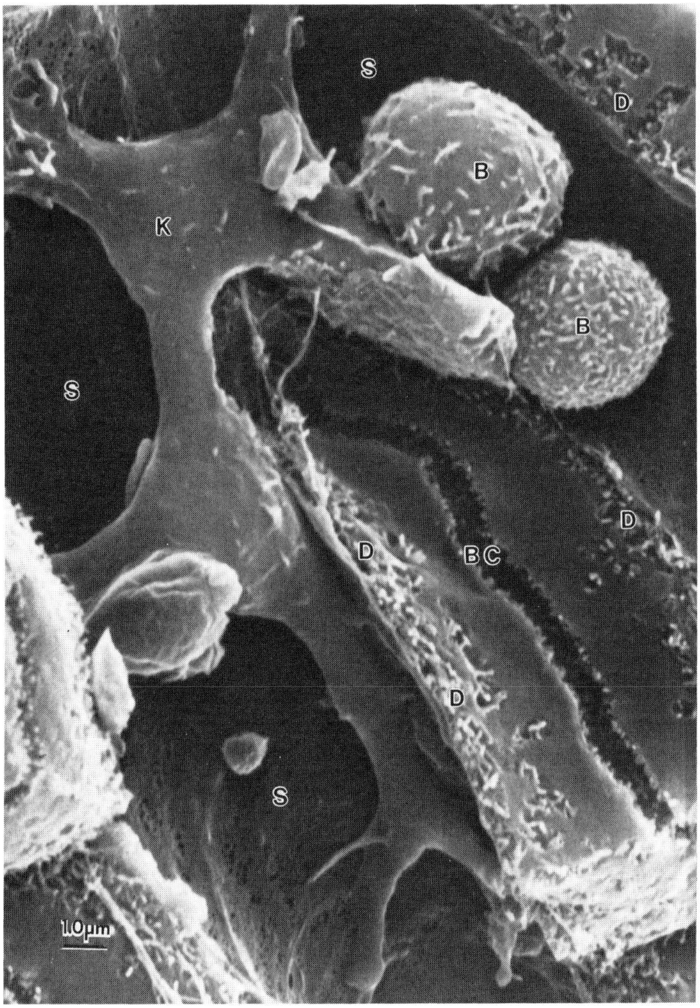

Figure 2-11
Scanning electron micrograph of a guinea pig liver. A large Kupffer cell, *K*, spans across two sinusoids with endothelial fenestrae. Notice the space of Disse, *D*, with its microvilli and the hemi-bile canaliculi, *BC*. Two blood cells are seen in the sinusoidal lumen, *B;* S, sinusoid. (From Wisse E et al: The liver sieve: considerations concerning the structure and function of endothelial fenestrae, the sinusoidal wall and the space of Disse, Hepatology 5:683-692, 1985.)

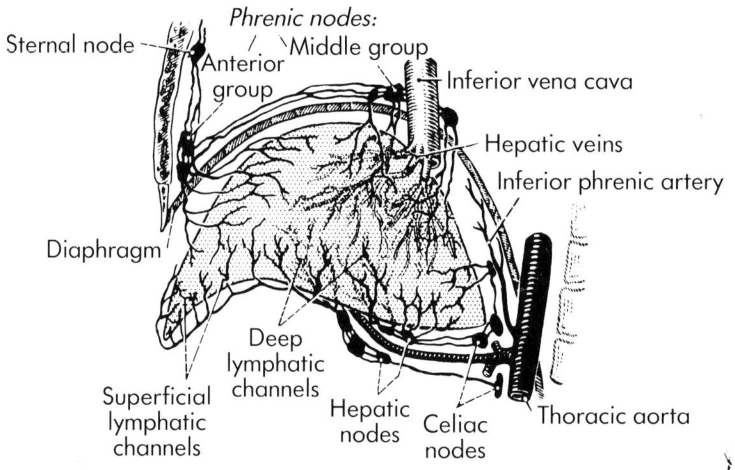

Figure 2-12
The lympatic drainage of the liver. (Reproduced with permission from Woodburne AM: Essentials of human anatomy, ed 8, London, 1965, Oxford University Press, p. 451.)

mal cells. Other cells along the sinusoids include lipocytes, pit cells (which apparently are cytotoxic T lymphocytes), and nerve cells. The lipocytes store vitamin A and may be the precursors of myofibroblasts, which play an important role in the development of hepatic fibrosis.

It is thought that the space of Disse is also the beginning of the lymphatic system in the liver. Fluid from this space reaches the space of Mall in the portal areas, where it flows into larger lymph vessels and is drained from the liver through multiple sites (Figure 2-12).

HEPATOCYTE ULTRASTRUCTURE

Hepatocytes are unrivaled by any other parenchymal cell type in functional diversity and complexity (Figure 2-7). They secrete bile salts into the intestine, thereby facilitating emulsification and absorption of dietary fat. They take up digested material from the afferent blood and store carbohydrates, protein, vitamins, and some lipids, releasing these compounds often in association with a carrier, e.g., triglyceride molecules complexed to a protein. Hepatocytes synthesize albumin and other plasma proteins, glucose, fatty acids, cholesterol, and phospholipids. They metabolize, detoxify, and inactivate exogenous compounds, such as drugs and insecticides, and endogenous compounds, such as steroids and other hormones. Liver cells can convert substances into more active forms, e.g., T4 to T3. Furthermore, it has been shown that in certain rodents, liver cells play a major role in the intestinal immune system by sequestering circulating immunoglobulin A

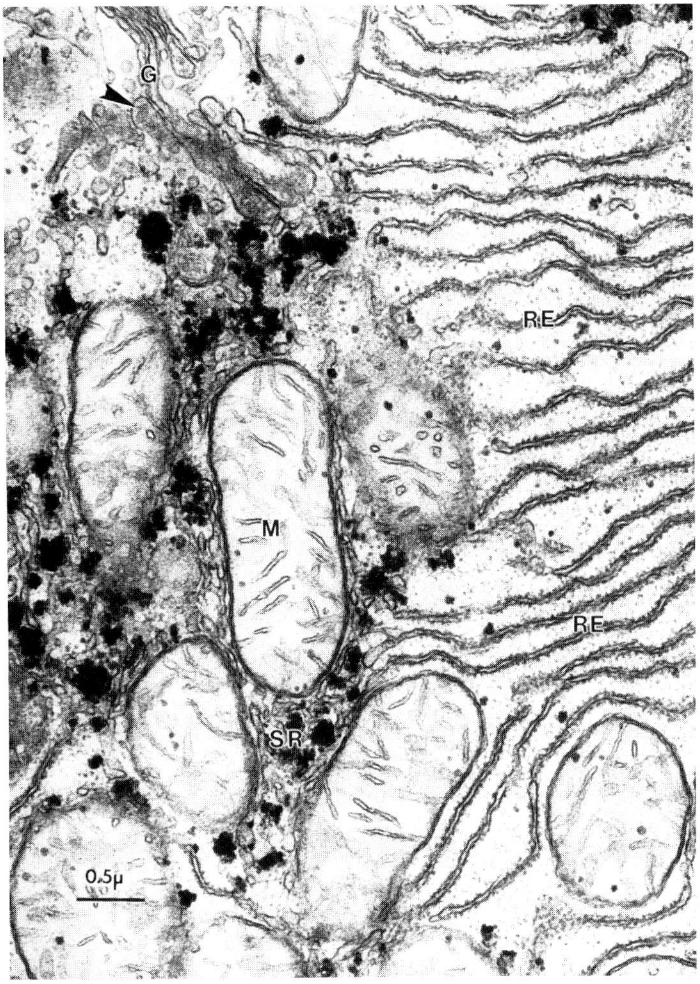

Figure 2-13
High-magnification electron micrograph of a portion of a liver cell. Note the continuity between the rough-surfaced endoplasmic reticulum, *RE,* and the smooth-surfaced endoplasmic reticulum *SR*. The osmiophilic (dense staining) spherical bodies within the Golgi, *G,* vesicles are very low density lipoprotein (arrowhead). *M,* mitochrondria.

(IgA) and secreting it into the intestine via the bile. Mitochondria are ubiquitous organelles but are especially numerous in liver cells (800/cell, Figures 2-7 and 2-13). They participate in oxidative phosphorylation and oxidation of fatty acids. Changes in mitochondrial structure, i.e., swelling or loss of intramitochondrial granules (calcium), are nonspecific changes that indicate early hepatic injury. The general function of lysosomes appears to be the disposition and catabolism of exogenous and endogenous substances. Microbodies occupy 4% of the total cell volume and are specialized for β-oxidation of long-chain fatty acids.

The endoplasmic reticulum is composed of a minute system of membrane-limited canals. Unlike cells in most tissues, both the rough-surfaced endoplasmic reticulum (RER) and smooth-surfaced endoplasmic reticulum (SER) are well developed in hepatocytes (Figure 2-13).

In transmission electron micrographs, the protein-synthesizing RER usually appears as aggregates of ribosome-studded, flattened cisternae arranged in parallel profiles scattered randomly throughout the cytoplasm (Figures 2-7 and 2-13). The SER consists of minute membrane-limited tubules without ribosomes (Figure 2-13).

The endoplasmic reticulum (microsomes) probably is involved either directly or indirectly in essentially every function of the hepatocytes. Evidence suggests that hepatic drug-metabolizing enzyme activities, rate-limiting steps in the conversion of cholesterol to bile acid (7α-hydroxylase), and microsomal steps in cholesterol biosynthesis are confined to the SER. The surface area of this membrane system is extraordinary. Morphometric data indicate that the liver of a 70 kg man would contain enough SER to cover a football field. The liver can rapidly increase SER in response to the need to metabolize xenobiotics.

GOLGI COMPLEX

In most mammalian hepatocytes, the Golgi complex is composed of three to five closely-packed, parallel, smooth-surfaced cisternae; varying numbers of large and small vesicles; and occasionally lysosomal elements (Figures 2-7 and 2-13).

It consists of cis and trans elements. Secretory vesicles are associated with the concave or trans region of the Golgi and are filled with very low-density lipoproteins destined for secretion. Within the Golgi complex are enzymes largely responsible for glycosylation of proteins.

INCLUSIONS

Large fat droplets without a limiting membrane can be seen in most liver cells (Figure 2-7). During fasting they become most abundant in zone 1 cells, but after ethanol consumption, they increase markedly in zone 3 (centrolobular).

Glycogen deposits, appearing as electron-dense granules under most tissue-preparation techniques, are scattered throughout the SER (Figure 2-7, 2-8, and 2-13). During fasting they disappear first from zone 3. After refeeding, they appear first in zone 1.

BILE CANALICULI AND PERICANALICULAR CYTOPLASM

The smallest branches of the biliary tree are the bile canaliculi. These extracellular areas are located between two or more adjacent hepatocytes (Figure 2-7). The bile canaliculi are isolated from the remainder of the intercellular space, and thus from the sinusoidal lumen, by junctional complexes. Perhaps the most important component of the junctional complex is the tight junction, which is always located immediately adjacent to and completely surrounding the canalicular lumen. Under physiologic conditions, this junction has been considered impervious even to small molecules. The 1 μm-wide area of cytoplasm immediately surrounding the bile canaliculus is the pericanalicular cytoplasm. During times of enhanced bile secretion, this area of cytoplasm contains many vesicles indicating a role for vesicles in bile secretion. The most prominent structural alterations during cholestasis are at the canalicular level: (1) dilatation of the bile canaliculi, (2) blunting of microvilli, and (3) changes in surrounding microfilaments. Tight junctions may rupture following bile-duct ligation but will recover their morphologic integrity during the postcholestatic regenerative phase.

VESICULAR TRANSPORT OF BILIARY PROTEINS

Bile contains many proteins and polypeptides. One of the major proteins in bile is secretory component, the receptor for IgA. Secretory component is found both free and linked to polymeric IgA by disulfide bonds. Secretory IgA is the major immunoglobulin in bile. Other intact proteins, such as albumin, insulin, EGF, and apolipoproteins, are also found in the bile.

The hepatocyte accomplishes biliary protein transport by using subcellular structures common to many cells: membrane receptors, vesicles, microtubules, Golgi complexes, multivesicular bodies, and lysosomes. Tight junctions between adjacent hepatocytes prevent regurgitation of biliary components from the bile into blood.

Proteins that are taken up by liver- receptor-mediated endocytosis are degraded, secreted intact into bile, or utilized by the cell. Receptors on the hepatocyte sinusoidal plasma membrane determine which proteins are specifically taken up, but once endocytosis has occurred, the mechanism determining which of the above pathways will result is completely unknown.

MICROFILAMENTS AND MICROTUBULES

Both microfilaments (90Å in diameter) and microtubules (250Å in diameter) have been implicated in the process of bile secretion. Microfilaments contain actin, and their location surrounding the bile canalicular membrane has invoked speculation that they (1) provide and maintain bile canalicular tonus, (2) exert a contractile force that facilitates secretion of bile into the canalicular lumen, (3) maintain the high pressure found within the biliary tree, and (4) account for some of the energy dependence of bile secretion by subcellular organelles involved in endocytosis, cytoplasmic transport, and exocytosis of certain biliary substances.

Several recent studies have shown that microtubules are absolutely essential for the vectorial movement of transport vesicles within liver cells. Many studies have shown that disruption of normal microtubule function, such as is caused by alcohol, will result in toxic injury to the liver cell, i.e., fatty liver, because of inability to move lipoproteins in and out of the liver.

LIPID METABOLISM

The hepatic synthesis of very low-density lipoprotein (VLDL) in response to a fatty acid load was first demonstrated morphologically in the isolated perfused rat-liver preparation. The liver also plays a prominent role in removing lipoproteins from plasma. Chylomicrons and VLDL remnants rely entirely on the liver for their removal. They are taken up by receptor-mediated endocytosis and are destroyed by multivesicular bodies and lysosomes. Low-density lipoproteins (LDLs), a result of incomplete VLDL remnant removal, are also removed from the circulation by the liver (and other cells).

Failure to remove any of these lipoproteins because of a genetic disorder, or secondarily because of toxic liver injury, results in a marked rise in circulating triglycerides and cholesterol. The final result is an increased risk of heart disease and stroke and/or premature aging.

EXTRAHEPATIC BILE DUCTS

The cells that line the extrahepatic biliary space are similiar in morphology to those of the intrahepatic ducts, except that the cells in the extrahepatic biliary space are columnar and the surrounding vasculature is not as well developed. PAS-positive cells are found in tubular glands, which are seen occasionally within the epithelium.

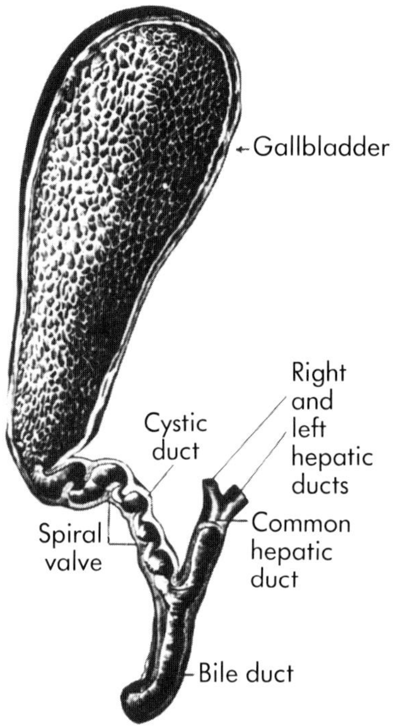

Figure 2-14
Interior of the gallbladder and bile ducts. (From Warnich R and Williams PR: Gray's anatomy, ed 35, Philadelphia, 1973; WB Saunders Co, p. 1310.)

GALLBLADDER

The mucosa of the gallbladder comprises a single layer of columnar cells that contain an extensive supranuclear Golgi complex, RER, numerous vesicles, and small mitrochondria. Junctional complexes are found in the apical region of the cells. The microvilli are numerous, and the lateral plasma membranes are thrown into a series of convoluted folds. During active absorption of fluid from the bile, these intercellular spaces become markedly distended. Autonomic nerve fibers are observed in the serosa, and goblet- cell-containing glands, which are sparse in the normal gallbladder, are frequently observed in patients with chronic gallbladder inflammation. A spiral fold of mucosa keeps the cystic duct open (Figure 2-14).

CHOLEDOCHODUODENAL JUNCTION

The junction of the common bile duct, pancreatic duct, and duodenum is an anatomic area of medical and physiologic importance. It regulates the flow of bile and pancreatic enzymes into the duodenum and governs the filling of the gallbladder.

During passage through the intestinal wall, the associated bile and pancreatic

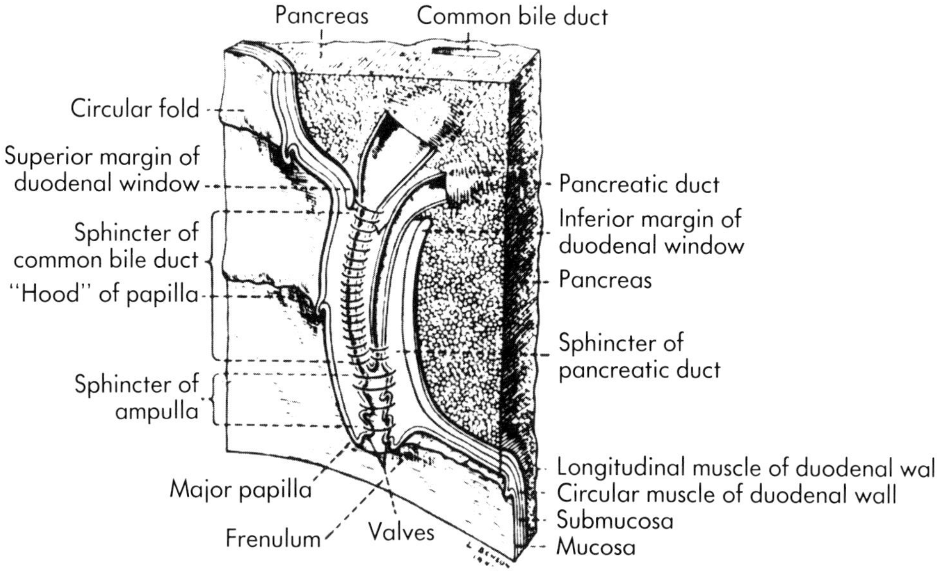

Figure 2-15
From Lindner HH: The muscular apparatus at the terminal end of the common bile duct. In Way LW and Pelligrini CA, eds: Surgery of the gallbladder and bile ducts, Philadelphia, 1987, WB Saunders Co, p. 3.

ducts are invested by a common musculus proprius, termed the sphincter of Oddi (Figure 2-15).

LIVER DEVELOPMENT

The first indication of the liver's appearance from the foregut is at 3 weeks gestation. A small endodermal epithelial lining thickens, rapidly becomes hollow, and develops into hepatic and pancreatic portions. The hepatic portion eventually forms the liver and hepatic bile ducts, and the gall bladder and cystic duct. The hepatic diverticulum invades the septum transversum, as thick cords growing between two vitelline veins, and a capillary network begins to form. Initially liver parenchymal cells are in cords. Eventually these cells become two cell-layered plates, and by 5 years of age human liver cells form a monocellular plate of cells.

LIVER REGENERATION

The liver has a remarkable ability to regenerate. Removal of 70% of the liver results in turning liver cells from Go to S-phase with complete and rapid restoration of the liver size. Similarly, infectious agents and chemicals that damage the liver also stimulate liver regeneration. However, the processes are different in that regeneration following partial hepatectomy does not induce α-fetoprotein secretion but toxic injury regeneration does.

In the case of partial hepatectomy, parenchymal cells regenerate, but toxic injury may stimulate stem cell (oval) proliferation as well. Growth factors, both autocrine and pericrine, appear to be important. Perhaps the best-known growth factor is EGF. Its regulatory control is changed immediately after partial liver removal, and it is directed into the cell nucleus. Intracellular pH, Ca^{++}, polyamines, and inositol trisphosphate all increase. This increase is followed by the development of S-phase. Of great interest is that when regeneration is complete, these events are shut down as fast as they began. TGF-β, a factor produced by liver endothelial cells, may participate in the cessation of the regeneration response.

SUGGESTED READINGS

Blouin A, Bolender RP, and Weibel ER: Distribution of organelles and membranes between hepatocytes and nonhepatocytes in rat liver parenchyma, J Cell Biol 72:441, 1977.

This is a definitive work giving the precise quantitative analysis of liver organelles and cells.

Ito T: Cytological studies on stellate cells of Kupffer and fat-storing cells in the capillary wall of the human liver, Acta Anat Nippon 26:42,1951.

This is the original description of fat-storing cells.

Jones AL, Ruderman NB, and Herrer MG: Electron microscopic and biochemical study of lipoprotein synthesis in the isolated perfused rat liver. J Lipid Res 8:429,1967.

The first morphologic discovery of the synthesis and secretion of VLDL in liver is described in this article.

Jones AL and Burwen SJ: Pathways and function of biliary protein secretion. In Forte LC, ed: Handbook of physiology: the gastrointestinal system III, New York, 1989, Oxford University Press, p. 663.

This is a modern review of bile protein secretion.

Jones AL, Schmucker SL, Mooney JS et al: Morphometric analysis of rat hepatocytes after total biliary obstruction, Gastroenterology 71:1050,1976.

A careful quantitative analysis of liver cell changes during cholestasis is presented.

Mall FP: A study of the structural unit of the liver, Am J Anat 5:277,1906.

This is a classic paper describing the liver lymph system.

Rappaport AM: Anatomic considerations. In Schiff L, ed: Diseases of the liver, Philadelphia, 1969, J B Lippincott Co, p. 1.

A detailed description of the zones of the liver lobule as they are related to disease is presented.

Wisse E, DeZanger RB, Charles K et al: The liver sieve: concerning the structure and function of endothelial fenestrae, the sinusoidal wall and the space of Disse, Hepatology 5:683,1985.

This is the most clearly written and informative description of sinusoidal fenestrae and their functional significance.

3 Basic Function of the Liver

Neville Basman *and* ***Alfred Baker***

METABOLISM OF BILIRUBIN

Bilirubin is an end product of heme degradation that has no known physiologic function. However, knowledge of its metabolism is important because jaundice is such an important clinical occurrence and because the liver plays a central role in bilirubin metabolism. A summary of clinically important abnormalities of bilirubin metabolism is given in Table 3-1, and an overview of bilirubin metabolism is depicted in Figure 3-1.

Assay Methods

The development of new, reliable clinical tests for bilirubin has accounted for advances in the ability of physicians to understand jaundice. Measurement of bilirubin involves the reaction with Ehrlich's reagent (diazotized sulfanilic acid) to form a colored product. The portion that reacts without any other additions is referred to as direct bilirubin. A second portion reacts only in the presence of an organic compound (usually ethanol) and thus is referred to as the indirect fraction.

Development of the "Kodak Ektachem" technology allows for a simultaneous, rapid, and reliable measurement of both the unconjugated and conjugated fractions. This method also permits accurate measurement of covalently bound or δ-bilirubin. Bilirubin binds to albumin by noncovalent, Van der Waals forces. However, with prolonged conjugated hyperbilirubinemia, a variable and increasing fraction may be tightly and covalently bound to albumin. This fraction is referred to as δ-bilirubin.

This third type of bilirubin helps explain several previously confusing clinical phenomena, including the slow disappearance of bilirubin from the plasma despite improving liver function. δ-bilirubin is not excreted by the kidneys, and its half-life approximates that of albumin, to which it is tightly bound: approximately 14 days. δ-Bilirubin may also account for discrepancies that can be seen between the total bilirubin and the sum of the unconjugated and conjugated fractions. Finally, it helps to explain why some patients with marked hyperbilirubinemia may have minimal bilirubinuria. This phenomenon is usually noted late in the course of conjugated hyperbilirubinemia when liver function has improved. The δ-bilirubin that remains is not filtered by the kidney and thus does not appear in the urine.

Table 3-1 Clinicopathologic classification of jaundice

	Defect	Bilirubin (mg/dl)	Liver enzymes	Diagnosis	Treatment	Prognosis	Inheritance
Unconjugated							
Hemolysis							
Acute Chronic	Raised pigment load	Variable, may be markedly raised <5	Normal	Blood smear Hemolytic workup	—	—	—
Gilbert's	Lowered hepatic uptake	<3		Exclude hemolysis	None needed	Excellent	Autosomal dominance
	Lowered glucuronyltransferase activity 50% associated mild lowered red blood cell count	Conjugation < 0.4	Normal	Raised bilirubin with fasting			
Crigler-Najjar							
Type I	Absent glucuronyl transferase activity	Mostly >20	Normal	Exclude other causes. No response to phenobarbital	None effective	Usually death due 20 to kernicterus	Autosomal recessive
Type II	Markedly lowered glucuronyl transferase activity	Usually < 20	Normal	Exclude other causes. Responds to phenobarbital	Phenobarbital	Usually good. Rare cases of kernicterus	Autosomal dominant

Conjugated							
Dubin-Johnson	Defective biliary secretion	Variable (usually <10)	Normal	BSP retention. 45 min retention <20% often secondary rise after 90 min. Urine coproporphyrin type I rise with normal total	—	Good	Autosomal recessive
Rotor	Defective biliary secretion	Variable (usually <10)	Normal	45 min BSP retention 30% to 50%. No secondary rise Moderate rise in urine. Total coproporphyrin	—	Good	Autosomal recessive
Postoperative cholestasis	Multifactorial raised pigment load Hypoglycemia, Hypotension, drugs, sepsis, renal insufficiency	Variable (may reach 40 mg/dl) Mostly conjugated	Variable, often markedly raised alkaline phosphatase. Mildly raised transaminase (<200)	Exclude extrahepatic obstruction	Treatment of underlying conditions	Poor. Related to severity of underlying conditions	—
Sepsis	Bacterial products interfere with secretory mechanisms	Variable, often markedly elevated	Variable, often raised alkaline phosphatase Mildly raised transaminases	Exclude obstruction, clinical scenario	Treat underlying sepsis	Poor. Related to severity of infection	

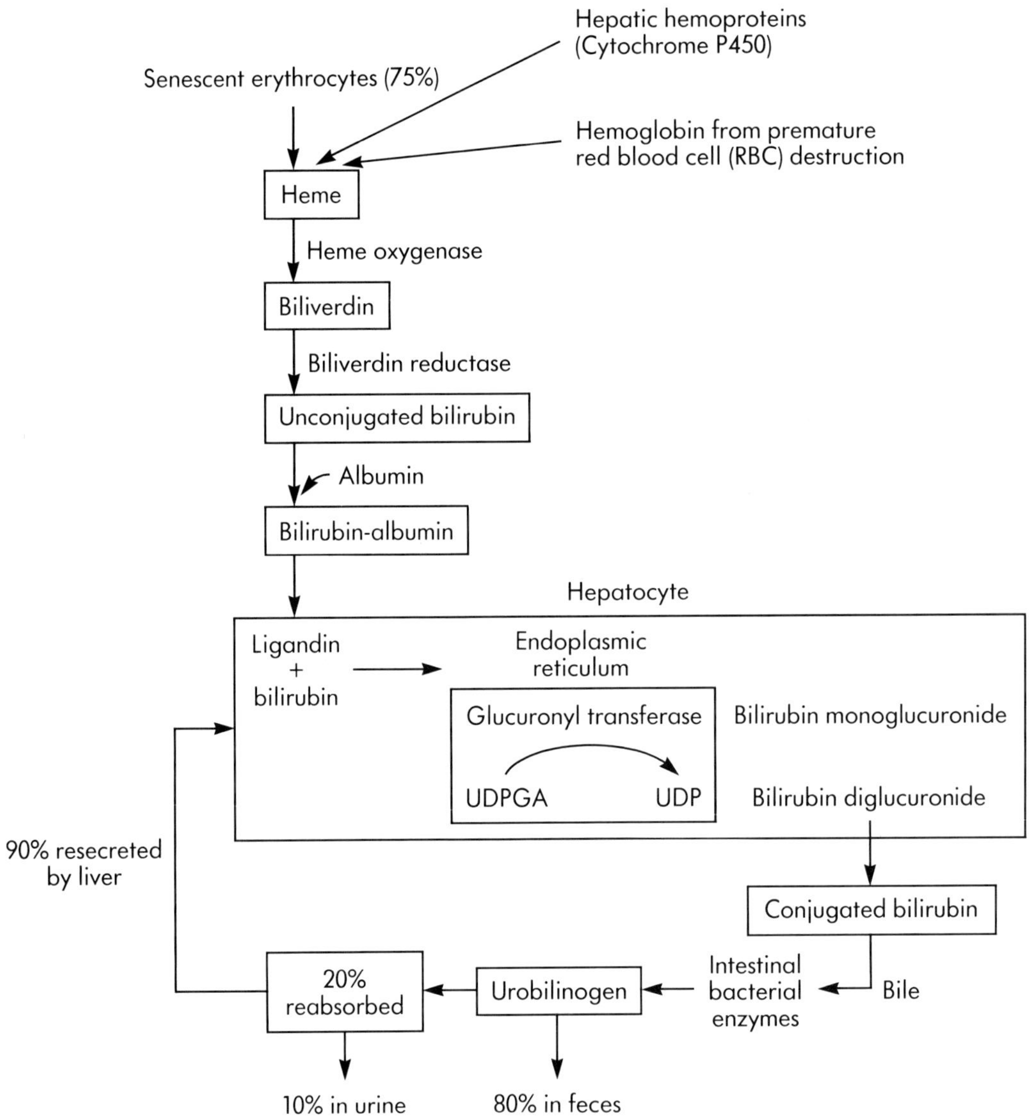

Figure 3-1
Overview of bilirubin metabolism.

Bilirubin Formation

Approximately 75% of bilirubin production occurs through degradation of the heme moiety of hemoglobin in the reticuloendothelial system (RES). The remaining 25% results from the breakdown of nonerythrocytic hemoproteins, of which the cytochrome P-450 system is the most important. A minor fraction of bilirubin production results from premature destruction of newly formed erythrocytes in the RES.

Heme is first oxidized to biliverdin (so called because of its green color) by the microsomal heme oxygenase system. This heme-cleaving enzyme is most abundant in tissues involved in heme degradation. Its activity may be increased by three to five times in response to an increased heme load, such as hemolytic anemia. The biliverdin is rapidly converted to bilirubin by the enzyme biliverdin reductase. The chemical conversion from heme to bilirubin is rapid and occurs within several minutes. Thus biliverdin itself is not readily detectable either in the serum or the bile.

Approximately 250 mg (3.8 mg/kg) of bilirubin is formed a day, but the system can accommodate at least a twofold rise in pigment load before jaundice occurs. With hemolysis or ineffective erythropoiesis, the increased production may exceed the hepatic excretory capacity and result in unconjugated hyperbilirubinemia. With chronic hemolytic states, e.g., hereditary spherocytosis, the serum bilirubin level does not exceed 5 mg/dl because the bone marrow cannot increase production of red blood cells more than eightfold. Therefore a serum bilirubin level more than 5 mg/dl suggests associated underlying hepatic dysfunction. However, with acute hemolytic states, e.g., an incompatible blood transfusion, marked bilirubin elevations may occur.

Bilirubin Transport

The unconjugated bilirubin is transported to the liver tightly but reversibly bound to albumin. Provided the molar ratio of bilirubin to albumin is 1:1 or less, the bilirubin remains bound to a single high-affinity site. However, when the 1:1 ratio is exceeded (equivalent to a bilirubin concentration of approximately 35 mg/dl), binding occurs at two additional lower affinity sites. It is then susceptible to displacement by other organic anions, e.g., sulfonamides, furosemide, and contrast media, and by changes in pH.

Free or unbound bilirubin in plasma can be transported across the blood-brain barrier and produce neonatal kernicterus. The bilirubin level at which kernicterus occurs has not been determined, but the commonly accepted level for exchange transfusion is 20 mg/dl.

Hepatic Uptake

The hepatic uptake of bilirubin and other organic anions such as sulfobromophthalein (SBP) is a carrier-mediated saturable process. The system operates well below saturation and exhibits high first-pass effects. It is not a rate-limiting factor in bilirubin metabolism. Reflux may approximate 40% of the bilirubin removed by the liver in a single pass. In unconjugated hyperbilirubinemic states, such as Gilbert's syndrome, the hepatic uptake is considered to be normal, but because of defective intracellular binding of bilirubin, increased reflux into plasma occurs.

The albumin-bilirubin complex passes through fenestrations in the sinusoidal-lining cells into the space of Disse for direct contact with the hepatocyte's plasma membrane. Binding proteins on the plasma membranes appear to dissociate the unconjugated bilirubin from albumin before uptake. Bilirubin then binds to cytoplasmic protein, especially ligandin, providing a major mechanism for transport to the endoplasmic reticulum. A small fraction of bilirubin is transported unbound. There also appears to be a separate channel for transport of bilirubin produced from hepatic heme degradation.

Conjugation

Conjugation of bilirubin results in formation of water-soluble derivatives that are readily excreted into the bile and urine. Carbohydrate moieties, especially glucuronic acid, esterify bilirubin in the endoplasmic reticulum. This is catalyzed by the enzyme uridine diphosphate-glucuronyl transferase (UDP-GT).

Gilbert's syndrome appears to be a heterogeneous entity in that some patients exhibit a defect in bilirubin and organic anion uptake but most patients have decreased glucuronyltransferase activity. Crigler-Najjar syndrome (congenital nonhemolytic jaundice) exhibits either an absence (type 1) of glucuronyltransferase activity or a marked decrease (type 2) in it, (see Table 3-1). Therefore these syndromes result in increased unconjugated hyperbilirubinemia.

Excretion

Conjugated bilirubin is excreted into the bile by a rate-limited, energy-requiring mechanism. This excretion occurs against a marked concentration gradient. Transport may be a carrier-mediated system. It appears to be shared by other organic anions but separate from bile acids.

Bilirubin excretion is the rate-limiting step for overall transport from blood to bile. A variety of conditions may inhibit the excretory mechanism and result in conjugated hyperbilirubinemia. Dubin-Johnson and Rotor's syndromes exhibit a defect in the bilirubin excretory mechanism.

A defect in the excretory mechanism caused by sepsis can result in jaundice (see Table 3-1). Bacterial products, such as endotoxins, have been implicated as inhibiting the bile excretory apparatus. Other factors, including hypoxia, blood transfusions, and drugs, probably play an additional role. Marked hyperbilirubinemia may develop, associated with elevated alkaline phosphatase, mild increases in transaminase, and a liver biopsy that reveals cholestasis and a nonspecific portal-tract infiltrate. The reactive liver dysfunction is in itself of minor clinical significance and reverses with adequate treatment of the sepsis. However, its presence usually reflects severe uncontrolled sepsis with its high mortality rate. A similar clinical picture is seen with the entity of benign postoperative intrahepatic cholestasis. In this syndrome, marked hyperbilirubinemia occurs after major surgery. Jaundice develops in 2 to 14 days and is accompanied by markedly increased conjugated bilirubin levels, as high as 40 mg/dl (see Table 3-1).

Enterohepatic Circulation

The conjugated bilirubin that is secreted in the bile is not a single compound. The major conjugate is bilirubin-diglucuronide, which accounts for approximately 80%, with small amounts of bilirubin monoglucuronide, xyloside, and glucoside. Following canalicular excretion, bilirubin is little changed as it passes through the biliary tree and small intestine. In the colon and terminal ileum, bacterial enzymes, such as β-glucuronidase, hydrolyze the bilirubin glucuronides to unconjugated bilirubin. These are then reduced by bacterial enzymes to a number of colorless tetrapyrroles, referred to as urobilinogens. Oxidation leads to formation of urobilin, which contributes to the normal color of the stool. Eighty percent of the urobilinogens are excreted in the stool. Of the remaining 20%, which is reabsorbed, 90% is promptly reexcreted by the liver, allowing only 10% to appear in the urine. Therefore of the 250 mg per day excreted in the bile, only approximately 4 mg appears in the urine, and the rest is excreted in the feces. In conditions associated with bacterial overgrowth (intestinal stasis), increased deconjugation of bilirubin occurs with subsequent increased absorption of unconjugated bilirubin. This proves to be of little clinical significance except possibly to contribute to the physiologic hyperbilirubinemia of neonates.

MECHANISMS OF LIVER INJURY AND REGENERATION

Despite the large number of factors that can injure the liver, this organ has a limited number of histologic patterns of response. A small number of mechanisms appear to explain most of the features of liver injury. In addition, hepatic regeneration is a unique response of this organ to injury. It sometimes permits the return of normal structure and function even after severe damage.

Liver Injury in Major Liver Diseases

Table 3-2 shows the mechanisms that underlie the morphologic features of some of the major liver diseases. The clinical and histologic picture of *viral hepatitis,* particularly hepatitis B, results mainly from immunologic injury to the liver. Hepatitis B does not appear to be cytopathic, and liver injury arises mainly from direct lymphocyte toxicity to infected cells. Display of hepatitis B core antigen

Table 3-2 The major mechanisms of liver injury in some types of liver disease

	Mechanism(s) of liver injury	Main histologic features
Viral hepatitis	Immunologic	Acidophilic bodies, spotty necrosis
Drug hepatitis	Immunologic	Acidophilic bodies, spotty necrosis, occasionally eosinophils
Drug hepatotoxicity	Metabolic activation	Zonal necrosis, fatty infiltration
Ischemia	ATP depletion, increased intracellular Ca^{++}	Perivenular necrosis
Cholestasis	Immunologic Hepatotoxic	Cholestasis Triaditis
Alcoholic hepatitis	Acetaldehyde Perivenular ischemia Fibrogenesis Lipoperoxidation	Hydropic change Perivenular ischemia Perivenular fibrosis Mallory bodies

(HBcAg) on the hepatocyte cell membranes along with human lymphocyte antigens (HLA) class 1 antigens appears to be necessary for lymphocytes to recognize infected hepatocytes. The severity of liver injury mainly reflects the patient's immune response. Patients with acute hepatitis B usually have a normal immune response; infected cells are destroyed rapidly, and few visible infected hepatocytes are present. Patients with chronic persistent hepatitis B may not display antigens for lymphocyte recognition on hepatocyte membranes or may have decreased lymphocyte responsiveness. Although infected cells persist, little hepatic damage occurs.

Drug hepatitis also results mainly from immunologic injury to liver cells. This form of drug-induced injury does not depend on the dose. Instead, repeated exposure to the offending agent is usually associated with rapid onset of severe liver damage. Although specific antigens have not been identified in the livers of patients with most types of drug hepatitis, lymphocytes from sensitized patients are transformed when tested with drugs such as halothane, suggesting that immunologic responses may be responsible. The histologic pattern resembles that of viral hepatitis, but a predominance of eosinophils in some biopsies may suggest a drug etiology.

Toxic hepatitis may be caused by exposure to a number of chemicals used in industry and to some drugs. This form of liver injury is dose-related, and reexposure does not ordinarily produce more severe damage. Carbon tetrachloride is metabolized by liver microsomes to reactive intermediates. These compounds bind covalently with cell macromolecules, including proteins and lipids, to produce liver injury. Some drugs are metabolized to free radicals that initiate lipoperoxidation. Glutathione and other cytoprotective substances deactivate these toxic compounds, but the levels often fall with this form of liver injury. Nutritional depletion and liver injury limit hepatic glutathione synthesis. Acetaminophen hepatotoxicity also results from metabolism of the drug by the liver to toxic intermediates that bind covalently with cell macromolecules. Liver injury does not occur unless a sufficient dose (usually more than 6 to 8 g) is taken. At this level the protective effects of glutathione are exceeded, resulting in liver injury.

Ischemia causes liver injury in several clinical disorders, including hypoxemia due to congestive heart failure and pulmonary failure. Ischemia may also contribute to the liver damage produced by drugs and toxins, such as alcohol, which cause centrilobular cell swelling, decreasing lobular blood flow. The marked enzyme release that occurs 1 to 3 days after liver transplantation has also been attributed to ischemia, probably exacerbated by reperfusion. Initially, cell ATP levels decline, and glycogen is metabolized by the tricarboxylic acid cycle for energy. This causes intracellular acidosis and results in membrane injury with failure to maintain cell membrane ionic gradients. Calcium influx appears to be a major factor leading to irreversible damage. Reperfusion may exacerbate cell injury by producing oxygen-free radicals resulting in lipoperoxidation. Mild ischemic injury is usually centrilobular, but when the lesion is severe, the entire lobule may be injured except for a few periportal hepatocytes. *Cholestasis* is discussed in the next section of this chapter.

A number of mechanisms have been

identified that may contribute to liver injury in patients with *alcoholic hepatitis*. Acetaldehyde, the metabolite of ethanol produced by liver alcohol dehydrogenase, is a reactive substance that binds covalently with liver cell macromolecules. Binding to tubulin, the protein that forms microtubules, is particularly avid. Therefore the exit of protein-containing substance from the liver is limited, increasing cell protein, fat, and water content. Hydropic change is a major consequence and is more marked in centrilobular hepatocytes, perhaps because of increased alcohol dehydrogenase activity. Glutathione content also falls, decreasing the cytoprotective capability against reactive metabolites, such as acetaldehyde. Ingestion of alcohol may result in increased collagen production in several cells in the liver, particularly myofibroblasts, contributing to the development of cirrhosis. Alcoholic hepatitis develops only in a minority of people who consume alcohol heavily, usually after many years of drinking, so the precise role of these mechanisms in the pathogenesis of alcoholic hepatitis remains uncertain.

Regulation of Hepatic Regeneration

Hepatic regrowth after resection, recovery from fulminant hepatic failure, and repair of the liver after acute and chronic hepatitis are examples of liver regeneration. The regenerative nodules that develop in cirrhosis may also reflect this process. Unfortunately, there is no clinically reliable way to monitor the regenerative response in humans.

The most important factors involved in hepatic regeneration are shown in Table 3-3. Two lines of evidence support a role for these substances. First, EGF, insulin, and glucagon have been extensively studied in animal models to document their effects on liver regeneration. Portal venous blood is necessary to maintain normal liver size and the proliferative response to hepatic resection. Portacaval transposition in dogs results in hepatic atrophy. The infusion of insulin into the lobes of livers deprived of portal blood prevents atrophy and preserves normal cell turnover. Heterotopic liver transplants in dogs atrophy unless perfused by splanchnic blood. In eviscerated rats the proliferative response after partial hepa-

Table 3-3 Substances that regulate hepatic regeneration

	Molecular weight	Source
Epidermal growth factor	6000	Submandibular gland, Brunner's glands, kidney
Insulin	6000	Pancreas
Glucagon	3500	Pancreas, GI tract
Insulinlike growth factor (IGF-I)	7600	Liver, fibroblasts, embryo, other
Insulinlike growth factor (IGF-II)	7500	Liver, ovaries, other

tectomy is decreased. But it can be restored to normal by infusion of both insulin and glucagon. Hepatic regeneration in rats after partial hepatectomy can be blunted by infusion of anti-insulin antiserum. EGF can initiate a proliferative response in unoperated animals without liver injury. This hormone binds to the hepatic remnant after partial hepatectomy, consistent with the role for EGF in hepatic regeneration.

The second line of evidence includes studies using rat hepatocyte cultures, which also provide evidence that insulin, glucagon, and EGF are involved in hepatic regeneration. The addition of either insulin or glucagon to resting hepatocyte cultures results in little proliferation, but a marked increase is observed when they are added along with EGF. Insulinlike growth factors resemble insulin in many biologic properties, but the effects are not suppressed by anti-insulin antiserum. These substances also add to the proliferative response in hepatocyte cultures.

Understandably, hepatic regeneration in humans has been less well-studied. Evidence of liver regeneration can be detected as early as 2 weeks after partial hepatectomy using liver-spleen scans. The regenerative response involves hyperplasia of residual hepatic lobes and, as in animals, the resected lobes do not regrow. The growth response is slower in elderly patients, even those with normal residual liver histology, and usually is not apparent after hepatic resection in patients with cirrhosis. As in animals, portal blood seems to be necessary to maintain normal human liver size and function. For this reason heterotopic liver transplants have been used only as a temporary solution to treat liver failure in patients.

CHOLESTASIS

Cholestasis is a term initially used by pathologists to describe the microscopic finding of bile stasis in the liver. For the clinician it refers to a spectrum of diseases in which there is interference with intrahepatic or extrahepatic bile flow.

Cholestasis has two major consequences. First, there is defective excretion of substances that are normally eliminated in the bile. These substances then accumulate in the serum and tissues. Second, there is defective secretion of bile salts needed for fat absorption. The clinical consequences of cholestasis are depicted in Figure 3-2.

Bile Flow

Bile formation begins in the canaliculi, where the secretion of solute into the bile establishes an osmotic gradient. This osmotic gradient is the driving force for movement of fluid and electrolytes into the bile. The bile ducts can alter the canalicular bile through further absorption and secretion of solutes.

The major determinant of canalicular bile flow is secretion of bile acids into the canaliculi. This is referred to as bile acid-dependent flow. A separate bile acid-independent component of bile flow also exists, but it is quantitatively less important.

Bile Acid-dependent Flow

Bile acids are quantitatively the most abundant solute in bile (comprising approximately 55%), and their secretion is the major mechanism promoting bile flow. On the other hand, certain bile acids may act to inhibit bile flow and thereby contribute to cholestasis. Thus bile-acid metabolism is a key factor in the pathophysiology of cholestasis.

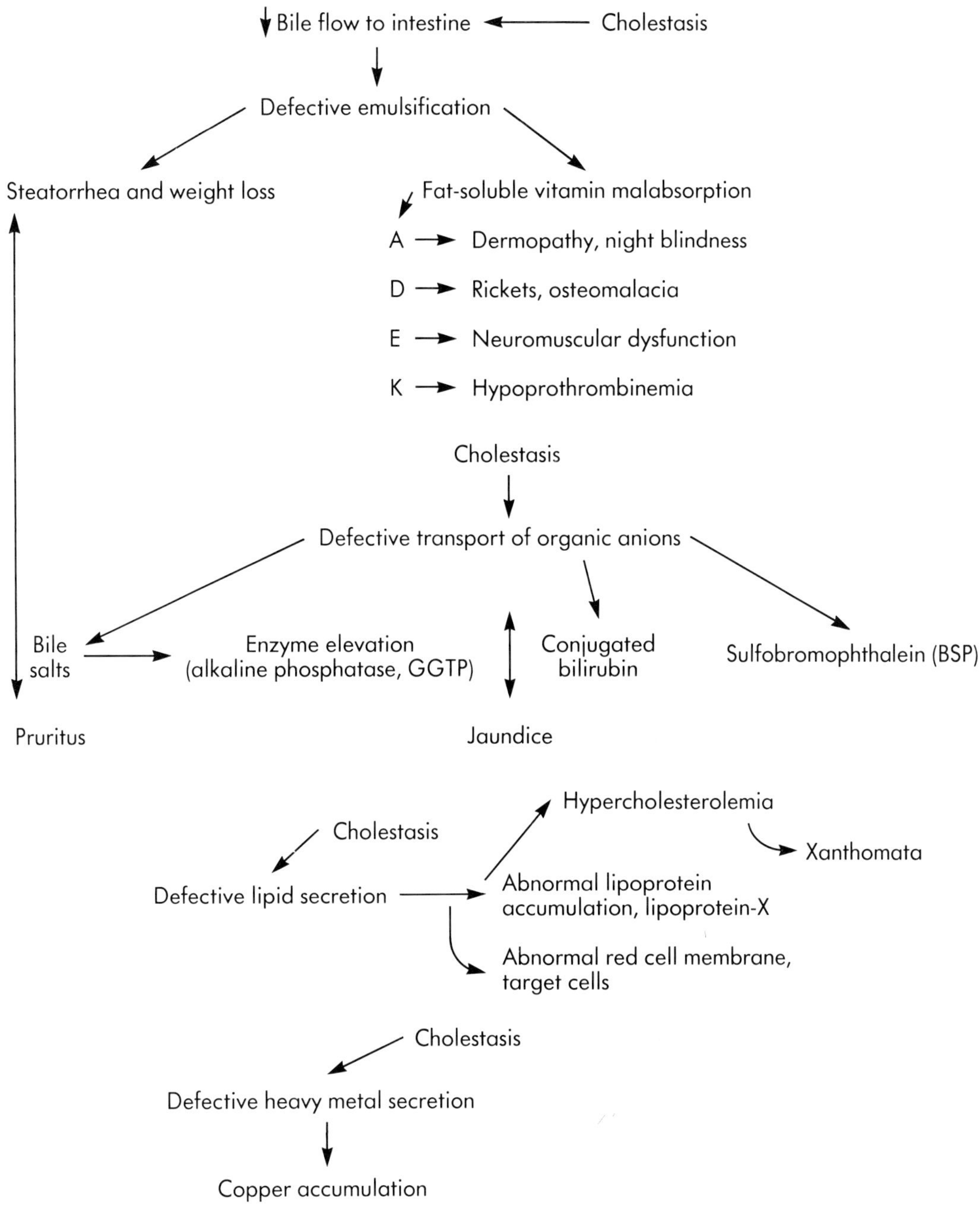

Figure 3-2
Clinical consequences of cholestasis.

Bile acids are produced in the liver as the major products of cholesterol metabolism. The two principal bile acids formed in humans are cholic acid and chenodeoxycholic acid, referred to as the primary bile acids. They are conjugated with an amino acid, gylcine or taurine, before being secreted into the bile canaliculi. The primary bile acids are metabolized in the intestine by bacterial action to secondary bile acids, including deoxycholic and lithocholic acid. Except for lithocholic acid, bile acids are efficiently reabsorbed in the terminal ileum, allowing only approximately 5% to escape in the stool. The reabsorbed bile acids enter the enterohepatic circulation and are efficiently extracted by the liver. Hepatic synthesis of bile acids occurs to replace the fraction lost in the stool, thereby maintaining a constant bile-acid pool. A synthetic rate of 50 to 600 mg a day is able to maintain a bile acid pool of approximately 2 to 3 g and to secrete 20 to 30 g a day in the bile.

Bile-acid uptake and secretion by the hepatocyte is an energy-dependent active process involving intracellular organelles and carrier-mediated mechanisms. A linear relationship exists between the rate of bile-acid secretion and the rate of bile flow.

The periportal (zone 1) hepatocytes are the major sites of bile acid-dependent secretion, but the pericentral (zone 3) hepatocytes are relatively deficient. Thus a lobular gradient is created, promoting the flow of bile in the portal direction. Some forms of cholestatic liver injury may interfere with this gradient and thereby promote cholestasis. The zonal differences in bile-acid transport predispose to a predominant centrilobular distribution of bile plugging, which is characteristic of cholestatic conditions.

Although bile acids are important in promoting bile flow, under certain circumstances they may inhibit flow. Most bile acids at high concentrations can produce or aggravate cholestasis. Lithocholic acid produced from chenodeoxycholic acid in the intestine may produce cholestasis in animals. Elevations of lithocholate have been reported in several cholestatic liver diseases, such as primary biliary cirrhosis and Byler's disease. Such elevations may play a role in pathogenesis. The exact mechanism by which lithocholate produces cholestasis is uncertain, but it may be related to the ability of lithocholate to alter membrane permeability.

Bile Acid-independent Flow

A component of canalicular bile flow is independent of bile acid secretion and is referred to as bile acid-independent flow. A sodium, potassium–adenosine triphosphatase (ATPase) (Na^+, K^+-ATPase) mediated sodium-transport system is responsible for maintaining a chemical and electrical gradient, thereby acting as a driving force for bile flow. Stimulation of this mechanism by phenobarbital accounts for this agent's choleretic action. A bicarbonate transport system and glutathione secretion have also been implicated as possible mediators of bile acid-independent flow.

Ductular Bile Flow

Bile entering the ductules and larger bile ducts continues to be modified by secretion and absorption. Little is known about the specifics of the transport mechanisms, except that a bicarbonate-rich secretion that is stimulated by secretin occurs. The secretory action of bile ducts explains the choleresis associated with some liver disorders that have bile-duct proliferation.

Mechanisms of Cholestasis

Cholestasis occurs when there is mechanical obstruction to the extrahepatic bile flow, destruction of intrahepatic bile ducts, or a disturbance of the hepatocyte bile secretory mechanisms.

Extrahepatic cholestasis caused by mechanical obstruction occurs with conditions such as bile-duct strictures, stones, and ampullary and pancreatic tumors. Extrahepatic cholestasis is relatively easy to diagnose using modern radiographic imaging techniques, such as ultrasound, computed tomography (CT) scans, endoscopic retrograde cholangiopancreatography (ERCP), or percutaneous transhepatic cholangiogram (PTC).

Cholestatic disorders resulting from primary defects in the intrahepatic bile ducts occur in the group of disorders referred to as vanishing bile duct syndrome (see box below). The etiologic factor responsible for the bile-duct destruction is often unknown. An infection with Reovirus 3 has been implicated in neonatal biliary atresia. Immunologic mediators have been implicated as playing a role in conditions such as primary biliary cirrhosis (PBC), primary sclerosing cholangitis (PSC), rejection, and graft vs. host disease.

The pathogenesis of cholestasis originating at the hepatocyte level often involves impairment of several components of the bile-secretory mechanism. These impairments include disturbances of intracellular organelles, membrane transport systems, and structural changes. The specific disturbance that occurs at a molecular level continues to be sought.

VANISHING BILE-DUCT SYNDROMES

Developmental/congenital

Biliary Atresia

Syndromatic paucity of intrahepatic ducts (e.g., Alagille syndrome)

Nonsyndromatic paucity of intrahepatic ducts

Ductal-plate Malformations (polycystic, Caroli's, congenital hepatic fibrosis)

Acquired

Primary biliary cirrhosis (PBC)

Primary sclerosing cholangitis (PSC)

Allograft liver rejection

Graft vs. host disease (GVHD)

PROTEIN METABOLISM

The serum contains a large number of proteins, the major source of which is the liver. Hepatocytes synthesize albumin, coagulation factors, and most of the α- and β-globulins. Notable exceptions are γ-globulins and factor VIII, which are produced in the reticuloendothelial system. Measurement of the serum albumin concentration and the prothrombin time (PT) is used to assess hepatic synthetic capacity. However, determination of albumin and clotting factors is limited by a lack of sensitivity and specificity. The values are normal in patients with mild liver disease, but abnormal results may be obtained in nonhepatic diseases, such as nutritional deprivation.

Albumin and Globulin Metabolism

Albumin synthesized by the liver is not stored in the hepatocyte but is rapidly secreted. Because it is not a high-priority protein (necessary for organism protection), it is synthesized only during periods of adequate nutritional intake, but production is stopped during nutritional deprivation. The serum albumin level is the net result of hepatic production, distribution, and degradation. The liver synthesizes albumin at a rate approximately equal to 200 g/kg body weight per day. Synthesis may be affected by several factors. Nutritional deprivation adversely affects albumin production and rapidly results in decreased albumin synthesis. Infections, burns, or surgery may result in hypoalbuminemia. This deficiency is multifactorial, representing direct losses through the burn or surgical wound, an increased metabolic requirement, nutritional deprivation, and cytokine release during stress. Interleukin-1 and tumor-necrosis factor (TNF) appear to inhibit albumin synthesis. Hepatic secretion of albumin may also be inhibited by drugs, such as colchicine, and by acetaldehyde, a metabolic product of alcohol. Changes in intrahepatic colloid osmotic pressure also appear to regulate the rate of hepatic synthesis.

Following delivery into the plasma, albumin is widely distributed in the intravascular and extravascular spaces. The concentration in the plasma is above that in the extravascular spaces, thereby maintaining the integrity of the colloid osmotic pressure.

The turnover of albumin is fairly stable, and degradation occurs at a very slow rate (approximately 3% per day). Serum albumin has a half-life of approximately 17 days. Little is known about the mechanism of albumin degradation.

The decreased albumin level seen in patients with nonascitic cirrhosis probably represents depressed protein synthesis. However, in the presence of ascites the albumin pool is actually increased, and high rates of synthesis have been observed. The explanation is uncertain but may be secondary to changes in the hepatic colloid osmotic pressure. These changes stimulate protein synthesis and direct losses of newly synthesized albumin into the ascitic fluid.

Serum albumin helps to maintain plasma colloid osmotic pressure. This pressure counteracts the hydrostatic pressure acting to move fluid out of the intravascular space. Therefore a decreased serum albumin concentration contributes to the formation of edema. Serum albumin also serves to transport a variety of substances, such as hormones, drugs, ions, fatty acids, and bilirubin. Hypoalbuminemia results in decreased binding of these substances and, consequently, abnormal free plasma levels with a variety of metabolic derangements. The fraction of a drug bound to albumin acts as a circulating reservoir, leaving the unbound or free portion as the metabolically available fraction. Because only the free fraction of a drug is available to the tissues, hypoalbuminemia and the subsequent increase in the free fraction enhances the effect of the drug.

When the serum albumin falls in patients with liver disease, the γ-globulin level often rises. This increase may occur in any hepatic disease that is severe and prolonged. Synthetic disturbances usually appear earlier in the course of hepatocellular dysfunction than cholestatic disorders. A decreased albumin level usually reflects severe hepatic injury. In acute viral hepatitis the aminotransferases and bilirubin elevations do not correlate with outcome, but a decreased albumin level usually reflects severe hepatic involvement.

The explanation for the increased γ-globulin is not clear, but it may be due to the shunting of antigens normally cleared by the liver. These antigens then become available to the rest of the RES and stimulate γ-globulin production. It is also possible that the immune system in liver disease patients shows increased responsiveness. High globulin levels are especially common in patients with alcoholic hepatitis and autoimmune chronic active hepatitis. The pattern of immunoglobulin elevation is not diagnostic, but elevations of immunoglobulin M (IgM) are common in primary biliary cirrhosis, elevations of IgG are common in chronic active hepatitis, and elevations of IgA are common in alcoholic cirrhosis.

Clotting Factors

The liver plays a central role in coagulation homeostasis. It synthesizes clotting factors, including fibrinogen, prothrombin, factors V, VII, IX, X, XI, and XII, proteins C and S, prekallikrein, and high-molecular-weight kininogen. It is also responsible for production of coagulant inhibitors (antithrombin 3) and fibrinolytic proteins (plasminogen). The liver also serves as a major site for clearance of circulating anticoagulants and activated fibrinolytic substances. Liver disease also is often associated with a decrease in platelet number secondary to sequestering in the spleen, as well as a disturbance of platelet function. Therefore pathogenesis of bleeding during liver disease is complex, involving disturbances of coagulation-factor production, platelet deficiencies, and defective function and failure to clear activated fibrinolytic substances.

Measurement of the prothrombin time (PT) and partial thromboplastin time (PTT) is useful to assess abnormalities of clotting that occur with liver dysfunction. These measurements do not reflect a specific defect but a generalized decrease in protein synthesis.

The vitamin K-dependent factors prothrombin and factors VII, IX, and X are required for blood-coagulation regulation. Vitamin K is required for formation of γ-carboxyglutamic acid, an amino acid that confers coagulation activity to precursor proteins. A disturbance of vitamin K metabolism may result in prolonged PT.

A prolonged PT is not specific to liver disease; it occurs with vitamin K deficiency, congenital coagulation factor deficiency, or consumptive coagulopathy. Some drugs, particularly antibiotics, may cause vitamin K depletion.

Administration of vitamin K may help to differentiate patients with obstructive jaundice from those with parenchymal disease. In obstructive jaundice, vitamin K absorption is disturbed because bile salts required for absorption fail to enter the intestine. Thus repletion through parenteral vitamin K administration improves PT. In parenchymal disease, PT is prolonged because of a synthetic disturbance and thus is not corrected with vitamin K administration.

The PT is of some prognostic value, especially in acute liver disease. A PT prolonged more than 3 seconds is associated with significant hepatic damage and a poor outcome. However, this prognosis also depends on the reversibility of the hepatic insult.

METABOLISM OF CHOLESTEROL AND LIPOPROTEINS

Cholesterol Metabolism

Cholesterol is an essential constituent of biologic membranes and an important precursor of steroid hormones, vitamins, and bile acids. On the other hand, its atherogenic potential has been well established, making hypercholesterolemia an important risk factor for coronary artery

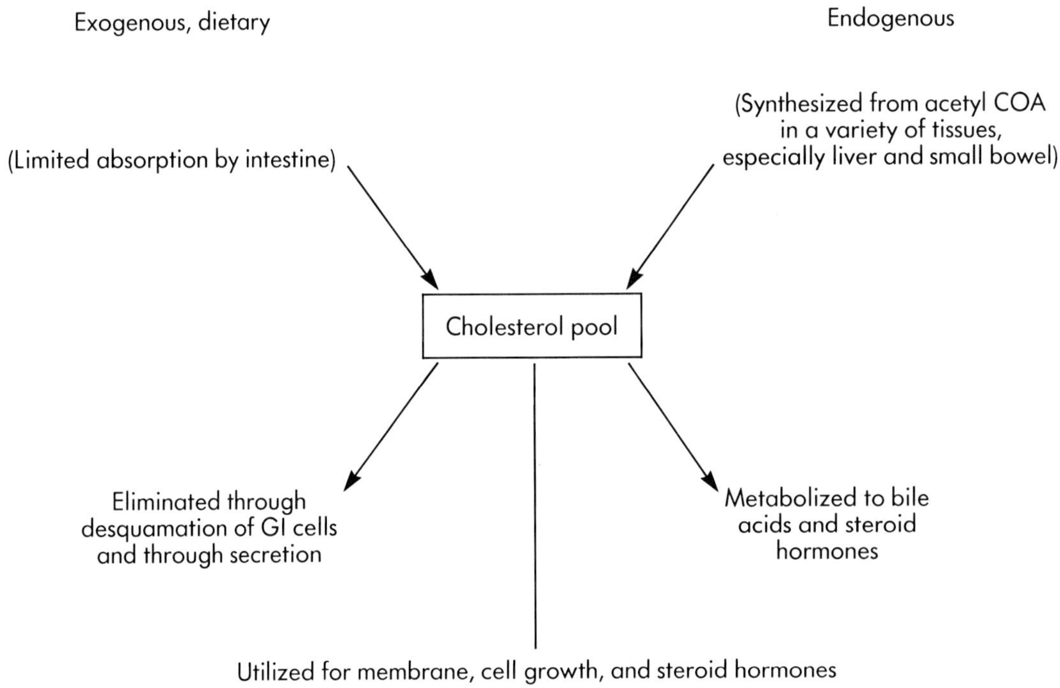

Figure 3-3
Cholesterol metabolism.

disease and stroke. Furthermore, increased cholesterol secretion in the bile can result in supersaturation of the bile, a prerequisite for the formation of cholesterol gallstones. Therefore a complex metabolism exists to meet the continuous need for cholesterol while counteracting the tendency toward dangerous accumulation.

The body pool of cholesterol in the adult remains fairly constant by balancing absorption and endogenous synthesis with metabolism and excretion (Figure 3-3). The liver plays a central role in regulating cholesterol balance. First, hepatic LDL receptors have been established as playing a central role in regulating the uptake of cholesterol from the plasma. Second, biliary secretion of cholesterol and its degradation product, bile acid, represents the major mechanism for elimination of cholesterol from the body. Finally, the liver (and intestines) synthesize the various lipoprotein particles needed to transport cholesterol between tissues. Therefore it is not surprising that liver dysfunction may result in significant disturbances of cholesterol and lipoprotein metabolism.

Lipoprotein Metabolism

Lipoproteins are particles consisting of lipid and specific proteins called apoproteins. Lipoproteins are typically classified on the basis of electrophoretic mobility and hydrated density (Table 3-4).

Table 3-4 Features of major lipoproteins

Type	Density	Lipid compositions
Chylomicrons	0.95	Triglycerides (exogenous)
VLDL	0.95-1.04	Triglycerides (endogenous)
IDL	1.005-1.019	Esterified triglycerides, phospholipids
LDL	1.019-1.063	Triglycerides, esterified cholesterol
HDL	1.063-1.210	Cholesterol, phospholipids

The function of the lipoprotein classes is to transport lipids in the plasma. Triglycerides are transported from synthetic sites in the intestine (chylomicrons) and liver (VLDL) to peripheral tissues, where the liberated free fatty acids are used as an energy source. Cholesterol is transported from the liver and intestines to peripheral tissues, largely as cholesterol ester in the core of LDL, where it is used for cell-membrane and steroid synthesis. Excess tissue cholesterol is transported back to the liver (HDL) for excretion in the bile or for reuse. An overview of the lipoprotein pathway is depicted in Figure 3-4.

Chylomicrons consisting of triglycerides and exogenous cholesterol are produced in the intestine from dietary lipids. The function of chylomicrons is to transport dietary lipids and fat-soluble vitamins from the intestine to the tissues and liver. The triglyceride in the chylomicron core undergoes lipolysis by lipoprotein lipase (LPL), an enzyme attached to capillary endothelium. This breakdown releases free fatty acids, which are used as an energy source. The chylomicron remnants so formed are efficiently taken up by high-affinity receptors on the liver. The liver secretes endogenous cholesterol and triglycerides into the plasma in the form of VLDL. The triglycerides are removed by LPL, resulting in the formation of a cholesterol-rich particle called intermediate-density lipoprotein (IDL). Some of these particles are cleared from the plasma by the liver, but most IDL particles are converted to LDL. A second hepatic enzyme, hepatic lipase, is thought to be involved in the conversion of IDL to LDL. LDL is then removed from the plasma by LDL receptors on the liver and peripheral tissue. Thus LDL is the major source of cholesterol for the peripheral cells. Excess cholesterol in the peripheral cells is transported back to the liver, mainly in the form of HDL. Cholesterol within HDL may also be exchanged into VLDL and LDL and thereby transported back to the liver. The process of transport from the periphery back to the liver is called "reverse cholesterol transport" but generally is only partially understood. Esterification of cholesterol results in the production of spherical HDL particles, which contain a core of cholesteryl ester. This reaction is mediated by lecithin-cholesterol acyltransferase (LCAT), an enzyme produced by the liver. This enzyme plays a key role in lipoprotein metabolism, specifically reverse cholesterol transport. The principal protein component of HDL, apolipoprotein A-I (apo A-I), is a major cofactor for LCAT activation. Thus the liver plays a major role in HDL metabolism by direct synthesis and reac-

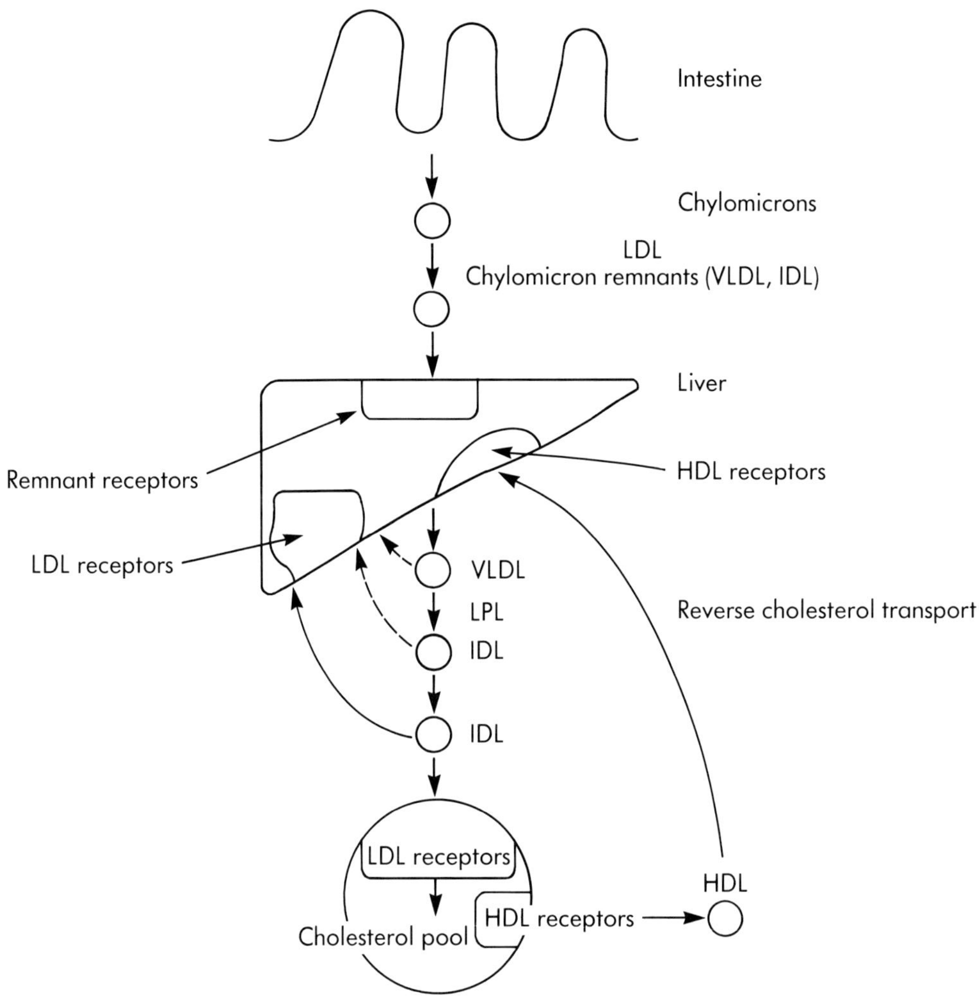

Figure 3-4
Lipoprotein cascade.

tion of apo A-I and HDL and by production of LCAT.

Lipid Disturbances in Liver Disease

Cholestatic liver disease. Cholestatic liver diseases, such as primary biliary cirrhosis, are commonly associated with striking hyperlipidemia. Marked increases in total serum cholesterol occur, but elevations of phospholipid and triglyceride also occur. Most of the excess cholesterol occurs in the form of an abnormal particle called lipoprotein-X (LP-X). It is thought that LP-X rises either because of regurgitation of bile into the plasma or because of deficient LCAT activity, resulting in accumulation of phospholipid and cholesterol in the serum. Secondary cholesterol deposits may occur, resulting in cutaneous xanthomata and xanthelasma.

Parenchymal liver disease. Both acute and chronic parenchymal liver disease may be associated with lipid abnormalities. The changes are similar but are usually less pronounced with chronic disease. The most characteristic alteration is a decrease in the percentage of cholesterol esters and HDL. This decrease is primarily due to an inability of the damaged hepatocyte to produce LCAT and apo A-I, resulting in deficient esterification of cholesterol and decreased HDL. This inability usually is resolved with clinical improvement.

Hypertriglyceridemia (usually less than 500 mg/dl) occurs commonly in parenchymal liver disease. It is transient and returns to normal with improvement in liver function. Evidence suggests that a deficiency in hepatic triglyceride lipase occurs, possibly accounting for the raised triglyceride.

Summary

The liver plays a central role in the complex cholesterol and lipoprotein metabolism. It regulates uptake and excretion of cholesterol and synthesizes the various enzymes and apoproteins needed for cholesterol transport. Therefore disturbances of lipid concentrations and compositions commonly accompany liver dysfunction.

DRUG CLEARANCE AND HEPATIC METABOLISM

Some Pharmacokinetic Principles

Clearance, generally the most useful description of experimental and human drug disposition, refers to the quantity of blood completely cleared of a drug or xenobiotic in a set time. The main determinants of clearance (Cl) are the blood flow (Q) and the effectiveness of the removal of the drug from the circulation, or extraction ratio (E), according to the following formula:

$$Cl = Q \times E$$

Other descriptions are used to refer to some aspects of hepatic drug metabolism, include $t_{1/2}$, the time required for the concentration of a test substance to fall to half its maximal concentration. Thus half-life is frequently used to refer to the disposition of some drugs. The half-life of some benzodiazepines is increased more than twofold in cirrhotics. The following description is dependent on clearance and the initial volume of distribution of the test substance, V_D. It represents a more indirect parameter:

$$t_{1/2} = \frac{V_D \times 0.693}{Cl}$$

The formula above shows that the extraction ratio is a major factor in determining the clearance of drugs by the liver. Drugs with a high extraction ratio (greater than 0.6) exhibit high first-pass effect; that is, a large proportion of the drug will be eliminated on the first passage of blood through the liver. In addition, drugs with a high first-pass effect show little systemic availability when administered by mouth. Orally administered drugs first pass by way of the portal blood to the liver before reaching the general circulation, so only a small quantity of a drug with a high extraction ratio would be expected to reach the systemic circulation.

Nitroglycerin is an example of such a drug. Because of its high extraction ratio, most of the drug is eliminated from the blood during the first passage through the liver, so little of the drug is available for a systemic effect. Sodium valproate, a drug for the treatment of seizures, also exhibits a high first-pass effect. However, when administered to cirrhotics systemic levels of sodium valproate are considerably higher, and the cardiac side effects, as reflected in electrocardiographic changes, are greater. The altered pharmacokinetics of sodium valproate in cirrhosis illustrates the effect of liver disease on drugs with a high extraction ratio. Cirrhosis is accompanied by the development of extrahepatic and intrahepatic shunts. Thus nutrient hepatic blood flow declines, and drugs ordinarily removed by the liver pass without interruption to the systemic circulation. The net result is that even drugs with a high extraction ratio exhibit pharmacokinetics like drugs with low extraction ratios. Liver enzyme activity rather than blood flow becomes the main determinant of drug elimination.

Quantitative Liver-function Tests

In healthy subjects the clearance of drugs with a low extraction ratio also reflects mainly hepatic enzyme activity. Antipyrine and aminopyrine have received extensive study as model drugs with low extraction ratios. Clearance of both drugs is decreased in experimental animal cirrhosis and in humans with chronic liver disease compared with healthy control subjects, but decreased hepatic blood flow alone does not change clearance greatly. In addition, inducers of hepatic drug metabolizing enzymes, such as phenobarbital, increase the clearance of these drugs, whereas inhibitors of hepatic drug metabolism decrease the clearance.

These characteristics have led some investigators to use the clearance of model drugs that have low extraction ratios to quantitate liver function. Considerable attention has been devoted to the aminopyrine breath test, an easy and convenient test that does not require multiple blood samples as do most conventional clearance measurements. In this test, aminopyrine is labeled with a stable isotope of carbon, and a measured dose is administered by mouth to a test subject. The drug is absorbed into the portal circulation and taken up by the liver, and the labeled carbons are removed in a rate-limiting reaction by aminopyrine N-demethylase, a component of the microsomal drug-metabolizing system. Labeled carbon atoms equilibrate in the body's CO_2 pool and are expired in the breath. Breath samples are collected, and stable isotopic enrichment is measured by differential isotope ratio spectrometry. Appearance of the isotope in breath reflects hepatic N-demethylase activity.

A number of studies have shown that the aminopyrine breath test can reliably discriminate between cirrhotic and noncirrhotic patients, as documented by liver biopsy findings. Compared with other noninvasive tests, the aminopyrine breath test appears to be useful in detecting the early stage of alcoholic cirrhosis, and it provides a useful indicator of short-term prognosis in this population. The aminopyrine breath test also discriminates reliably between patients with mild and severe chronic hepatitis. In contrast, findings in the aminopyrine breath test are not necessarily abnormal in patients with primary biliary cirrhosis, in which there is preservation of functional hepatic mass, as well as hepatic enzyme activity until late in the course of the disease. As expected with drugs with a low extraction ratio, alterations in hepatic blood flow alone appear to have little effect on the aminopyrine breath test.

Alcohol and Drug Metabolism

Elimination of drugs from liver cells is mediated by the hepatic microsomal drug-metabolizing enzyme system. Many drugs require initial metabolism by the cytochrome P-450 drug-metabolizing system located in the microsomes (phase 1 reaction). This enzyme system catalyzes the oxidation of a wide range of substrates and is usually followed by a conjugation reaction (phase 2 reaction), often with glucuronide, sulfate, or glutathione. These reactions render the compounds water-soluble, permitting biliary or urinary excretion. In general, phase 1 reactions are more markedly impaired by liver disease than phase 2 reactions. Thus the clearance of benzodiazepines, such as lorazepam, requiring only a phase 2 reaction, is much less affected by the presence of liver disease than is the clearance of oxazepam, which requires both phase 1 and phase 2 reactions.

The hepatic metabolism of a number of drugs is inhibited in humans by acute ingestion of alcohol. The clearance of phenobarbital, meprobamate, and other sedative-hypnotics is decreased after acute ingestion of alcohol. The mechanism probably involves competition with ethanol to bind to microsomal drug-metabolizing enzyme sites. Ingestion of phenobarbital with alcohol is particularly dangerous because ethanol markedly reduces the lethal dose of phenobarbital.

Chronic ethanol consumption also alters the hepatic metabolism of drugs and xenobiotics. Chronic alcohol consumption carries an increased risk for development of carcinoma of the lung, oropharynx, esophagus, and pancreas. Studies using the liver microsomes of rats that were repeatedly fed alcohol demonstrate an increased capacity to activate potential carcinogens, some of which give positive results in the Ames test. Thus the liver, the major site of xenobiotic metabolism, appears to play an important role in development of several carcinomas.

METABOLIC HOMEOSTASIS

Receiving blood from the intestine through the portal vein, the liver is ideally situated to play a major role in the regulation of carbohydrate, protein, and lipid metabolism. In addition, the organ is the main site of catabolism of a variety of hormones involved in regulating hepatic metabolism and preserving metabolic homeostasis. These hormones include insulin, glucagon, glucocorticoids, thyroxin, and growth hormone.

Carbohydrate Metabolism

After a meal the liver prevents wide swings in blood-glucose levels and serum osmolality by extracting glucose from portal blood. Insulin, which is released into the portal vein during feeding, is the major hormone mediating this response. The liver is extremely sensitive to the effects of insulin, and small increases in portal blood concentrations cause substantial increases in hepatic glucose uptake. Hepatic autoregulatory mechanisms also modify glucose uptake.

Excess hepatocyte glucose is stored mainly as glycogen, which can be mobilized rapidly to maintain blood sugar levels during periods of fasting. Glucose may also be metabolized in glycolysis or the hexose monophosphate shunt. These pathways may lead to increased lipid synthesis by the liver, often accompanied by increased VLDL synthesis and secretion.

During fasting a critical function of the liver is to maintain blood-sugar levels for the brain and peripheral nerves, tissues that can use only this substrate for fuel during periods of fasting lasting up to several weeks. Glycogenolysis is the main source of blood sugar during short periods of fasting, lasting up to 24 hours. However, as the period of starvation lengthens, the liver's glycogen stores are depleted, and most tissues in the body quickly adapt to use of ketone bodies and fatty acids as fuels. But the brain and peripheral nervous system require several weeks to adapt to use of nonglucose sources of energy.

Gluconeogenesis, a key function of the liver, also helps to meet the need for blood sugar during short periods of fasting. Glucogenic amino acids undergo molecular rearrangement in the liver, creating carbon skeletons that can be used for net glucose synthesis. Lactate from muscle glycogenolysis can also be used by the liver to help support the blood sugar.

Hypoglycemia

Considering the involvement of the liver in modulating the blood-sugar concentration, it is surprising that hypoglycemia is not more common in patients with acute and chronic liver disease. Because maintenance of blood sugar is such a critical liver function, it is preserved even in most patients with advanced liver disease. The kidney can also contribute to gluconeogenesis and may prevent hypoglycemic complication in some patients with liver disease.

Most investigators have suggested that impaired glycogen metabolism, probably decreased glycogen storage, is the major factor resulting in hypoglycemia in patients with acute and chronic liver diseases. Thus patients with fulminant hepatic failure, viral hepatitis, and cirrhosis usually display a subnormal rise in blood glucose concentration after parenteral glucagon administration. Patients with large tumors, including hepatocellular carcinomas, may have hypoglycemia because of increased glucose uptake by the tumor. Some toxins, such as acetaminophen and phosphorus, may be associated with hypoglycemia. A variety of mechanisms, such as impaired glycogen storage, glycogenolysis, and gluconeogenesis, may be involved in these situations of fluctuating blood glucose.

Acute ethanol ingestion occasionally produces profound hypoglycemia in fasting persons, regardless of the presence of liver disease. During fasting, liver glycogen levels become depleted. Ingested alcohol is metabolized mainly by alcohol dehydrogenase, and if the ingested quantity is large enough, the NAD/NADH ratio in the liver falls. This change in redox potential results in inhibition of gluconeogenesis, leading to hypoglycemia. This problem is more frequent in chronic alcoholics, probably because of their poor nutritional state and decreased hepatic glycogen stores. Some investigators have reported death rates as high as 10% for patients with alcohol-induced hypoglycemia.

Protein and Amino Acid Metabolism

In healthy adults, up to 10 kg of body mass is composed of protein. This important structural element of the body is constantly being remodeled. Therefore protein turnover may be as much as 300 g/day. Up to 250 g of protein, from both endogenous protein catabolism and dietary sources, are broken down and eliminated from the body daily. As with carbohydrate metabolism, the liver is a key organ in protein trafficking, both after a meal and during fasting.

After ingestion of a meal containing protein, portal vein amino acids rise markedly, but peripheral blood amino acids rise only modestly. Although the liver is a major site for amino acid uptake, branched chain amino acids (valine, isoleucine, and leucine) are less avidly removed from portal blood and passed to the periphery, where they are taken up mainly by muscle. Depending on the size of the meal, up to 50% of ingested protein may be catabolized through the urea cycle, but smaller quantities are used for synthesis of new protein.

During fasting, some protein equivalents continue to return to the liver through the portal vein because of enterohepatic cycling and exfoliation of intestinal cells. Nonetheless, protein balance becomes negative, mainly because of the necessity of gluconeogenesis. Thus alanine and other glucogenic amino acids are released from muscle and travel to the liver for glucose production. However, serum proteins undergo little short-term catabolism, and they serve to preserve serum osmolality and normal cardiovascular function.

The Urea Cycle

The liver is also the unique site of detoxification of excess nitrogen equivalents in the body, which result mainly from protein breakdown. Two moles of ammonia enter the urea cycle, and for each rotation, a mole of urea is produced. Approximately 75% of the resultant urea is excreted through the kidneys, but a small quantity is eliminated through the gastrointestinal tract.

In acute and chronic liver injury the liver's capacity to eliminate nitrogen equivalents through the urea cycle may be limited. In addition, protein catabolism may add to the nitrogen load if malnutrition is present. Consequently, the serum ammonia level rises, contributing to the development of hepatic encephalopathy, one of the major clinical effects of severe liver injury. In addition, a number of deficiencies of the enzymes that make up the urea cycle have been described. Patients with these deficiencies have similar clinical presentations, which include marked hyperammonemia, seizures, and mental retardation, as well as death in infancy.

SUGGESTED READINGS

Brown MS and Goldstein JC: Lipoprotein receptors in the liver, J Clin Invest 72:743-747, Sept 1983.

This review emphasizes the central role of liver in lipoprotein metabolism.

Brewer HB et al: Apoliproproteins and lipoproteins in human plasma: an overview, Clin Chem 34(8):B, B4-B8, 1988.

An overview of serum apolipoprotein and lipoprotein metabolism and classification is presented.

Fenster LF: Reactive hepatopathy, Postgrad Med 76:62-68, 1984.

This is an article on hyperbilirubinemia occurring as a result of sepsis and surgery.

Gollan JL and Schmid R: Bilirubin update. In Popper H and Schaffner F, eds: Formation, transport, and metabolism, vol 7, Progress in liver diseases, New York, 1982, Grune & Stratton.

The authors present a detailed update on bilirubin metabolism.

Oelberg DA and Lester R: Cellular mechanisms of cholestasis, Ann Rev Med 37:297-317, 1986.

This is an article on the molecular mechanism of various cholestatic disorders.

Rothschild MA, Oratz M, and Schriber S: Serum albumin, Hepatol 8:385-401, 1988.

This is an overview of serum albumin, emphasizing the role of the liver.

Weiss JS et al: The clinical importance of a protein-bound fraction of serum bilirubin in patients with hyperbilirubinemia, N Engl J Med 309:147-50, 1983.

An overview of the significance of δ-bilirubin is presented.

SECTION TWO

Evaluation of Injury and Repair

4 Mechanisms of Liver Injury

Stephen B. Sinclair** and **Gary A. Levy

Liver damage can occur following viral infection or exposure to drugs and toxins. Drugs and toxins can injure cells through direct damage to cell membranes or through the release of reactive intermediary metabolites with resultant release of oxygen free radicals and lipid peroxidation. Viruses can damage the liver directly, as in hepatitis A, δ-agent, or hepatitis C infection, or through immunologically mediated mechanisms, as in hepatitis B infection. The immunologic injury can occur either through a cellular-mediated or humoral-mediated mechanism, or through the release of cytokines. This chapter deals with mechanisms of liver injury as they are currently understood.

IMMUNOLOGICALLY MEDIATED LIVER INJURY

The Immune System

The immune system consists of lymphocytes, macrophages, neutrophils, and a series of related cells, including the dendritic cells of the spleen and the epidermal Langerhan's cells, as well as specialized epithelial cells, such as those found in the thymus, bone marrow, and other lymphoid organs (Figure 4-1). Individual lymphocytes are specialized in that they respond to a limited group of structurally related antigens. This commitment exists before the first contact of the immune system with a given antigen and is expressed by the presence on the lymphocyte membrane of receptors specific for determinants of that antigen. Individual lymphocytes possess a population of receptors, and one lymphocyte clone will differ from another in the structure of the combining regions of its receptors. The ability of the organism to respond to virtually any antigen occurs through the existence of a very large number of different lymphocyte clones.

Cellular Constituents

Lymphocytes differ from one another not only in their receptor specificity but also in their functional properties. Two broad classes of lymphocytes are recognized: the B lymphocytes, which are precursors of antibody-secreting cells, and the T, or thymus-dependent, lymphocytes. T lymphocytes consist of a series of subtypes, some of which mediate important regulatory functions, such as the ability to help or suppress the development of immune responses, including antibody production. Other T lymphocytes are involved in ef-

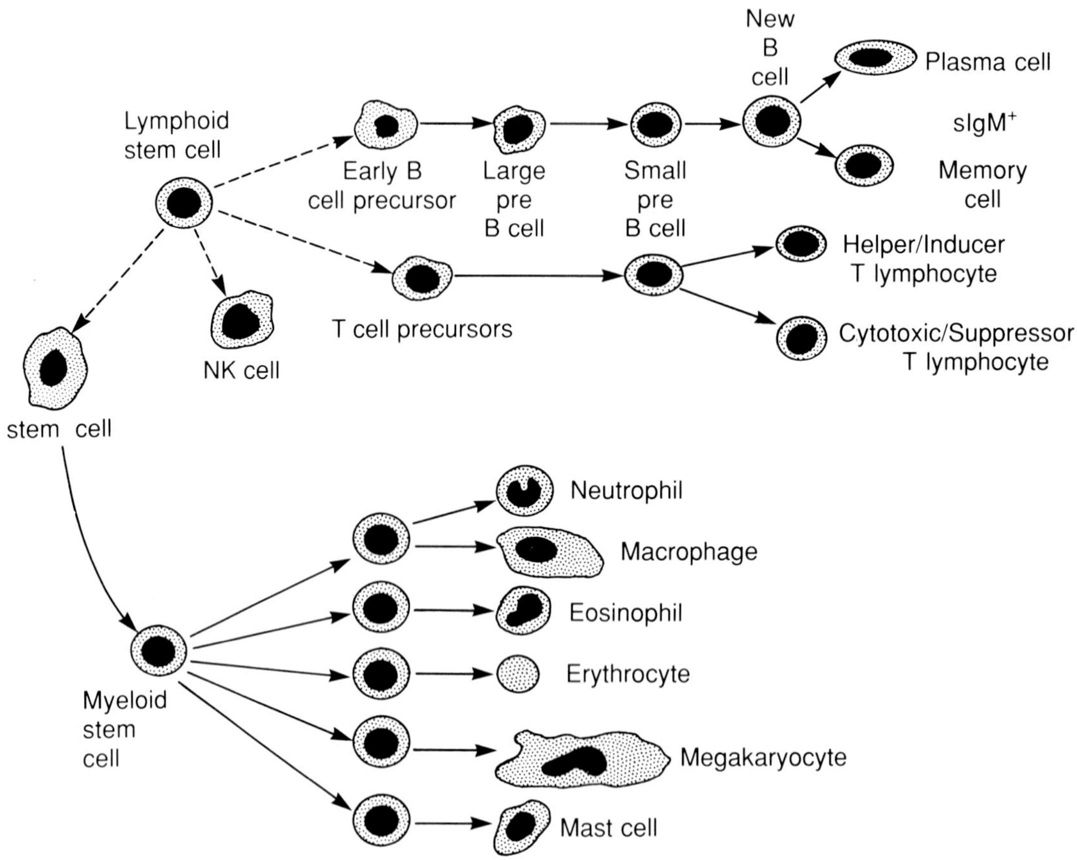

Figure 4-1
Cellular constituents of the immune response.

fector functions, such as the direct destruction of agents bearing antigenic components. Thus, we recognize groups of helper T cells, suppressor T cells, killer T cells, and T cells involved in delayed hypersensitivity and related immune phenomena.

In addition to these two major lymphocyte classes, lymphoid cells that mediate certain nonspecific cytotoxic responses have been defined. These cells include natural killer (NK) cells, which are involved in tumor-cell surveillance. A second type of nonspecific killing of target cells is antibody-dependent cellular cytotoxicity (ADCC), capable of killing antibody-coated target cells after recognition of the antibody bound to that target cell.

Another cell important in the inflammatory response is the mononuclear phagocyte, or macrophage. The macrophage can initiate and amplify the immune response through its ability to process and present antigens and to produce cytokines. The macrophage in turn becomes the target of a positive-feedback loop when it is activated by lymphokines elaborated during the specific immune response. Therefore the tissue macrophage has two major roles. It becomes activated by interferon-γ (IFN-γ) and has a critical role as an effector cell, with heightened capacity for ingestion and killing. In addition, macrophage factors initiate coagulation, cause chemotaxis of leukocytes, and promote wound healing through stimulation of fibroblast replication and secretion of collagen and glycosaminoglycans.

The initial activation of helper T cells in the course of the primary immune response probably depends on T cell corecognition of a complex consisting of an antigen and a major histocompatibility-complex molecule on an antigen-presenting cell. Such antigen-presenting cells include macrophages, Langerhan's cells, and dendritic cells. The activation of T cells by antigen-presenting cells depends not only on the antigen-major histocompatibility complex displayed on the surface of the antigen-presenting cell but also on the accessory-cell function mediated by the antigen presenting-cell. In humans, IL-1 may mediate such accessory function. Some T helper cells (Th1) appear insensitive to the action of IL-1, and the accessory signals may involve an uncharacterized molecule.

Suppressor T cells. In addition to the stimulation of the immune response, specialized T cells designated as suppressor T cells have the capacity to suppress immune responses. A substantial body of research indicates the existence of circuits of suppressor cell activity involving both suppressor-inducer cells and suppressor-effector cells. Furthermore, it must be recognized that suppressive regulatory events in the immune system can be caused by inhibitory actions or by secretory products of helper or inducer cells. A good example is the capacity of IFN-γ to inhibit many of the functions of IL-4 on murine B cells.

Cytotoxic T lymphocytes (CTL). T cells act as important effectors of immune responses. This action occurs through lysis of target cells bearing foreign antigens. Cytotoxic T lymphocytes (CTLs) generally recognize antigen associated with class I major histocompatibility complex (MHC) molecules and express CD8. However, there are now examples of $CD4^+$, CTL cells that corecognize antigen and class II MHC molecules. The molecular mechanism by which CTLs cause target cell lysis is the production of cytoplasmic granules that contain lytic molecules (perforins). CTLs appear to play an important role in the destruction of virus-infected cells, and in the allogeneic response.

Other T Cell-Dependent Immune Responses

T cells play critical roles in a series of important immune responses, including the delayed-type hypersensitivity reaction and contact sensitivity. An analogue of delayed-type hypersensitivity is the activation of macrophages, which occurs under the influence of T cell products. T cell activation of macrophages is mediated through the production of lymphokines and has obvious importance in immunity to many types of infectious agents and tumor cells.

The Major Histocompatibility Complex

The MHC plays a central role in many aspects of immunity, both in encoding histocompatibility (or transplantation) antigens and in regulating immune responses against conventional antigens. The MHC is a complex of genes that is found on chromosome 6 in humans and on chromosome 17 in mice. The constituent genes of MHC molecules specify class I MHC molecules, class II MHC molecules, certain complement components (often designated class III MHC), and a series of other proteins, including the lymphokines TNF-α, and lymphotoxin (TNF-β).

Class I MHC molecules. Class I molecules are membrane glycoproteins expressed on virtually all cells. They consist of an α-chain of approximately 45,000 daltons in noncovalent association with β_2 microglobulin, a 12 kd molecule not encoded in the MHC. Both the MHC-encoded α-chain and β_2 microglobulin are members of the immunoglobulin supergene family. α-Chain polymorphism is responsible for the antigenic differences of class I molecules found among different individuals of the same species.

In humans, three distinct loci have been identified in coding highly polymorphic class I MHC molecules: HLA-A, HLA-B and HLA-C.

2 Class II MHC molecules. Class II molecules are membrane glycoproteins that consist of two chains, α and β, both of which are encoded in the MHC and are members of the immunoglobulin super gene family. In mice, class II MHC molecules are coded by the genes in the I region and thus are referred to as I-region-associated (Ia) antigens. In humans, there are three major sets of class II molecules encoded in the DR, DQ, and DP regions of the MHC. In contrast to mice, in which each Ia antigen contains a single α and single β gene, the class II regions in humans can express more than one α or β gene.

Class II molecules have a more restricted tissue distribution than class I molecules. They are found on B cells, macrophages, epidermal Langerhan's cells, dendritic cells, thymic epithelium cells, and human-activated T cells. The levels of class II expression are regulated by IFN-γ and in the B cells by IL-4. Furthermore, IFN-γ can induce cells that normally lack class II molecules to express these molecules. This suggests that immunologically mediated inflammation can result in an increased expression of class II MHC molecules and enhance the expression of class I molecules.

Lymphokines

Lymphokines, the molecular mediators of many T cell functions, are a set of potent polypeptides (Table 4-1). Among the currently recognized T cell–derived lymphokines are interleukin 2 (IL-2), interleukin 4 (IL-4), interleukin 5 (IL-5), IFN-γ, lymphotoxin, granulocyte-macrophage colony-stimulating factors (GM-CSF), and interleukin 3 (IL-3). In addition to these factors, interleukin 6 (IL-6) is produced by lymphocytes although it can be made by many other cell types.

Effector Mechanisms of Immunity

The ultimate purpose of the immune system is to develop responses that protect the individual against infections with pathogenic microorganisms and against the development and spread of malignant tumors. The elements responsible for this effector function include the cytotoxic T cells, cells that destroy antibody-coated target cells (ADCC), and cells that kill tumors and other target cells nonspecifically (NK). A second important set of effector mechanisms is the engagement by products of the immune system of potent in-

Table 4-1 Cytokines

Cytokine	Other name	Cell source	Function
Interleukin-1 (IL-1)	Lymphocyte activating factor	Macrophage	T and B cell growth regulation
Interleukin-2 (IL-2)	T cell growth factor	Lymphocyte	T cell growth regulation and regulation of Ig synthesis
Interleukin-3 (IL-3)	multicolony stimulating factor	Lymphocyte	Stimulation of hematopoietic precursors
Interleukin-4 (IL-4)	B cell stimulating factor	Lymphocyte	Ig class switching T cell growth regulation B cell growth factor
Interleukin-5 (IL-5)	B cell growth factor Eosinophil differentiation factor	Lymphocyte	Stimulation of B cell growth
Interleukin-6 (IL-6)	B cell stimulating factor Interferon B2 Hepatocyte stimulatory factor	Lymphocyte	Control of Ig synthesis
Interferon γ (IFN-γ)		Lymphocyte	Macrophage activation Ig class switch
Lymphotoxin (LT)	Tumour necrosis factor β (TNF-β)	Lymphocyte	Inhibition of cell growth
Tumor Necrosis Factor (TNF-α)		Macrophage	Inflammation
Interferon α and β (IFN-α and β)		Macrophage	Inhibition of antibody production
Transforming Growth Factor β (TGF-β)		Macrophage	Increase in collagen Inhibition of proliferation of T and B cells and hepatocytes

flammatory processes. These processes include the activation and attraction of macrophages, neutrophils, eosinophils, basophils, and related cell types. A third critical effector mechanism of immunity flows from the activation of the complement system as a result of antigen-antibody interactions. The complement system is a cascade of proteins that produces inflammatory mediators and that leads to the direct lysis of antigen-bearing cells, including bacteria, virus-infected cells, and tumor cells.

Regulation of the Immune Response

The elements of the immune response relate to one another in a complex but orderly manner, ensuring that no individual clone of cells comes to dominate completely the lymphocyte population under normal circumstances. To achieve this balance, there need to be regulatory mechanisms, which are of several general types. These mechanisms include the physical state of the antigen, the absence of certain cofactors at the time of interaction with antigen, and the immaturity of the cell at the time of antigen contact. Tolerance induction is critical in avoiding autoimmune phenomena.

A second important system preventing clonal dominance is provided by a system of regulatory controls often referred to collectively as suppression. Suppression reflects a specific or nonspecific inhibition of the action of an antigen-specific helper T cell. In some circumstances the magnitude of expression is determined by the amount of help available, suggesting a type of feedback inhibition related to the size of the immune response itself. The inability to analyze the cells that participate in suppression and the molecules that control suppression has made it difficult to characterize the specific nature of this suppressor response.

Another regulatory system is based on the existence of antibodies and on T cell receptors of unique antigenic determinants associated with the variable regions of such molecules. These determinants are called *idiotypes.* The fact that essentially all antibodies and all T cell receptors express idiotypes implies the existence of the antibody repertoire of immunoglobulins that can recognize the variable region of any immunoglobulin T cell receptor molecule. The interactions of anti-idiotype antibodies with the variable regions of antibodies prevent those antibodies from binding the antigen for which it is putatively specific, suggesting that the interaction of idiotype and anti-idiotype involves an antigenic determinant in or near the antibody combining site. The existence of complementary idiotypes and anti-idiotypes leads to a dynamic equilibrium.

VIRAL HEPATITIS

A number of viruses, including hepatitis A, hepatitis B, and hepatitis C, can produce either acute or chronic liver injury. Hepatitis A and C are thought to cause hepatic injury primarily through the cytopathic nature of the virus, whereas hepatitis B produces injury primarily through immune-mediated mechanisms.

Hepatitis A Virus

Hepatitis A virus (HAV) has many biochemical and biophysical characteristics like those of the enteroviruses and therefore has been classified as a picornovirus (Table 4-2). It is difficult to adapt to growth in cell culture and usually replicates very slowly without cytopathic effect. As first described by Finestone, HAV is a nonenveloped 27 to 32 nm virus that is morphologically indistinguishable from other picornoviruses. By electron microscopy, full and empty particles appear to be spheric and featureless, but fine structural analysis has demonstrated an eicosahedral symmetry. The virion is composed of a genome of linear single-stranded RNA of 7.5 kilo base pair (kbp) and a capsid containing multiple copies of three or four proteins. The virion has an RNA genome that is linear and alkali sensitive. The genome of HAV can be divided into 3 parts: (1) a 5′ noncoding region that accounts for 10% of the genome; (2) a single open-reading frame that appears to encode all of the viral proteins, with regions designated as P1 for

Table 4-2 Characteristics of hepatitis A virus

Primary host	Human
Host range and tissue tropism	Narrow
Primary habitat	Liver
Sensitivity	
Acid	Stable
Heat	Stable
Guanidine	Resistant
Biophysical	1.32 - 1.34
Buoyant density (g/cm^3 in CsCl)	
Sedimentation coefficient	155 - 160
Viral proteins (Mr × 10.$^{-}$)^{n}	
VP1	33.2
VP2	24.8
VP3	27.8
VP4	≤2.5
VPg	2.4
Genome	7.48
Length (kb)	38.0
% (G + C)	

capsid proteins and P2 and P3 for nonstructural proteins; and (3) a 3′ noncoding region.

The capsid proteins (VP1, VP2F, and VP3) have been detected by polyacrylamide gel electrophoresis. There is also evidence of the presence of an additional structural protein, VPg linked to the 5′ terminus of the genome.

Although most HAV proteins are unlike those of other picornaviruses, minor similarities within the group exist. For example, the predicted amino acid sequences of HAV show less identity with those of polio virus type I than with those of encephalomyocarditis virus or rhinovirus type II. Homology has been demonstrated in the functional regions of proteins 1B, 2C, 3C, and 3D. Protein 2C, a nonstructural protein, probably functions in transcription of the genome.

Pathogenesis and pathology. Natural infection with HAV usually follows ingestion of material contaminated with feces containing HAV. However, the sequence of events that begins with entry via the GI tract and ultimately results in hepatitis is not well understood. It is also not clear whether injury to the liver is the result of an immunopathologic process or if the virus is directly cytopathic and capable of destroying the hepatocyte without any contribution by the host's immune system. Because mature virions of other picornaviruses exit the cell by infection-mediated disintegration of the host cell, it seems reasonable to assume that HAV may be directly cytotoxic to hepatocytes. Although some correlation has been seen between severity of disease and virus shedding in the stool, fecal excretion is in most cases greatest before the onset of illness. In addition, viral antigen is first detected in the liver parenchyma of experimentally infected primates within 1 to 2 weeks of intravenous inoculation and may persist there throughout the acute phase. Cytopathology is unimpressive during this early phase of maximal viral replication, although a direct viral effect may occur when inocula of high doses of HAV are administered. No significant in vitro virus-induced cytopathic effect has been observed by light microscopy, but damage to cellular organelles has been detected by electron microscopy.

These findings suggest that virus-induced cytopathology may not be responsible for the pathologic changes seen in HAV infection. They also suggest that host-mediated immunologic responses may contribute to the pathogenesis of hepatitis A. The deposition of hepatitis with the appearance of IgM anti-HAV, immune complexes, and reduced levels of serum complement may be coincidental or relevant to the clinical pathology.

In vitro studies have shown evidence of cell-mediated lysis of HAV-infected target cells by natural killer cells and by cytolytic T cells, release of macrophage-migration inhibition factor from sensitized cells in response to HAV antigen, and production of interferon by immune lymphocytes that were stimulated with HAV. Although it has not been possible to correlate these findings with events in vivo, they suggest that liver disease may result primarily from cellular immune mechanisms.

Hepatitis B Virus

HBV belongs to a group of viruses now known as the hepadnaviruses (Table 4-3). Members include the woodchuck hepatitis virus (WHV), which was discovered in a *Marmota monax* colony in the Philadelphia Zoo in the serum of animals commonly found to have hepatitis and hepatocellular carcinoma. Ground squirrel hepatitis virus (GSHV) was discovered in 1980 in the serum of wild *Spermophilus beecheyi* in Northern California, and duck hepatitis B virus (DHBV) was discovered in 1981 in the sera of domestic ducks from a geographic region in the People's Republic of China. Hepatocellular carcinoma is common in these animals from this region. Recently hepadnaviruses have been described in tree squirrels in the United States and in herons in Germany. Less well documented findings in studies of other rodents, marsupials, and cats have suggested that other hepadnaviruses also may be present in nature.

Table 4-3 Hepadna viruses

Virus	Species affected
Hepatitis B virus (HBV)	Humans, baboons
Woodchuck hepatitis virus (WHV)	Marmata monax
Ground squirrel hepatitis virus (GSHV)	Spermophilus beecheyi
Duck hepatitis B virus (DHBV)	Domestic ducks

Hepadnaviruses share the following unique features: (1) virion size and ultrastructure with an envelope surrounding an electron-dense spheric nucleocapsid or core; (2) characteristic polypeptide and antigenic composition; (3) common virion DNA size, structure, and genetic organization; and (4) an unusual mechanism of viral DNA replication that includes reverse transcription. Another characteristic feature is the moderately narrow host range. HBV appears to infect only humans naturally; however, successful experimental infections of chimpanzees and a few other high primates have been performed. All of the hepadnaviruses exhibit striking tropism for hepatocytes although infection of some other cell types, including lymphocytes and macrophages, has been demonstrated. Infections with hepadnaviruses have been shown to be associated with acute and chronic hepatitis, immune complex–mediated disease, and hepatocellular carcinoma. Furthermore, the hepadnaviruses appear to serve as helper viruses for the hepatitis delta virus (HDV) and provide the virion envelope polypeptide for this defective RNA virus.

The virions of HBV are spheric particles approximately 42 to 47 nm in diame-

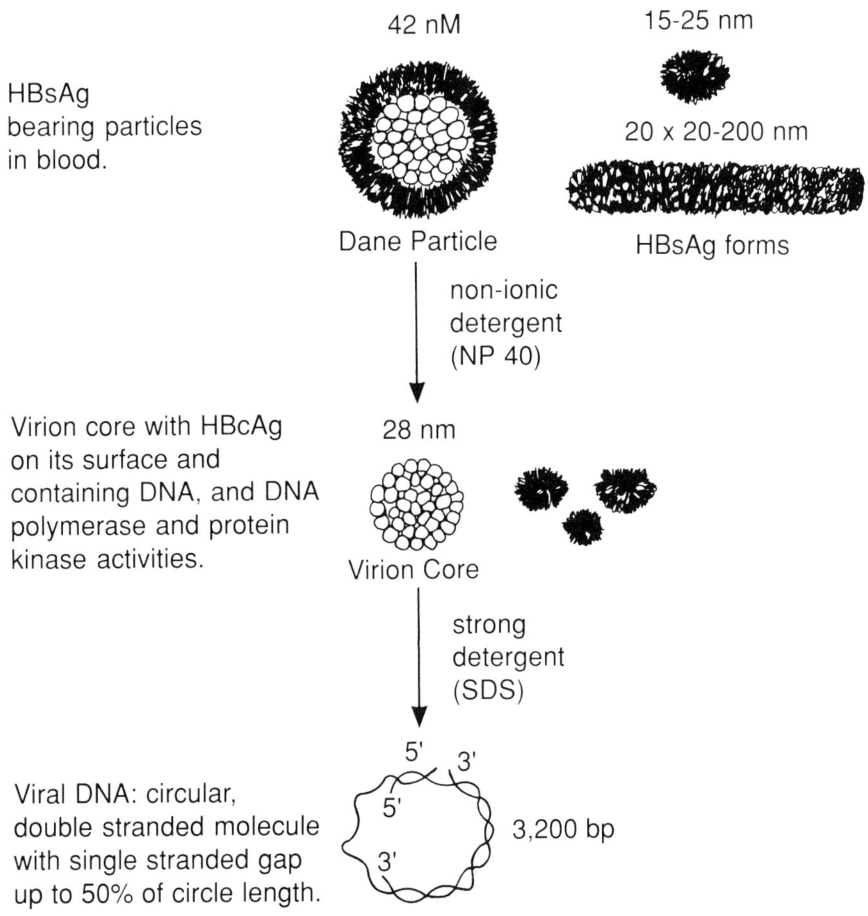

Figure 4-2
A schematic representation of the hepatitis B virus (HBV) forms found in the blood of patients.

ter (Figure 4-2). They exhibit an electron-dense spheric inner core with a diameter of approximately 20 to 25 nm and an outer shell, or envelope, approximately 7 nm in thickness. The spheric 20 nm diameter inner core particles, which can be released from the virions by detergent treatment, bear the viral core (c antigen, HBcAg), the viral e antigen (HBeAg) and the viral DNA, DNA polymerase activity, and a protein kinase activity that phosphorylates the major structural polypeptide of the virion core. Virus concentrations in sera of HBV-infected humans can exceed 10^9/ml although no virions are detectable in the sera of some HBsAg-carrier patients.

In addition to complete virus (virions), there are more numerous particulate forms that bear viral surface antigen in

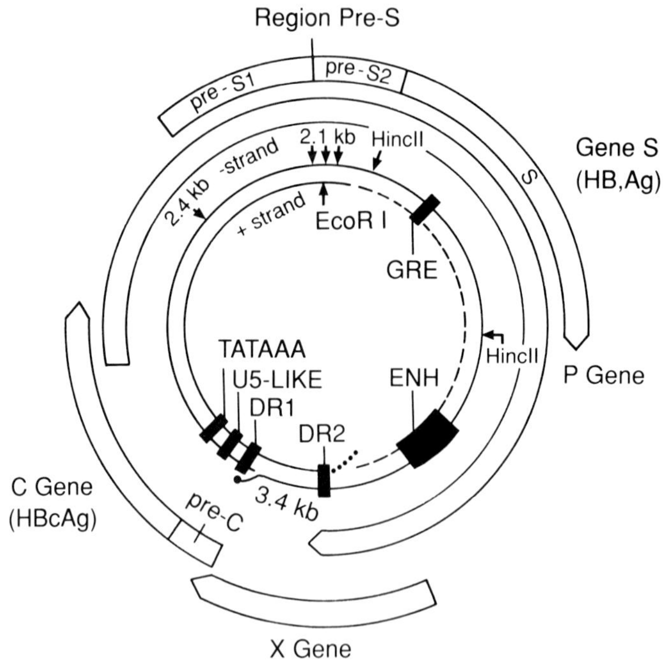

Figure 4-3
The viral genome of HBV. The small arrows on the negative strand indicate the 5′ ends of the three major transcripts (3.4, 2.4, and 2.1 kb) which are terminated near the poly (A) signal (TATAAA). The map position of the first nucleotide of the glucocorticoid-responsive element (GRE), DR2, DR1, the U5-like sequence, and the poly (A) addition sequence (TATAAA) are indicated, and the general region exhibiting enhancer activity (ENH) is also shown. (From Robinson W. In Fields B and Knipe D, eds: Virology, New York, 1990, Raven Press.)

the serum of infected hosts. These forms consist of spheric particles and filamentous forms approximately 20 to 25 nm in diameter. They are considered to be incomplete viral envelope forms (HBsAg).

Molecular biology. The viral genome of the hepadnaviruses is a small, circular, partially double-stranded molecule approximately 3200 bases in length (Figure 4-3). The complete or negative strand (L) is nearly full length, lacking only a few nucleotides. In contrast, the positive strand (S) is incomplete and may lack up to 50% of its full length. The circular configuration is maintained by base pairing over the region of the gap in the negative strand, called the cohesive (cos) region, and is the major coding strand from which the major RNA molecules are produced. Four open reading frames have been identified in the hepadnavirus genome. They have been labeled the S, C, X, and P regions. The S, C, and X reading frames contain the genes for the HBsAg, the core antigen HBcAg, and the X protein. The P region is the gene for the viral DNA polymerase.

Several other functionally important elements have been identified in the hepadnavirus genome. These elements include an 11 base pair direct repeat sequence, designated DR1 and DR2, which play a role in viral DNA replication and the integration of viral DNA into the host genome. Four promoter sequences have now also been described. One sequence, called the pre-S1 promoter, upstream from the start of the pre-S1 sequence, appears to initiate the synthesis of a messenger RNA for a protein containing the pre-S1, pre-S2, and S sequences. Another sequence, called the pre-S2 promoter within the pre-S1 region, appears to direct the synthesis of an RNA transcript that functions as a messenger for the pre-S2 and S gene-specified polypeptides. Both of these promoters fall within the coding sequence of the P gene, and their action does not appear to be cell specific or tissue specific. A sequence upstream from the start of the C gene and within the coding region of the X gene directs the synthesis of an RNA transcript, which may function as messenger for the synthesis of C gene- and P gene-specific polypeptides. This appears to serve as a template for the synthesis of the virus-negative DNA strand by reverse transcription. The C promoter appears to exhibit some specificity for liver cells. A fourth promoter element has been described upstream from the X gene and within the P open reading frame.

A transcriptional enhancer element has now been defined upstream from the C gene promoter. The C promoter and other HBV promoters appear to be under control of this HBV enhancer. This control has been shown to be much more active in differentiated liver than in any other cell types. Another hepadnavirus genomic region, within the S coding region, has been shown to account for the fivefold enhancement of gene expression in the presence of glucocorticoids. An 18-nucleotide sequence in HBV that is similar to other known glucocorticoid response of DNA elements has been identified in this region. A polyadenylation signal that appears to be used by all of the major transcripts lies within the C gene upstream from the 3′ end of the DNA strand.

Viral proteins. *Envelope (surface) proteins.* The HBsAg's specificities are contained in 3 HBV-encoded envelope polypeptides. The 2 smallest polypeptides (24,000 and 27,000 daltons) are present in greatest amounts in HBsAg preparations. They represent the 226 amino acid polypeptides in a glycosolated form of the same polypeptide encoded by the S region, designated p24 and gp27. Two sets of larger polypeptides are minor components found in HBsAg preparations containing virions. They are a 33,000 dalton polypeptide encoded by the pre-S2 and the glycosylated form of the same polypeptide (36,000 daltons), designated p33 and gp36, respectively, and a 39,000 dalton polypeptide encoded by the pre-S1 region and its glycosylated form (42,000 daltons), designated p39 and gp42, respectively.

Analyses of preparations of different HBsAg particle types have shown that the 20 nm spheric particles contain almost exclusively small polypeptides (p24 and gp27), that filamentous particles contain mostly small polypeptides and small pre-S2–containing polypeptides (p33 and gp36), and that virions contain all surface antigenic polypeptides in nearly equal molar amounts. Thus the virion has antigenic specificity not present in other HBsAg particles. After infection with HBV, patients develop anti-pre-S1, anti-pre-S2, and anti-S responses, indicating that all of these antigenic specificities are expressed during the primary infection.

It is now recognized that the surface of HBsAg-bearing particles is antigenically complex. At least five antigenic specificities have been described on HBsAg particles. A group-specific determinant (a) is shared by all HBsAg preparations and by two pairs of subtype determinants (d, y and w, and r). These usually behave independently as alleles. Antigenic heterogeneity of the w determinants and of additional determinants has also been described. Seven HBsAg subtypes (ayw, ayw2, ayw3, ayr, adw2, adw4, and adr) have now been described. Unusual combinations of HBsAg subtype determinants, such as awr, adwr, and adyr, have been described in the Far East. The subtype determinants in these cases, which are found on the same particles, suggest that phenotypic mixing or unusual genetic recombinants may have formed during mixed infections. Although there are no recognized biologic differences between the HBV viruses of different antigenic subtypes, HBsAg subtypes are unevenly distributed around the world and have provided useful markers for epidemiologic studies of the spread of the virus in humans.

An important property of the small polypeptide encoded by the S region and of its glycosolated form (p24 and gp27) is the ability to assemble into 20 nm spheric membrane particles without the pre-S sequences. This property has been exploited to produce highly immunogenic HBsAg particles in yeast in mammalian cells as HBV vaccine antigens. Pre-S2 sequences also contain an antigen that can elicit protective immunity and a sequence that binds polymerized human serum albumin. Immunization with a synthetic peptide with a sequence corresponding to amino acids 120-153 of the pre-S2 coding region protected chimpanzees against HBV challenge, and antibody raised against this peptide in rabbits prevented infection of chimpanzees on subsequent inoculation, suggesting that this peptide contains an antigen that can elicit a protective immune response and HBV neutralizing antibody. Human serum albumin polymerized by glutaraldehyde binds HBsAg and the synthetic peptide corresponding to amino acids encoded by the pre-S2 region. This data suggests that this pre-S2 sequence may represent a virion receptor for binding HBV to hepatocytes. Pre-S1–encoded polypeptides have been implicated in HBsAg binding to hepatocytes, and antibody to a pre-S1 synthetic peptide blocks binding of HBsAg particles to HepG2 cells. The pre-S1–encoded polypeptide also exerts a significant effect on envelope protein secretion and affects virus assembly. When pre-S1 polypeptides (p39 and gp42) are expressed alone in cells, they are not secreted. The biologic significance for regulation of virus assembly and release from cells is not known at present.

Nucleocapsid (core) proteins. The virion core protein is found in the blood of infected hosts only as an internal component of the virus. No free HBcAg has been demonstrated in serum. HBeAg is known to be physically and antigenically distinct from both HBsAg and HBcAg particles in serum.

HBcAg and HBeAg now are known to be different antigenic specificities of protein encoded by the viral C gene. The HBcAg polypeptide has an apparent size of 22,000 daltons (p22), and the polypeptide containing HBeAg specificity in serum is approximately 16,000 daltons and appears to be a truncated form of the p22 polypeptide. HBeAg exists in serum but avidly and specifically binds albumin, alpha$_1$ anti-trypsin, and immunoglobulins. This binding is thought to mask the HBcAg determinants. When the p22 polypeptide is assembled in core particles, the HBeAg determinants are masked and only exposed to antibody by disruption of core particles and release of free polypeptide chains.

The pre-C sequence within the C open reading frame appears to affect the fate of the C-encoded polypeptides in cultured cells. Expression of pre-C sequences leads to accumulation of C protein in membranes and secretion of HBeAg.

Protein kinase activity has been found in the virion core and HBcAg particles from HBV-infected hepatic tissue. P22 can be cleaved to form p16. It has been suggested that p22 may have protease activity and may undergo self-cleavage under certain conditions. Whether this protein kinase activity is a virus-encoded protein or is of cellular origin is not yet clear, and its role in HBV infection and replication has not been defined.

The P gene product. The P open reading frame has been found to contain a sequence that shares homology with sequences in the pol genes of retroviruses. Thus this gene has been considered likely to encode the protein with the reverse transcriptase activity found in virions and corelike particles in infected liver. The antibody to a synthetic peptide corresponding to an N-terminal region of the P-gene products of duck hepatitis virus (DHV) has now been shown to react with the polypeptide covalently attached to the 5′ end of the negative DNA strand, suggesting that the P gene encodes this protein primer for synthesis of the DNA strand.

The X-gene product. The X open reading frame encodes for a polypeptide of 154 amino acids. The only functional property shown for the X protein of HBV expressed in cells in culture is activation of transcription controlled by enhancer elements of β-interferon, the human immunodeficiency virus (HIV), and SV40 virus. The isolated X gene does not appear to activate HBV transcription or gene expression. However, it is not known whether the X gene activates a cellular gene that plays a role in HBV replication.

Virus replication. A receptor on the HBV virion surface required for attachment of the virus to cells has not been identified although a sequence in the pre-S1 protein that apparently binds HBsAg to HepG-2 cells has been identified. Three major unspliced transcripts with lengths of approximately 3.4, 2.4, and 2.1 kb have been detected in HBV-infected liver tissue. The 5′ end of the 3.4 kb transcript of HBV has been mapped to the pre-C region and is approximately 6 nucleotides upstream of the DR1 sequence. The C promoters are thought to regulate its synthesis. The terminal redundancy of this transcript indicates that during its synthesis, RNA polymerase II must first read through the *cis*-acting DNA sequence that functions to terminate transcription when the sequence is reached a second time. The large transcript appears to function as a template for viral DNA synthesis and to serve as messenger RNA for the major core protein (p22) and the P-gene product. The 5′ end of the 2.3 kb transcript in HBV-infected liver has been mapped in the viral genome upstream of the initiation codon for the pre-S1 sequence. This transcript (pre-S1 transcript) appears to serve as mRNA for synthesis of the pre-S1 containing HBsAg polypeptide (p39). The 5′ end of the 2.1 kb transcript in HBV-infected liver has been mapped to a position within the pre-S1 region and is referred to as the pre-S2 transcript. It functions as the mRNA for pre-S2 (p31) and S (p24) polypeptide synthesis. The transcript from which the X protein is translated is unknown at present.

Closed circular DNA is the first viral DNA form detected after infection and is the only form found in the nucleus, making it the best candidate as template for viral transcription during viral replication. It has also been demonstrated that sequences integrated in cellular DNA can be transcribed in hepatocellular lines in culture and probably in hepatocytes containing only integrated HBV DNA.

The mechanisms that regulate hepadnavirus transcription are not well known. Liver-specific factors are probably important and may explain the tropism for the liver; however, none of these factors has been identified. Expression of the 3.4 kb transcript has been observed only in cells of hepatic origin. The 2.1 kb pre-S2 transcript has been detected in several nonhepatic cell lines, suggesting that expression of this transcript is not liver-cell dependent. Furthermore, recent work in transgenic mice has demonstrated that expression of HBsAg occurs in liver cells while showing lower expression in a few other tissues, again demonstrating liver tropism of this virus. Four cellular factors that bind specific sequences in the HBV-enhancer region have now been described. Although they appear to be related to transcription factors, none of these appears to be liver specific. The apparent liver cell requirement for the large (3.4 kb) transcript expression suggests that the tropism of hepadnaviruses for hepatocytes may be determined at the level of transcription.

Little is known about the synthesis of the P-gene and X-gene products. The HBcAg polypeptide (p20) and the P-gene product appear to be translated from the 3.4 kb transcript. Because their transcription frames are different, it is not clear whether they are translated as separate discrete proteins or as a single fusion protein that is subsequently cleaved into the two products. A 35 kd protein with both HBcAg and P-gene polypeptide specificities presumed to represent a fusion protein has now been observed in extracts of hepatocellular carcinoma tissue. The HBcAg is detected only in the nucleus and cytoplasm of HBV-infected livers. The three HBsAg polypeptides appear to be translated as discrete polypeptides from at least two overlapping mRNAs of different sizes. These polypeptides are first detected intracellularly within membrane vesicles in the cytoplasm of infected liver cells.

Genomic replication. Genomic replication of the hepadnaviruses involves a reverse transcriptase step as indicated by the recent findings of Summers and Mason in the DHV-infected system. After the virus enters the cell, the infecting genome is converted to a closed circular viral DNA (ccDNA), which is first detected in the cell nucleus. The conversion of the virion DNA to ccDNA requires completion of the DNA positive-strand synthesis, removal of the protein primer from the negative DNA strand and removal of the oligonucleotide primer from the positive

DNA strand and elimination of the terminal redundancy of the negative DNA strand, and ligation of the DNA ends. The viral ccDNA is the template for the synthesis of the 3.4 kb transcript. This transcript is the template for reverse transcription and mRNA for the major structural protein for the virion core (p22), the reverse transcriptase protein, and the polypeptide primer for the synthesis of the negative strand. Synthesis of the negative DNA strand is initiated within the DR1 sequence.

The primer for synthesis of the viral DNA positive strand is a 19 kd oligoribonucleotide with a sequence corresponding to that of the 5′ terminal fragment of the RNA template containing the DR1 sequence. DNA positive-strand synthesis is initiated at the last nucleotide of DR2 near the 5′ end of the negative DNA strand template.

Core hepadnaviruses are assembled into complete virions with HBsAg and cell membrane lipid-containing envelopes. The secretion of complete virions can be found in blood containing DNA-RNA hybrid molecules or complete negative DNA strands without associated positive DNA. Hepatitis B viral DNA can exist in two forms intracellularly. It can exist as an episomal viral DNA involved in virus replication or as integrated viral DNA in infected cells. Nonintegrated forms of viral DNA have recently been found not only in liver cells but also in lymphocytes from the blood of chronic HBV carriers.

Evidence of integrated HBV DNA sequences in at least some patients with infected livers and in many patients with hepatocellular carcinoma has been obtained by restriction of endonuclease digestion of tissue DNA and by Southern blot analysis. Both integrated and episomal viral DNA have been found in tissue from patients with hepatocellular carcinoma. Restriction endonuclease Hind III digestion of the tumor DNA and Southern blot analysis have revealed DNA fragments that contain viral DNA sequences larger than the unit length of the viral DNA (3.2 kb). This suggests that viral DNA may be integrated at a few specific cellular DNA sites in some tissues from some patients with hepatocellular carcinoma but it is always integrated at different sites in different tumors. These results suggest that cells in these tumors are of clonal origin and that when multiple sites of integration exist, they probably arise through DNA rearrangements of an original single integration site. Cloning and sequence analysis of integrated viral DNA with flanking cellular DNA sequences have suggested that the clone-flanking cellular sequences are not the same for any two integrations. Furthermore, integration has been found in many different chromosomes. Thus the following conclusions can be derived with regard to hepadnavirus integrations: they appear to be sporadic, they accumulate in the liver during long periods of persistent infection, they may be promoted with liver injury and regeneration, and rearrangements and deletions appear to be the rule in the integrated viral genomes.

Hepatocellular cell lines in cultures containing HBV in only an integrated form have been found to express only the S-gene with no expression of other viral genes. Furthermore, livers of chronically infected patients in which integrated viral DNA and no episomal or replicating viral DNA forms can be detected have been shown to contain HBsAg in some cells but no HBcAg. The blood of such patients contains HBsAg particles but no Dane particles. Thus HBsAg can be expressed without complete virus replication. Expression of the S-gene in cells with only an integrated virus occurs probably because the intact S-gene, its promoter, and the viral enhancer are preserved in a number of integrations.

Mechanisms of injury. Primary HBV infection may be associated with mild or subclinical hepatitis or with more severe acute hepatitis. Persistent infection also is associated sometimes with a histologically normal or near-normal liver (the carrier state) and sometimes associated with chronic hepatitis, which can be severe and can progress to cirrhosis. Pathologic features of acute and chronic HBV infection include hepatocellular necrosis, lymphocyte inflammation, and, when progressing to cirrhosis, regenerative nodules with diffuse fibrosis.

The clinical manifestations of acute and chronic HBV infection appear to reflect the host's immune response to the virus rather than a direct cytopathic effect. It has been difficult to define the role of different effector cell populations in the pathogenesis of HBV-related chronic active hepatitis. Most previous studies have examined only the effector function of cells from peripheral blood, which may not reflect events occurring in the liver. Postulated mechanisms for disease have included the direct action of cytotoxic antibodies, antibody-dependent cellular cytotoxicity, NK cell activity, delayed-type hypersensitivity reactions, and specific T cell– mediated cytotoxicity.

Current evidence supports the concept that HBV is not a cytopathic agent. Infection of hepatocytes by this virus does not appear to injure the cell directly to a degree sufficient to explain the histologic injury associated with clinical hepatitis. A considerable body of evidence has accumulated, and it appears that some of the characteristics of the resulting diseases may be a consequence of the host's immune response.

A major limitation of studies on the specificity of liver damage in chronic active hepatitis has been the absence of human cell lines capable of sustaining HBV replication in vitro. Studies of classical MHC-restricted cytolytic T lymphocyte function have been hindered by the lack of target cells expressing appropriate class I or class II HLA antigens and viral antigens. Despite these difficulties, considerable circumstantial evidence supports a role for HBcAg-specific cytolytic T lymphocytes in chronic active hepatitis (Figure 4-4). Peripheral blood mononuclear cells from patients with chronic active hepatitis have been shown to have direct cytotoxicity for autologous hepatocytes expressing HBcAg but not HBsAg, and this cytotoxicity is blocked by antibodies to the HBcAg antigen. The immunogenicity of HBcAg has also been studied in inbred strains of mice to define the epitopes to which antibody responses are directed and the epitopes for T cell recognition. In these studies HBcAg was found to be much more immunogenic than HBsAg. HBcAg can function as a T cell independent antigen in mice, and all mouse strains responded to it in studies. HBcAg-specific T cells have been shown to be capable of priming an antibody response to HBsAg and can overcome genetically determined nonresponsiveness to S-epitopes. Furthermore, studies in inbred strains of mice have defined important B cell and T cell epitopes of pre-S, S, c, and e antigens for that species. The surface phenotypes of liver-infiltrating cells

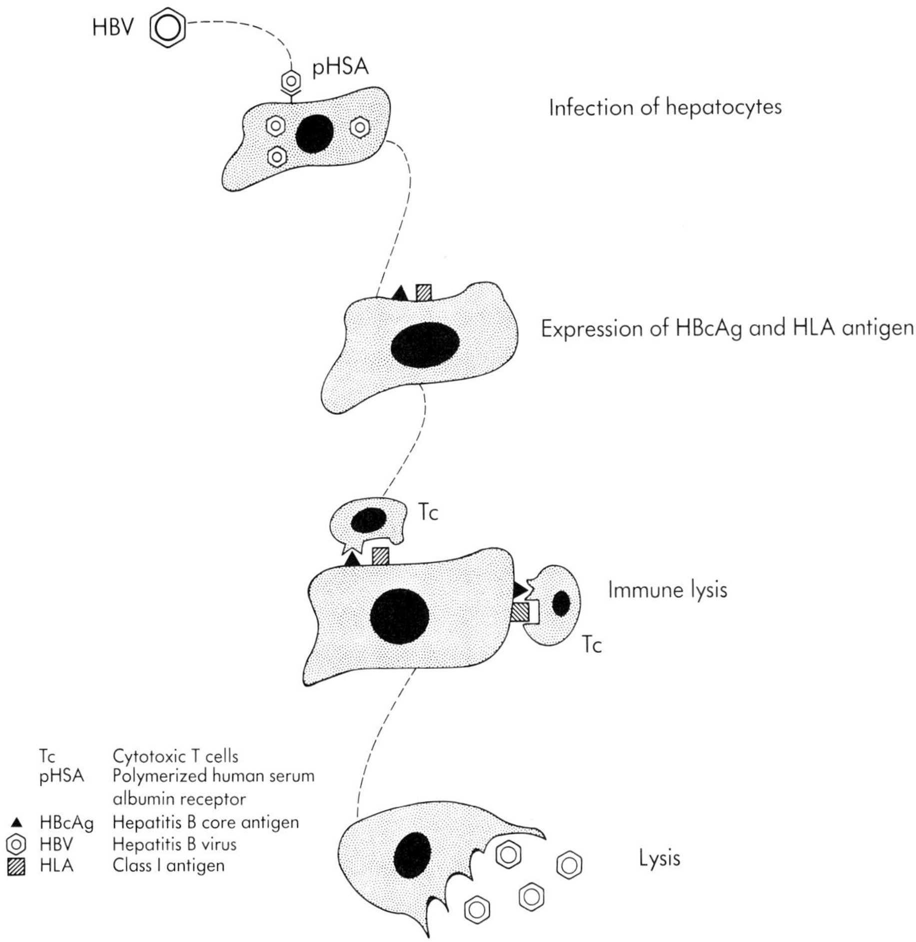

Figure 4-4
Mechanisms of immunologic injury in HBV infection.

have been characterized extensively in patients with chronic active hepatitis, and the majority of cells express the $CD8^+$ phenotype of class I-restricted cells. Disease activity in chronic active hepatitis has also been shown to correlate with the presence of HBcAg on the hepatocyte membrane. The disease appears to become quiescent when HBV DNA is integrated into the hepatocyte genome with loss of HBcAg expression despite continued expression of HBsAg.

More direct evidence for the involvement of HBcAg-specific cells in chronic active hepatitis has come with the isolation of proliferative $CD4^+$ T lymphocyte clones from liver biopsy material. These clones were specific for HBcAg, and they produced γ-interferon in response to antigenic stimulation. They also provide an

HBcAg-specific help to autologous B cells. Analysis of HBcAg-specific cytolytic T lymphocyte activity has not been performed because of the lack of suitable HLA-compatible target cells. Antigen recognition by the $CD4^+$ clones was restricted by class II HLA antigens. These studies suggest that the cells probably had regulatory rather than effector functions because hepatocytes were thought to express only class I antigens and thus would not be targets for $CD4^+$ effectors. However, recent studies using immunoelectron microscopy have confirmed that a proportion of HBcAg-expressing hepatocytes in chronic active hepatitis do express class II antigens, possibly induced by γ-interferon. Therefore, these $CD4^+$ clones may have class II-restricted delayed-type hypersensitivity or cytolytic T lymphocyte effector function against HBcAg-expressing hepatocytes.

There is little evidence to support a role for humoral immunity in the pathogenesis of liver injury following HBV infection. Antibody responses appear no different in chronic HBV infection with or without significant hepatitis. In addition, severe, acute, and chronic viral hepatitis can occur in patients with agammaglobulinemia. On the other hand, it has been demonstrated that HBsAg-anti-HBsAg complexes are found more often in the circulation of patients with significant chronic hepatitis B than in those with little or no liver disease.

A possible alternative mechanism for liver cell injury is a direct cytopathic effect of the virus when HBcAg is expressed. It has been shown recently that when HBcAg was expressed in a cell line in culture not impaired by HBsAg expression, a significant cytopathic effect was produced, suggesting that HBcAg expression can be toxic to cells. The association of HBeAg in serum and HBcAg in the liver with active hepatitis would be consistent with such a mechanism. Another possible mechanism for liver cell injury in HBV infection is very high expression of HBsAg in hepatocytes, leading to cell injury. This mechanism has recently been postulated as operative in transgenic mice carrying an HBV genome fragment encoding pre-S and S under control of a strong liver-specific mouse-albumin promoter. These mice developed chronic hepatitis, cirrhosis, and hepatocellular carcinoma apparently related to high-level expression of HBsAg in the liver and resulting in direct hepatocyte necrosis. It seems unlikely that this is a major mechanism of liver injury during natural infection in humans.

δ-Agent Induced Hepatitis

The hepatitis δ-virus consists of an RNA genome and two virus-specific forms of the structural protein hepatitis δ-antigen (HDAg) that are encapsulated by the surface antigen of the helper HBV. The RNA genome of HDV is approximately 1680 bases in length, the smallest genome of any known animal virus. It was described in southern Italy but has now been found in HBsAg-positive drug addicts and hemophiliacs in England, Canada, and the United States. Its importance lies not only in its high infectivity but also in its association with continuing inflammatory activity, rapid development of cirrhosis, and death.

Although the mechanism for δ-agent-induced hepatitis is not clearly understood, the δ-agent appears to be directly cytopathic to the hepatocyte. Inoculation of chimpanzees with δ-agent results in severe acute hepatitis in all animals as opposed to the results seen with HBV inoculation. Moreover, all chimpanzees expressing δ-antigen in liver biopsies have severe liver damage. A healthy carrier state for δ-agent does not appear to exist in humans. Furthermore, when liver tissue from human patients with δ-infection is studied, little or no inflammation is found. This finding further suggests that the virus itself is directly cytopathic and that the damage is not immunologically mediated.

Hepatitis C

Hepatitis C virus (HCV) infection is the most common cause of post-transfusion hepatitis. Patients infected with HCV commonly develop chronic hepatitis and cirrhosis although the clinical disease is often milder than that seen with HBV infection. Isolation and identification of the HCV virus was facilitated by the availability of blood from a chronically infected chimpanzee. Following extensive ultracentrifugation of the plasma to recover the virus, random priming of the extracted nucleic acid was performed to create a cDNA library in λ gt11. Screening of the resultant recombinant phage culminated in the identification of antigen-producing clones that had a common open reading frame. The open reading frame has been expressed in yeast as a fusion polypeptide with expression of a protein. A radioimmunoassay and enzyme-linked immunoabsorbent assay that have high sensitivity for blood-borne hepatitic C have been developed. HCV shares many virion characteristics with the *Flaviviridae* genus and *Togaviridae* families. However, clinical evidence does suggest that HCV may not account for all post-transfusion hepatitis and/or episodic hepatitic C.

Little is known about the mechanism of HCV-induced liver disease although it has been suggested that the virus is directly cytopathic in contrast to HBV infection. Histologic examination shows less lymphocytic infiltrate in areas of hepatocyte damage, and the response to interferon shows a prompt improvement in transaminases, suggesting that the interferon is antiviral.

Fulminant Viral Hepatitis

Fulminant hepatitis is a consequence of hepatitis A, B, and C infection. It is a rapidly fatal disease worthy of special mention. The incidence of fulminant hepatitis (FH) is 0.1% to 1.0% of all cases of acute viral hepatitis, and the mortality varies with the severity of hepatic encephalopathy from 60% in stage II to more than 90% in stage IV encephalopathy. Although the pathogenesis of FH is not well known, it has been suggested that the injury may be immune mediated.

Vigorous immune responses to HBsAg have been reported in fulminant hepatitis B infection. HBsAg was cleared from the serum significantly faster in patients with FH than in serum from patients with nonfulminant hepatitis. The presence of both antigen and antibody (immune complexes) in patients with FH may be responsible for the severe liver disease that ensues. Furthermore, it has been demonstrated that antibodies to the translation products of the pre-S1 and pre-S2 regions of the envelope gene of HBV occur early during the course of fulminant hepatitis B and may participate in the severe hepatic injury and account for the inability to detect the virus either in serum or in the liver, which is characteristic of FH.

Cellular immune mechanisms may also be responsible for the hepatocellular in-

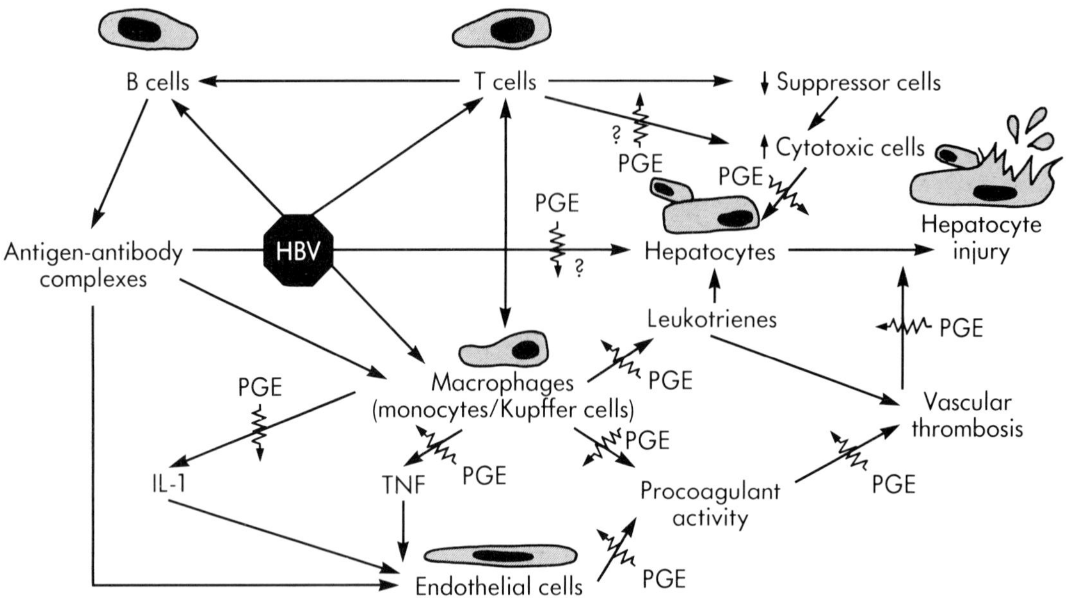

Figure 4-5
Postulated mechanisms for hepatocyte injury and HBV-induced fulminant hepatitis. *PGE,* prostaglandin E; *IL-1,* interleukin 1. (From Sinclair S, Wakefield A, and Levy GA. In Springer: Semin Immunopathol 12:33-45, 1990.)

jury in FH (Figure 4-5). An elevation in CTL and a reduction in suppressor T cells have now been reported in the peripheral blood of patients. Serial studies have shown an imbalance of these two subsets of T cells in the acute phase of infection but not in the recovery phase. Analysis of cells in liver histology has again demonstrated an increase in CTL.

About 50% of cases of FH are associated with a moderate to severe consumption coagulopathy or disseminated intravascular coagulation (DIC). Histopathologic studies in humans have revealed severe and extensive hepatic cell necrosis as the most conspicuous and common abnormality seen in the liver. This necrosis morphologically resembles hepatic necrosis produced experimentally in the rabbit by a Schwartzman reaction using *Escherichia coli* endotoxin. This resemblance has led to the hypothesis that the acute, severe, and extensive hepatic cell necrosis seen in patients with FH is probably the result of an anoxic state caused in most instances by intrahepatic circulatory disturbances. Thrombi formation has been noted in and around the necrotic areas in a significant number of cases of patients with FH. Further experimental evidence supporting a role for activation of the immune-coagulation system has been reported in a murine model of viral hepatitis (murine hepatitis virus [MHV]). Production of cytokines such as interleukin 1 (IL-1), TNF, and leukotrienes has been reported in animals that develop FH. These cytokines can induce the production of coagulants by endothelial cells. The endothelial cells subsequently express adhesion molecules (ELAM1), which promote adhesion of lymphocytes and neutrophils. Leukotriene infusion in animals also appears to produce FH, suggesting a possible role for these agents in liver injury. Treatment of animals and humans with exogenous prostaglandins and leukotriene inhibitors has resulted in marked clinical improvement in the setting of FH. Thus the imbalance in production of cytokines, including eicosanoids and leukotrienes, during FH may be important in the pathogenesis of FH.

AUTOIMMUNE HEPATITIS

A number of liver diseases, including primary biliary cirrhosis, sclerosing cholangitis, and lupoid chronic active hepatitis, have autoimmune features. These liver diseases are often associated with other autoimmune disorders, such as thyroiditis, sicca syndrome, and pernicious anemia. Autoimmune hepatitis tends to occur in young women and is often associated with multiple autoantibody markers, such as antismooth muscle antibodies and antinuclear antibodies. Autoimmunity represents a loss of tolerance to self-antigens although the exact mechanisms for this break in tolerance and autodestruction are not well known. The immunologic basis for autoimmune hepatitis is not clear, and it is not known whether it is a manifestation of cytotoxic T cells, NK cells, or K cell recognition and destruction of hepatocytes expressing specific membrane antigens. Two putative liver membrane antigens have been implicated in autoimmune hepatitis. One is liver-specific protein (LSP), a partially purified lipoprotein complex that contains both liver-specific and nonliver-specific antigenic determinants. A second antigen is liver membrane antigen (LMA). Patients with autoimmune hepatitis have been found to have antibodies to LSP in their serum, but the significance of these antibodies is not clear at present. A genetic predisposition to autoimmune hepatitis is suggested by disease sequestering within families and by the association with the HLA type B8/DR3. This haplotype is known to be associated with a wide variety of other autoimmune disorders and may be a marker of defective immunoregulation. Further evidence for support of immune disregulation in the pathogenesis of autoimmune hepatitis is the observation of a defect in suppressor T cell function in patients with autoimmune chronic active hepatitis (CAH).

PRIMARY BILIARY CIRRHOSIS

PBC is a chronic, nonsuppurative, and destructive cholangitis that possesses many features of an immunologically mediated disease. Evidence implicating immunologic mechanisms as causative of PBC includes a strong association with other putative autoimmune diseases, such as thyroiditis, ulcerative colitis, and sicca syndrome. A characteristic early histologic appearance is lymphocytic infiltration and granulomatous formation in and around the bile ducts. Furthermore, a number of abnormalities of the humoral and cellular immune system have been reported, including a disproportionate elevation in serum IgM and the presence of antimitochondrial antibodies (AMA). AMA are a heterogenous group of nonorgan-specific antibodies to mitochondrial antigens. The presence of antibodies is of considerable diagnostic importance because they are found in greater than 90% of patients with PBC. In PBC the antibodies recognize a cluster of four major mitochondrial inner membrane proteins, collectively designated M2. Several groups have now characterized the PBC specific antigen (M2) by western blotting and defined a number of subgroups according to their molecular weights. In PBC the major M2 autoantigen (74 kd) is the E2 component of the pyruvate dehydrogenase complex.

The mechanism of immune-mediated tissue damage in PBC is not known. It has been suggested that a primary immunoregulatory defect may allow for an autoimmune reaction to the biliary duct epithelial antigens (M2). The observation that PBC is associated with diseases of other exocrine glands suggests that the putative antigen may be common to duct epithelium in a number of different sites. The clinical, histologic, and immunologic similarities between PBC and graft vs. host disease has led to the postulate that there may be similar immunopathogenetic mechanisms operative in both of these disorders. It has been postulated that PBC may be the result of a T cell-mediated immune attack on native or altered histocompatibility (HLA) antigens present on biliary and other duct epithelium. Whether the expression of the antigens is a primary event or follows a viral infection is not known at present. Attempts to recover specific cytotoxic T cells from liver biopsies of patients with PBC are now underway. It is hoped that these experiments will provide evidence to define the pathogenetic mechanisms important in PBC.

DRUG-INDUCED LIVER INJURY

Drugs are a significant cause of hepatic injury. Although they account for a relatively minor portion of cases of acute hepatic disease (5%), up to 25% of cases of FH may be the result of adverse reactions to medical agents. They are also important causes of chronic liver diseases, including fatty liver, CAH, cirrhosis, and vascular and neoplastic lesions of the liver.

The susceptibility of the liver to damage by chemical agents may be related to its primary role in drug metabolism or may be a consequence of hypersensitivity reactions. Susceptibility to hepatic injury by drugs is influenced by genetic factors, age, sex, nutritional status, exposure to other drugs, and systemic diseases. Although genetic factors are clearly important in determining vulnerability of laboratory animals to hepatotoxins, the effect of genetic factors is less clear in humans. However, patients who have a genetically limited capacity to convert aryl epoxides to nontoxic dihydriols seem predisposed to develop hepatic injury from phenytoin and halothane. Susceptibility to contraceptive steroid-associated cholestasis appears to have a strong genetic component. Susceptibility to some agents, including methyldopa, nitrofurantoin, and halothane leads to hepatic injury more frequently in females than in males. Age has also been reported to affect susceptibility. The incidence of isoniazid-induced hepatic injury increases with age. Aspirin-associated liver injury appears to occur only in children, and valproic- acid-induced liver injury occurs mainly in patients less than 20 years old. Nutritional status introduces several relevant factors. High-protein diets can enhance the cy-

Table 4-4 Patterns of drug-induced liver injury

Liver injury	Drugs
Cytotoxic	
Direct or toxic metabolite	Acetaminophen, CCl_4
Hypersensitivity	Isoniazid, halothane
Cholestasis	
Canalicular	Anabolic steroids
Hepatocanalicular	Chlorpromazine
Vascular lesions	
Veno-occlusive disease	Estrogens Pyrrolizidine alkaloids
Neoplasms	
Adenomas	Estrogens
Hepatocellular carcinoma	Anabolic steroids

tochrome P-450 system and increase the potential for converting a drug to its toxic metabolites, and the reverse is true for low protein intake. Insufficient intake of protein and sulfur-containing amino acids can lead to depleted glutathione stores and enhanced toxicity. Drugs such as cimetidine, which diminish cytochrome P-450 activity, may prevent formation of toxic metabolites. Initial reports suggest that such drugs may be useful therapeutic agents.

There are three broad categories of drug-induced liver injury (Table 4-4). A number of drugs are directly cytotoxic to liver cells or injure the liver through the production of toxic metabolites. A variant of direct toxic injury is the classic idiosyncratic or hypersensitivity reaction, which usually appears within 1 to 5 weeks of initiation of drug therapy. Fever, rash, and eosinophilia are hallmarks of this reaction. The degree of injury is unrelated to drug dosage. Generalized hypersensitivity caused by some drugs (e.g., penicillin) almost never results in liver injury, but generalized hypersensitivity caused by phenytoin leads to liver disease with appreciable frequency. Cholestatic indirect hepatotoxins produce jaundice or impaired liver function by selective interference with hepatic mechanisms for excretion into the bile canaliculus or injury to the bile ducts. A third form of injury is injury to the vascular endothelium with resultant hepatic vein thrombosis. The lesions observed are characterized by cellular intimal proliferation with or without fibrin deposition.

Normally, withdrawal of the offending drug is the only therapy required; however, in instances when FH ensues, aggressive medical therapy, including liver transplantation, may be required.

Mechanisms of Drug-Induced Hepatic Injury

Hepatotoxic agents. A number of drugs are hepatotoxic and can produce hepatic injury by two distinct mechanisms. One group of agents produces liver injury by direct chemical attack or by production of a toxic metabolite. These drug reactions are usually dose-dependent and also affect organs other than the liver.

Although the exact mechanism of hepatotoxicity is uncertain, the products of reductive metabolism are highly reactive species that bind to cellular macromolecules and cause lipid peroxidation and inactivation of drug-metabolizing enzymes and other enzymes. The membrane injury provokes the release of calcium from mitochondria and SER. Furthermore, the injury appears to interfere with the calcium-ion pump, which normally prevents cytosolic accumulation of calcium. The deleterious effect on cell metabolism with resultant calcium accumulation, the loss of potassium and enzymes from the cytoplasm, and the loss of essential energy that results from mitochondrial injury all contribute to the necrosis.

In most instances a metabolite rather than the parent drug is the toxic species. The centrilobular localization of drug-induced hepatic necrosis can be attributed to the higher concentration of the biotransforming enzyme systems in the central zone. The liver contains several enzyme systems with broad substrate specificity. These enzymes usually inactivate the parent drug, but in some cases they convert the drug to a toxic metabolite. The drug-metabolizing enzymes of the microsomal P-450 family are particularly likely to produce potent alkylating, arylating, or acylating compounds that bind covalently to molecules essential to the viability of the hepatocyte, and necrosis ensues. Within the P-450 gene superfamily are three families that transcribe the major xenobiotic-metabolizing enzymes found in liver and other tissues. It is now possible by molecular cloning to isolate, identify, and characterize practically all of the P-450 enzymes. The differential expression of these enzymes or the genes involved in their regulation may account for the varying degrees of susceptibility to drug injury.

A second category of drugs includes activated compounds, antimetabolites, and related compounds that produce hepatic injury by selective interference with a specific metabolic pathway or structural process. The structural injury produced by indirect hepatotoxins is presumably initiated by membrane injury but is primarily due to selective blockage of key metabolic pathways required to maintain the intact hepatocyte.

Many drugs unpredictably produce hepatic injury in a small portion of recipients. These drugs have been referred to as causing hypersensitivity reactions, a designation that suggests the mechanism of hepatic injury to be drug allergy. In some instances the injury probably is a manifestation of hypersensitivity, but in other situations the mechanism of injury is unknown and may represent aberrant metabolism in susceptible patients that permits the production or accumulation of hepatotoxic metabolites. The term "hypersensitivity" should be reserved for hepatic injury for which there is clinical evidence of drug allergy, including rash, fever, and eosinophilia with a prompt recurrence to rechallenge of the drug. Some drugs seem to produce hepatic injury by either mechanism. For example, most cases of liver damage induced by isoniazid appear to result from toxic metabolites. However, in a few cases the liver damage is accompanied by fever and eosinophilia and may be presumed to result from hypersensitivity.

Efforts to demonstrate a role for cellular or humoral immunity in clinical cases have yielded variable and inconclusive results. Antibodies to phenytoin have been found in patients experiencing reactions to the drug. Lymphocytes from patients with reactions to some drugs have been reported to undergo lymphoblastic transformation and to release macrophage migration inhibitory factor, or kinins, that inhibit bile flow, but such reports have not been consistent. Furthermore, efforts to establish an immunologic basis for drug-induced hepatic disease have been hampered by the probability that the putative antigen is an unknown metabolite of the suspected drug. Nevertheless, the circumstantial evidence seems sufficiently compelling to support the view that hypersensitivity plays a role in the hepatic injury provoked by some drugs.

Microfilament Dysfunction as a Mechanism of Cholestasis

The cholestasis associated with drug administration can take several forms. Centrilobular cholestasis is accompanied by portal inflammatory changes. Bile duct changes have been reported with some drugs, such as erythromycin. Pure canalicular cholestasis is characteristic of other drugs, such as the anabolic steroids. Chronic cholestasis has been linked to such drugs as methyltestosterone and estradiol.

Bile canalicular changes are frequent, especially dilatation, loss of microvilli, and pericanalicular ectoplasmic thickening, usually accompanied by bile retention. In several cholestatic drug reactions, phospholipid membranous structures have been observed in the pericanalicular region and in lysosomes and plugging the bile canaliculi. The finding of phospholipidosis in a biopsy is a frequent ultrastuctural indicator of a drug effect. With amphiphilic drugs, such as amiodarone, the cell tries to secrete the drug-membrane complexes via lysosomes into bile canaliculi, which become plugged, producing micromechanical canalicular cholestasis. The cytoskeleton of the liver cell is also affected by failure of the pericanalicular microfilaments to contract. A growing list of pharmacologic agents has been implicated in cholestatic liver disease. Cholestasis is usually dose-dependent and reversible even if large doses of the drug have been taken over many years. Some drugs, although primarily cholestatic, can also produce hepatotoxicity. The liver injury that these drugs cause is mixed.

Drug-Induced Vascular and Sinusoidal Lesions of the Liver

A number of important vascular lesions of the liver can be produced by drugs. These lesions include thrombosis of the hepatic veins, occlusion of the hepatic venules, and peliosis hepatis. In addition, other lesions, including sinusoidal dilatation, perisinusoidal fibrosis, and hepatoportal sclerosis can occur. Midzonal and pericentral sinusoidal dilatation was first reported as a complication of oral contraceptive therapy. It has also been described with intake of azathioprine, which may have a direct effect on the sinusoidal cells (endothelium) with resultant thrombosis and fibrosis in the space of Disse. Peliosis hepatis is a condition characterized by large, blood-filled cavities that may or may not be lined with sinusoidal cells. It results from leakage of red blood cells through the endothelial barrier followed by perisinusoidal fibrosis. It has been described in patients taking oral contraceptives, anabolic steroids, azathioprine, and danazol. Hepatic vein thrombotic occlusion leads to Budd-Chiari syndrome, which has been reported in patients taking oral contraceptives. Although the mechanism is not known, the syndrome has been attributed to the thrombogenic effects of contraceptive steroids. Injury and occlusion of the central hepatic venules is also known to be related to the ingestion of pyrrolizidine alkaloids (bush teas). The initial lesion is central necrosis accompanied and followed by a progressive decrease in venule caliber. All of these lesions may be only partially reversible when the drug is stopped. Cirrhosis also can develop. Several types of benign and malignant hepatic neoplasms can result from the administration of drugs. Adenomas, lesions occurring in females in the childbearing years, are related to the use of contraceptive steroids. The risk increases with duration of use and diminishes if the drug is withdrawn. An increased risk of hepatocellular carcinoma is found in patients taking oral contraceptives for 8 years or more. This tumor may develop in the absence of cirrhosis, and it rarely metastasizes. Hepatocellular carcinoma may also be seen in patients taking androgenic hormones for aplastic anemia or hypopituitarism and in athletes taking them to increase muscle mass. Angiosarcoma may follow administration of androgens, exposure to vinyl chloride, thorotrast, and inorganic arsenic.

ALCOHOL AND THE LIVER

Alcohol causes a broad spectrum of liver disease, from fatty liver to cirrhosis. In the United States cirrhosis from alcohol is the fourth most common cause of death in adults. Not all individuals who drink excessive amounts of alcohol develop liver damage. In fact, the incidence of cirrhosis among alcoholics at autopsy is only 10% to 15%. Females have a predisposition to alcoholic liver disease. This has recently been attributed to a lack of alcohol dehydrogenase in the gastric mucosa, which accounts for higher blood ethanol values following a standard dose of ethanol.

Mechanisms of Liver Injury

Fatty liver is the only liver injury produced by alcohol in rodents, and there have been no good animal models to study alcohol-induced cirrhosis. The major pathogenetic mechanism for alcohol-induced liver injury is probably a direct hepatotoxic effect of alcohol. The capacity of acetaldehyde to cause liver peroxidation has been demonstrated in isolated perfused livers. Ethanol administration results in inhibition of glutathione production with depression of glutathione levels in the liver, reducing the scavenging effect of toxic free radicals that are generated during alcohol ingestion. Furthermore, the increased activity of microsomal NADPH oxidase after ethanol consumption results in enhanced superoxide and hydrogen peroxide production favoring lipid peroxidation.

A number of investigators have suggested a role for the immunologic system in alcohol-induced liver injury. Antibodies against ethanol-altered components of liver cells have been detected in the serum of patients with alcohol-induced liver disease. Alcoholic hyalin, an abnormal cytokeratin, has been postulated to trigger an immune response. Cytotoxic activity of mononuclear cells has been demonstrated against autologous liver cells in alcoholics. Acetaldehyde has recently been suggested to serve as a neoantigen and shown to elicit an immune response when injected into mice, and antibodies against acetaldehyde have been detected in patients with alcoholic hepatitis. Therefore these antibodies, which do not serve as specific markers of alcoholism, can contribute to the aggravation or perpetuation of the liver injury. One can conclude that the mechanism of injury in alcohol-induced liver disease is toxic metabolic but that secondary immune events can contribute to the disease.

SUMMARY

In this chapter we described the current concepts of the pathogenesis of viral, drug, alcohol and toxin, and immunologically mediated liver injury. We further described the molecular biology of the hepatitis A, hepatitis B, and hepatitis C viruses.

Injury of the liver may be due to the direct cytopathic effect of a virus (such as hepatitis A, δ, and hepatitis C) or activation of the immune system with resultant production of cytotoxic T cells, NK cells, and K cells. Involvement of cytokines has now been postulated as being through either their action as direct toxins or their ability to activate the immune-coagulation system with subsequent damage to endothelial cells and ischemic necrosis.

Drug-induced injury can be either direct, indirect, or cholestatic. Production of toxic metabolites with lipid peroxidation accounts for the majority of direct and indirect toxic injury, and disturbances in the canalicular microfilament system results in cholestasis.

Further work is required to gain understanding of the immunologic processes leading to tissue damage. Our understanding of molecular events will aid in this process.

SUGGESTED READINGS

Choo QL et al: Isolation of a cDNA clone derived from a blood-borne non-A, non-B viral hepatitis genome, Science 244:359, 1989.

In this recent article the authors describe the molecular biology of the hepatitis C virus.

Fields BN and Knipe DM: Virology, ed 2, New York, 1989, Raven Press.

This is a textbook of basic and applied virology with sections on the molecular biology and pathophysiology of hepatitis A, B, and C.

Kuo G et al: An assay for circulating antibodies to a major etiologic virus of human non-A, non-B hepatitis, Science 244:362, 1989.

This article describes the relevance of circulating antibodies to hepatitis C.

Leiber CS: Biochemical and molecular basis of alcohol-induced injury to liver and other tissues, N Engl J Med 319(25):1639-1650, 1988.

A review on the biochemical and molecular aspects of alcohol-induced liver injury is presented.

Mackay IR and Gershwin ME: The molecular basis of mitochondrial autoreactivity in primary biliary cirrhosis, Immunology Today 10(9):315-318, 1989.

This review article explores recent advances in our understanding of mitochondrial antibodies and their relationship to PBC.

Paul WE: Fundamental Immunology, ed 2, New York, 1989, Raven Press.

This is a complete textbook of basic immunologic processes.

Sinclair SB et al: Biochemical and clinical response of fulminant viral hepatitis to administration of prostaglandin E: a preliminary report, J Clin Invest 84:1063-1069, 1989.

This recent article describes the role of prostaglandins in the treatment of fulminant viral hepatitis.

Sinclair SB and Levy GA: Drug induced hepatic injury, Textbook of internal medicine, Kelley WN, ed., Philadelphia, 1991, J B Lippincott Co.

This is a recent review on drug-induced hepatic injury.

Sinclair SB, Wakefield A, and Levy GA: Fulminant hepatitis: Springer Semin Immunopathol 12:33-45, 1990.

A review on the immunopathology of fulminant viral hepatitis is presented.

Thomas HC, Pignatelli M, and Scully LJ: Viruses and immune reactions in the liver, Scand J Gastroenterol 114:105, 1985.

This is a review on the immunopathology of hepatitis B infection.

Weiner AM et al: Detection of hepatitis C viral sequences in non-A, non-B hepatitis, Lancet 335:1-3, 1990.

This is a recent article on the molecular biology of HCV.

5 Pathophysiology of Liver Fibrosis

Marcos Rojkind and Patricia Greenwel

Cirrhosis is the end stage of many diseases that affect the liver chronically. It is produced by several chemical and biologic agents. These agents include chemicals normally present in the body, such as copper and iron; substances ingested for pleasure, such as alcohol; and chemicals administered as therapy for other diseases, such as methotrexate. The biologic agents include the viral agents (hepatitis B, C, and non-A, non-B viruses) and the parasites of the *Schistosoma* family. Anatomically, cirrhosis is characterized by generalized liver damage, attempts of the hepatocytes to regenerate, and excess deposition of connective tissue. This deposition occurs in a disorganized manner and it causes a complete distortion of the liver architecture. As a result of the anatomic alterations, functional and hemodynamic changes also occur. Liver dysfunction can be mild but can be as severe as to cause encephalopathy and coma. The hemodynamic alterations include portal hypertension with development of extensive collateral circulation and esophageal varices (the latter can rupture and cause death). The prognosis for patients with the disease is generally poor. The 5-year survival rate of patients without complications is over 70%. However, when complications develop, the survival rate can be lower than 30%. There is no specific therapy for liver cirrhosis, and treatment is applied for individual complications of the disease. However, the disease can be prevented when the causative agent is reduced or eliminated. Recent developments in therapy indicate that anti-inflammatory and antifibrogenic agents can ameliorate the disease and in some cases decrease or even reverse liver fibrosis.

THE CELLS

The liver comprises at least five different classes of cells. They are the hepatocytes, fat-storing (Ito), endothelial, Kupffer, and pit cells. In the normal liver, and for each species, the volume occupied by each cell type and the actual number of cells is a constant. For example, it has been estimated that there is one fat-storing cell for every 5 to 10 hepatocytes. Each cell has a specific function and can influence the biologic activities of the other cells. This influence occurs through the production of metabolites, which are essential for other cells, and/or through the release of cytokines and growth factors, which can either stimulate or inhibit the proliferation of the other cells. Accordingly, liver function results from the multiple interactions among the different cells. Thus in disease states, when one cell is injured, the ratio of cells is changed, altering the function.

THE EXTRACELLULAR MATRIX

Collagens

The normal liver contains approximately 5 mg of collagen per gram of fresh tissue. Five of the 12 distinct genetic types of collagen have been found in the liver. Of these, type I and type III collagen are the most abundant; they account for up to 70% of total liver collagen. The other genetic types, mainly types IV, V, and VI, are present in smaller quantities and make up the remaining 30%. The ratio of collagen type I to type III is 1:1 (Table 5-1). Each type of collagen has a unique distribution although more than one type is present in the same location. Although tissue fibrils are made of a single collagen type, recent evidence indicates that some fibrils may contain mixtures of at least two distinct genetic types of collagen.

Table 5-1 Collagen content and synthesis in normal, regenerating, and cirrhotic livers

	Normal	5 days after hepatectomy	11 days after hepatectomy	Cirrhosis
Content				
mg/g	1.0	0.5	1.0	5.2
Type I collagen (% total)	45.5	52.5	30.8	63.6
Type III collagen (% total)	47.7	23.9	56.3	27.8
Type V collagen (% total)	6.6	23.6	12.8	8.4
Ratio I/III	1:1	>2:1	<1:1	>2:1
Synthesis				
dpm × 10^{-3} ^{3}H-hypro/g fresh tissue	2.2	9.5	1.9	30.2
Type I collagen (% total)	44.0	48.0	32.0	52.4
Type III collagen (% total)	41.7	21.3	57.2	41.8
Type V collagen (% total)	14.1	29.7	10.6	5.7
Ratio I/III	1:1	>2:1	<1:1	>1:1

The distribution and specific location of each collagen type has been investigated using immunocytochemical techniques (Table 5-2).

Noncollagenous Proteins

The connective tissue contains several proteins that do not have the glycine-proline-hydroxyproline sequence that is characteristic of collagen molecules. Therefore they are referred to as noncollagenous proteins. Some of them are found primarily in the loose connective tissue and include proteins such as thrombospondin, fibronectin, and tenascin. Others, such as laminin and entactin, are present in basement membranes. In addition to their structural role, the proteins have important biologic properties. They possess cellular binding domains of the arginyl-gly-

Table 5-2 Distribution of collagen

	Cirrhotic liver		
Normal liver	**Early (fatty liver)**	**Intermediate (fibrosis)**	**Advanced (cirrhosis)**
Type I collagen			
Portal stroma around central veins; space of Disse in direct contact with the hepatocyte plasmalemma; along the sinusoidal wall, particularly at point of branching.	Changes are apparent until week 4 of CCl_4 treatment. Deposition starts in regions adjacent to central veins, usually near areas of hepatocyte necrosis.	Deposition is more prominent. Thin deposits are present in central regions. In the space of Disse, dense deposits become prominent.	Most prominent extracellular matrix component in the fibrosis septa. Thin bundles separate hepatocytes from the capillary basement membrane in the regenerating nodules.
Type IV collagen			
All basement membranes: ductular, neural, and vascular; small discontinuous deposits along the entire length of the sinusoids; absent from stroma.	After 2 weeks of treatment, deposits become apparent, and they increase as the process advances. Continuous deposits join some central veins.	Deposition becomes more prominent. In many regions continuous subsinusoidal deposits are found.	The subendothelial deposits become continuous, forming a true basement membrane also containing laminin. The hepatic exchange vessels are transformed from sinusoids into capillaries. In the fibrous septa cirrhosis is confined to vascular and ductal basement membranes.

cine-aspartate (RGD) type that were originally described in fibronectin. In addition to the RGD domains, laminin contains other cellular binding sites. Through these binding domains, cells possessing receptors of the integrin family can interact and attach to the noncollagenous proteins of the extracellular matrix. In addition, some of the noncollagenous proteins have binding domains for collagen and glycosaminoglycans (GAGs), forming an extensive meshwork that connects the cells to the extracellular matrix. These multiple interactions are important for the cells to maintain their polarization and to express their function. It has been shown that the extracellular matrix modulates the phenotypic expression of cells in culture.

The noncollagenous proteins and the core proteins of some GAGs contain repeats that resemble the cysteine-rich domains of EGF. One could speculate that these domains, which may be exposed when the extracellular matrix proteins are cleaved during tissue injury, possibly could initiate the proliferative response before the arrival and/or local production of cell growth factor.

The β-subunit of the integrin class of proteins possesses a sequence corresponding to a phosphorylation site for protein

Table 5-3 Production of GAG by cultured fat-storing cells

	Type of GAG	Effect of transforming growth factors (TGF)-β	Effect of 100 mM ethyl alcohol (ETOH)	Effect of 375 mM acetaldehyde
Cell bound (20% to 40%)	Heparan sulfate	Slight inhibition in synthesis	No effect	No effect
Secreted 60% to 80%)	Chondroitin sulfate	Stimulation	No effect	Causes 25% inhibition
	Dermatan sulfate. Increases with time in culture and corresponds to 60% of the total secreted GAGs	No effect	No effect	Causes 75% decrease in dermatan sulfate formation. Effect can be overcomed by β-D-xylosides (artificial initiators of polysaccharide chain elongation)
	Hyaluronic acid. Decreases with time in culture	Stimulation	Not determined	Not determined

kinase C activity. Therefore interaction with extracellular matrix components could generate signals and modify gene expression in the responding cell. It has been shown that interaction of fibronectin-derived peptides with its receptor induces the expression of collagenase and stromelysin genes by cultured synovial cells. A similar mechanism could occur with fat-storing cells or hepatocytes because both cell types interact with fibronectin.

Glycosaminoglycans

Liver GAGs are localized to the extracellular matrix and the plasma membrane of cells. They are produced by both epithelial cells and mesenchymal cells. Table 5-3 contains a summary of the production of GAGs by fat-storing cells in the liver. In addition to their structural role, GAGs in general and heparins in particular sustain the expression of a normal phenotype by cultured rat hepatocytes. The mechanism by which the GAGs express their biologic activity is not known. It has been indicated that the plasma membrane core protein interacts with actin filaments through the protein *talin*. However, whether this type of interaction generates the signal transduction that induces change in phenotypic expression will have to be determined.

ALTERATIONS IN LIVER CIRRHOSIS

The liver can respond to injury in two distinct ways. It can either regenerate and restore normal structure and function, or it can start a repair process that leads to cirrhosis. The factors that determine the outcome of the injury are unknown. It has been shown that when the injury is acute and single and when it removes a substantial amount of functional liver mass, the liver regenerates. However, when the injury is small and repetitive, it may not be sufficient to induce regeneration; thus fibrosis and cirrhosis develop. In most cases of cirrhosis, regeneration and scarring occur simultaneously, although fibrosis predominates. Therefore it is possible to detect nodules of cells that had regenerated that are surrounded by connective tissue septa.

Changes in Cell Populations

Throughout the development of liver cirrhosis, alterations occur in cell populations and in matrix composition and distribution. Initially changes in cells are due to the arrival of inflammatory cells and the removal of dead hepatocytes. In addition, there is local proliferation of both parenchymal and nonparenchymal liver cells in response to injury. The maximal number of nonparenchymal cells is obtained 48 to 72 hours after injury. In general, hepatocyte proliferation precedes the proliferation of nonparenchymal cells. In addition to the changes described above, transformation of fat-storing cells into myofibroblasts also occurs. Although there is no direct evidence for this occurrence in vivo, the presence of transitional cells, which contain features of both fat-storing cells and myofibroblasts, strongly supports this suggestion. Further evidence to support that fat-storing cells are precursors of myofibroblasts has been obtained in vitro: cultured fat-storing cells lose their vitamin A droplets and develop an enlarged ER and abundant actin fibrils. In the late stages of the disease, the number of myofibroblasts decreases, there are fewer inflammatory cells, and the predominant feature is the scar.

How do the Inflammatory Cells Arrive?

The exact mechanism of cell migration into or within the liver is not known. However, several chemotactic substances have been described. They vary from leukotrienes to collagen and fibronectin fragments. In general the production of any chemotactic substance during liver injury can promote the attraction of inflammatory cells and the migration of cells within the liver. The changes in cell populations alone can disturb the balance of cytokines and growth factors and further promote cell proliferation and/or collagen production. Moreover, the inflammatory cells that arrive are "activated" and produce larger quantities of cytokines and growth factors, further changing the balance. However, it is also possible that the "activated" cells stop the production of cytokines that inhibit cell proliferation and regulate collagen production. This also alters the balance of cytokines and induces proliferation of fat-storing cells and deposition of excess collagen.

As a consequence of the production and release of growth factors, mesenchymal cells proliferate. Proliferation depends on, among other factors, the presence of receptors on the plasma membrane of target cells. It has been suggested that fat-storing cells in the liver are heterogeneous populations of cells; therefore, not all the cells can respond equally to cytokines and growth factors. Thus the cell population that increases its number most rapidly and significantly is the highly responsive cell. One could then speculate that, among other things, cirrhosis will develop faster in those patients who possess fat-storing cells that respond more readily to growth factors. Alternatively, cirrhosis will develop in those patients who respond to injury by producing larger quantities of cytokines or those who have fat-storing cells that respond more efficiently to cytokines, increasing the expression of extracellular matrix components (see below).

Alteration of Extracellular Matrix

It has already been established that the extracellular matrix is increased in liver cirrhosis. Excess deposition of connective tissue results from the imbalance of synthesis and deposition. Collagen synthesis is increased, and collagen degradation is either normal or decreased.

Excess collagen production alone is not sufficient to explain the alterations observed in cirrhosis. Therefore modifications in the types of collagen produced and changes in the sites of collagen deposition play an important role in cirrhosis. During physiologic growth, such as occurs during liver regeneration after hepatectomy, increased collagen deposition occurs. However, the types of collagen produced are those needed to reform the sinusoids and restore normal liver architecture. Therefore, during liver regeneration the needed amounts and types of collagen are produced by the right cells and deposited in the correct sites. The orderly deposition of extracellular matrix is a coordinated process in which many liver cells are involved. In contrast to regeneration, the main collagen produced in cirrhotic livers is type I. Matrix organization is lost because of disorderly synthesis and deposition of the various components of the extracellular matrix. Accordingly, the wrong extracellular matrix is produced in abnormally large quantities and is being deposited in the "wrong" places. The sinusoids are transformed into capillaries, and a basement membrane is formed in

Table 5-4 Distribution of noncollagenous components of the extracellular matrix

	Cirrhotic liver		
Normal liver	**Early (fatty liver)**	**Intermediate (fibrosis)**	**Advanced (cirrhosis)**
Fibronectin			
Portal stroma around central veins, along the full length of the sinusoids in direct contact with the hepatocyte microvilli; absent in basement membranes; most prominent component in the space of Disse.	After 2 to 4 weeks of treatment it increases in the space of Disse. Deposition is pronounced in areas adjacent to central veins. Deposits increase as the process advances. Nodular appearance.	Long septa radiate from central veins. As fibrosis progresses, the fibronectin-containing septa become wider. Eventually these septa extend from central vein to central vein.	Sinusoidal deposits remain prominent, although at this stage they are deposited below the endothelial basement membrane. Fibronectin staining has its maximum intensity at the interface between fibrous septa and hepatocytes.
Laminin			
Codistributes with type IV collagen in all basement membranes. Absent in the sinusoidal wall.	After 4 weeks of treatment, traces are demonstrable in some sinusoids. It codistributes with type IV collagen.	It becomes more prominent in the space of Disse.	Same distribution as type IV collagen within the hepatic lobule. Groups of hepatocytes are surrounded by continuous basement membrane also containing type IV collagen. In the fibrous septa it has the same distribution as type IV collagen.

the Disse space. When comparing the differences in collagen production between physiologic growth and scar formation, one could say that in the former, the process is highly regulated and the increase in collagen production is modulated by the newly formed cells. Accordingly, when growth has been completed, collagen production returns to normal levels. During scar formation, excess collagen production is not modulated, and matrix deposition occurs at the sites of injury. Furthermore, collagen production is sustained by either the initial injurious stimulus or secondary mechanisms triggered in response to injury.

The noncollagenous proteins of the extracellular matrix also increase during chronic liver injury. It has been shown that laminin and fibronectin are increased in liver cirrhosis (Table 5-4). In an animal model of skin wound healing, there is a shift in the type of fibronectin produced in the basal portion of the wound. It has been shown by in situ hybridization that a fetal type of fibronectin is being expressed. This fibronectin contains the cellular binding domain; therefore, fibronectin produced may remain at the site of injury and bind to cells. As indicated above, because fibronectin is a chemoattractant for various cell types, it can help in recruiting the various cell types at the injury site. Although the nature of fibronectin produced in cirrhotic livers is not known, it is known that part of the fibronectin produced remains in close association of cells localized at the injury site.

Which Cells are Involved in Fibrogenesis?

Hepatocytes, endothelial cells, and fat-storing cells produce collagen in vivo and in vitro. Either each cell type produces a different genetic type of collagen, or the ratios of types of collagen produced vary. However, the three cells have the capacity to produce extracellular matrix in the normal liver. In cirrhosis the cells may change phenotype, and different types of collagen may be produced. It has already been shown by immunocytochemical methods that fat-storing cells produce collagen type IV. However, in culture the fat-storing cells resemble the phenotype of cirrhotic fat-storing cells and produce mainly collagen type I. Recently, in situ hybridization methods have been used to determine the localization of collagen (Table 5–5) and laminin (Table 5-6) transcripts in various liver cells. Although the data indicate that no transcripts of type I collagen are present in hepatocytes, other evidence suggests that hepatocytes contain type I collagen mRNA and express

Table 5-5 Expression patterns of procollagen mRNA

Normal liver	CCl_4-induced cirrhosis	Experimental biliary fibrosis
α-2(I) and α-1(III) procollagen mRNA is present in some stromal cells of the portal tracts, in few cells around the central veins, and in some sinusoidal cells homogeneously distributed in the lobule. Absent in hepatocytes. α-1(IV) procollagen mRNA is not detected except in a very small number of portal tract stromal cells.	α-2(I), α-1(III), and α-1(IV) procollagen mRNA is detected in the sinusoidal spaces in close proximity to the central vein walls and in the portal tract stroma. Present in perivenular, septal, and perisinusoidal nonparenchymal cells. The number of cells positive for α-2(I) and α-1(III) transcripts is increased. Absent in hepatocytes.	α-2(I) and α-1(III) procollagen mRNAs are detected on portal tracts, mesenchymal cells, and perisinusoidal cells in proximity to portal tracts. α-1(IV) procollagen transcripts are found in some periductular nonepithelial cells and in the epithelial cells of proliferating bile ducts. Absent in hepatocytes.

Table 5-6 Laminin mRNA expression in normal and fibrotic human livers

Normal liver	Fibrotic liver
Expression is localized in nonepithelial cells of the portal field stroma mainly in close proximity to hepatocytes and around vessels and bile ducts. Transcripts are found along sinusoids and around central veins. Some vascular endothelial cells and bile duct epithelia are positive. Absent in hepatocytes.	Positive signal in many nonepithelial cells, epithelial cells of the fibrotic septa, and cells surrounding proliferating bile ducts and portal veins. Increased levels observed in epithelial cells of proliferating bile ducts. Transcripts are found in groups of cells localized along sinusoids and fibrotic bands adjacent to hepatocytes of regenerating nodules. Absent in hepatocytes.

the protein. The relative contribution of each cell type to overall collagen production is still debatable. However, excess deposition of collagen results from increased production of collagen by hepatocytes, endothelial cells, and fat-storing cells and from a decrease in collagen degradation. The decrease in collagen degradation can result from a lack of enzyme or can be due to the increased production of collagenase inhibitors.

ROLE OF CYTOKINES AND GROWTH FACTORS

Throughout the past few years, great emphasis has been given to the role of cytokines and growth factors in the development of liver cirrhosis. Although they are important and their production is increased during cirrhosis, the role of each cytokine and/or growth factor in the development of cirrhosis remains to be determined.

TGF-β 1 is a cytokine produced by many cells, including monocytes, macrophages, and Kupffer cells. It inhibits the proliferation of cultured hepatocytes that had been stimulated with EGF and insulin or with TGF-α. TGF-β inhibits the proliferation of fat-storing cells and induces the production of collagen and fibronectin by cultured mesenchymal cells. In addition, TGF-β stimulates the expression of fibronectin receptors in cultured fibroblasts. It has been suggested that TGF-β is the main mediator of collagen production in cirrhosis.

IL-1 is a cytokine produced by peripheral blood monocytes during the acute phase response. It is also produced by macrophages and Kupffer cells. It is involved in, among other things, decreasing the expression of the albumin gene and stimulating the induction of some acute phase proteins. Serum IL-1 levels are increased in cirrhotic patients of various etiologies. IL-1 can stimulate the production of collagen and collagenase by cultured cells. Therefore it could also play an important role in the development of cirrhosis. However, further work is needed to determine how myofibroblasts and fat-storing cells respond to IL-1.

TNF-α is another cytokine produced by monocytes and macrophages. Serum levels of TNF are increased in patients with cirrhosis of various etiologies. TNF is a mediator of the acute phase response and is the cytokine responsible for muscle wasting (cachexia) that occurs in chronic inflammatory diseases. TNF has several effects on matrix deposition. It not only stimulates the production of collagen in cultured fat-storing cells but also induces collagenase production by various cell types. The increase in collagen is not associated with changes in steady-state levels of type I collagen mRNA. Therefore regulation of collagen production by TNF is a translational or post-translational event. This is in contrast with the effect of TGF-β, which induces the steady-state levels of type I collagen mRNA. The induction of collagenase activity by TNF occurs secondary to the induction of the oncogenes c-fos and c-myc. Because of these multiple activities of TNF, it is important to determine whether increased collagen production is secondary to the increased degradation of extracellular matrix by the release of collagenase.

Interferon-γ and other interferons affect extracellular matrix production by several cultured cells. Interferon-γ specifically decreased the expression of α-2 (I) collagen mRNA in primary cultures of rat hepatocytes. When given in vivo to animals infected with cercaria of *Schistosoma mansoni,* mRNA levels for collagen type I and type III were significantly decreased. However, these results must be taken with caution. The decrease in collagen mRNA levels could result from the modulation of the immunologic events that occur in this animal model. It has already been established that increased cell proliferation and excess collagen production result from mediators produced by either the eggs of the parasite or the inflammatory cells that compose the granulomas. Furthermore, it has been shown that destruction of the parasites by praziquantel is followed by a reduction in liver collagen content.

TREATMENT OF CIRRHOSIS

Traditionally, cirrhosis has been considered an irreversible, therefore incurable, disease. Most therapy developed in the past has been related to the treatment of complications of the disease. Although it is still debatable whether cirrhosis is curable, the disease is treatable. In recent studies, it has been shown that colchicine treatment is beneficial for cirrhotic patients. The 10-year survival in the colchicine-treated group was more than 50%, compared with 30% survival in the placebo group. From the different reports in the literature, it is apparent that, with a few exceptions, patients included in double blind trials do much better clinically and biochemically than the average cirrhotic patient treated in the same institution but not included in a specific therapy protocol. This improvement is irrespective of whether the patient receives the placebo or the experimental drug. This "placebo effect" indicates that when the physician is interested in the patient for personal reasons, the physician takes special care of the patient. The patient is monitored more frequently, and complications of the disease are prevented.

What kind of therapy can we provide for the patient with cirrhosis? Until now, there has been a lot of magic in the development of therapy because the concept of antifibrogenic therapy was quite narrow and was associated only with inhibition of collagen production. However, according to the pathophysiologic mechanisms of liver cirrhosis described above, five major areas can be selected as important targets for therapy: (1) the elimination of the etiologic factor that produces liver damage, (2) the protection of liver cells from the various injurious agents, (3) the modulation of inflammation with modification of cytokines and growth factors that lead to cell proliferation and collagen production, (4) the selective inhibition of collagen deposition, and (5) the removal of collagen already present in the scar tissue.

Ideally, the best treatment for liver cirrhosis is not to treat but rather to prevent the causes of chronic liver injury that lead to cirrhosis. However, realistically, preventive medicine will be possible in some but not all the causes of liver cirrhosis. Proper education, improvement of people's socioeconomic status, and development of vaccines could perhaps eradicate schistosomiasis and hepatitis. The incidence of the inherited alterations that lead to liver cirrhosis could be diminished through proper genetic counseling of members of families that carry the abnormal genes. The incidence of alcoholism and alcoholic liver disease will continue to increase until the chemical alterations that lead to alcohol addiction are established and proper counseling can be offered to subjects at risk. However, even then, alcohol will continue to be one of the major causes of chronic liver disease.

If we fail at the preventive medicine level, we will have to rely on noninvasive methods of diagnosis that will allow us to detect early stages of liver disease. Patients diagnosed early could have more dramatic responses to therapy and develop fewer complications than patients diagnosed later.

When the mechanisms that lead to an increased number of cells within the liver are unraveled, it will be possible to develop chemicals to prevent either the arrival of inflammatory cells and/or the proliferation of myofibroblasts. If the arrival of the inflammatory cells that stimulate myofibroblast proliferation and excess collagen deposition is prevented, liver fibrosis could be prevented.

Within the next decade we expect many exciting developments with regard to therapy. These developments may include a large variety of drugs to remove the etiologic agent, to protect the hepatocyte, or to modulate the deposition of connective tissue. We may even see successful introduction of normal genes that will prevent iron and copper accumulation. The most difficult task, convincing physicians that cirrhosis is a treatable disease, has been accomplished. Antifibrogenic therapy is not a dream; it has become a reality.

SUMMARY

This chapter presents the chain of events that lead to excess collagen deposition in the liver. The cells that participate in the processes and their relative contributions to collagen deposition are analyzed. The mediators that stimulate cell proliferation and/or excess collagen deposition are discussed. Finally, the general strategies for treatment of liver fibrosis are reviewed. This treatment-strategy review is not intended to convince the readers that cirrhosis can be cured but to encourage physicians and researchers to take a more positive attitude toward this disease to develop and explore new ways to prevent and treat liver cirrhosis.

SUGGESTED READINGS

Armendariz-Borunda J, Seyer JM, Kang AH et al: Regulation of TGF-β gene expression in rat liver intoxicated with carbon tetrachloride, FASEB J 4:215-221, 1990.

In this article the authors demonstrate that increased transcripts of TGF-β are associated with increased collagen deposition. They suggest that this cytokine may play a key role in liver fibrogenesis.

Bachem MG, Riess U, Melchior R et al: Transforming growth factors (TGF-α and TGF-β 1) stimulate chondroitin sulfate and hyluronate synthesis in cultured rat liver fat-storing cells, FEBS Lett 257:134-137, 1989.

This article describes the effects of cytokines on GAGs produced by rat liver fat-storing cells.

Buck CA and Horwitz AF: Cell surface receptors for extracellular matrix molecules, Ann Rev Cell Biol 3:179-205, 1987.

This review analyzes the groups of receptors for extracellular matrix components with special emphasis on the integrin family. The authors discuss the cells that contain integrins, the nature and size of subunits, and some of the functional implications of cell matrix interactions.

Chojkier M: Hepatocyte collagen production in vivo in normal rats, J Clin Invest 78:333-339, 1986.

Chojkier M, Lyche KD, and Filip M: Increased production of collagen in vivo by hepatocytes and nonparenchymal cells in rats with carbon tetrachloride-induced hepatic fibrosis, Hepatology 8:808-814, 1988.

The authors describe an excellent method to measure which liver cells are involved in collagen production in vivo. They show that in vivo at least 80% of the collagen produced in the liver is made by hepatocytes. They also show that in liver cirrhosis, the hepatocytes also contribute, with a large proportion of collagen deposited in the liver.

Czaja MJ, Weiner FR, Flanders KC et al: In vitro and in vivo association of transforming growth factor-β 1 with hepatic fibrosis, J Cell Biol 108:2477-2482, 1989.

In this article, the authors demonstrate that increased transcripts of TGF-β are associated with increased collagen deposition. They suggest that this cytokine may play a key role in liver fibrogenesis.

Dinarello CA and Savage N: Interleukin-1 and its receptor, CRC Crit Rev Immunol 9:1-20, 1989.

This review discusses the chemistry and biology of IL-1, a cytokine that stimulates the acute-phase response and that may play a role in liver fibrosis.

Fujita M, Spray DC, Choi H et al: Glycosaminoglycans and proteoglycans induce gap junction expression and restore transcription of tissue-specific mRNAs in primary liver cultures, Hepatology 7:1S-9S, 1987.

This article describes the importance of the extracellular matrix and GAGs in cell function. It specifically shows that GAGs induce the expression of gap-junction proteins.

Gressner AM and Althaus M: Effects of ethanol, acetaldehyde, and lactate on proteoglycan synthesis and proliferation of cultured rat liver fat-storing cells, Gastroenterology 94:797-807, 1988.

This article describes the effects of cytokines, alcohol, and acetaldehyde on the production of GAGs by fat-storing cells.

Gressner AM and Haarmann R: Hyaluronic acid synthesis and secretion by rat liver fat-storing cells (perisinusoidal lipocytes) in culture, Biochem Biophys Res Commun 151:222-229, 1988.

This article describes the GAGs produced by fat-storing cells.

Heinrich PC, Castell JV, and Andus T: Interleukin-6 and the acute phase response, Biochem J 265:621-636, 1990.

This review discusses the biology and regulation of IL-6 production with special emphasis on CIS acting elements of acute-phase protein genes.

Kershenobich D, Vargas F, Garcia-Tsao G et al: Colchicine in the treatment of cirrhosis of the liver, N Engl J Med 318:1709-1713, 1988.

In this article the authors describe their 15 years of experience in the treatment of liver cirrhosis with colchicine. They show significant differences in survival of colchicine-treated patients as compared with survival of placebo-treated patients.

Martinez-Hernandez A: The hepatic extracellular matrix. I. Electron Immunohistochemical studies in normal rat liver, Lab Invest 51:57-74, 1984.

Martinez-Hernandez A: The hepatic extracellular matrix. II. Electron immunohistochemical studies in rats with CCl_4-induced cirrhosis, Lab Invest 53:166-186, 1985.

These articles describe the distribution of connective tissue components in normal and cirrhotic livers.

Massague J, Cheifetz S, Ignotz RA et al: Multiple type-β transforming growth factors and their receptors, J Cell Physiol 5:43-47, 1987.

This review discusses the chemistry and biology of TGF-β and of its receptor molecules.

Milani S, Herbst H, Schuppan D et al: Cellular localization of laminin gene transcripts in normal and fibrotic human liver, Am J Pathol 134:1175-1182, 1989.

This article demonstrates the cellular localization of mRNA transcripts of extracellular matrix proteins in normal and cirrhotic livers.

Milani S, Herbst H, Schuppan D et al: In situ hybridization for procollagen types I, III and IV mRNA in normal and fibrotic rat liver: evidence for predominant expression in nonparenchymal liver cells, Hepatology 10:84-92, 1989.

This article demonstrates the cellular localization of mRNA transcripts of extracellular matrix proteins in normal and cirrhotic livers.

Milani S, Herbst H, Schuppan D et al: Procollagen expression by nonparenchymal rat liver cells in experimental biliary fibrosis, Gastroenterology 98:175-184, 1990.

This article demonstrates the cellular localization of mRNA transcripts of extracellular matrix proteins in normal and cirrhotic livers.

Rojkind M: Extracellular matrix. In Arias IM, Jakoby WB, Popper H et al, eds: The liver: biology and pathobiology, ed 2, New York, 1988, Raven Press, pp. 707-716.

This article reviews the chemistry of extracellular matrix components and analyzes the changes in different types of collagen in cirrhosis.

Rojkind M, Gatmaitan Z, Mackensen S et al: Connective tissue biomatrix: its isolation and utilization for long-term cultures of normal rat hepatocytes, J Cell Biol 87:255-263, 1980.

This article describes the importance of the extracellular matrix in cell function. It introduces the concept of biomatrix, a complex matrix extracted from tissue that contains in native form most of the different types of collagen and the noncollagenous protein originally present in the tissue.

Rojkind M, Giambrone MA, and Biempica L: Collagen types in normal and cirrhotic liver, Gastroenterology 76:710-719, 1979.

This reference describes the isolation and characterization of collagen in normal and cirrhotic liver. It shows that livers contain approximately equal amounts of type I and type III collagen. Although all the collagen types are increased in cirrhotic livers, type I collagen predominates.

Rojkind M and Greenwel P: The liver as a bioecological system. In Arias IM, Jakoby WB, Popper H et al: The liver: biology and pathobiology, ed 2, New York, 1988, Raven Press, pp. 1269-1285.

In this review article the liver is analyzed as an ecologic system. The authors explain that all the cells and matrix components are important for the structural and functional organization of the organ. It is emphasized that cytokines and growth factors produced within the liver are responsible for the fine regulatory control of cells and the matrix. Cirrhosis is described as an alteration in the homeostatic mechanisms that maintain the ecologic system.

Rojkind M, Rojkind MH, and Cordero-Hernandez J: In vivo collagen synthesis and deposition in fibrotic and regenerating rat livers, Coll Relat Res 3:335-347, 1983.

This article compares the changes in collagen types in normal, fibrotic, and regenerating livers. It demonstrates that collagen synthesis is increased in regenerating and fibrotic livers but that the types of collagen produced differ. In the regenerating liver the predominant types of collagen produced are types III and V; in cirrhosis, type I is predominant.

Schafer S, Zerbe O, and Gressner AM: The synthesis of proteoglycans in fat-storing cells of rat liver, Hepatology 7:680-687, 1987.

This article describes the GAGs produced by fat-storing cells.

Seyer JM, Hutcheson ET, and Kang AH: Collagen polymorphism in normal and cirrhotic human liver, J Clin Invest 59:241-247, 1977.

This reference describes the isolation and characterization of different types of collagen in normal and cirrhotic livers. It shows that livers contain approximately equal amounts of type I and type III collagen. Although all the collagen types are increased in cirrhotic livers, type I collagen predominates.

Sherry B and Cerami A: Cachectin/tumor necrosis factor exerts endocrine, paracrine and autocrine control of inflammatory responses, J Cell Biol 107:1269-1277, 1988.

This review discusses the chemistry and biology of the different cytokines that have been suggested to play a role in liver fibrosis and in stimulation of the acute phase response.

Werb Z, Tremble PM, Behrendtsen O et al: Signal transduction through the fibronectin receptor induces collagenase and stromelysin gene expression, J Cell Biol 109:877-889, 1989.

In this article the authors describe that interactions of either antibodies to fibronectin receptor (integrin) or fibronectin fragments with the fibronectin receptor specifically induce the expression of collagenase and stromelysin. The authors measured the changes in specific mRNA transcripts, immunoprecipitable proteins, and the enzymatic activity of the two enzymes.

SECTION THREE

Evaluation of Liver Status

6 Clinical Evaluation of Liver Status

Carlo H. Tamburro

The art and skill of history taking continues to be a symbol of the physician despite all the technologic advances in medicine. However, the type of patient information obtained during a medical examination has changed in scope and form. The use of this information goes beyond the basic need for diagnoses and treatment management. There are now economic, social, ethical, legal, and regulatory needs for these data. Presently the staff, time, and money needed to handle these data almost equals that needed for medical care delivery.

This chapter illustrates information collection, storage, and retrieval techniques, which link traditional medical examination processes with data base formats for computerization and analyses. These computer-oriented formats are necessities for modern clinical care and problem solving. In the near future their use for the evaluation of new, rapidly developing treatment modalities and for analytic assessment of the outcomes of medical care will be commonplace.

Computerized handling of medical data along with skillful history taking, careful physical examination, and detailed study of laboratory findings are and will continue to be essential requirements for the clinician.

HISTORY

Chief complaint. One third of patients referred to hepatologists have no complaints attributable to the hepatobiliary system. Abnormal liver tests or incidental radiologic abnormalities are the major reasons for referral. The original complaint(s) or reason(s) for performing the test or procedure may identify subtle clue(s) relevant to the underlying hepatobiliary abnormality or disease. Nevertheless, all such incidentally discovered hepatobiliary abnormalities require follow-up study.

The major presenting symptoms and signs of patients with hepatobiliary disorders are listed in Table 6-1 and discussed individually, beginning on p. 98.

Present illness. In taking the history of a present illness (PI), the chronology of symptoms not only provides an assessment of duration and severity but also allows characterization of the illness, thus aiding in disease recognition or exclusion. Therefore the data format of the PI allows the patient's unique chronologic story to be recorded while providing for computerization of all essential common facts (negative and positive). Appendices A-1, A-2, and A-3 provide examples of a problem list and initial history.

Past medical data. Past medical illnesses and social, familial, occupational,

Table 6-1 Common presentation of hepatobiliary disease

Major symptoms	Major signs
Fatigue	Jaundice
Abdominal pain	Edema
Increase in abdominal girth	Ascites (abdominal swelling)
Yellow eyes	Vascular skin changes
Pruritus	Enlarged liver
Weight change	Enlarged spleen
Anorexia	Abnormal extremity finding
Nausea	Neurologic changes
Vomiting	Muscle wasting
Hematemesis	Hemorrhoids
Melena	Endocrine abnormalities
Hematochezia	Cardiac-pulmonary findings
Diarrhea	Fever
Constipation	Fetor hepaticus
Fever	
Epistaxis	
Impotence	
Abnormal menses	

environmental, and nutritional histories can be effectively organized in a data base format for computerization. The completion of a detailed past medical history by the patient (or a relative) before the initial visit provides the doctor with clues for further inquiries. This information maximizes efficiency while enhancing the quality of direct patient inquiry and the amount of time allowed for it. The Health Assessment Survey/Screen, Appendix A-4, is an example. These histories and the review of systems generally follow an anatomic sequence or a physiologic process and are structured for ease of adaptation and change.

The following areas require special attention because of their frequent causal relationship to liver disease.

Alcohol Consumption

Excessive and prolonged consumption of alcohol remains the leading cause of liver injury in most industrialized societies. The quantity and duration of alcohol intake have important diagnostic and prognostic implications. However, most individuals are notoriously inaccurate when answering the question, "How much alcoholic beverage do you drink?" Patients who provide the most accurate answers are the extremes—total abstainers and overt alcoholics; most other people will admit to drinking, "but not much" or "socially." "Much," i.e., the quantity, is the key word. Table 6-2 outlines the alcohol content of various beverages, and the box on p. 97 provides a relatively easy-to-remember clinical guide to toxic levels of alcohol consumption. Even an estimate of quantity and duration is useful and should be determined based on the best available historical data.

Although quantity and duration are essential factors in the development of alcohol-related liver injury, genetic predisposition is also important. A family history is essential because only 25% to 30% of 80 gm per day alcohol consumers develop serious liver disease.

Drugs/Medications

Hepatotoxicity caused by prescribed medication and illicit drugs is rapidly becoming the third most frequent cause of abnormalities in liver-test results with and

Table 6-2 Ethanol content* of alcoholic drinks

Type	Proof (percentage of ETOH)	Amount	Grams (average)
Whiskey	80-100 (40%-50%)	Per ounce	10-13
		Average drink (2 oz)	20-25
		Per quart/liter	300-400
		Fifth	250-300
Liquor	50-80 (25%-40%)	Per ounce	6-10
		Average drink (2 oz)	12-20
		Pint/½ liter	100-160
Wine	20-28 (10%-14%)	Per ounce	3-4
		Average drink (4-6 oz)	12-24
		Pint/½ liter	40-55
		Quart/liter	80-110
Beer	6-12 (3%-6%)	Per ounce	1-2
		Average drink (12-16 oz)	10-24
		Six-pack (12 oz cans)	60-150
		Quart/liter	23-49

*Expressed in ounces for clinical use and grams† for scientific reading.
†100% alcohol contains 24 gm/oz (30 ml).

CLINICALLY USEFUL GUIDE TO ESTIMATE ALCOHOL TOXICITY

"Drink" measure: 1 oz whiskey or 4 oz wine or 12 oz beer = 13 gm alcohol

One drink per day or less is nontoxic.
Between one and four drinks per day may be injurious under special circumstances (e.g., pregnancy).
Five drinks per day or more (on average) is associated with toxicity in organs, glands, and systems.*
Occurrence of serious alcoholic liver injury, especially alcoholic hepatitis, increases significantly when 80 gm or more of alcohol is consumed per day.

*Including the liver, pancreas, heart, peripheral/central nervous system, and gastrointestinal tract.

without symptoms. The multiplicity of drugs (over the counter and prescribed) enormously complicates differential diagnosis. Accurate knowledge of the drug(s) used, amount used, frequency of use, and times and dates of use is required to differentiate effectively drug hepatotoxicity from other forms of hepatotoxicity.

A simple method for initial and subsequent documentation of drug/medication use is illustrated in Appendix A-5. This chart provides a concise, ongoing, accessible record that is easily reviewed and transferred and lends itself to computerization.

Environmental and Occupational Exposure

The increase in exposure to synthetic chemicals continues to raise serious concerns about health risks. Even though serious liver injury caused by environmental toxins is uncommon (<5% in high-risk populations), incidental human exposure frequently occurs. In modern occupational health screening programs, liver-test abnormalities have been identified in 5% to 25% of "healthy" industrial workers. Even though these individuals are asymptomatic, their potential exposure to toxic material requires further medical evaluation. Accurate histories of their exposure from occupational and other sources are obviously essential. However, because viral hepatitis and alcoholism are the two major confounding factors in incidental exposure in industrialized countries, knowledge of blood products received, needles, alcohol, drugs and medications used, and life-styles greatly assists in developing the correct clinical interpretation.

PHYSICAL EXAMINATION

Physical examination findings are more easily computerized. Sample data formats for an initial physical examination and a short combined patient history and physical examination follow-up report are shown in Appendix A-6 and A-7. These particular formats are designed for the common findings of hepatobiliary disease most frequently seen in urban areas. They are easily adaptable for specific patient and disease characteristics in other locations, regions, or practices.

CLINICAL APPROACH

Presenting Symptoms

The more common symptoms with which patients with hepatobiliary disease present are listed in Table 6-1. These symptoms may present themselves individually or in combination with others, or they may be the most prominent among many symptoms. The following symptoms are discussed in the approximate order of their occurrence.

Fatigue, lassitude, and listlessness. Fatigue and its sister symptoms, including tiredness, lack of energy, and malaise, are the most frequent (>80%)* and abstruse symptoms of liver disease (LD). These symptoms are clearly related to the LD even though the exact mechanism causing them is unknown. Recovery from the liver illness is associated with disappearance of these symptoms, and recurrence or exacerbation of the illness causes these symptoms to reappear or worsen. In acute liver disease, e.g., acute viral hepatitis, these symptoms precede the clinical manifestation (jaundice) and follow the biochemical parameter (enzyme elevations). In chronic disease these symptoms are more correlated with the synthetic function of the liver (albumin, prothrombin, and cholesterol levels) and the severity of its architectural distortion (micronodular > macronodular).

However, the illnesses of many patients with liver disorders who complain of chronic fatigue or lassitude have psychologic and psychiatric components. Because of the subjective nature of these symptoms, the physician is often uncertain whether their origin is psychic or organic. Table 6-3 summarizes the characteristics that differentiate liver disease–induced symptoms from psyche-related causes.

Abdominal pain. Up to 70% of patients with clinical or subclinical hepatobiliary disease complain of abdominal

*Percentage represents an approximate numeric frequency of occurrence in patients with hepatobiliary disorders.

Table 6-3 Hepatic vs. nonhepatic characteristics of fatigue/lassitude

	Chronic liver disease	Psychic disorders
First appearance	Gradual or acute with disease onset	After an unpleasant event, grief reaction, medical/surgical illness
As day wears on	Worsens	Improves
Relation to activity	All physical types	More to some than others
Related to degree of organ injury	Yes	No
Improved by physical rest	Yes	Usually not
Interferes with mental activities	Only with encephalopathy	Yes
Impaired sleep	Reversed sleeping pattern (sleepless nights, naps during day)	Rest provides neither sleep nor relief
Highest spirit and energy	Best in morning	Worse in morning
Associated disorders	Anemia Nutritional deficiency Metabolic disorders Musculoskeletal disease Neurologic disease	Usually no objective evidence of disease or associated disorders

pain, especially in the right upper quadrant (RUQ), right flank, and/or epigastric area. Complaints of left upper quadrant (LUQ) and lower abdominal pain occur less often (in approximately 20% of patients). Abdominal pain is conveyed by two nervous system pathways. The visceral pathways (visceral afferent fibers of sympathetic nerves) are sensitive to stretch and spasm and insensitive to nerve section or temperature. The somatic pathways (somatic fibers of sympathetic nerves), which innervate abdominal cavity walls, parietal peritoneum, and mesenteric and peripheral parts of the diaphragm, are sensitive to pressure, tension, traction, toxins (chemical and bacterial), enzymes, infiltrative processes, and edema. The central parts of the diaphragm and biliary tract have axon fibers that accompany the phrenic nerve and are responsible for referred pain in the shoulder area.

The causes of abdominal pain in patients with hepatobiliary disease are similar to the causes of such pain in individuals without hepatic disease. Table 6-4 lists the more common sources of abdominal pain by anatomic location and their common clinical characteristics. The asterisk

Table 6-4 Differential characteristics of common causes of abdominal pain

Anatomic location†	Temporal pattern‡	Prevalent characteristic	Probable etiology
Upper quadrants			
RUQ	Recurrent attacks	Nocturnal	Duodenal (peptic) ulcer
RUQ (subcostal)	Periodic episodes	Radiates to shoulder	granulomatous bowel (GB) disease*
RUQ	Continuous	Organ tenderness	Liver enlargement*
Epigastric	Recurrent attacks	Worse when supine	Reflux disease
LUQ	Continuous	Local tenderness with pressure	Splenic enlargement*
Supraumbilical	Recurrent attacks	Increases with food, radiates to back	Pancreatitis*
Supraumbilical	Continuous	Radiates to back	Pancreatic cancer
Supraumbilical	Recurrent	Exacerbated by food	Gastritis ulcer
Supraumbilical	Continuous	Early satiety	Gastric cancer
Diffuse	Continuous	Rebound tenderness	Abdominal peritonitis*
Diffuse	Periodic episodes	Nonspecific	Metabolic (porphyria)*
Lower quadrants			
RLQ	Periodic episodes	Bloating	Crohn's disease
Changing	Recurrent attacks	Lifelong, crampy with loose stool	Irritable bowel*
LLQ	Periodic episodes	Fever, chills, peritoneal signs	Diverticulitis
Periumbilical	Continuous	Abdominal distention	Small bowel ileus/obstruction*
Periumbilical	Recurrent attacks	No distention Occurs in older adults	Small bowel ischemia
Nonspecific	Continuous	Positive hemoccult Pencil-like stool	Colorectal cancer

*More frequent in patients with hepatobiliary disease.
†RLQ = Right lower quadrant
LLQ = Left lower quadrant
‡"Continuous" = Pain that remains constant from inception.
"Recurrent attacks" = Pain episodes of hours or a few days, frequent unpredictable recurrence.
"Periodic episodes" = Pain episodes of prolonged time (days) with interspersed long (months) asymptomatic periods.

identifies those causes more frequently occurring with hepatobiliary disease; these causes are given further comment.

Intestinal pain. The most common cause (>80%) of chronic or recurrent abdominal pain is bowel related. Pain in the right upper quadrant, right flank, and right subcostal region is frequently due to large bowel (hepatic flexure) distention or small bowel ileus with spasm or cramp caused by disordered motility. Pain in the left upper quadrant is similarly caused by colon distention in the splenic flexure area. Colonic pain is usually central and infraumbilical. Small bowel pain is paraumbilical, and very low abdominal or suprapubic pain is more likely of urinary bladder or rectal origin.

Liver pain. Liver pain or tenderness in the right upper quadrant is due to liver (Glisson) capsule distention because the liver's capsule, but not the parenchyma, has pain receptors. Rapid increases in organ size caused by inflammation (e.g., viral or alcoholic hepatitis) or a tumor are the most common (>70%) causes of liver pain. In chronic liver disease, in which the liver is small, scarred, and shrunken, hepatic capsular distention is rarely the cause of RUQ pain.

Biliary system pain. Although gallbladder pain is located in the epigastric or RUQ, spasms of the biliary tract can radiate to the right shoulder and subscapular area. Inflammation of the gallbladder walls with contact to the parietal peritoneum can cause localized subcostal pain with both point (visceral) and rebound (peritoneal) pain.

Asymptomatic gallstones are commonly associated with chronic liver disease. Often, nonspecific abdominal complaints or biochemical liver test abnormalities lead to ultrasound or x-ray evaluation with the incidental discovery of gallstones or nonvisualization of the gallbladder. More often than not in these cases, the gallstones are due to the liver disease and secondary changes in hepatic cholesterol and bile acid secretions and are not the cause of the abdominal complaints or the abnormal liver tests.

Pancreatic pain. Pancreatic disease is frequently associated with alcoholic and viral liver disease. As a retroperitoneal organ, the pancreas stimulates somatic nerve endings, causing severe pain that radiates to lateral quadrants, back and left shoulder, often going through to the back. It is made worse by lying down and improved by bending forward or lying in a knee-to-chest position. Even though chronic alcohol consumption and biliary tract calculi are the most common causes (>95%), trauma, lipid disorders (i.e., Zieve syndrome), family history, and elevated calcium should be checked or tested for. Nondescript abdominal pain caused by subclinical pancreatitis, which can occur without nausea and vomiting, can be identified by an elevated serum amylase and/or lipase level.

Porphyria-induced pain. Probably the most frequently missed causes of abdominal pain are the porphyrias. Porphyria causes nonspecific coliclike abdominal pain, which is somatic and is difficult to differentiate from pain of biliary tract, gallbladder, and pancreatic origins. Patients experiencing chronic or recurrent abdominal pain without accountable cause should always have urinary porphyrins checked during acute pain.

Splenic pain. Spleen-related pain occurs only with splenic enlargement (99%) or infarctions (1%). This pain is usually due to splenic congestion and distention and occurs mainly in the LUQ. In such

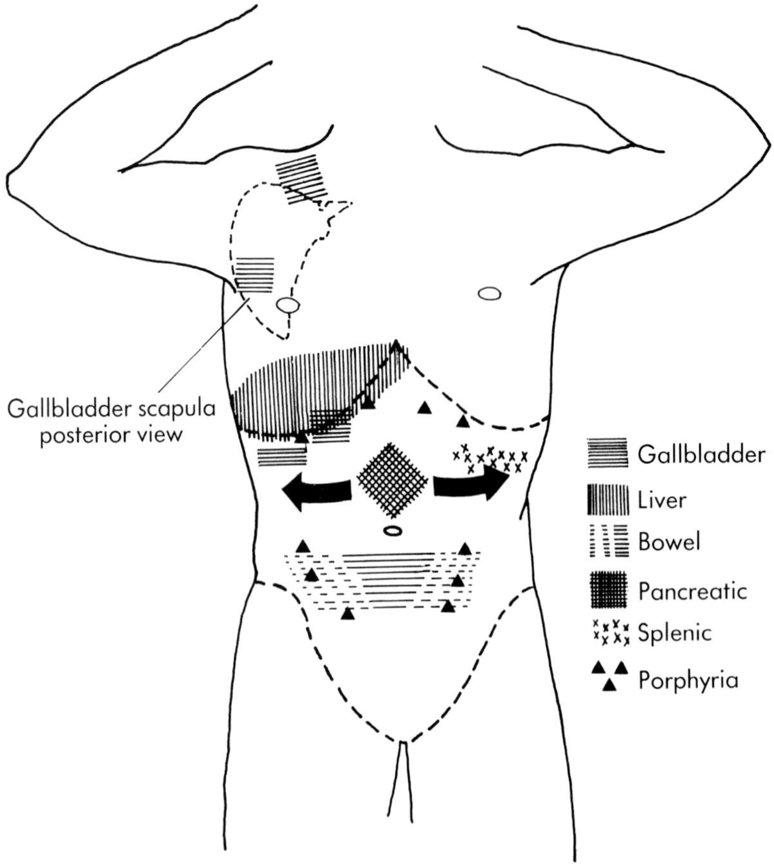

Figure 6-1
Characteristic location of abdominal pain from various causes.

cases palpation of the LUQ while the patient takes a deep inspiration will elicit left subcostal pain and tenderness.

Figure 6-1 illustrates the common locations of the hepatobiliary related pains described above.

Special note post–liver biopsy pain. Pain is frequently encountered after liver biopsy. Initially, it occurs in the epigastric region or involves pain referred to the right shoulder and the neck. This is believed to be reflex gastrointestinal (GI) or biliary tract spasm, respectively. Pleuritic RUQ pain, which develops later (within hours or the next day), most likely is due to blood irritating the peritoneal pleura and diaphragm. In contrast, severe RUQ pain with rebound tenderness immediately after the biopsy is usually due to leakage of bile from puncture of the gallbladder.

Enlargement of abdominal girth (abdominal swelling). Progressive distention, swelling, or enlargement of the abdominal cavity is the first manifestation of latent liver disease for 5% to 10% of patients. Patients relate a need to wear looser or larger garments or to let out their belts by a notch or two. The abdominal distention is more prominent after meals, is related to the amount of food ingested, and is not relieved by the expulsion of gas or feces, belching, or vomiting.

The most frequent (90%) cause of abdominal swelling is fluid accumulation (ascites). This type of abdominal swelling is almost always (98%) associated with a gain in weight. Lower extremity edema or decreased frequency of urination appears in 40% and 10% of patients, respectively. Other causes of abdominal swelling are intestinal distention, paralytic ileus, aerophagia-induced gastric dilatation, and reflux ileus associated with biliary colic. Only 5% to 10% of abdominal swelling is secondary to solid organ enlargement (liver and/or spleen). Very rarely (<1%) abdominal aneurysms manifest themselves as abdominal fullness and are identified by the presence of a bruit or pulsations. In the female patient a careful gynecologic history, especially the date of the last menstrual period, is an absolute necessity because such swelling can be due to pregnancy or tumor(s) of pelvic organs.

Yellow eyes/jaundice. Although jaundice is not a symptom of hepatobiliary disease, it is not uncommon for the patient to first seek medical attention after noticing skin or eye (sclerae) discoloration before symptoms become troubling. The historical characteristics of the different common causes of jaundice are shown in Table 6-5. Changes in the color of urine and/or feces are sometimes noticed before clinical jaundice. Early darkening of urine is characteristically seen in patients with viral and drug hepatitis.

Pruritus. Itching is a distinct and very disagreeable cutaneous dysesthesia that characteristically occurs in patients with acute or severe intrahepatic and extrahepatic obstruction. It is anatomically diffuse, may be intermittent, typically interferes with sleep, and is associated with mild to severe excoriations. In cholestatic jaundice, the itching is associated in some patients with excessive bile acid content in the skin. Vasodilation caused by heat and sweating exacerbates this form of pruritus, and cold relieves it. All forms of hepatic cholestasis may be associated with pruritus. In PBC and primary sclerosing cholangitis, pruritus often precedes clinical jaundice.

Weight change. Complaints of an unintentional body weight gain or loss of more than 5 kg (10 lbs) or 10% of usual body weight within 3 to 6 months should be considered abnormal. This degree of weight change exceeds the normal week-to-week or month-to-month weight variation. In hepatobiliary disease such weight changes are mainly caused by accumulation of fluid or body fat and/or muscle wasting. Therefore inquiries into the patient's nutritional history, GI symptomatology, chronic or recurrent infections (e.g., viral, bacterial, fungal, or parasitic), drug/alcohol abuse, and/or other symptoms or signs of latent malignancy and extrahepatic disorders involving the pancreas and GI tract (often associated with the same etiologic agents, e.g., viruses, alcohol, or drugs) are warranted.

Anorexia. Loss of the desire to eat is a common (>80%) accompaniment of acute liver injury (e.g., viral) and a universal one with advanced or end-stage active liver disease. The patient either

Table 6-5 Differential characteristics of the common types of jaundice by history

	Acute viral hepatitis	Cholestatic drug jaundice	Common bile duct gallstones	Carcinoma, ampullary region	Chronic viral hepatitis	Chronic alcoholic hepatitis	PBC PSC*
History							
Antecedent history	Contacts, injections, transfusions, unknown	Taking a drug	Dyspepsia, previous attack	None	Transfusion, injection, contact, unknown	Drank alcohol	None
Pain	None or ache over liver	None	Constant, epigastric biliary colic or none	Constant, epigastric, back, or none	None RUQ soreness	Usually none	None
Pruritus	Transient	Can occur	Occurs	Occurs	Can occur	Can occur	Occurs characteristically or frequently†
Itching develops	Rapidly	Rapidly	Slowly	Slowly	Gradually	Slowly	Gradually
Type of jaundice	Rapid onset, slow fall with recovery	Variable, usually mild	Fluctuating or persistent	Usually but not always progressive	Progressive	Progressive, very slow recovery	Progressive
Weight loss	Slight	Slight	Slight to moderate	Progressive	Slight	Progressive	Slow, progressive
Feces color	Variable, light or dark	Pale	Intermittently pale	Alcoholic	Lighter	Lighter to pale	Lighter to alcoholic

*PSC = Primary sclerosing cholangitis. PBC = Primary biliary cirrhosis.
†Pruritus is characteristic only in the late stages of PBC although it can be a presenting symptom in earlier stages.

avoids eating or finds eating a tasteless activity. Associated weight loss occurs with all serious hepatic-related anorexia. The sudden onset of anorexia in a cirrhotic patient who previously enjoyed eating frequently heralds developing hepatocellular carcinoma.

Nausea. Although closely associated with vomiting, there are conditions in which nausea is present in the absence of vomiting. This is common (60% to 70%) in acute liver disease, especially of viral and alcoholic origins. Medications dependent on hepatic metabolism occasionally (2% to 5%) are associated with nausea. Chronic nausea is occasionally reported by patients with advanced liver disease and chronic obstructive lung disease (smoking-induced). The nausea is resistant to treatment and is believed to be related to medications for bronchodilation. Neither the mechanism causing nausea nor its etiology is clearly understood.

Vomiting. Vomiting is usually associated with prior nausea and is most commonly (>70%) seen in association with acute hepatitis, cholecystitis, and biliary colic. In chronic liver disease, the more frequent underlying causes (>70%) include upper GI bleeding from rupture of varices and excessive alcohol ingestion and as a side effect of certain medications.

Hematemesis. Vomiting of blood is a result of hemorrhage in the upper GI tract (proximal to the ligament of Treitz). Ninety percent of hematemesis in patients with hepatic disease is caused by alcoholic gastritis; rupture of esophageal varices; use of drugs, such as aspirin, indomethacin, and nonsteroidal anti-inflammatory drugs (NSAIDs); Mallory-Weiss tears; and reflux gastritis. In advanced stages of liver disease, blood dyscrasias secondary to hepatic clotting and platelet abnormalities contribute (5% to 10%) to spontaneous hemorrhages.

Melena. Darkening of the stool color, or melena (coal black, sticky, and smelly stool), indicates bleeding from anywhere in the GI tract. Although the classic view is that the melena is caused by blood exposed to gastric acid, it is more likely due to prolonged transit time and bacterial action on the red blood cells. In hepatobiliary disease the most common causes of melena (>95%), in descending order, are gastritis (alcohol/drug), esophageal varices, peptic ulcer, and Mallory-Weiss tears. Less common (<5%) but serious causes include colonic polyps, telangiectasias, colonic varices, and epistaxis.

Hematochezia. Bright-red blood covering the stool is likely to be from the lower segment of the GI tract (rectal area) or anus. In chronic liver disease the presence of blood in or covering the stool, on the toilet paper, or on garments is most often a manifestation of hemorrhoidal bleeding caused by increased portal pressure and/or coagulation disorders associated with chronic liver disease. Brisk bleeding in the small intestine or from higher colonic lesion, e.g., polyps, tumor, and angiodysplasia, can also produce this symptom and must be excluded.

Diarrhea. The frequent or intermittent passage of watery stool in patients with hepatobiliary disease occurs more often in up to 25% of patients than it is reported. It is caused by varied mechanisms. Osmotic diarrhea is caused by large amounts of poorly absorbable, osmotically active substances that retard water and electrolyte absorption, e.g., lactulose. Altered motility caused by delayed intestinal transit promotes stasis of fluid and food contents in the gut lumen and allows overgrowth of intestinal bacteria, which deconjugate bile. These unconjugated bile acids may lead to impairment of micelle formation, inhibit intestinal mucosal absorptive processes, and contribute to poorly formed, diarrhealike stools in larger volumes.

In contrast, classic steatorrhea is uncommon in chronic liver disease, even in the presence of pancreatic disease. However, the loss of bile acids (e.g., in PBC, PSC, and alcoholic hepatitis) can impair micelle formation in the duodenum, causing increased fatty acids in the colon, increased fecal water, and a chronic low-grade diarrhea.

Constipation. A decreased frequency of defecation or the passage of excessively hard or dry stool may precipitate hepatic encephalopathy in cirrhotic patients. Patients often complain of lower abdominal discomfort, distention, and flatulence. This is most likely related to a blunted defecation reflex or ineffective propulsive motility of the colon caused by the use of certain drugs, such as anticholinergics, antacids containing aluminum or calcium and analgesics (e.g., codeine).

Fever. Fever occurs in both the acute and the chronic stages of hepatobiliary disease. In acute stages, viral hepatitis, cholecystitis, secondary hepatic microabscesses, and intermittent obstruction with ascending cholangitis (Charcot's biliary fever) should be excluded. In chronic stages, alcoholic hepatitis, granulomatous and tuberculous infections, pyogenic abscesses, and primary hepatocellular carcinoma with necrosis account for more than 75% of the causes.

Epistaxis. Nasal bleeding frequently occurs with chronic liver disease because of focal (dryness, irritation, and nose blowing, wiping, and picking) or systemic factors (clotting defects caused by platelet dysfunction, decreased clotting factor production, or a cofactor deficiency, e.g., vitamin K. Occasionally (<2%) epistaxis can be a serious source of blood loss.

Impotence. Loss of libido and/or erectile dysfunction are frequent complaints (40% to 60%) in men with moderate to advanced LD. When associated with alcohol or drug abuse, the etiology is related more to the individual's general health and psychosexual problems than liver injury. Cessation of alcohol and drugs is more important than replacement hormonal therapy.

Abnormal menses. Cessation of menses or abnormal menses is found early in women with developing chronic liver disease. It is a more prominent feature in alcohol-related liver disease. Abnormal findings of plasma estradiol−17, follicle-stimulating hormone (FSH), and leutinizing hormone (LH) are associated with this symptom.

Presenting Signs

The most commonly occurring signs of hepatobiliary disease are listed in Table 6-1. In the early stages of liver disease, few if any of these physical findings are identifiable. As liver disease progresses, an increased number of signs develop. If looked for carefully, one or more of these common signs can be discovered in more than 75% of patients with histologic cirrhosis. The following signs are discussed in the approximate order of their occurrence.

Jaundice (icterus). Jaundice, or yellow eyes, is most easily detected by examination of the conjunctivae of the eyes in natural daylight. Mild icterus is frequently (15% to 20%) overlooked in artificial light. Conjugated bilirubin is clinically detectable at levels of 2 to 3 mg/dl because of its water solubility. Free or unconjugated bilirubin, which is more lipid soluble, less readily stains skin or elastic tissue and becomes clinically apparent at 3 to 4 mg/dl. Bilirubin's affinity for tissue accounts for the disparity between the depth of the skin jaundice and serum bilirubin levels during the stages of recovery, i.e., skin pigmentation remains after serum levels return to normal.

Dark- or black-skinned individuals often have increased melanin pigmentation in their conjunctivae that may simulate jaundice. This confusion can be avoided by examining the mucosal undersurface of the tongue for jaundice because the sublingual mucosa is not affected by subconjunctival fat or conjunctival pigment. This examination is done by having the patient touch the roof of the mouth with the tip of the tongue while the physician examines the mucosal undersurface. Fluorescent lighting decreases one's ability to identify the milder degrees of jaundice, so examination is best done in daylight.

A patient with a normal bilirubin level may appear icteric because of pallor, subconjunctival fat (5% to 10%), or, rarely, carotene or carotenoid pigments, Atabrine, picric acid, acriflavine, or fluorescein (0.5%) medications. These rare cases of increased skin pigmentation can be differentiated by examination of palms and soles. Carotenoid pigments, drugs, and chemicals cause generalized increased pigmentation of the palms and soles, as well as the dorsum of the arms, hands, and feet while having little or no effect on the scleral color. The urine foam test can confirm the presence of carotenoid pigments. To perform this test, collect urine in a transparent container and shake until foam is formed. White foam is concentrated or has pigment of another source. Yellow foam identifies bile pigments. Hemolysis and blood loss should also be considered in patients with hepatic disease who present with both pallor and icterus.

Complaints of darkening urine in individuals with chronic liver disease can be mistakenly attributed to bile pigments, but the cause can be verified by using the urine foam test. In acute disease, e.g., acute viral hepatitis or an early obstructive lesion, this procedure is useful because bile pigments appear in the urine before they occur in the skin or the mucosal membranes.

The differential physical characteristics of the common causes of jaundice are shown in Table 6-6.

Edema. A common manifestation of chronic liver disease is excess interstitial body fluid. Edema can occur in severe acute injury as the liver goes into failure. The earliest indication of edema development is unexplained weight gain, even in the absence of "swelling."

Any detectable edema is abnormal and pathologic. It most often manifests itself as swelling, either locally (e.g., in the abdomen), multicentrically (e.g., in the feet or ankles), diffuse (e.g., in the arms, legs, and abdomen), or radiologically, as unilateral or bilateral pleural effusion (R > L, Figure 6-2). There are three major physiologic mechanisms for edema formation: (1) elevated hydrostatic portal systemic pressure, (2) reduced oncotic (colloid osmotic) pressure, and (3) impaired lymphatic flow. Reduced colloid osmotic pressure (low albumin) and expanded plasma volume (sodium and water retention) are the major factors. Urine sodium levels are less than 10 mEq/L, serum so-

Table 6-6 Differential characteristics of the common types of jaundice by physical examination

	Acute viral hepatitis	**Cholestatic drug jaundice**	**Common bile duct gallstones**	**Carcinoma, ampullary region**	**Chronic viral hepatitis**	**Chronic alcoholic hepatitis**	**PBC PSC**
Findings							
Diathesis	Young, usually <35 years old	Often female, psychiatric patient	Frequently female, obese	>40 years old	Older, usually >35 years old	Mostly male (5:1)	PBC: mostly women (7:1) PSC: mostly men (5:1)
Depth of jaundice	Variable	Variable, rash sometimes	Moderate	Deep	Mild to severe	Mild to deep	Mild to severe
Ascites	If severe and prolonged	None	None	Rarely with metastases	Occurs	Occurs frequently	Occurs
Liver	Enlarged and tender	Slightly enlarged	Enlarged, slightly tender	Enlarged, not tender	Normal or small	Enlarged or small	Normal or small
Palpable gallbladder	None	None	None	Can occur	None	None	None
Tender gallbladder	None	None	Can occur	None	None	None	None
Enlarged gallbladder	About 20%	None	None	Occasionally	Can occur	Can occur	Can occur
Fever	Onset only	Onset	Frequent	Not usually	None	Low grade, common	None

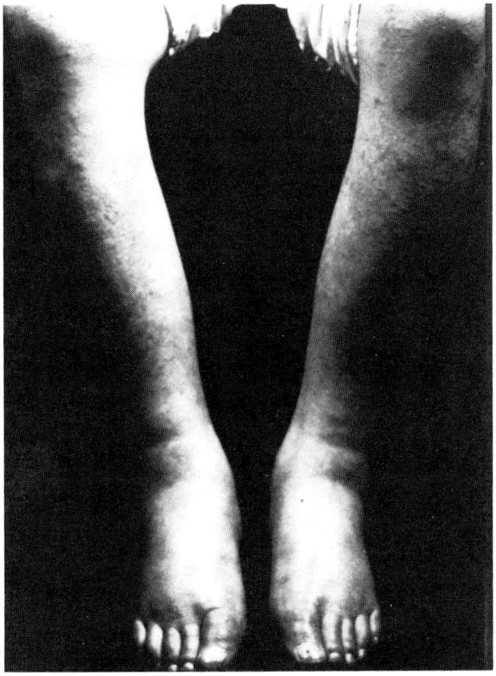

Figure 6-2
Typical peripheral edema in cirrhotic patient.

dium levels are low or decreased, and plasma osmolality is decreased.

Differential clinical characteristics of hepatic vs. nonhepatic edema are outlined in Table 6-7.

Abdominal findings

Ascites. Increased abdominal fluid is more difficult to ascertain when confounding conditions are present (e.g., obesity or exaggerated spinal lordosis). Significant intra-abdominal fluid accumulations (>2 L) can change the external contour of the abdomen. When the patient is in the upright position, fluids migrate to the lower abdomen, causing lower abdominal protuberance; in the su-

Table 6-7 Clinical Differentiation of Hepatic vs. Non-Hepatic Edema

Hepatic	Nonhepatic (e.g., heart, kidney, nutritional)	Metabolic (e.g., hyperthyroidism, hyperaldosteronism)	
First Manifestation	Abdomen Ankles Feet Pleural space	Feet	Eyelids,(peri-orbital) Pretibial area
Postural dependency	Yes	Yes	No
Progression	Remains local	Progresses feet upward with increasing severity	None
Lower-extremity discoloration	None	Yes, bluish (vascular)	None
Pigmentation	Lower extremity (status dermatitis)	Lower Extremity (status dermatitis)	Diffuse if present*
Serum albumin	Low	Normal	Normal
Urine Na	Low	Low/Increased	Normal/Increased

*Except with heart or kidney failure.

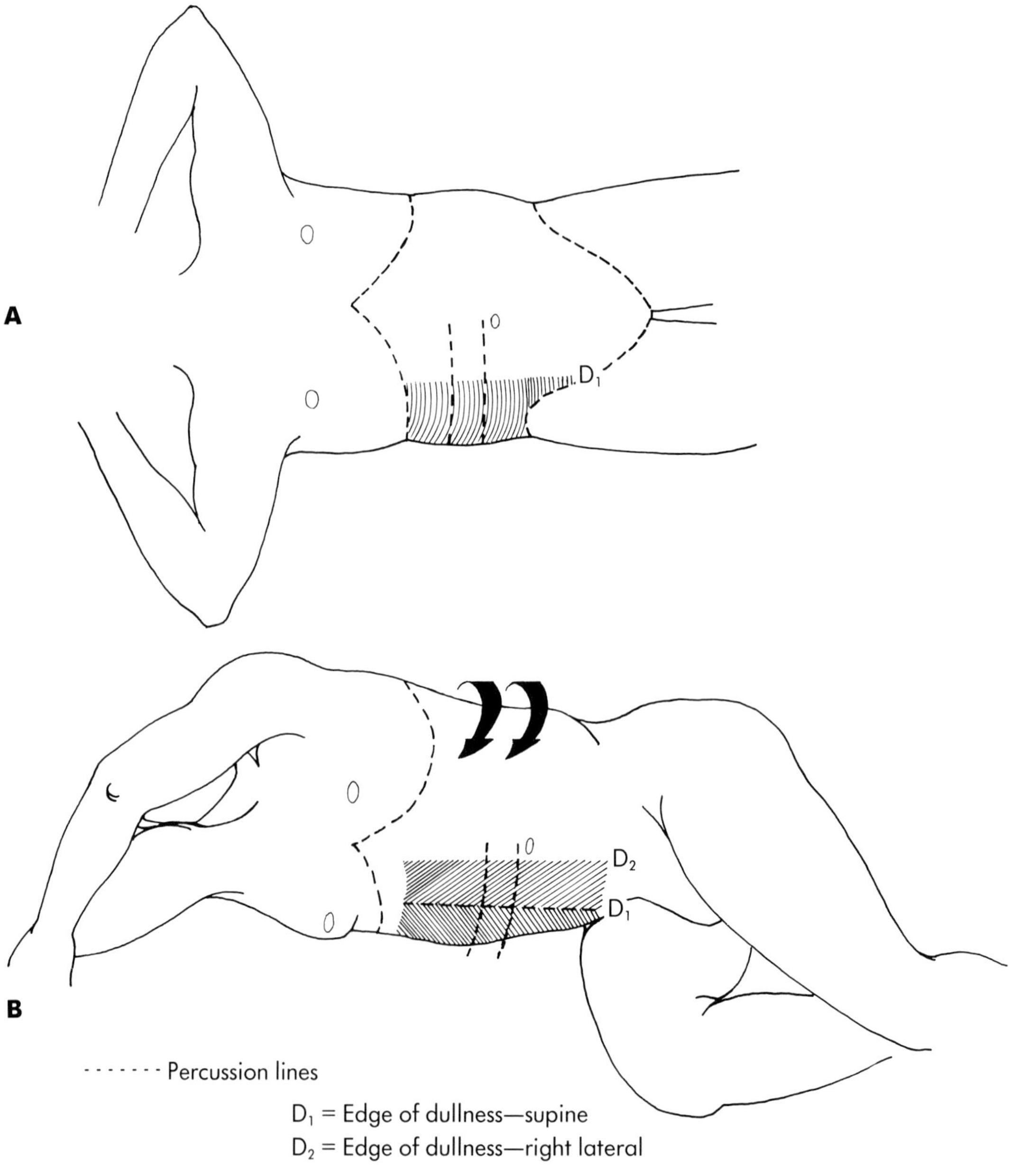

Figure 6-3
Characteristic location of abdominal dullness in patient with ascites **(A)** in supine position, **(B)** in lateral position.

pine position, fluid migration causes bulging flanks.

The two standard methods for detecting abdominal fluid during physical examination are described below.

1. "Shifting dullness": Abdominal percussion with the patient in supine position. This action elicits dullness in the lower half of the flanks (Figure 6-3, *A*), which shift when patient is rolled to a lateral position. Dullness is now detected in the dependent side of the abdomen, and tympany is present in the superior side (Figure 6-3, *B*). When patient is returned to supine position, dullness returns to the flank areas, thus "shifting dullness."

2. "Fluid wave": Abdominal palpation with the patient in supine position. The patient indents the midabdomen with a hand (Figure 6-4, *A*) while the examiner taps on the flank and palpates the opposite flank for the pulsation of the fluid wave (Figure 6-4, *B,* see insert).

A third technique is "ballottement" of the liver or spleen. When a palpable organ is pushed downward by a thrust of the hand, the organ will float back up and bump the hand, held in place on the abdominal wall because of the fluid-filled

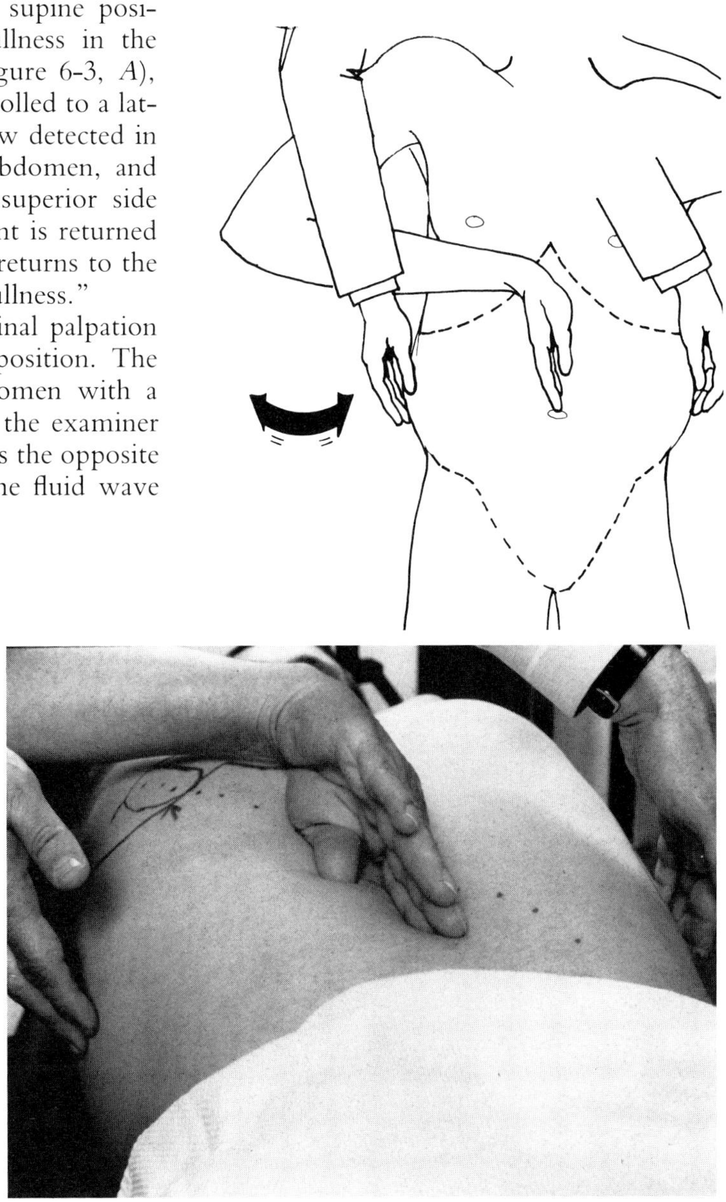

A

B

Figure 6-4
(A) "Fluid wave" technique illustrated, **(B)** Demonstration of a "fluid wave" in patient with ascites.

abdomen. The percussion method is most sensitive but can be misleading in overweight individuals. The fluid wave technique requires another person's assistance and is less sensitive. Ballottement is least sensitive (seen only in large amounts of ascites) but most accurate.

Liver enlargement. Depending on the body habitus (Figure 6-5), the lower edge of a normal liver can be palpated 1 to 3 cm below the right costal margin in the midclavicular line (lateral to the right rectus muscle). A normal liver may be displaced downward by a low diaphragm, emphysema, or kyphosis of the spine. The box below lists the most common

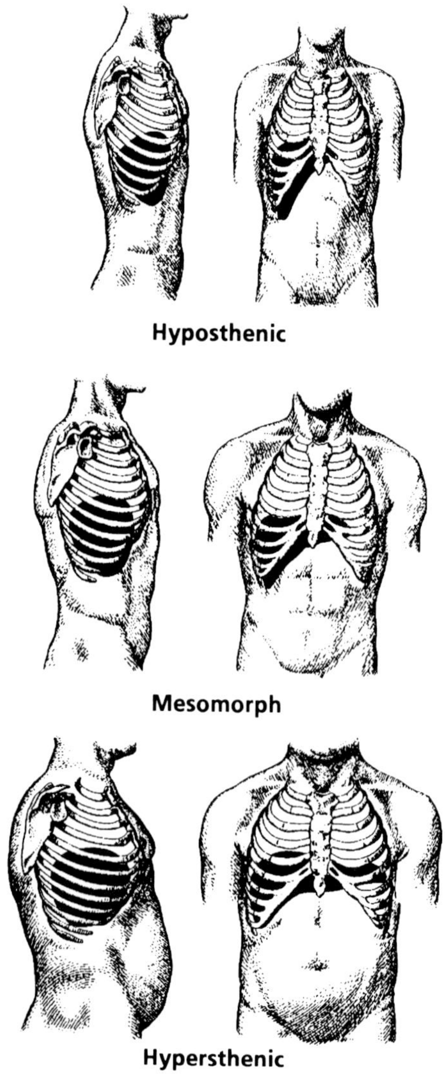

Figure 6-5
Body habitus and the liver. Anterior and lateral views of the position of the liver in persons with different body configurations. (From Leevy CM: Evaluation of liver function in clinical practice, ed 2, Indianapolis, 1974, The Lilly Research Laboratories.)

CAUSES OF CLINICAL DETECTABLE CHANGES IN HEPATIC SIZE

Excessive enlargement (to umbilicus or below)

Metastatic malignant masses
Polycystic liver disease
Hodgkin's disease (leukemic infiltration)
Amyloidosis
Severe chronic congestive heart failure
Severe fatty metamorphosis of liver
Constrictive pericarditis
Hepatic vein thrombosis

Rapid enlargement (hours to days)

Acute congestive heart failure
Acute cholestatic jaundice
Severe uncontrolled diabetes
Acute alcoholic steatosis

Progressive reduction (small) in size

Chronic active disease (all forms)
End-state cirrhosis (all forms)

Rapid reduction in size

Fulminant hepatic necrosis (all forms)

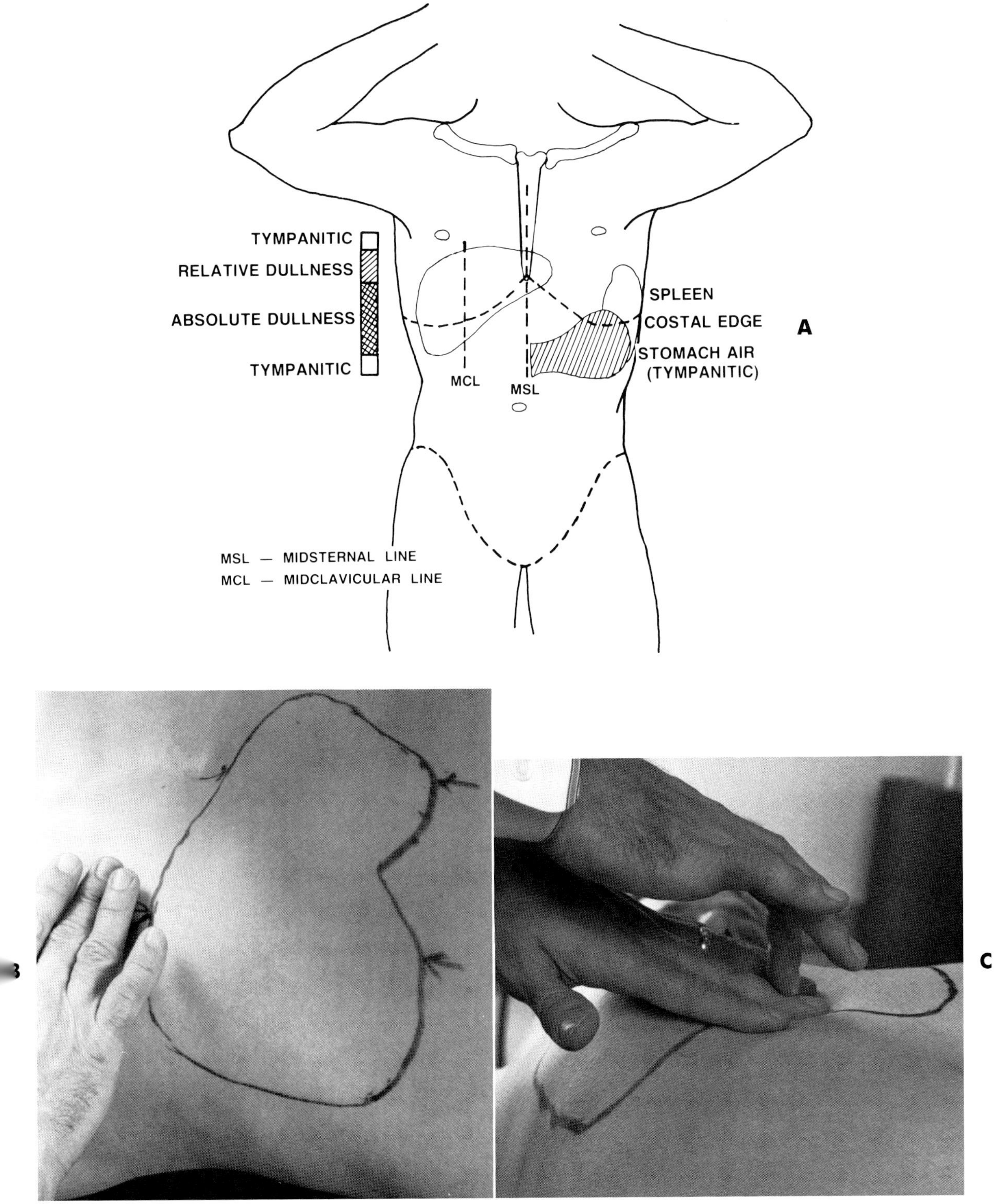

Figure 6-6
(A) Clinical determination of liver size by percussion. **(B)** Examination technique: one-handed method, **(C)** Examination technique: using two-handed method.

causes of marked liver enlargement and rapid changes in liver size. Preferential enlargement of the left or caudal lobe is seen in cirrhotic patients with focal nodular regeneration and in patients with Budd-Chiari syndrome. A pulsating liver is rare but has been reported with intrahepatic aneurysms and marked tricuspid valve regurgitation.

The most accurate clinical manner for determining liver size is percussion. Physical examination of the liver is conducted with the patient in the recumbent position with head and lower extremities in the same plane. The span of liver dullness is estimated by percussion during quiet breathing in both the right midclavicular line (MCL) and the midsternal line (MSL, Figure 6-6, *A*). The MCL is a perpendicular line from the middle of the right clavicle and is usually slightly medial to the nipple line. The MSL is at the xiphoid process. Percussion of the upper border of liver dullness, in the MCL, is begun at the lung resonance downward toward the liver (Figure 6-6, *B*, see arrows). The beginning of relative dullness (beginning change in resonance) is considered to be the dome of the right lobe.

The lower edge of the liver may be determined by either palpation or percussion. Percussion is started at a level below the umbilicus, percussing upward in the MCL (Figure 6-6, *C*). Palpation can be used for confirmation and determination of the liver texture. The distance (in centimeters) from the upper border of relative dullness to the lower edge of dullness, or palpation, is the midclavicular length of liver (i.e., right lobe measurement).

The MSL measurement is obtained in similar fashion of percussion in the midline and constitutes the midsternal measurement (i.e., left lobe measurement). The upper border of the MSL is determined when absolute dullness is reached because of the heart's location.

NOTE: Measure the width of your hand at the proximal interphalangeal (PIP) joints and the width of each finger (usually 1.5 to 2 cm). This measurement provides the examiner with a permanent ruler accurate within 2 cm (Figure 6-7, *A*). Description of hepatic size as fingerbreadths

A

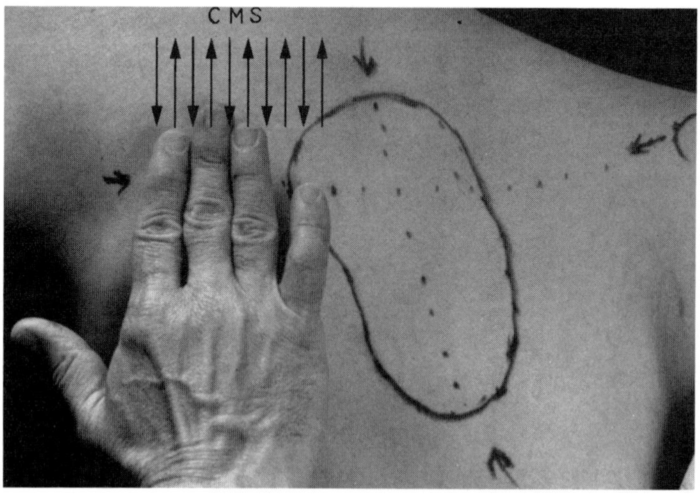

Figure 6-7
(A) Clinical hand measurement of organ size and top view of one-handed percussion technique.

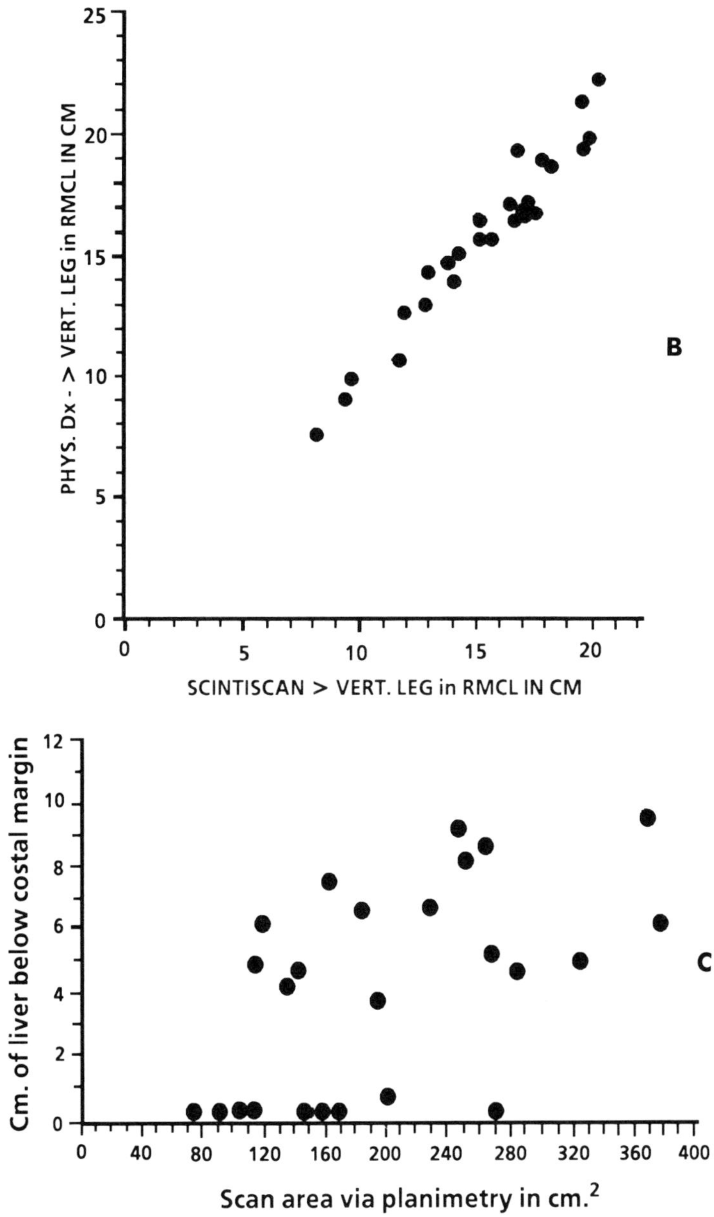

Figure 6-7, cont'd.
(B) Lack of correlation of liver projection below thoracic cage as determined by physical examination and anterior surface projection established by photoscans, **(C)** Correlation of linear surface projection as determined by means of physical examination and photoscans. (From Leevy CM: Evaluation of liver function in clinical practice, ed 2, Indianapolis, 1974, The Lilly Research Laboratories.)

below the right costal margin is inaccurate and should not be used (Figures 6-7, *B* and 6-7, *C* and box on p. 117).

A friction rub over the liver may be palpable or audible. The most common causes of a friction rub are excessive bleeding after a liver biopsy, a surface tumor, perihepatitis, or intrahepatic abscess. An audible murmur over the liver usually indicates a primary hepatocellular carcinoma, arteriovenous (A-V) malformation, or severe alcoholic hepatitis. A venous hum of portal hypertension is best heard in the MSL between the xiphoid and the umbilicus.

Spleen enlargement. A normal spleen is rarely (<1%) palpable in an adult, even with deep inspiration (exception: very short, thin individuals or adolescents). It is the body's largest "lymph node," situ-

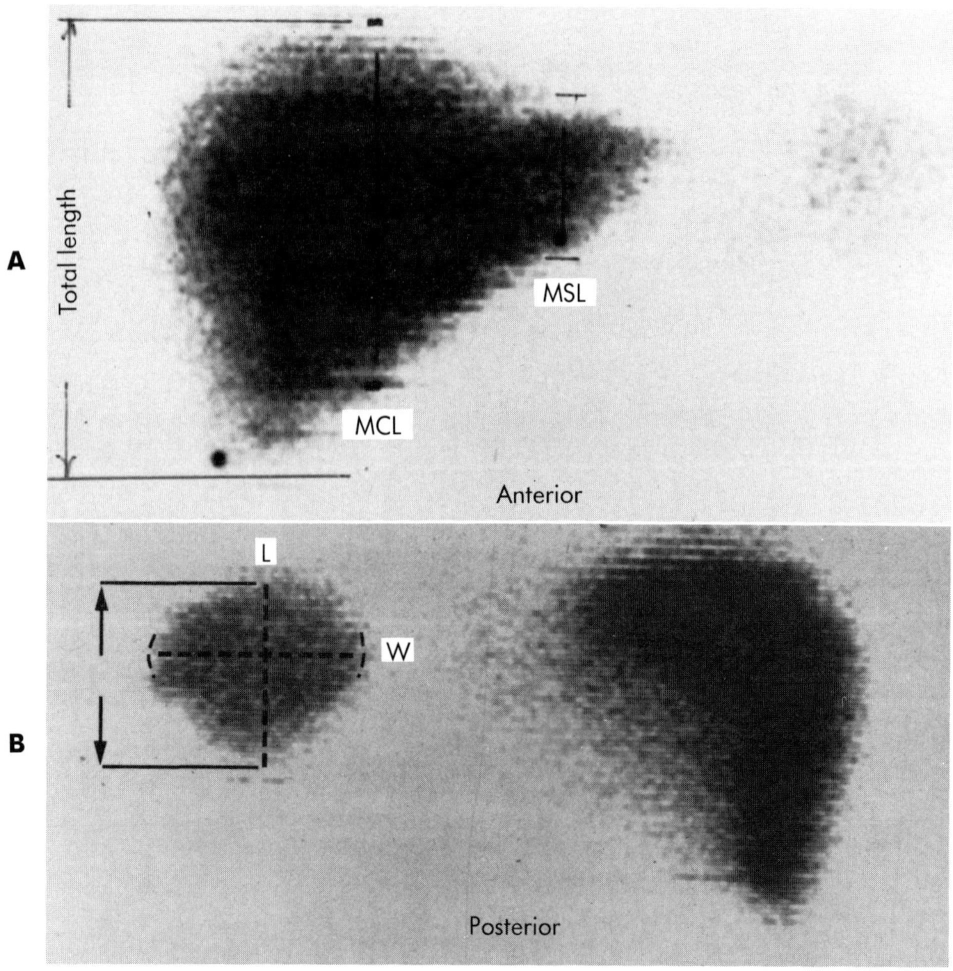

Figure 6-8
(A) Determination of hepatic size from radioisotopic scan, anterior view, **(B)** Determination of spleen size from radioisotopic scan, posterior view.

METHOD OF DETERMINING LIVER SIZE FROM SCAN

Liver-scan measurement at the MCL is obtained by drawing a vertical line from the uppermost border to the lowermost border of radioactivity at a point midway between the anterior axillary, or outer rib cage marker, and the midsternal, or xiphoid process marker. The length of the MSL is obtained by measuring the length of line drawn from the uppermost border to the lowermost border of radioactivity in MSL at the xiphoid process (Figure 6-8, *A* and 6-8, *B*).

ated in the posterior aspect of the left upper abdomen behind the stomach and covered by the diaphragm. To palpate the spleen, the patient should be lying face up with knees flexed. The examiner should begin at the left lower abdomen and palpate upward just below the costal margin using the fingers in a cupped manner while the patient takes deep inspirations with mouth open (Figure 6-9, *A*). Bimanual palpation of the spleen can be done with the patient turned slightly toward the examiner and using the examiner's left hand to exert pressure upward in the patient's left flank while palpating for the spleen edge, using the right-handed method as indicated above.

Following are the two validated percussion methods for determining spleen size

1. The percussion sign (Castell's method): the patient is in a supine position, and the examiner percusses over the patient's lower left intercostal space in the anterior axillary line. If the spleen is normal in size, the resonant note is produced and persists with full inspiration. If the spleen is enlarged, a change in the percussion note from resonance to dull occurs during full inspiration, i.e., a positive percussion sign. This change may be present even if the spleen is not palpable. When the spleen is greatly enlarged, the dull percussion note may be present in both inspiration and expiration.

2. The determination of the actual spleen size by percussion is done in a manner similar to that used for the liver. The clothing is removed to allow complete examination of the abdomen, left flank, and back. The patient lies on the right side with hands above the head and the left knee and hip partially flexed (Figure 6-9, *B*). The spleen is percussed along two main axes: the long axis, an imaginary line running from the left scapular to the left anterior superior iliac spine, and the short axis, an imaginary line perpendicular to the long axis and running from the left nipple toward the sacrum (Figure 6-9, *C*, see insert).

Long axis percussion is started just below the lower border of the left scapula, proceeding toward the anterior superior iliac crest until the area of absolute dullness is reached (Figure 6-10). Percussion of the inferior border is begun just above the iliac crest, percussing upward along the long axis until the area of absolute dullness is reached, being careful not to confuse the rib border (relative dullness) with the inferior border of the spleen (absolute dullness). When the inferior border of the spleen is palpable, it is used as the lower border of the long axis (Figure 6-10, *lower arrow*).

The minor (width) axis percussion is started from just below the left nipple toward the posterior iliac crest in a line perpendicular to the long axis. The distance between ink marks identifying percussion

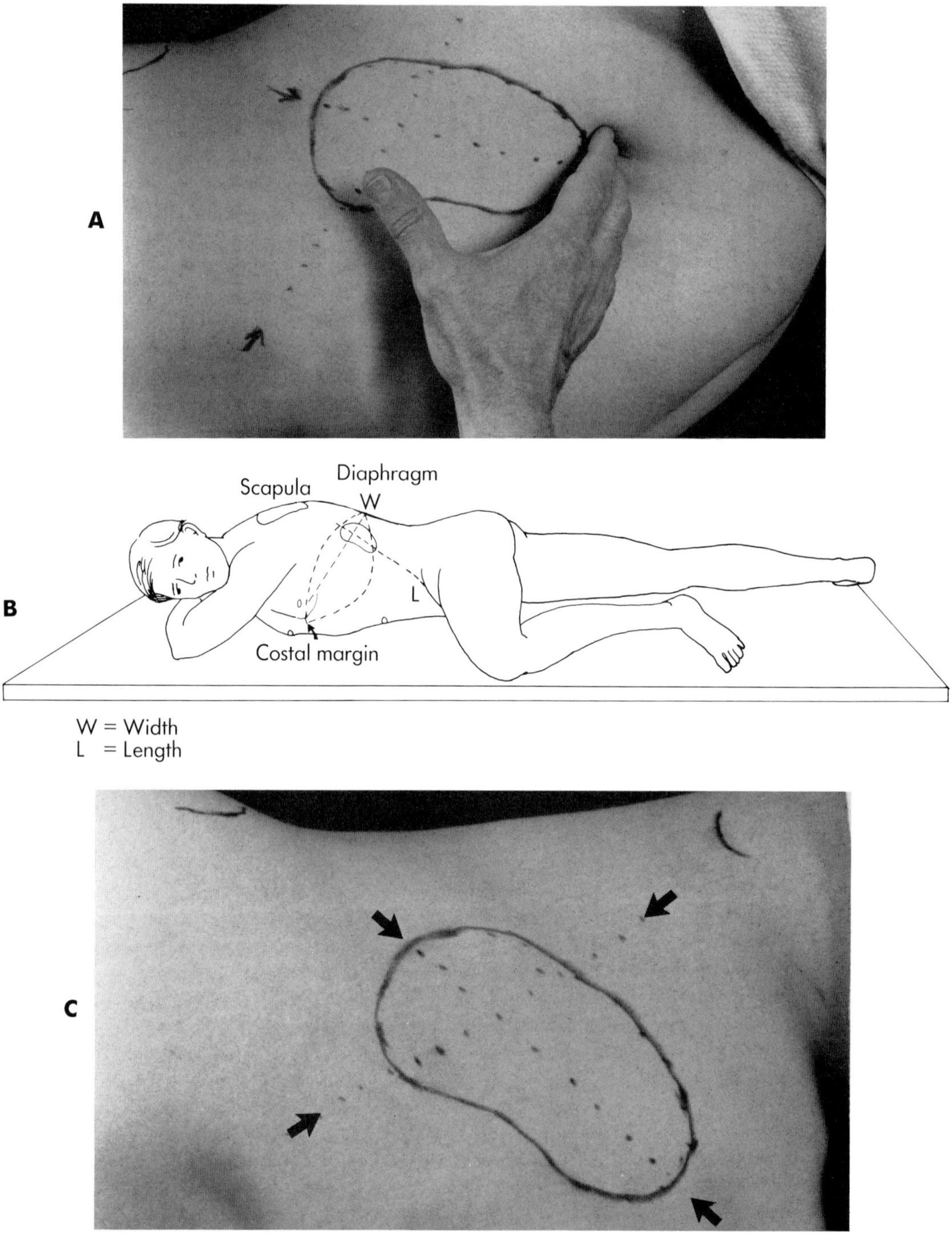

Figure 6-9
(A) Palpation of spleen, **(B)** Clinical determination of spleen size by percussion, **(C)** Lines of percussion for the spleen.

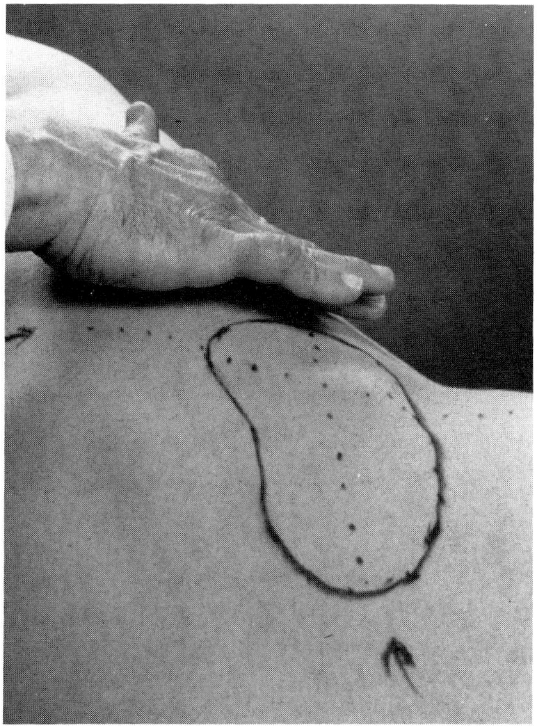

Figure 6-10
One-handed spleen percussion technique (side view).

Table 6-8 Normal ranges of liver and spleen size in adults

Liver	MCL	MSL
Mean	13	7
range*	7-17	3-10
90%	8-15	4-9
Spleen	**Length**	**Width**
Mean	11	7
Range*	8-15	4-10
90	9-14	5-9

*100% of 667 healthy industrial workers.

> **METHOD OF DETERMINING SPLEEN SIZE FROM SCANS**
>
> Spleen length is determined using the posterior view of Technetium-99m (Tc) sulfur colloid scans and measuring the maximum length from the upper to lower border of radioactivity. Spleen width is a similar measurement of the maximum radioactivity along a perpendicular (to long axis) line across the upper half of the spleen. (see Figure 6-8, *B*).

changes on the axes determines length and width.

NOTE: Percussion is best done by tapping the patient with the pads of three fingers (index, middle, and ring) while feeling and listening for resonance and absolute dullness (see Figure 6-7, top view and Figure 6-11 side view. See also the box at left).

This one-hand clinical percussion method for organ size will reflect actual scan measurement of liver size to within 2 cm in more than 95% of the patients and of spleen size within 2 cm in more than 75% of patients. Obesity (>25 lbs over ideal weight) and ascites interfere with the accurate determination of both the liver and spleen size. Table 6-8 provides normal ranges for liver and spleen size by percussion.

Gallbladder enlargement. In most individuals (<85%), the gallbladder fundus lies at the outer border of the right rectus abdominus muscle at its junction with the right costal margin just inside the MCL (Figure 6-11, *A, larger arrow*). An alterna-

A

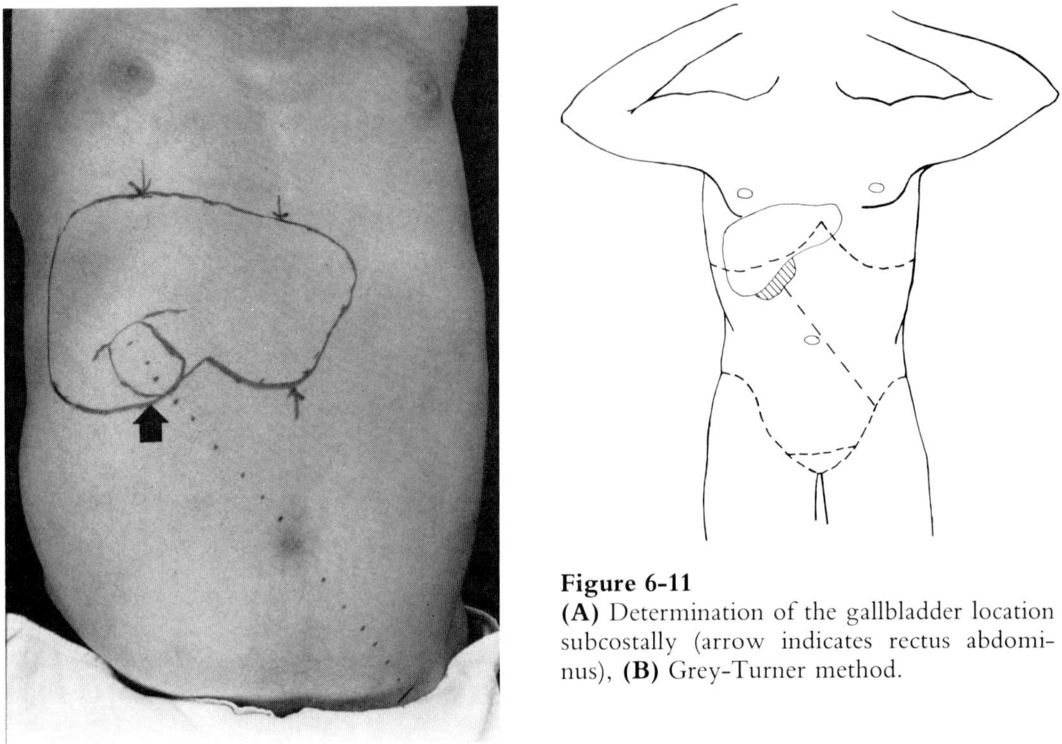

B

Figure 6-11
(A) Determination of the gallbladder location subcostally (arrow indicates rectus abdominus), **(B)** Grey-Turner method.

tive method of identifying gallbladder location is to draw a line from the left anterior iliac spine through the umbilicus to the right costal margin. At the intersection of the costal margin, or the lower edge of the liver, should be the site of the gallbladder fundus (Grey-Turner method, Figure 6-11, *B*). Obesity and extensive ascites interfere with the accuracy of both methods.

The gallbladder is normally not palpable. The presence of palpability implies enlargement or distention. When palpable, the gallbladder is a pear-shaped cystic mass that can sometimes be seen through the right anterior abdominal wall in thin individuals. It moves with respiration and is moveable laterally. Gallbladder swelling is dull to percussion and continuous with the liver.

An inflamed gallbladder causes abdominal tenderness during examination. Murphy's sign (pain during deep inspiration) can be elicited by having the patient take a deep breath when the examiner's fingers are placed below the liver edge or at the costal margin. The gallbladder is driven against the fingers, and the pain causes the patient to catch his or her breath. Liver regenerative nodules or malignant growths in the gallbladder region have a hard feeling and are rarely painful (1%).

Vascular skin changes. Spider angioma (arterial spiders and spider telangiectasias) are central arterioles in the skin from which radiate numerous small vessels re-

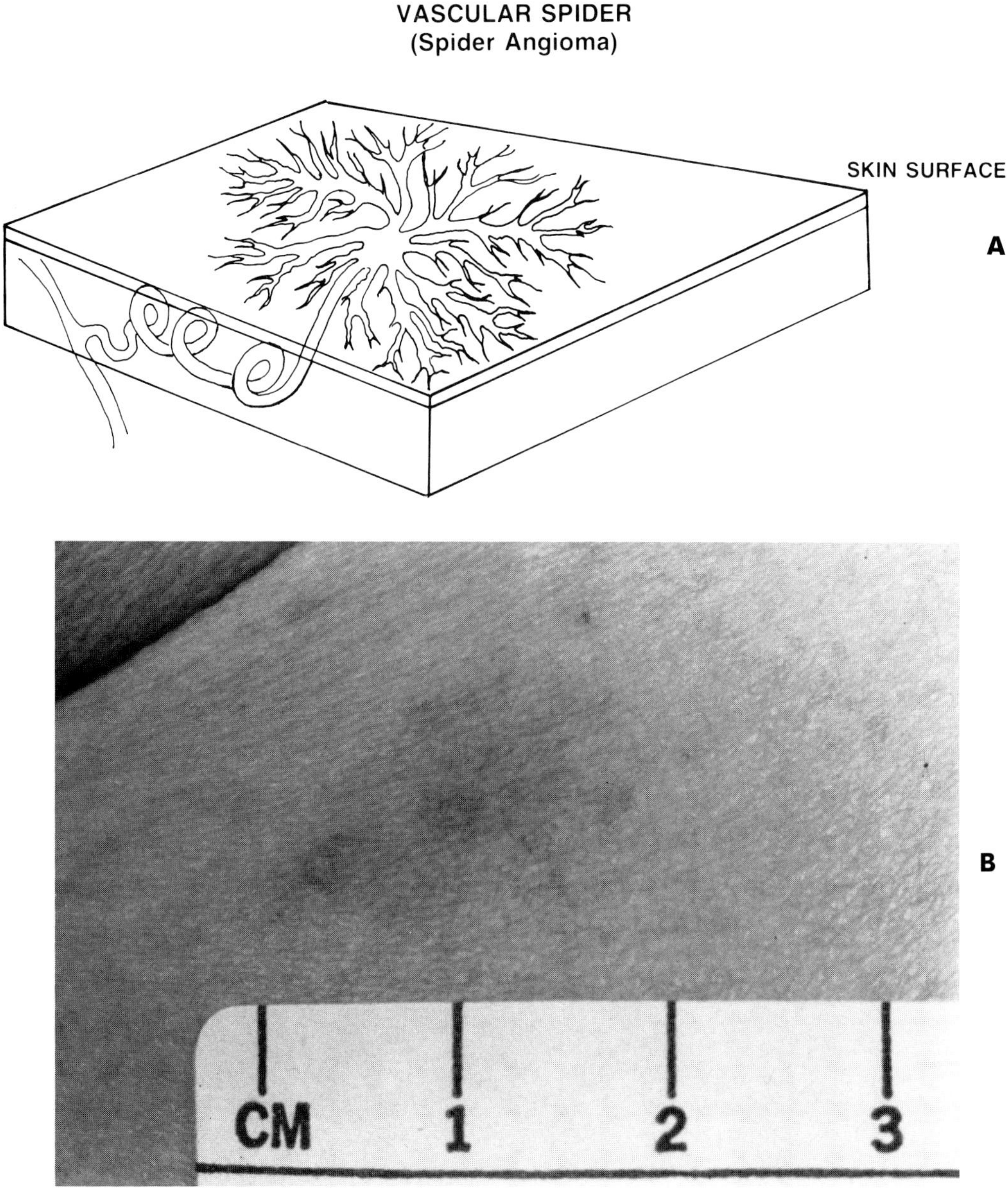

Figure 6-12
Vascular skin changes: **(A)** spider angioma architecture, **(B)** Spider angioma.

C 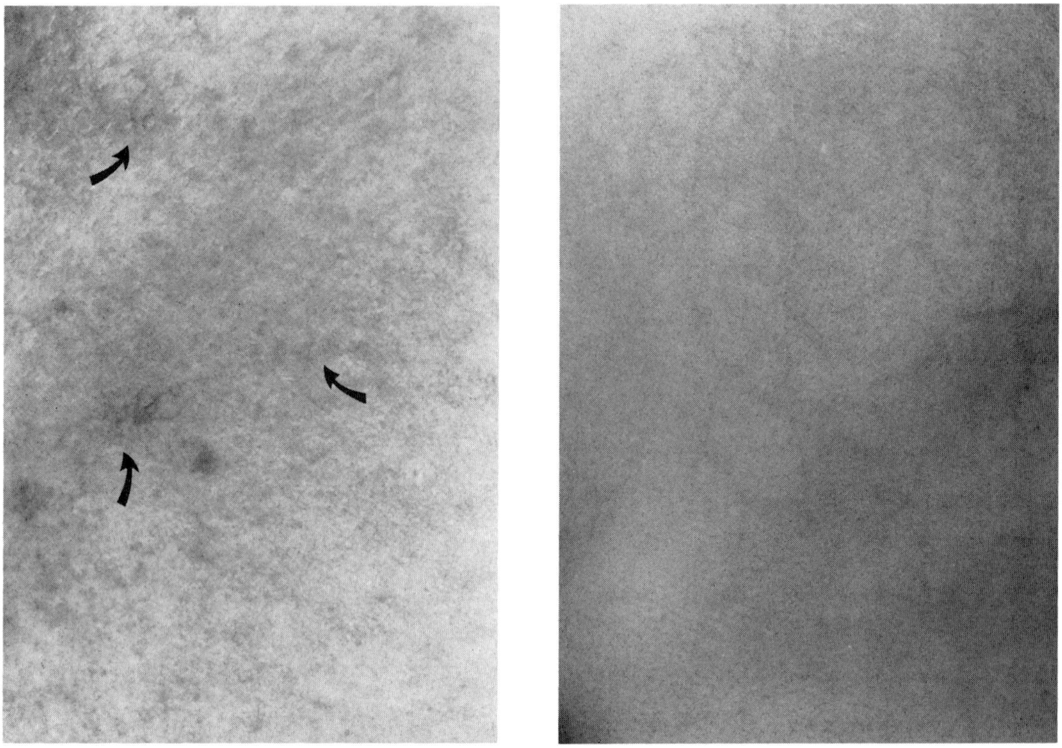 D

Figure 6-12, cont'd.
(C) Spider angioma and "paper money skin" (see curved arrows), **(D)** Abdominal wall vascular pattern.

sembling a spider's legs (Figure 6-12, *A*). They range in size from a pinhead to 0.5cm in diameter. They can be seen or felt to pulsate, and when pressed on the center prominence with a pencil or pen point, the entire lesion blanches. These lesions are found above the waistline, most commonly around the neck, face, back, shoulders, chest, forearms, and hands (Figure 6-12, *B,* see insert). They disappear or fade with improvement of liver function and hypotension caused by blood loss and after death. The fresh appearance of spiders usually reflects an active progression of liver disease. They are especially common with chronic viral or alcoholic liver disease. They may appear transiently with acute viral hepatitis and are seen less commonly in primary biliary tract disease.

These lesions are rare (<0.5%) in the normal population. A few vascular spiders are not diagnostic of liver disease, but a large number or increasing numbers warrant investigation. They are seen during pregnancy, appearing between the second and the fifth months and usually disappearing within a few months after delivery.

Another vascular change seen with vascular spiders is scattered threadlike vessels in the skin. Their distribution is similar to

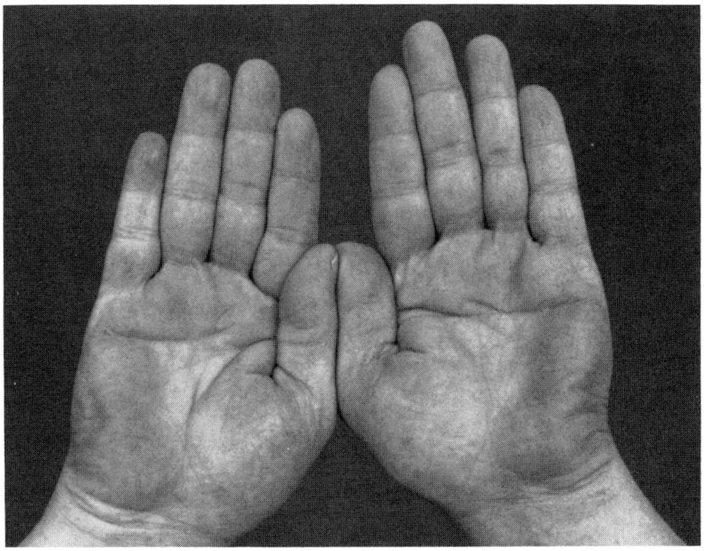

Figure 6-13
Palmar erythema.

that of the vascular spiders. Because of the resemblance to the red silk threads in the U.S. dollar bills, this phenomenon has been called "paper-money skin" (Figure 6-12, *C curved arrows*).

Hemorrhagic telangiectasias, which are hereditary, simulate vascular spiders. These lesions are usually on the upper body or on mucosal surfaces (e.g., nose, tongue, lips, palate, or pharynx) and frequently involve nail beds in addition to the palmar surface and fingers. Telangiectasias are punctiform, flat, and slightly elevated with sharp margins. Their connections with several vessels give them a resemblance to vascular spiders. Pulsations are very unusual. These lesions are associated with cirrhosis, especially PBC.

Circulatory and pulmonary changes associated with liver failure are manifested by a variety of clinical skin signs. Flushed extremities, bounding pulses, and capillary pulsations are due to an increase in blood flow to the skin and are major components of increased peripheral blood flow. These effects occur in addition to the more common abdominal portal system venous changes seen in cirrhotic patients (Figure 6-12, *D*).

Palmar erythema. In "liver palms" the hypothenar and thenar eminences and pulps of the fingers are bright red and warm (Figure 6-13). Islets of erythema are found at the bases of the fingers. This mottling blanches under pressure, but the color rapidly returns. Some patients complain of mild throbbing and tickling of the palms. Similar findings can be seen on the soles of the feet. Palmar erythema is frequently (80%) seen with spider angiom but may appear independently. Similar palmar erythema is seen in pregnancy and in patients with familial palmar flushing without liver disease, prolonged rheumatoid arthritis, chronic febrile illnesses, leukemia, and thyrotoxicosis.

Breast. Breast enlargement (gynecomastia) occurs in 30% to 40% of men

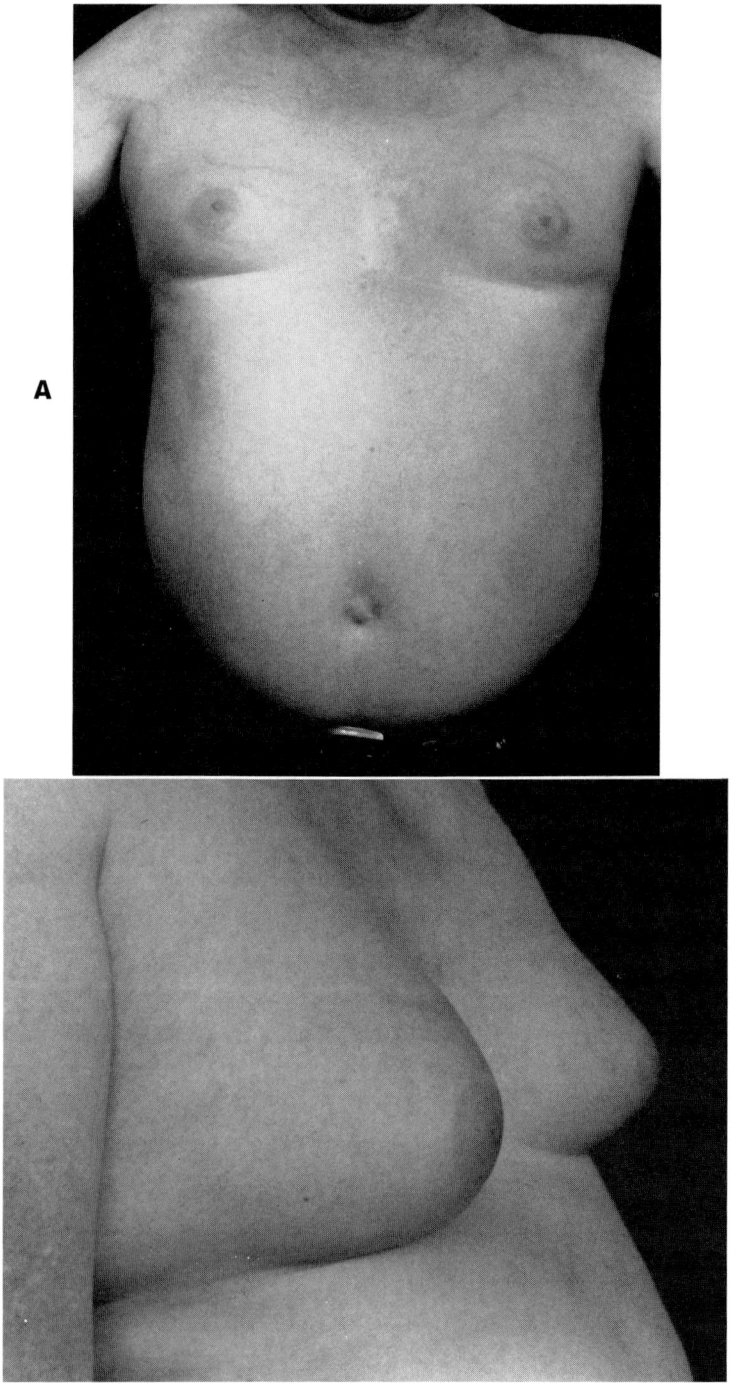

A

B

Figure 6-14
Gynecomastia, **(A)** Front view, **(B)** Side view.

CLINICAL STAGES OF HEPATIC ENCEPHALOPATHY

Stage I

Altered mood and/or behavior
Disorders of sleep
Irritability
Hypersomnia
Inversion of sleep rhythm 4
Reduction of spontaneous movement, apathy
Personality changes
Childishness
Frequent jocularity
Euphoria
Overly pleasant or cooperative nature
Slightly impaired organic mental function

Stage II

Fixed stare
Monotonous voice
Slowness and brevity of response
Loss of concern for personal matters or family
Slow, slurred speech
Flapping tremor*
Constructional apraxia*
Impaired writing*
Defecation in inappropriate places

Stage III

Excessive appetite
Perseveration
Dysphasia
Disorders of vision
Obedience of only simple commands
Marked confusion
Delirium
Reaction only to intense or noxious stimuli
Deep stupor

Stage IV

Sucking and grasping reflexes
Muscle twitching
Reflex response to noxious stimuli
Coma resembling normal sleep
Increased muscle tone, rigidity, ankle clonus, extensor plantar response

Stage V

No response to any stimuli
Coma—complete unresponsiveness

*See Figure 6-15.

with chronic liver disease (CLD) and is caused by hyperplasia of the glandular elements (Figure 6-14, *A* and 6-14, *B*). Breast lumps can also occur (<5%) but are mostly benign (>90%). Gynecomastia can be unilateral. Breast tenderness is frequently seen (10% to 20%) with the concomitant use of spirolactone therapy.

Neurologic changes. The interrelationship of hepatic disease with mental function has been recognized since Babylonian times. As liver disease progresses, all forms of neuropsychiatric signs and symptoms can be seen. Liver failure may affect all parts of the brain. Variability and fluctuation of these physical manifestations are more characteristic than any particular sign or symptom. Individual features depend on the severity and the pathogenic factors of the disease process. The box above lists these features and their usual progressive appearances during liver failure.

Asterixis, "hepatic flap" or "flapping" tremor, is the most characteristic neurologic abnormality in hepatic decompensation. This sign is due to impaired flow of afferent information to the brainstem reticular formation, causing lapses in posture or inability to maintain a position. This is best demonstrated by having the patient stretch out the arms, hyperextend the wrists with forearms fixed, and separate the fingers. A rapid extension-flexion movement occurs at the metacarpophalangeal and wrist joints (Figure 6-15, *A*). This tremor disappears with coma and is bilateral but not necessarily synchronous, absent at rest, changed by intentional movement, and maximized by sustained flexion or posture. In the most severe form the flapping tremor can affect the head, jaws, tongue, and the arms and other limb joints. A flapping tremor can be seen in all forms of metabolic encephalopathy, e.g., renal failure and hypokalemia.

Intellectual impairment or impaired organic mental function can vary from slight to gross confusion. Following are some of the easiest methods of detection:

Constructional apraxia: Tests measure the inability to reproduce simple designs (Figure 6-15, *B*) such as a five-pointed star or continuous, concentric circles.

Writing impairment: Tests measure the ability to complete a signature or sentence in a legible manner or form continuous circles (Figure 6-15, *C*).

Reitan Trail Making Test: the patient is timed on the ability to connect randomly placed numbers sequentially on a page. There are four types to minimize proficiency with repeat uses (Figure 6-16, *A*, type I and 6-16, *B*, type III).

These clinical findings are also associated with slow and often slurred speech, monotonous voice, slow response to questions, and short attention span.

Body habitus. Feminization of the male body habitus also occurs in chronic

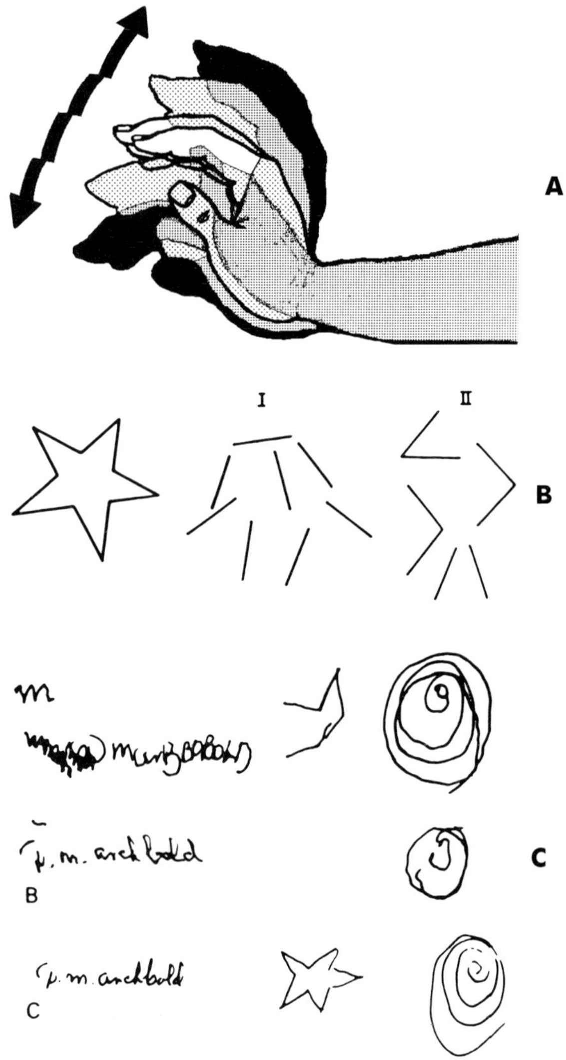

Figure 6-15
(A) Asterixis flapping tremor. (From Leevy CM: Evaluation of liver function in clinical practice, ed 2, Indianapolis, 1974, The Lilly Research Laboratories.) **(B)** Construction of five-point star. (From Davidson EA and Summerskill WHJ: Psychiatric aspects of liver disease, Postgrad Med J 32:487-494, 1956.) **(C)** Writing impairment. (From Conn HO and Lieberthal MM: The hepatic coma syndrome and lactulose, ed 1, Baltimore, 1979, Williams & Wilkins.)

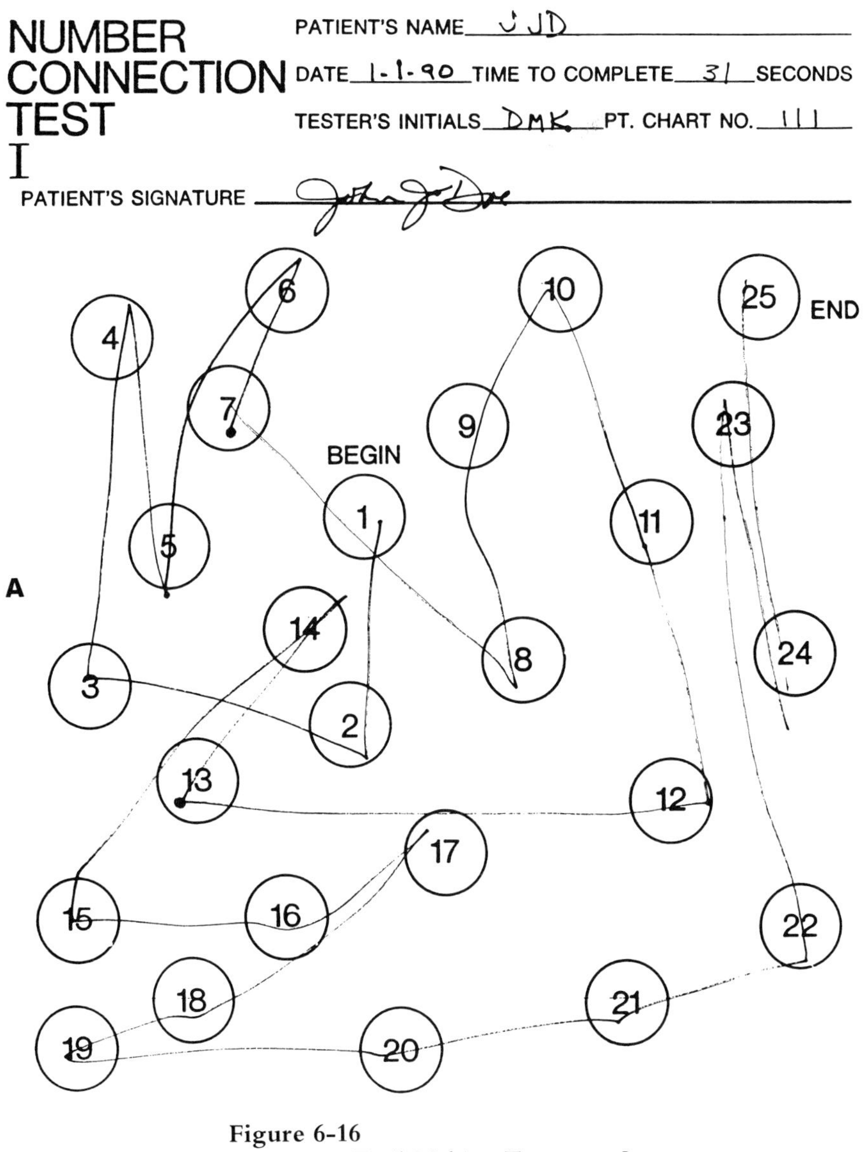

A

Figure 6-16
(A) Reitan Trail Making Test, type I.

Continued.

NUMBER CONNECTION TEST III

PATIENT'S NAME________________

DATE 3-27-96 TIME TO COMPLETE 63 SECONDS

TESTER'S INITIALS DK PT. CHART NO. 303

PATIENT'S SIGNATURE________________

B

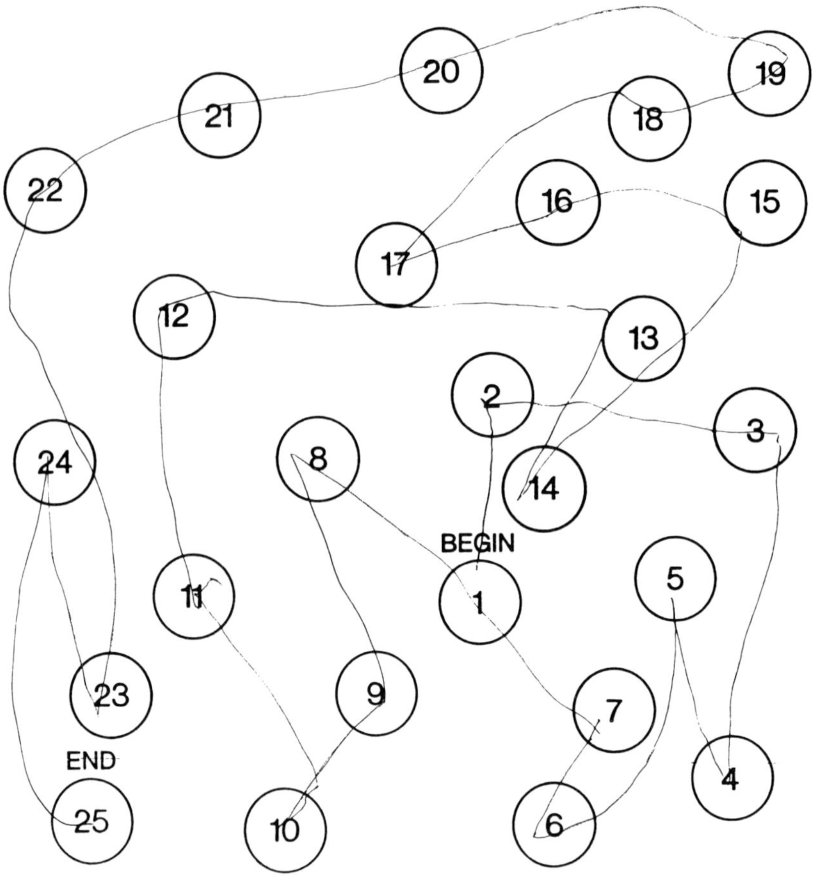

Figure 6-16—cont'd.
(B) Reitan Trail Making Test, type III.

liver disease, especially alcohol related. More common changes are female body habitus and escutcheon.

Muscle wasting. Easy fatiguability and weakness are the most (90%) common features of both acute and chronic liver failure. Loss of muscle mass is associated with the chronically injured liver's difficulty in synthesizing tissue proteins. Secondary anorexia and the accompanying poor dietary habits contribute to this malnutritional state (Figure 6-17, *A*).

Another common manifestation of protein malnutrition associated with cirrhosis is the development of a midline diathesis hernia. This condition is easily identified by having the patient lie in a supine position and raise the head so that the chin touches the chest. This will tighten the abdominal muscles, causing a midline bulge (Figure 6-17, *B,* see curved arrow).

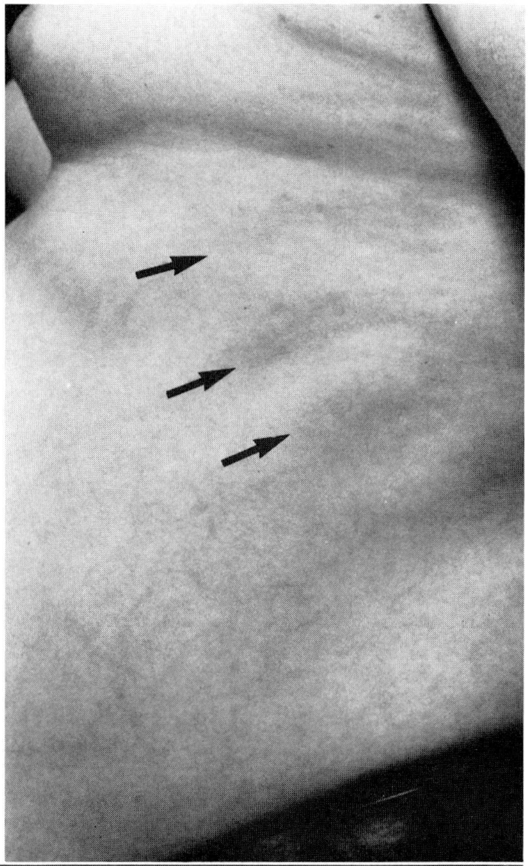

A

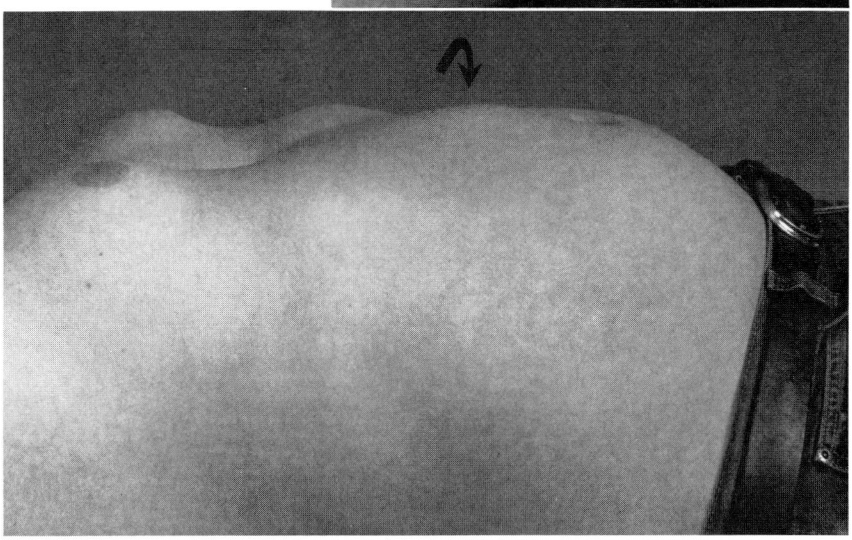

B

Figure 6-17
(A) Intercostal muscle wasting in obese cirrhotic patient (see arrows), **(B)** Midline hernia bulge (see curved arrow).

A

B

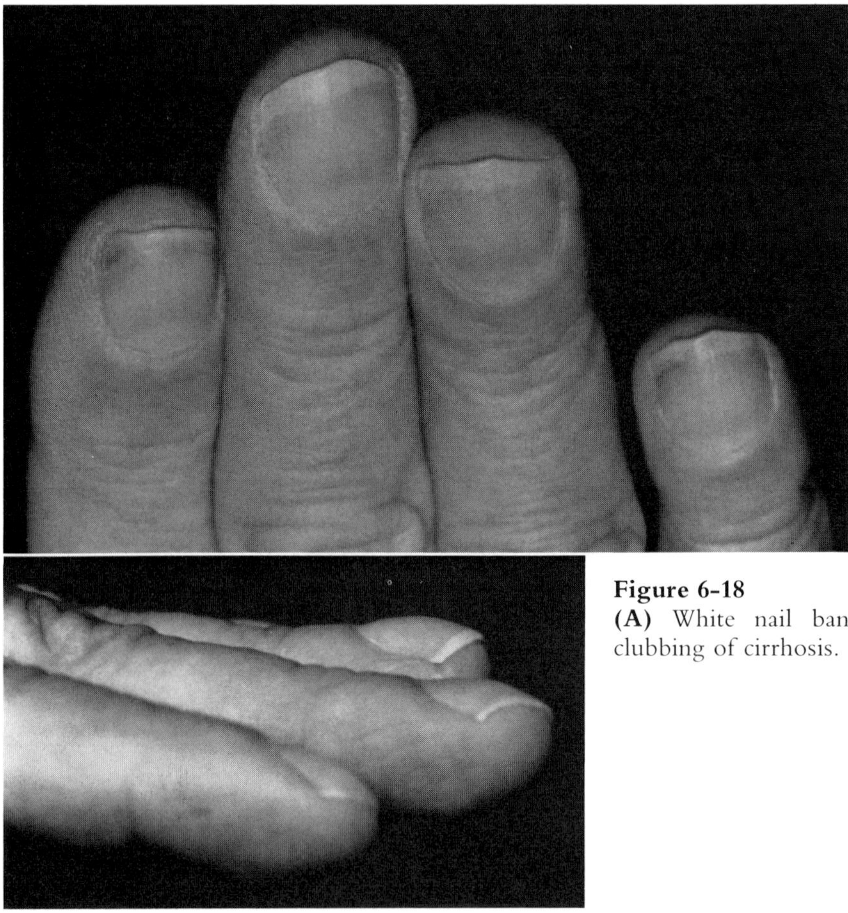

Figure 6-18
(A) White nail bands, **(B)** Digital clubbing of cirrhosis.

Fingernails. White nails (opaqueness of the nail bed) are a common finding in cirrhotic patients, and often the lunulae cannot be distinguished. These findings are bilateral and are noted especially in the nails of the thumb and forefinger.

In advanced cirrhosis the fingernails also manifest signs of associated protein deficiency. Horizontal white bands may develop across the fingernails, and there can be loss of the white lunar area of the fingernail bed (Figure 6-18, *A*).

Clubbing of fingers and hypertrophic osteoarthropathy are found in cirrhosis, especially in PBC (Figure 6-18, *B*). In hepatocellular failure with intrapulmonary shunting (hepatopulmonary syndrome), clubbing of fingers is often associated with cyanosis and increased cardiac output.

Hemorrhoids (piles). Hemorrhoids, varicosities of the hemorrhoidal venous plexus, are common in cirrhosis and portal vein thrombosis because of increased portal venous pressure and weakness in the supporting anal tissues. Hemorrhoidal

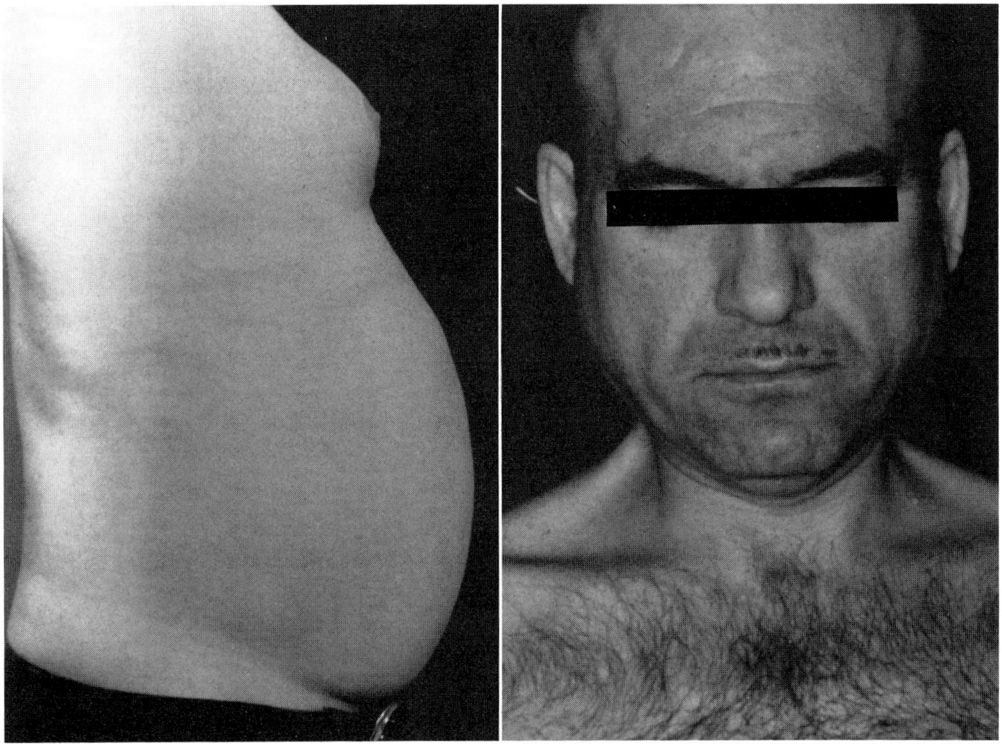

Figure 6-19
(A) Feminization of the male cirrhotic patient: sexual hair loss, smooth skin, and enlarged breasts. **(B)** Bilateral parotid enlargement.

bleeding can be a major cause of blood loss (<5%). Hemorrhoidal bleeding in chronic liver disease (CLD) is associated with abnormal clotting factors, low, dysfunctional platelets, nutritional deficiencies (vitamin C and folic acid), and increased abdominal pressure caused by ascites.

Endocrine changes. Commonly associated endocrine changes in CLD (cirrhosis) include body feminization; diminished libido and potency, impotence, sterility, soft, small testes; abnormal seminal fluid; lower incidence of prostatic hypertrophy; secondary sexual hair loss or the need to shave less often; enlarged or painful breasts; and parotid swelling (Figure 6-19).

In females the gonadal changes are not as clinically conspicuous. However, individuals complain of lower libido; infertility; erratic menstruation, either diminished or absent but rarely excessive; breast atrophy; occasional cyst hyperplasia; and atrophic uterus.

Cardiopulmonary. Tachycardia is often (25%) present because of increased cardiac output. Systolic ejection murmurs and even active precordial impulses can be present. Heart failure is rarely due to

Table 6-9 Cardiopulmonary manifestations of CLD

Finding cause	Cause
Cyanosis, hypoxia	Arteriovenous shunts, pulmonary vasodilation, ventilation perfusion mismatch
Tachypnea, hypocapnia	Increased central nervous system (CNS) sensitivity to NH_3, hypoxia, increased organic acids (lactate and pyruvate), hypokalemia (caused by diuretic or other electrolyte disturbances)
Pleural effusion (usually R > L)	Protein malnutrition, poor tissue repair, leak from the abdominal to the pleural cavity
Elevated right diaphragm	Abdominal ascites, phrenic nerve injury
Dilated pulmonary artery	High cardiac output, hyperdynamic circulatory state, splenic blood diversion to pulmonary circulation, primary hepatocellular tumor emboli

these circulatory changes. Table 6-9 lists common cardiopulmonary manifestations of CLD and their causes.

Blood pressure. As hepatocellular disease progresses, blood pressure decreases. At advanced stages it contributes further to reduced renal function (increased blood urea nitrogen [BUN] and creatinine), reduced cerebral blood flow (mental changes), and liver failure (increased bilirubin and decreased protein). Cardiovascular response varies with the type of liver disease and is related to the portal collateral circulation. Vasomotor tone is decreased. The vasculature fails to constrict in response to mental excitement, Valsalva maneuvers, and vertical tilting. This may be due to a combination of activations of normally present but functionally inactive arteriovenous anastomoses in the lung, skin, and other peripheral tissue. The diseased liver may be failing to remove vasodilating substances or may be producing them because of failed regulatory feedback. Ferritin is touted as a candidate vasodilator, as is an over-active sympathetic nervous system with resulting loss of the circadian rhythm.

Fever. Up to one third of patients with advanced alcoholic hepatitis have low-grade fevers, which rarely exceed 38° C (102° F). This fever is unaffected by antibiotics or a change in dietary protein. Fever is thought to be due to active necrosis associated with alcoholic hyaline.

Hands and feet. In chronic alcoholic cirrhosis, a diffuse bilateral defoliation of the palms of the hands (Figure 6-20, *A*) and soles of the feet (Figure 6-20, *B*) can occur (5%). The skin peels off in layers and is dry though no redness or evidence of fungal disease exists. These findings are associated with peripheral neuropathy and slowly are resolved with hepatocellular improvement.

Fetor hepaticus. Fetor hepaticus is found in 3% of patients with advanced stages of liver disease. It is a sweet, slightly fecal smell of the breath. Improved treatment of hepatic failure and use of a wide spectrum of antibiotics have reduced its occurrence.

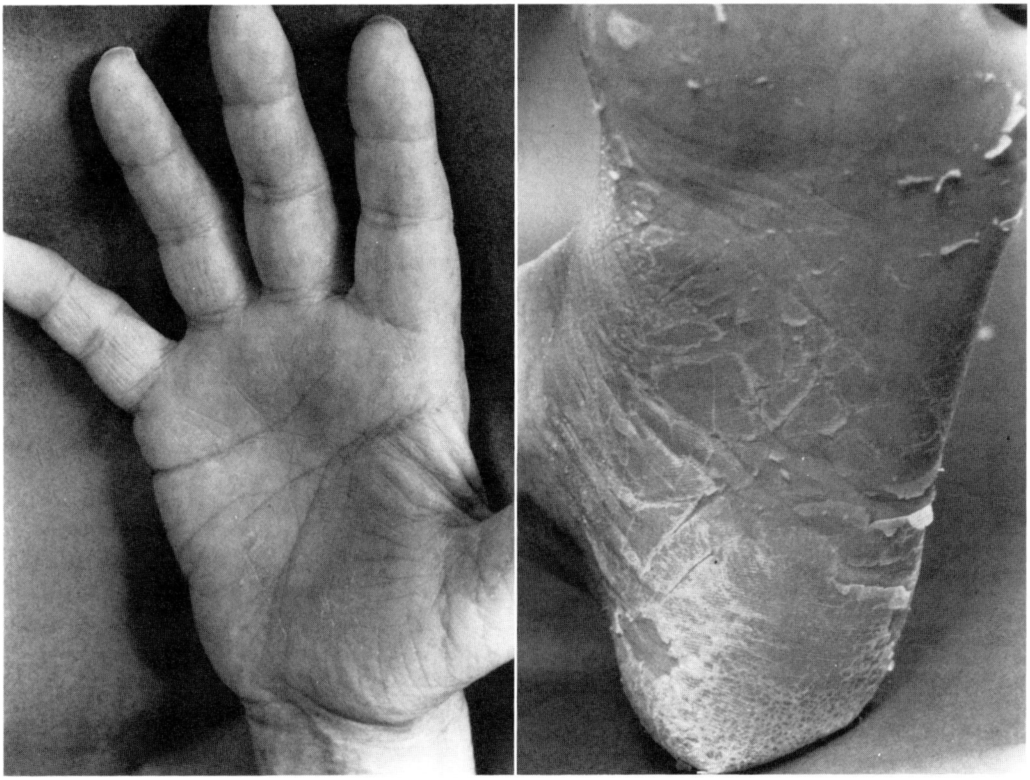

Figure 6-20
Defoliation of the **(A)** palms and **(B)** soles of the cirrhotic patient.

SUMMARY

This chapter on the clinical evaluation of liver status provides an introduction to the examination of the patient with liver disease for those without previous training and a review for those who wish to hone or update their clinical skills. This chapter addresses the signs and symptoms most commonly associated with liver disease and the manner in which these signs and symptoms most frequently present themselves. The manner of presentation described is more characteristic of those patients with liver diseases common in developed countries. Nonetheless, the descriptions of symptoms, their characteristics, and techniques of physical examination are applicable worldwide. The tables and illustrations are structured to enlarge the clinician's skill in symptom evaluation and interpretation. More precise and reproducible methods of clinical determination of liver and spleen size are also demonstrated. The illustrated format of these techniques should aid in the methodical and thorough performance of the physical examination.

The history-taking section is directed at assisting the physician in uncovering something about not only the illness but also the patient. The physical examination section provides more advantageous means of assessing any functional or structural change(s) suggested by the patient's symptoms. It is hoped that this chapter will provide a way of thinking as much as a way of doing.

ACKNOWLEDGMENT

Appreciation to the Veterans Administration Medical Center (VAMC) Louisville, Kentucky, medical illustration department, especially to Ms. Luann Rierdon for excellent photography and Mr. Hal Marquette for creative illustrations and artwork.

SUGGESTED READINGS

Castell DO: Spleen percussion sign: a useful diagnostic technique, Ann Intern Med 67:1265-1267, 1967.

This paper describes the clinical method for qualitative determination of spleen size.

Cattau EL, Benjamin SB, Knuff TE, and Castell DO: The accuracy of the physical examination in the diagnosis of suspected ascites, JAMA 247:1164-1166, 1982.

Careful study of examination methods and their accuracy in clinically determining the presence of abdominal fluid is presented.

Conn HO: Trail-making and number-connection tests in the assessment of mental states and portal systemic encephalopathy, Am J Dig Dis 22:541-550, 1977.

These tests were the first objective demonstrations of reproducible methods of quantitation of clinical neurologic and mental dysfunction in patients with liver disease.

Conn HO: A peek at the Child-Turcot classification, Hepatology, 1:673-676, 1981 (editorial).

This is a short, excellent review of the most frequently used clinical methods of classification of the severity of a patient's liver disease.

Elstein AS, Schulman LS et al: Medical problem solving: analysis of clinical reasoning, Cambridge, Mass, 1978, Harvard University Press.

A systematic, analytic examination of clinical decision making in the processes of patient evaluation and diagnosis is presented.

Galambos JT: Cirrhosis, Philadelphia, 1979, W B Saunders Co.

This is an excellent clinical monograph designed for the practicing physician who cares for patients with diseases of the liver. It is presented in a concise, very readable manner with clarity, thoroughness, and logic.

Gilchrest BA: Pruritus, pathogenesis, therapy, and significance in systemic disease states, Arch Intern Med 142:101, 1982.

The author presents an excellent review of the most troublesome symptom in patients with liver disease, which is "itching" for resolution.

Guyton AC, Cowley AW, Coleman TG et al: Regulation of interstitial fluid volume and pressure, Adv Exp Med Biol, 33:111-118, 1972.

This is a review and study of regulatory factors in extracellular tissue fluid volume and pressure.

Holdstock DJ, Misiewicz JJ, and Waller SL: Observations on the mechanism of abdominal pain, Gut, 10:19-31, 1969.

A clinical study of abdominal pain related to changes in intraluminal pressures of the small and large intestines is presented.

Howard CS, Sandoz JP, and Tamburro CH: A clinical determination of spleen size in human adults. Clin Res, 26:332A, 1978.

This was the first description of a quantitative method of determining spleen size.

Hurst JW: How does one develop a defined data base? Who collects the data? In Walker HK, Hurst JW, and Woody MF, eds: Applying the problem-oriented system, New York, 1973, Medcom pp. 25-27.

This is a practical summary of the methodology for development and operation of a defined data base.

Kassirer JP and Gorry GA: Clinical problem solving: a behavioral analysis, Ann Intern Med 89:245-255, 1978.

The authors examine the physician's thorough process in the evaluation of the patient relative to the factual bases on which many decisions are made.

Leevy CM and Tygstrup N, eds: Diseases of the liver and biliary tract: standardization of the nomenclature, diagnostic criteria and diagnostic methodology for diseases of the liver and biliary tract, 1976 Thasal S. Karger

This is an authoritative guide to international consensus on the proper terminology, criteria, and methods for diagnosis of diseases of the hepatobiliary system.

Morgan WL, and Engel GL: The clinical approach to the patient, Philadelphia, 1979, W B Saunders Co.

This classic text is designed to guide the beginner and reacquaint the practitioner. Therefore excellent detailed illustrations.

Naftalis J, and Leevy CM: Clinical evaluation of liver size, Am J Dig Dis 8:236-243, 1963.

This is the original description and verification of quantitative determination of liver size.

Peternel WW, Schaffer JW et al: Clinical evaluation of liver size and hepatic scintiscan, Am J Dig Dis 11:346-350, 1966.

A very good review of the comparison of clinical vs. hepatic scintiscan-determined liver size is presented.

Scharschmidt BF, Goldberg HI, and Schmid R: Approach to the patient with cholestatic jaundice, N Engl J Med 308:1515, 1983.

This is an excellent authoritative review, both clinically applicable and comprehensive, of the approach to clinical jaundice.

Sherlock S and Summerfield JA: Color atlas of liver disease, Chicago, 1979, Year-book Medical Publishers.

An outstanding comprehensive collection of physical signs and illustrative results of investigative procedures with comparative histopathology is presented.

Summerskill WHJ, Davidson EA, Sherlock S et al: The neuropsychiatric syndrome associated with hepatic cirrhosis and extensive portal collateral circulation, Q J Med 25:245, 1956.

This is an excellent, classic description and characterization of clinical neuropsychiatric findings in patients with advanced liver disease and portosystemic shunting.

Swarbrick ET, Hegarty JE et al: Site of pain from the irritable bowel, Lancet 2:443, 1980.

This is a detailed study and clinical documentation with illustrations of the distribution of abdominal pain induced by balloon inflation.

Walker HK, Hall WD, and Hurst JW: Clinical methods: the history, physical and laboratory examinations, 1990, Butterworth Publishers.

This is the most outstanding, thorough, and comprehensive multiauthored book directed at mastering the art and skill of total interpretation of history, physical examination, and laboratory results. This book is "must" reading for medical students and residents and an excellent review for practicing physicians.

7 Laboratory Evaluation of Liver Disease

Carlo H. Tamburro

Patients with liver disease present with and without clinical manifestations. In either situation, we are faced with the same four basic questions. Does the patient have liver disease? If present, what is its etiology? How severe is it? What is the treatment and prognosis? The patient's clinical manifestations and nonclinical abnormalities are presumably due to changes in hepatocellular function. Evaluation of hepatic function, especially that of the hepatocytes, is obviously essential. However, the liver is in a particularly unfavorable position. It is clinically an introverted organ, that is not easily accessible. Because of the organ's vast cellular reserve, adverse effects on the liver are often clinically imperceptible until the more advanced stages of injury are reached. Therefore the next step after completion of the history and physical examination is a systematic, step-by-step laboratory investigation to answer the four basic questions given above.

Laboratory summary data. Because hepatobiliary disease is often chronic, requiring a multitude of varied laboratory studies, laboratory summary data sheets are vital. Appendixes B-1 through B-3 contain examples of comprehensive data summary forms with sections for standard hematology, chemistry, and hepatobiliary, immunologic-serologic, and urinary studies. A-4 and A-5 contain diagnostic procedure sections. All are suitable for the computerized medical data base.

A laboratory test's efficacy is usually judged by its ability to assist in diagnosis. However, laboratory tests of hepatic function are not primarily diagnostic. Functional evaluation in principle is quantitative, in contrast to diagnostic testing, which is qualitative, i.e., either confirming or rejecting a specific diagnosis. For example, cirrhosis is defined by liver biopsy histology, and viral hepatitis is defined by serology. Albumin and serum transaminase levels reflect the synthetic function and membrane integrity, respectively, of the hepatocyte, but not the specific diagnosis.

The common clinical concept of "liver function" presumes that the liver's functions are associated. Clinical experience quickly confirms that dissociation of liver function is the more common manifestation. This is exemplified in the case of drug cholestasis (jaundice), in which the

TYPES OF INJURY IN HEPATIC DISEASE

- Cellular necrosis
  - Acute
  - Chronic
- Steatosis
  - Microvesicular
  - Macrovesicular
- Inflammation
  - Acute
  - Chronic
- Cholestasis
  - Biochemical
  - Chemical
- Vascular changes
  - Arterial
  - Venous
  - Sinusoidal
- Fibrosis
- Cirrhosis
- Tumor formation
  - Benign
  - Malignant

excretory function is impaired (elevated bilirubin) while synthetic function remains normal (normal albumin).

Therefore the multiple functions of the liver require a "battery" of tests for adequate evaluation. The purpose of functionally evaluating the liver is to characterize the patient with respect to the degree of hepatic impairment, if any, and to provide more precise predictions of prognosis and decisions regarding treatment and to monitor treatment outcome.

MAJOR FORMS OF HEPATIC INJURY AND METHODS OF EVALUATION

The liver responds to toxic agents, both synthetic and natural, in a limited number of ways (see box at left). These injuries have various etiologies and cause a variety of diseases and disorders, examples of which are listed in the box below.

ETIOLOGIC CLASSIFICATION AND COMMON EXAMPLES

Viral:	Hepatitis A, B, C, D, E, and EBV, CMV
Toxic:	Alcohol, drugs, chemicals, and poisons
Biliary tract obstructions:	Gallstones, strictures, tumors, atresia, and PSC
Metabolic:	Bilirubinemia, iron and copper overload, porphyrias, and lipid, protein, and carbohydrate disorders
Autoimmune:	Hepatitis, PBC, and PSC
Neoplastic:	Primary, and secondary
Bacterial:	Tbc, and pyogens
Parasitic:	Protozoal, and helminthic
Vascular:	Hepatic and portal vein thrombosis, and veno-occlusive disease
Congenital:	Polycystic, hepatic fibrosis
Cryptogenic:	Granulomatous, regenerative nodular hyperplasia
Secondary disorders:	Hypersplenism, pregnancy, trauma, and hepatorenal, endocrine, cardiopulmonary, and hematologic disorders

BIOCHEMICAL TESTS COMMONLY USED FOR EVALUATION OF LIVER DISEASE

Blood (serum/plasma)

Ammonia
Bile acids (BA)
Bile pigments
- Bilirubin
- Total (TB)
  - Conjugated/direct (DB)
  - Unconjugated/indirect (IB)

Coagulation tests
- PT
- PTT

Enzymes
- AP
- Aminotransferase
  - ALT
  - AST
- GGTP
- LDH
- 5′-Nucleotidase (5′ NT)

Lipid studies
- Cholesterol
- Triglycerides

Protein studies
- Albumin
- Amino acid profiles

Urine

Bile pigments
- Bile (conjugated bilirubin)
- Urobilinogen

Laboratory tests for the evaluation of these liver diseases fall into five categories: tests of biochemical activity (static tests), hepatic synthesis (synthesis tests) quantitative function (dynamic tests), anatomic structure (imaging studies), and morphology (histologic studies). The more conventionally used tests and profiles are shown in the box at left.

Static Tests

The static tests are the most frequently used and are conducted predominantly on biologic fluids of blood and urine. They are characterized as "static" tests because they reflect a level of disease at a point in time. These include tests for cellular injury, e.g., serum enzymes: alanine aminotransferase (ALT), aspartate aminotransferase (AST), γ-glutamyl transpeptidase (GGTP), and lactic acid dehydrogenase (LDH) and tests for cholestasis, alkaline phosphatase (AP), 5′-nucleotidase, total bilirubin, direct and indirect bilirubin, urine and bile (bilirubin), and urobilinogen. Serum enzyme studies best reflect acute injury and are the most useful for medical screening.

Synthesis Studies

Tests of hepatic synthesis, e.g., albumin, PT, clotting factors, and amino acids, as well as the less commonly used endogenous products, such as cholesterol, cholesterol esters, glycoproteins, transferrin, and α-globulins, are most useful in chronic or severe diseases that reduce the hepatic parenchymal mass. Tests of hepatic synthesis are the most specific and are the most effective in following disease progress. A major shortcoming is that extrahepatic factors interfere with many of the test values, thereby decreasing their specificity.

Dynamic Tests

Dynamic studies of the liver are "true" liver function tests because they provide qualitative or quantitative assessments of the functional capacity of the liver. These tests usually assess three functional capabilities: (1) hemodynamic (venous and arterial blood flows); (2) cellular (hepatocytic, biliary, and reticuloendothelial) uptake, transport, conjugation, and storage; and (3) metabolic (metabolism, detoxification, and excretion of substances). Although these tests are the most sensitive for early detection of subclinical liver injury, they generally are more complex and more costly to perform. Therefore they are not as suitable for routine or initial medical screening purposes.

Imaging Studies

The ability of structural studies (radiologic, radioisotopic, sonographic, and invasive procedures, e.g., endoscopic retrograde cholangiopancreatography [ERCP] and percutaneous transhepatic cholangiography [PTC]) to identify disease is inversely proportional to the stage of the disease process and degree of anatomic distortion. In screening programs of asymptomatic healthy workers, up to 12% of studies showed false positives, and 35% to 40% showed false negatives when compared with histologic verification. Structural studies are unsuitable for early detection or screening for liver disease even though they can be powerful tools for differential diagnosis in the clinical stages of disease.

Histologic Studies

Morphologic studies remain the gold standard for the diagnosis and evaluation of hepatic disease. Investigative liver biopsy has been an accepted clinical technique since it was first introduced by Iversen and Roholm in 1939. There are two nonoperative techniques: the aspiration technique of Manghini (using the Jamshiti needle), a suction method, and the core tissue technique of Vim-Silverman (using the Tru-Cut needle method). Both require training and experience for safe performance.

LABORATORY STUDIES FOR EVALUATION OF LIVER DISEASE

Presently, the clinician assessing the patient's liver status requires the results of a "battery" of tests. This profile provides essential information that an individual test cannot provide. Recognizing the characteristic pattern of these liver studies in different clinical situations provides a dynamic use of static tests because they change with time and treatment. Such liver test profiles have distinct clinical usefulness: (1) screening asymptomatic individuals for hepatic disease, (2) providing clues to the establishment of a diagnosis on the patient's first presentation (history and physical), (3) monitoring the response to therapy or disease progression, and (4) establishing the prognosis. Coupled with the initial clinical presentation, the standard liver tests provide the first step in differential diagnosis (Table 7-1 and Figure 7-1, Decision algorithm I).

Individual liver ("function") tests in the usual standard profile provide relatively limited quantitative information (i.e., information on the extent of liver damage). They are better suited for identifying pathophysiologic processes rather than the degree of liver injury. Because of their simplicity and ease of availability, these tests remain the first line of investigation in the day-to-day care of patients with liver disorders. However, limited awareness of their physiologic and pathologic interrelationships often leads to incorrect interpretation and serious clinical mismanagement. Other decision algorithms in this chapter will assist in diagnostic interpretation of these tests.

Table 7-1 Function of clinical presentation and standard liver tests in differential diagnosis of liver disease

Patient type	Clinical presentation	Probable liver condition(s)
I	Exposure screening Asymptomatic	Normal or subclinical disease
II	Asymptomatic Abnormal tests No physical findings	False positive test Metabolic disorder Subclinical disease
III	Asymptomatic Abnormal tests Positive physical findings	Active subacute disease
IV	Asymptomatic Normal tests Positive physical findings	Inactive structural disease Anatomic anomaly
V	Symptomatic Abnormal tests No physical findings	Early acute disease
VI	Symptomatic Abnormal tests Positive physical findings	Active disease
VII	Symptomatic >6 months Abnormal tests Positive physical findings	Chronic disease
VIII	Symptomatic Normal tests Positive physical findings	Anatomic abnormalities

Common Standard Studies

Standard (static) biochemical tests are most useful in identifying pathophysiologic abnormalities in three functional areas: hepatocellular integrity: ALT, AST, LDH, and GGT; the biliary tract: total and fractionated serum bilirubin, urine urobilinogen, AP, and 5′NT; hepatocellular synthesis: plasma proteins, total protein, albumin, globulin, and transferrins.

Bile pigment and fractionation

Serum bilirubin. Unconjugated bilirubin originates mainly from breakdown of RBC hemoglobin, which is transported to liver cells bound to plasma albumin. In the liver it is conjugated mainly with glucuronic acid and excreted through the biliary system. More than 95% of the normal adult population has a bilirubin concentration below 25 μmol/dl (1.2 mg/dl). When bilirubin concentration is above 50 μmol/dl (2.5 mg/dl), hyperbilirubinemia can be detected clinically as jaundice. The normal liver is capable of conjugating up to 1,500 mg/day. The higher concentrations of bilirubin, above approximately 1,000 μmol/dl (50 mg/dl), are seen when

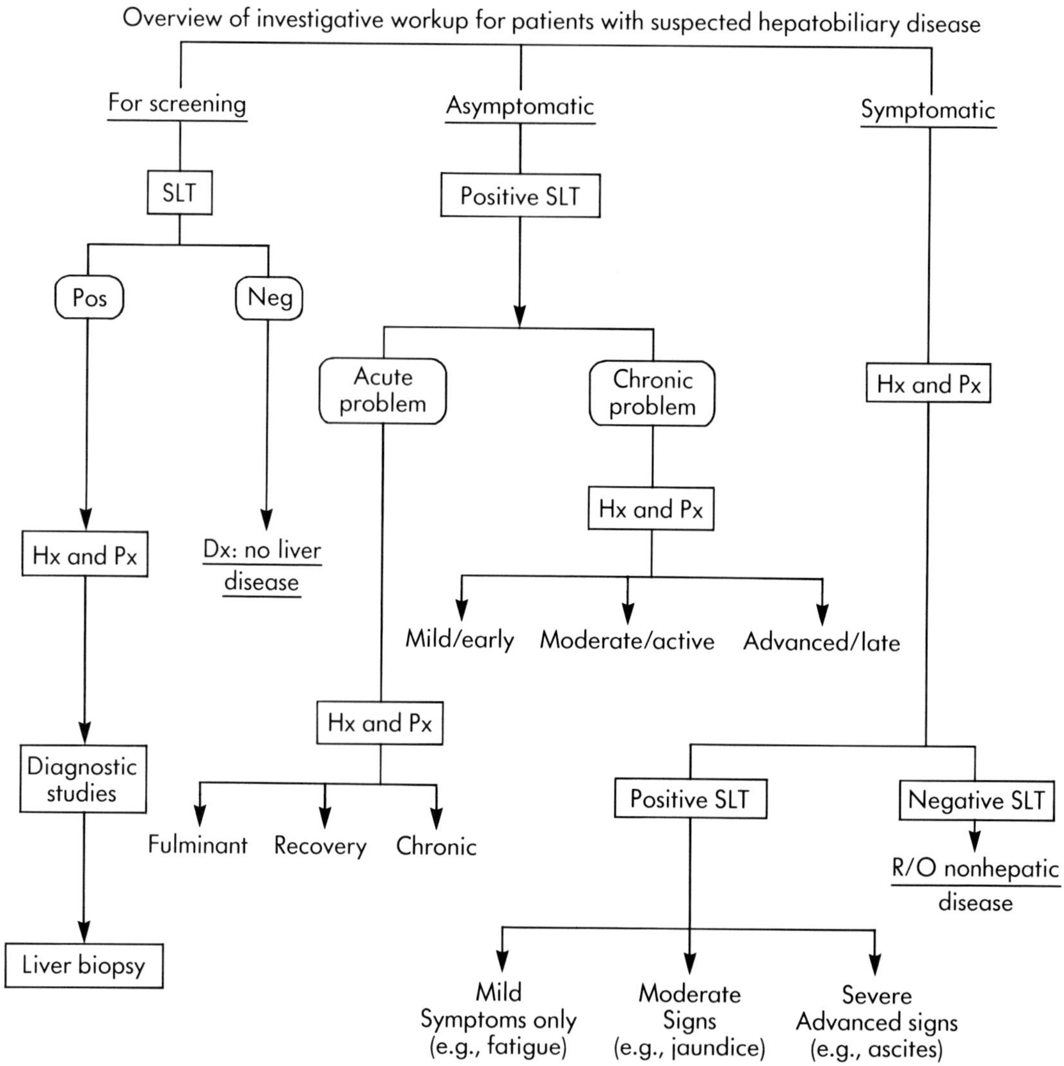

Figure 7-1
Decision algorithm I.

Table 7-2 Basis of tests for quantitation and fractionation of bilirubin

Metabolic components		
Total Bilirubin −	Conjugated bilirubin =	Unconjugated bilirubin
Test response		
	"Direct reacting"	"Indirect reacting"
Laboratory reaction		
Diazoreaction with alcohol	Diazoreaction without alcohol	

liver impairment is complicated by renal failure. As shown in Table 7-2, total bilirubin is determined by a diazoreaction with alcohol. The same chemical reaction without alcohol measures conjugated bilirubin. This measurement is referred to as "direct reacting." The difference between the conjugated bilirubin and the total bilirubin is the unconjugated fraction, referred to as "indirect reacting." This method of determining bilirubin concentration has been of great clinical value, but its limitations need to be recognized. Levels of bilirubin below 50 μmol/dl (2.5 mg/dl) do not permit accurate measurement of the two major fractions. Direct reacting levels overestimate conjugated bilirubin at low concentrations and underestimate it at high concentrations. The main indication for distinguishing the two fractions of bilirubin involves the differential diagnosis of hemolytic vs. obstructive jaundice and certain congenital hyperbilirubinemias.

Urinary bilirubin. Urinary bilirubin and urobilinogen can be detected reliably by using commercially available dipsticks. A positive test indicates hepatic or biliary tract dysfunction. Bilirubinuria can be present before the serum bilirubin level begins to rise. The accurate measurement of urinary urobilinogen is more difficult to test. The total absence of urobilinogen implies complete biliary tract obstruction and can be caused by malignant disease (e.g., pancreatic carcinoma and primary biliary tract tumors), cysts of the pancreatic or biliary duct, and severe alcoholic hepatitis. Determination of the definitive cause requires more direct diagnostic procedures, e.g., ultrasound (US), endoscopic retrograde cholangiopancreatography (ERCP) of the biliary tract, or transhepatic cholangiography (THC).

Hemolytic vs. nonhemolytic jaundice. The bilirubin level is a reflection of the balance between bilirubin production and clearance. The bilirubin production rate is directly related to the red cell's survival time. This time becomes shorter in hemolytic disorders, and the bilirubin level rises in direct proportion to the decrease in red cell survival time. The maximum compensatory RBC increase by the bone marrow is about eightfold and corresponds to a serum bilirubin level of approximately 75 μmol/dl (3.6 mg/dl) or less. There are only two situations in which hemolytic anemia will cause the serum bilirubin level to rise above 75 μmol/dl (3.6 mg/dl). The first is the presence of liver disease in which bilirubin clearance is impaired. The elevated biliru-

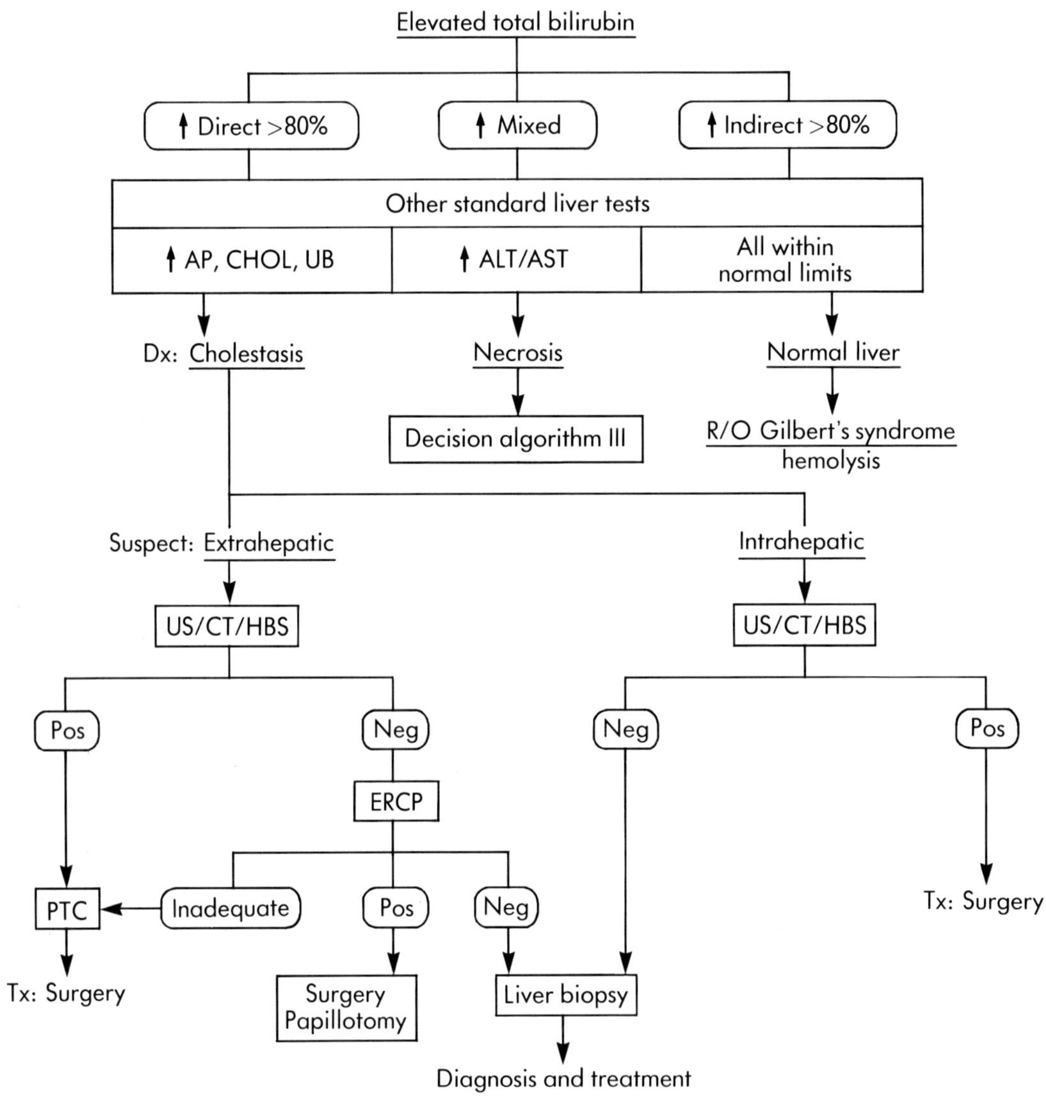

Figure 7-2
Decision algorithm II.

bin is predominantly of the conjugated fraction, e.g., Wilson's Disease with a hemolytic crisis, acute alcoholic hepatitis with severe hemolytic jaundice (Zieve's syndrome), or gram-negative sepsis. The second condition is acute hemolysis in the absence of clinical liver disease, e.g., sickle cell anemia or the thalassemias, in which the production rate exceeds the hepatic clearance. In these conditions the bilirubin will be increasingly conjugated. The distinction between conjugated and unconjugated bilirubin is most useful diagnostically in these complicated situations. Fractionation of the bilirubin is also useful in identifying congenital hyperbilirubinemia. Apart from Gilbert's syndrome, these conditions are rare but are differentiated in most cases when the results of other liver-function studies are normal (Figure 7-2, Decision algorithm II).

Clinical applications in the differential diagnosis of jaundice

Intrahepatic vs. extrahepatic. The term *cholestasis* implies impaired biliary secretion. Extrahepatic cholestasis refers to mechanical obstruction somewhere between the bifurcation of the hepatic duct and the ampulla of Vater in the duodenum. Intrahepatic cholestasis implies impairment of bile flow anywhere proximal to the bile duct, which is readily identifiable by cholangiography or ultrasonography. Conventional or standard liver tests do not readily permit the distinction between intrahepatic and extrahepatic cholestasis, but other laboratory tests do help in the differential diagnosis. Although in cholestasis there is a tendency for all substances secreted in the bile to accumulate in the serum, bilirubin levels do not always increase in the early stages of the disease process. Increases in the levels of serum alkaline phosphatase, GGTP, 5′NI and bile acids precede and correlate well with bilirubinuria, even in the absence of jaundice. In addition, major clinical correlations that sequentially follow these biochemical changes include pruritus, which often precedes the appearance of jaundice by days or weeks, light-colored stool caused by the absence of bile pigment, and dark urine caused by the presence of conjugated bilirubin in the urine. Bile duct patency is confirmed more effectively by ERCP, US, or radioactive imaging (RAI), using technetium(Tc)-labeled hepatobiliary imaging agents (e.g., iminodiacetic acid [IDA] derivatives: dimethyl [HIDA] and p-isopropyl [PIPIDA]). When combined with a liver biopsy, these tests give accurate results in more than 95% of cases. Table 7-3 illustrates the differential characteristics of laboratory tests of the common causes of jaundice. Figure 7-2, Decision algorithm II, illustrates the clinical approach to patient evaluation.

Serum enzyme studies. Plasma enzyme activity is mainly due to the release of enzyme proteins from tissue cells as a result of cell turnover or injury. Even though some enzymes are liver-specific, e.g., ornithine carbamyl dehydrogenase (OCD) or sorbitol dehydrogenase (SDH), they are less suitable for clinical evaluation of liver injury because of their low sensitivity.

Aminotransferases. The liver cells contain many enzymes referred to as transaminases. The two most widely used are the aspartate aminotransferase (AST), previously known as serum glutamic oxaloacetic transaminase (SGOT), and the alanine aminotransferase (ALT), previously known as serum glutamic pyruvic transaminase (SGPT). ALT and AST are found in liver, heart, bone, muscle, eryth-

Table 7-3 Differential characteristics of laboratory tests of the common causes of jaundice

Tests	Acute viral hepatitis	Drug cholestatis	Stones in common bile duct	Pancreatic carcinoma	Chronic viral hepatitis	Chronic alcoholic hepatitis	PBC and PSC
White blood cell (WBC) count	Decreased	Normal	Increased or normal	Increased or normal	Decreased	Increased	Normal
WBC	Increased lymphocytes	Eosinophilia initially	Increased polymorphs	Normal	Increased lymphocytes	Increased polymorphs	Normal
Occult blood	Negative	Negative	Negative	Positive	Negative	Positive	Negative
Urobilinogen	Negative early Positive late	Negative early Positive late	Positive	Negative	Increased late	Increased late	Increased late
Serum bilirubin (mg/dl)	Varies with severity	Variable	Usually 3-10	Steady rise to 15-30	Varies with severity up to 200	Varies with severity up to 60	Progressive up to 200
Serum AP (IU/dl)	<130	>130	>130	>130	>130	>130	>130
Serum transaminase units	>500 (early)	<100	<100	<100	>100	<100 low	<100
ALT/AST ratio	>1	Positive/negative	Positive/negative	Positive/negative	>1	<1	Positive/negative
Total serum cholesterol (mg/dl)	<300	>300	Variable	Variable	Low <200	Low <200	PBC: elevated PSC: progressive

rocyte, kidney, brain, and lung tissue. However, the ALT activity is much greater in the liver. The serum half-lives of ALT and AST are 18 and 48 hours, respectively.

These aminotransferases are sensitive tests of hepatic dysfunction, and their specificity increases with the enzyme level. Levels that are 10 times the upper limit of normal (10 × ULN) reflect primary hepatocellular damage in the form of either acute (viral, drug, or chemical) or chronic (viral, or autoimmune) forms of hepatitis. Occasionally, acute cardiac failure or shock and, less frequently, obstructive jaundice with ascending cholangitis cause AST levels in this range.

The etiology of serum levels <10 × ULN is less specific. Serum ALT/AST levels are only modestly increased in patients with alcoholic, drug, and chemical hepatitis compared with patients with viral hepatitis, in whom the ALT activity is markedly elevated. ALT/AST ratios <1 strongly suggest an alcoholic etiology. At these levels, etiologic inference is made by considering the relationship to the other liver studies, such as AP, GGTP, and bilirubin. Decision making in patients with ALT/AST ratios that are solely or predominantly elevated is shown in Figure 7-3, Decision algorithm III.

Alkaline phosphatase. Alkaline phosphatase (AP) is a group of enzymes that hydrolyze phosphate esters at alkaline pH. These enzymes are present in several kinds of tissue, including liver, bone, and intestinal, as well as in the placenta during pregnancy. The hepatic-derived AP is associated with the bile canalicular membranes' exterior surface and is believed to enter the bloodstream through the paracellular pathway, i.e., regurgitation from the canaliculus at the intracellular junction complex, as well as directly across the plasma membrane. AP may also be associated with the transport of bile acids into bile.

Increases in serum AP are seen in bile duct obstruction and are due neither to the liver cells' failing to clear AP from serum nor to the release of this enzyme from damaged hepatocytes, as in the case of the transferases. Impairment or obstruction of bile ductular flow appears to stimulate the hepatic synthesis of AP and to obstruct its excretion. Such obstruction may be at any level of the biliary tract, from the high intrahepatic ducts, e.g., in biliary cirrhosis or granulomatous disease, down to the common bile duct, e.g., gallstones, bile duct strictures, and pancreatic tumors. An increase in AP often precedes the onset of jaundice. In the absence of a concomitant increase in bilirubin concentration, such increased activity is highly suspicious for primary or secondary intrahepatic tumors causing biliary obstruction. Extrahepatic causes of increased AP occur during pregnancy, during the period of rapid bone growth in adolescence, in bone disease, and in certain malignant tumors. Such increases can be misinterpreted as evidence of liver disease. Fractionation of the AP enzymes by starch or polyacrylamide-gel electrophoresis can identify three distinct bands corresponding to liver, bone, and intestinal AP isoenzymes. Additional bands can be seen in pregnant women and in patients with malignant liver disease. Fractionation of the isoenzymes is only semiquantitative but is sufficiently sensitive to identify which isoenzymes are responsible for the increase in AP activity.

An older, alternative approach is heat fractionation of the AP. The standard AP assay is repeated after heating serum sam-

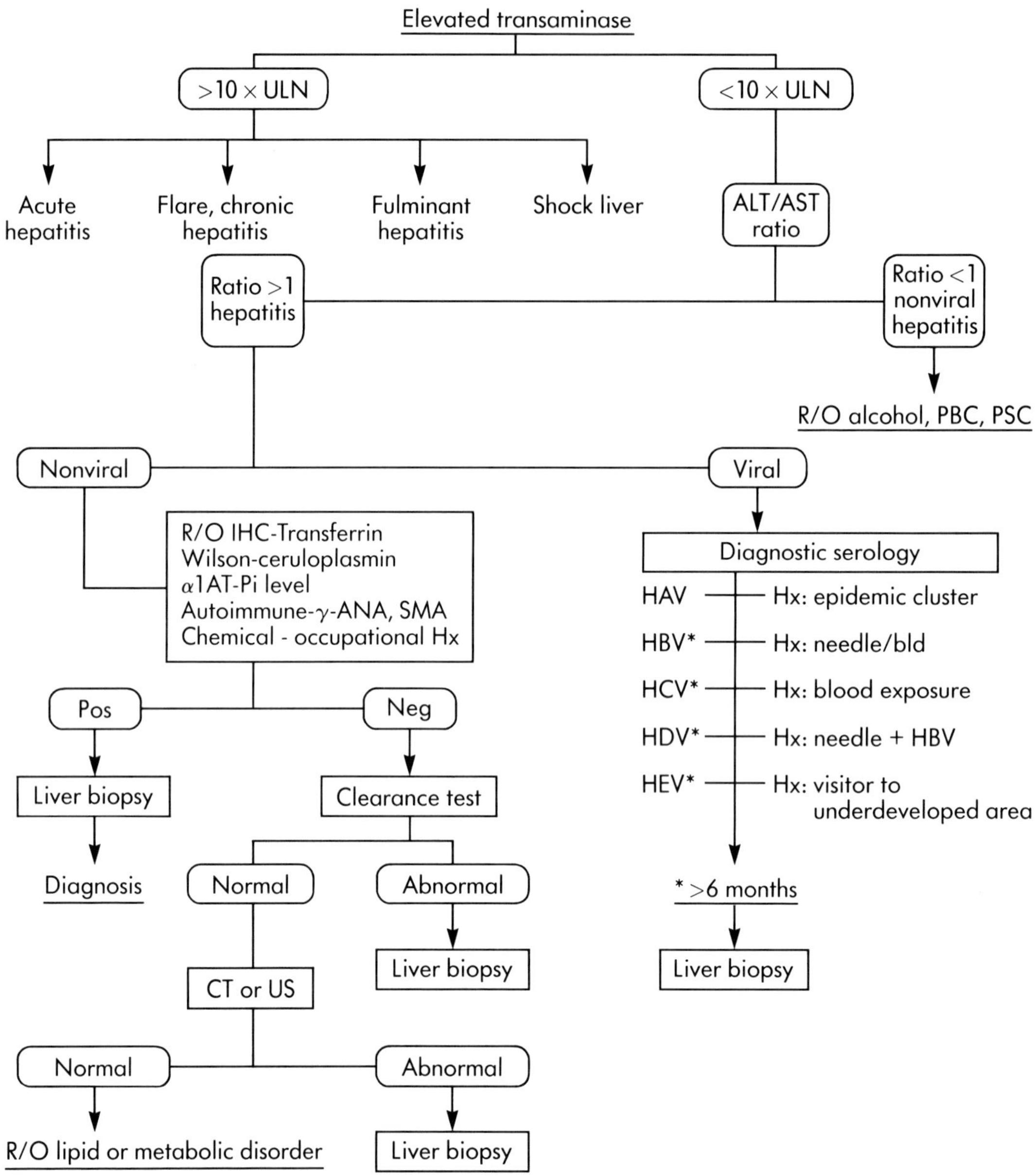

Figure 7-3
Decision algorithm III.

ples at 56° C for 15 minutes. The liver and bone isoenzyme phosphatase activities will be reduced to about 40% and 15%, respectively, of their original values. Placental isoenzymes remain unaffected. This method is not as discriminatory as electrophoresis but is easier to perform and can be used as a rough guide. Figure 7-4, Decision algorithm IV, deals with patients who demonstrate solely or predominantly elevated AP during laboratory examination.

γ-Glutamyl transpeptidase. γ-Glutamyl transpeptidase (GGTP) is a microsomal enzyme that transfers the glutamyl groups from γ-glutamyl peptides, other peptides, or amino acids. GGTP is widely distributed throughout the body tissues, but the serum levels are attributable mainly to the liver isoenzymes. In cholestasis the activity of GGTP parallels that of AP but is more sensitive. GGTP levels tend to rise in all forms of liver injury, and an elevated level is not always due to liver cell damage per se but can be induced by drugs, alcohol, and pancreatic, cardiac, and diabetic conditions. The major clinical usefulness of this test falls into two categories. First, in the presence of an elevated serum AP, a concomitant elevation of GGTP activity suggests that the AP originates in the liver. The second use of GGTP is in screening for alcohol abuse. GGTP is consistently elevated in alcoholics with liver disease but in only one quarter of those without liver disease. The absolute value does not correlate with the amount of alcohol consumed or the duration of drinking. Figure 7-5, Decision algorithm V, deals with solely or predominantly elevated GGTP.

Other serum enzyme studies. The 5′NT and leucine aminopeptidase (LAP) enzymes also parallel elevations of AP of liver origin. 5′NT catalyzes the hydrolysis of nucleotides and is located mainly on the canalicular membrane. Both 5′NT and LAP are increased in cholestatic conditions and are not elevated in patients with bone disease. The main advantage of 5′NT over ALT and GGTP is its liver specificity. Both of these serum enzyme activities mainly indicate the next most useful test rather than serve as the basis for diagnosis or therapeutic decisions. In most cases the combination of AST/ALT, AP, and GGTP provides satisfactory indications.

LDH is another frequently performed serum enzyme test, especially in automated chemistry panels. Clinically it has limited diagnostic value in either acute or chronic liver disease. A major exception is when it is the sole enzyme elevation or is disproportionately increased compared with other enzymes. Figure 7-6, Decision algorithm VI, deals with such cases.

Serum proteins. All plasma proteins are synthesized by the liver's hepatocytes except the immunoglobulins, which are synthesized by the reticuloendothelial system. The serum proteins most important in the diagnosis of various liver diseases include albumin, coagulation proteins, transferrin, ceruloplasm, and α-1 antitrypsin.

Serum albumin. Albumin is the major circulating protein. It is synthesized exclusively in the liver at about 12 gm/day. The total body pool is about 300 gm, with 60% in the extravascular pool and 40% in the vascular pool. The serum half-life is 21 days, and the liver is probably the primary site of breakdown. Albumin is the major factor in maintaining plasma oncotic pressure. It binds numerous hormones and ions, drugs, and fatty acids.

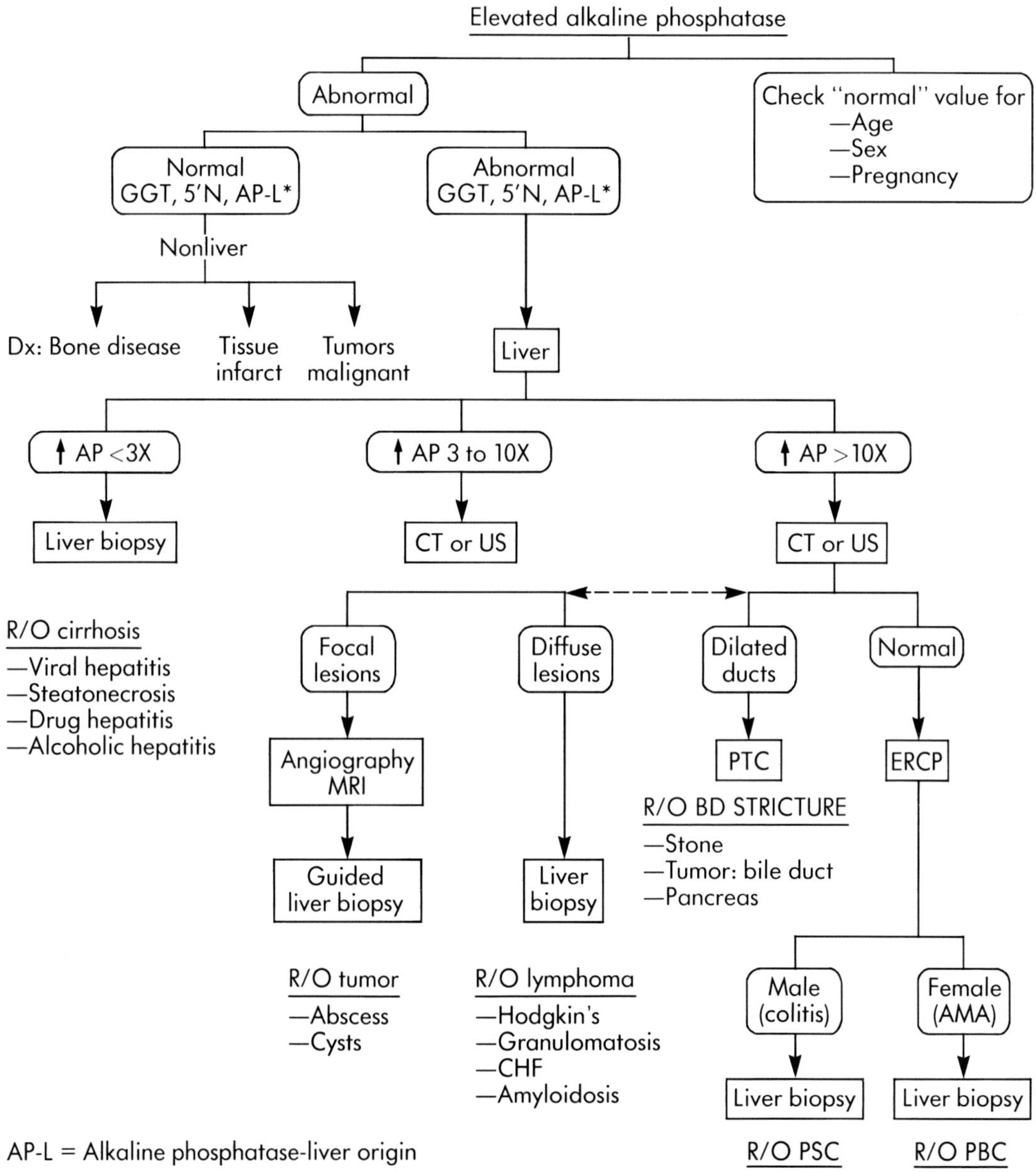

Figure 7-4
Decision algorithm IV.

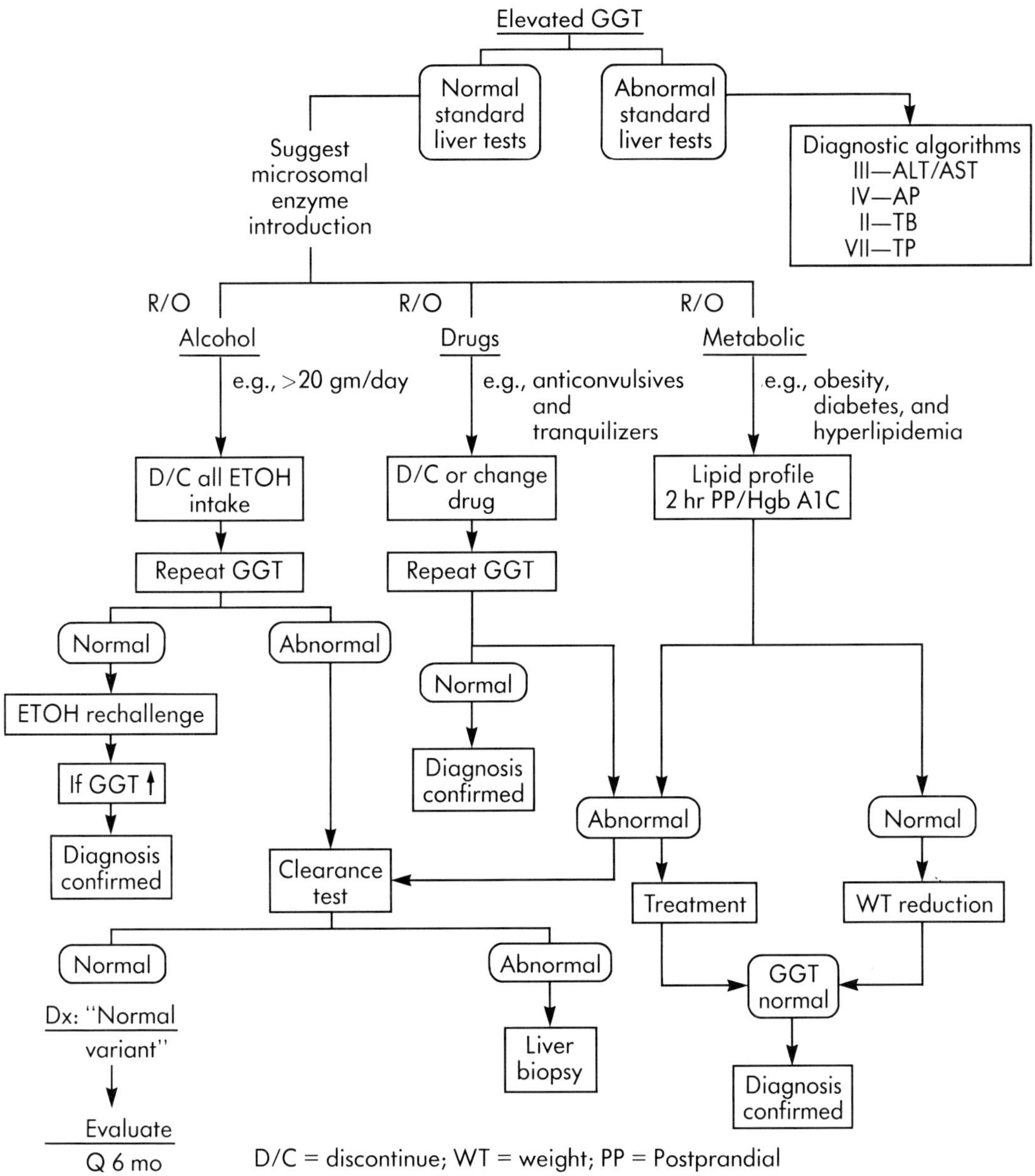

Figure 7-5
Decision algorithm V.

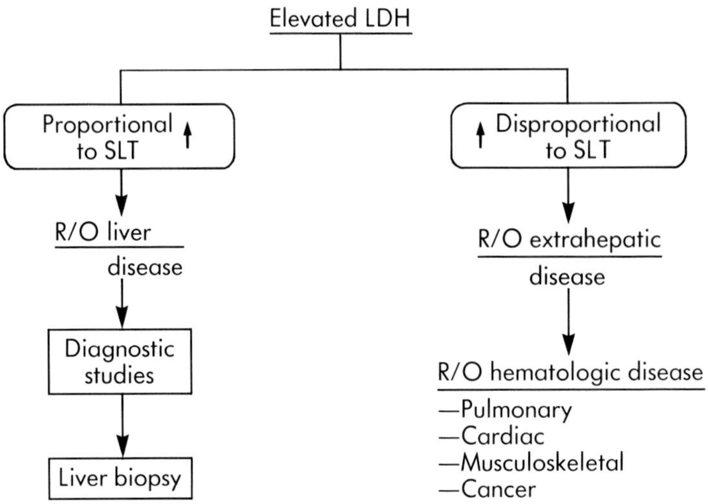

Figure 7-6
Decision algorithm VI.

The serum albumin level is regarded as an index of hepatic "synthetic function." However, several other factors influence the serum levels and must be taken into account: (1) an adequate protein intake; (2) decreased albumin levels caused by protein leakage into the lymph, abdominal cavity (ascites), or other extravascular compartments; (3) serum albumin dilution caused by salt and water retention; (4) drug or alcohol inhibition of albumin secretion from the hepatocytes despite normal synthesis; (5) concomitant compensatory reduction in degradation with impaired synthesis; and (6) slow change in serum levels caused by its long life (21 days), with serum levels mainly reflecting chronic changes.

Normal albumin levels in patients with cirrhosis are an indicator of good synthetic function. The majority of patients with mild cirrhosis have albumins in the normal range. However, only 15% of those with clinical evidence of cirrhosis are likely to have a normal serum albumin. Figure 7-7, Decision algorithm VII, deals with patients who have low serum albumin (<3.5 mg/dl [<35 g/L]).

Serum globulins. A fall in serum albumin is frequently associated with a compensatory rise in globulins. Extreme elevations (>50 gm/dl) are unusual except in autoimmune liver disease and severe CAH.

Prothrombin. The PT (indirect test for prothrombin content) is rapidly achieving status as a function test. In liver disease a prolongation of the PT indicates either a vitamin K deficiency (caused by malnutrition or obstructive jaundice) or poor utilization (caused by parenchymal liver disease). The prothrombin content is measured indirectly by a Quick's One-Stage PT measurement. This is the rate at which prothrombin is converted to thrombin in the presence of thromboplastin, calcium, and other coagulation factors. A prolonged PT in patients with chronic liver disease indicates advanced disease. This is most useful in the identification of impending subacute or acute FHF in patients with acute hepatitis. An

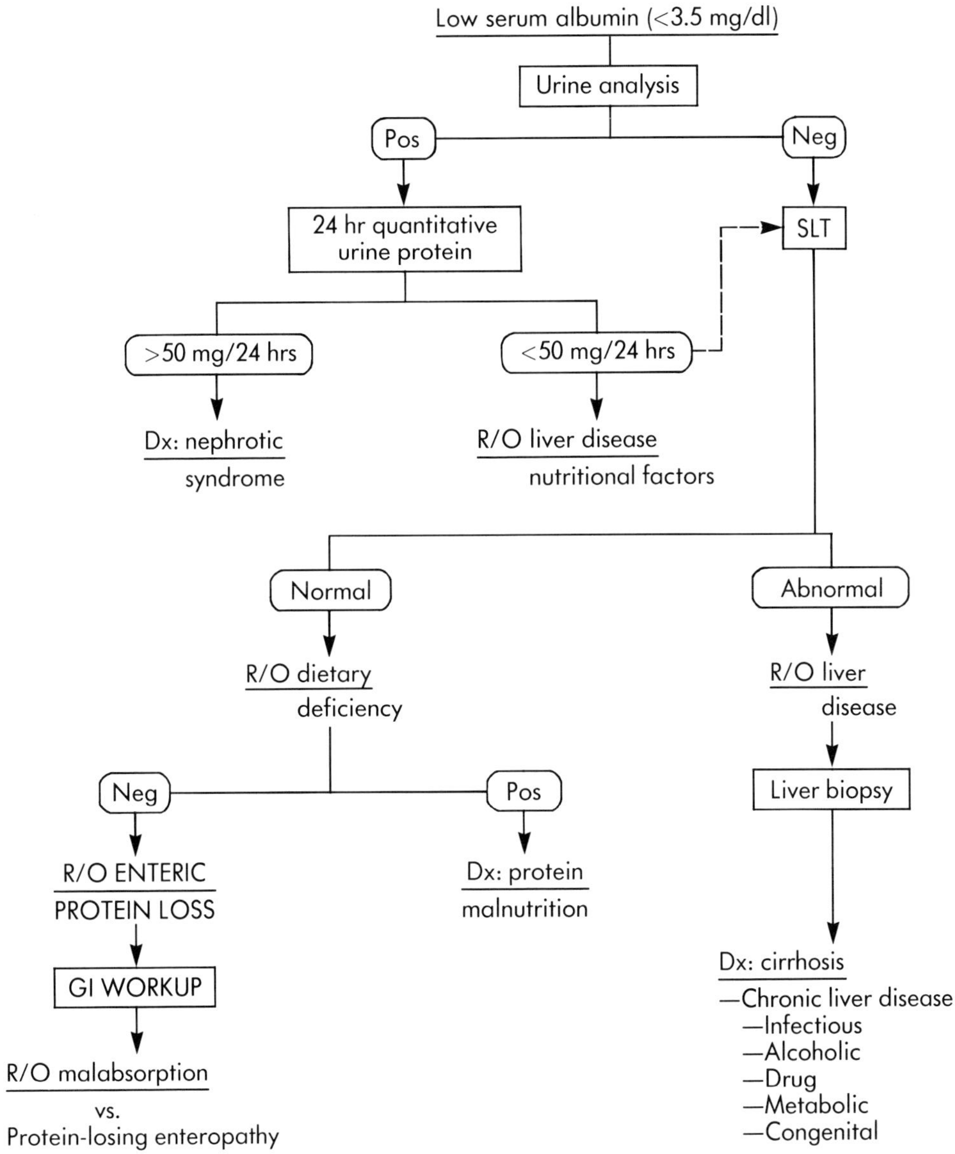

Figure 7-7
Decision algorithm VII.

Table 7-4 Use of PT in the identification of acute FHF

	Day 1	Day 2	Day 3	Day 4
PT	13	15	14	16
Standard control range	11-14	11-14	11-14	11-14
Difference	−1	+1	0	+2
Specific control value	12	13	11	11
difference	+1	+2	+3	+5

increasing prolongation of the PT is indicative of impending hepatic failure. Conversely, its return toward normal signals impending recovery. A prolonged PT in patients with chronic liver disease indicates advanced disease, and its progressive increase identifies potential candidates for hepatic transplantation.

In such cases the earliest and most accurate indicator of impaired prothrombin production is the difference in the PT and specific value of the control, *not* the control range. Table 7-4 illustrates this difference over a 4-day observational period in patients with severe liver injury. Using the difference between the control range and the patient's PT fails to identify progressive worsening of PT, but the time difference between the specific control value and the PT does identify worsening PT.

A prolonged PT in chronic liver disease (>3 seconds above control) also identifies individuals potentially at increased risk of hemorrhage after liver biopsy. PTs 3 to 6 seconds over control can be corrected by the use of fresh-frozen plasma or a 10-day course of anabolic steroids immediately preceding the liver biopsy.

Special Biochemical Studies

There are several biochemical tests that are not "routine" but are gaining acceptance or have special use in the diagnostic investigation of appropriate patients.

Bile acids. Serum bile acids (SBA) have a distinctive physiologic role, but their use as a diagnostic test was limited in the past because of the technical difficulty in measuring their serum levels. Now, simple, sensitive methods are available.

Bile acids are steroid molecules synthesized in the liver from cholesterol. Cholic acids (CA) and chenodeoxycholic acids (CDCA) are primary acids. Before being secreted in bile, they are conjugated with either taurine or glycine, thereby increasing their solubility. After passage into the small intestine (to facilitate fat absorption), most bile acids are actively reabsorbed from the ileum. Bile acids reaching the large bowel are partially deconjugated by the action of bacterial 7-α dehydroxylase to the secondary bile acids, deoxycholic acid (DOCA) and lithocholic acid (LCA). A third metabolite, ursodeoxycholate, a stereoisomer of CDCA, is a tertiary bile acid found in trace amounts. These bile acids are confined largely to the intrahepatic circulation with less than 1% being present in the peripheral blood. However, under pathologic conditions the hepatic clearance becomes important and is dependent on liver blood flow and the degree of portal systemic shunting.

Clinically, serum bile acid levels are elevated in most patients with chronic liver disease because of impaired hepatic uptake secondary to hepatocellular dysfunction or portal systemic shunting. Elevations of SBAs are remarkably specific for the presence of liver disease, with the only exception being bacterial overgrowth in the small intestine. The test is less sensitive in detecting early acute or mild liver disease. When combined with AST/ALT (more sensitive tests for mild liver disease), SBA permits mild and severe chronic liver disease to be distinguished. There is no advantage to the postprandial sample (take 2 hours after meals) over the fasting sample. Bile acid levels during fasting are an excellent second-level test in identifying patients suspected of having significant liver disease for whom conventional tests are normal or borderline.

Clearance tests

Quantitative evaluation of liver function. Clearance tests are quantitative studies of the ability of the liver to clear certain exogenous compounds from the body. Such test compounds are eliminated mainly or exclusively by the liver. Such tests reflect the functional hepatic mass and are affected in various ways by blood flow.

Indocyanine green is an anionic dye taken up solely by the liver and excreted unchanged, and without conjugation. Except for rare mild urticarial reactions, it is virtually nontoxic.

Galactose-elimination capacity is determined by the intravenous administration of galactose over the initial 15 minutes during zero-order clearance.

The aminopyrine breath test and the antipyrine and the caffeine clearance tests are quantitative tests of microsomal function based on the hepatic clearance of these compounds. Clearance is evaluated by either direct measurement or the determination of the concentration of radio-labeled CO_2 released from the compound into the breath. Aminopyrine breath samples are collected by a trapping solution of ethanol and hyamine at fixed times, either at multiple half-hour intervals or during a single, 2-hour sample. Results are expressed as a percentage of the total dose administered. In clearance studies, decreased fractional excretion reflects decreased functional hepatic mass, and the clearance of the substances is not significantly altered by hepatic blood flow. These clearance studies are becoming increasingly important in evaluating candidates for hepatic transplantation, by attempting to identify the patient's prognosis and rate of disease, progression, thus determining the ideal time for transplantation, while minimizing the associated risks.

Blood ammonia and amino acids. A major role for the liver is defending the brain against noxious nitrogenous compounds originating from protein breakdown in the gut. In cirrhosis, portal hypertension leads to portal systemic shunting: bypassing the liver and allowing these nitrogenous products to reach the brain, causing portal systemic encephalopathy (PSE). Patients with PSE characteristically exhibit increased concentrations of aromatic amino acids (i.e., phenylalanine and tyrosine) and reduced concentrations of branched-chain amino acids (leucine, isoleucine, and phenylalanine). Ammonia tolerance tests can be used to identify significant portal systemic shunting. This test involves the administration of an oral dose of 3 gm of ammonium chloride and the measurement of arterial ammonium 45 minutes after administration. A rise of >150 μgm/dl is abnormal and indicates significant portal systemic shunting.

Table 7-5 Differentiation of primary vs. secondary renal failure in liver disease

	Acute tubular necrosis	Primary renal disease	Secondary renal failure
Urine sodium meg/l	>20	<10	<10
Urine/Plasma (U/P) osmolality ratio	<1.1	1.1-1.15	>1.15
Osmolality	P > U	P < U	P << U

Tests of hepatic fibrosis. Presently, the only method for assessing fibrosis has been histologic examination of liver tissue. Despite the subjective nature of this test and the high potential for sampling error, there is no better test at the moment. However, considerable interest has recently developed in the immunologic methods for assaying aminoterminal procollagen type III peptides (PIIIP). Procollagen peptides are globular proteins that are cleaved from the ends of the procollagen molecule by procollagen endopeptidases to leave the helical part of the molecule to grow further. PIIIP shows promise for both diagnosing disease and monitoring its progression in response to treatment. The serum levels of PIIP appear to reflect fibrogenesis (rate of ongoing fibrosis) rather than the quantitative amount of fibrosis. This test is still under investigation.

Urine tests. Renal failure may also develop in cirrhotic patients who become fluid-depleted or septic. Tests of sodium and osmolality of urine and blood can be used to distinguish functional renal failure from primary renal disease. Table 7-5 identifies the means of differential diagnosis of renal failure in several liver diseases using urinary sodium and urine and plasma osmolalities. Only secondary renal failure (i.e., prerenal azotemia) effectively responds to volume expansion.

Peritoneal fluid analysis. In ascites, a frequent complication of hepatic disease, peritoneal fluid analysis can provide clinically significant information regarding its etiology. The appropriate locations for obtaining abdominal fluid for analysis are shown in Figure 7-8. Table 7-6 outlines the various characteristics of ascites and diagnostic follow-up.

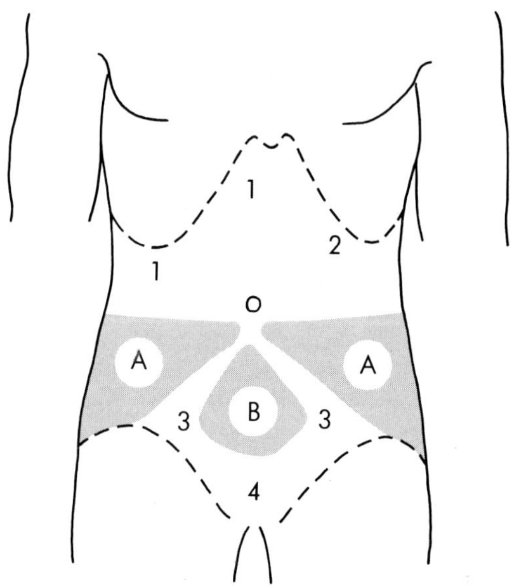

Figure 7-8
The best *(A)* supine and *(B)* upright sites to perform abdominal paracentesis. Locations and organs to avoid include *(1)* liver, *(2)* spleen, *(3)* inferior epigastric arteries, and *(4)* bladder.

Table 7-6 Ascitic fluid analysis

Appearance	Protein	Cells	Bacteria	pH	Diagnosis	Further tests
Clear	<25 mg/dl	<500 all mononuclear			Cirrhosis	
Turbid	>25 mg/dl				R/O tumor Possible fungus, venoocclusive disease	Cytology culture, US, Dopler
Turbid	>25 mg/dl	<500 polys; mono >50%	Yes†		R/O abdominal abscess, bowel perforation	Imaging studies
Turbid	>25 mg/dl	>500 polys; P/L ratio >1	No	?	R/O bowel infarction	Angiography
Turbid	>25 mg/dl	>500 polys; P/L ratio >1	Yes*	<7.3	SBP	Culture
Turbid	>25 mg/dl	>500 lymphs; P/L ratio <1			R/O TB	Culture
Turbid	>25 mg/dl	>100 mixed; P/L ratio ≥1	No	Acid	Pancreatitis	Amylase, lipase
Turbid	>25 mg/dl	>500 RBC			R/O cancer	Cytology
Milky	>25 mg/dl		None		Chylous ascites	Lipid content

* = Single organism.
† = Multiple organism.
P = Polys = neutrophils.
L = Lymphs = lymphocytes.
SBP = Spontaneous bacterial peritonitis.
TB = Tuberculosis.

DIAGNOSTIC TESTS FOR EVALUATION OF LIVER DISEASE

Virologic Studies

Developments in hepatitis virus serology are rapidly changing. There are now five viruses that can be identified immunologically as causing viral hepatitis: A, B, C, D, and E. Tables 7-7, 7-8, 7-9, 7-10, and 7-11 identify the various serologic studies available and the diagnostic patterns used in the diagnosis of each viral infection.

Immunologic studies

There is a variety of immunologically associated chronic liver diseases, which includes autoimmune CAH, PBC, PSC, and some forms of alcoholic liver disease. Immunologic investigation of these diseases involves the measurement of serum immunoglobulins, autoantibodies, and acute-phase reactants.

Serum immunoglobulins. Hyper-γ-globulinemia is a common finding in liver disease, particularly in chronic liver disorders. This condition is usually due to an increase in the γ-globulin fraction and is at least partially a consequence of enhanced antigenic stimulation of the immune system caused by inadequate phagocytic elimination in the liver of gut-derived antigens, which is caused by shunting. Hyper-γ-globulinemia is often indicative of an underlying inflammatory process involving the liver. Quantitative estimations of specific immunoglobulin classes (IgG, IgM) can be useful in the diagnosis of some liver disorders associated with preferential increases in levels of IgG, IgA, or IgM. Typical patterns of changes in the serum concentration of specific classes of serum immunoglobulins (IgA, IgM, and IgG) are shown in Table 7-12.

Autoantibodies. Circulating autoantibodies are immunoglobulins that recognize and bind to normal "self" constituents of tissue. These antibodies are generally classified as organ or non–organ-specific. They react with antigens that are present in one tissue or a limited number of tissues. Non–organ-specific antibodies frequently seen in liver disease include antinuclear antibody, anti–smooth muscle antibody, and antimitochondrial antibody. These antibodies have broader tissue distribution than other antibodies. Table 7-13 characterizes the various autoantibodies related to specific types of liver diseases and their most frequent association.

ANA. Antinuclear antibodies describe a spectrum of autoantibodies that react to a variety of nuclear antigens. Screening for ANAs is usually performed by indirect immunofluorescence (IF). Four distinct IF staining patterns are recognized: (1) homogeneous: diffuse staining of the nucleus, (2) peripheral: staining of the nuclear rim, (3) speckled: uniform fine or clumpy granular, and (4) nucleolar: stain-

Table 7-7 HAV serologic markers

Test results		
Anti-HAV total	**Anti-HAV IgM**	**Diagnosis**
+	+	A
+	−	B
−	+	C
−	−	D

Diagnoses:
A = Acute or recent infection. Infectious.
B = Previous exposure. Immune.
C = Probable false positive. Repeat both tests.
D = No prior exposure. Not immune.

Table 7-8 HBV serologic diagnosis

Test results							Diagnosis
		Anti-HBc					
HBsAG	HBeAG	Total	IgM	HBV/DNA	Anti-HBe	Anti-HBs	
+	+	+	+	+	−	−	A
+	−	+	+/−	+	−	−	B
+	−	+	−	−	−	−	C
+	−	+/−	−	−	+	−	D
+	−	−	−	−	+/−	+	E
−	−	+	+	−	−	−	F
−	−	+	+/−	−	+	−	G
−	−	+	−	−	−	+	H
−	−	+	−	−	−	−	I
−	−	−	−	−	−	+	J
−	−	−	−	−	−	−	K

Diagnoses:
A = Active infection, acute or chronic. Highly infectious.
B = If Igm is positive, early acute infection.† If IgM is negative, test for δ-hepatitis. Partial immune response.
C = Active disease, in recovery, partial immune response.†
D = Antigen (HBsAg) carrier state.
E = Carrier state with exposure to two HBV subtypes.
F = Recent infection, "core window," potentially infectious.
G = If IgM is positive, early recovery phase.* If IgM is negative, late recovery phase.
H = Prior exposure to HBV. Noninfectious. Immune.
I = Previous exposure or low risk of developing latent disease.
J = Vaccine recipient. Noninfectious. Immune.
K = No current disease or past exposure. No immunity.
*Potentially infectious. Low risk.
†Consider infectious. High risk.
‡Test for δ-hepatitis.

Table 7-9 HCV serologic markers

Test results		Diagnosis	Test results		Diagnosis
Anti-HCV	ALT/AST		Anti-HCV	ALT/AST	
Positive	Increased/ increased	A	Negative	Increased/ increased	C
Positive	Normal Increased/ increased	B	Negative	Normal	D

Diagnoses:
A = Active infection. Infectious.
B = Previous exposure or dormant disease.
C = R/O NANB hepatitis, other type(s).
D = No previous or present infection.

Table 7-10 HDV serologic markers

Test results									Diagnosis
HBsAg	Anti-HD		HD Ag	HBeAg	Anti-HBc		Anti-HBe	Anti-HBs	
	Total	IgM			Total	IgM			
+	+	+	+	+/−	+	++ +	−/+	−	A
+	+	+	+	−/+	+/−	+/−	+/−	−	B
+	++	++	+	−/+	+/−	+/−	−/+	−	C
+	+	−	−	−	+	+/−	+/−	−	D
−	+	+/−	−	−	+	+	+/−	+	E
+	−	−	−	+/−	+	−/+	−/+	−	F

Diagnoses:
A = Acute δ-coinfection. Highly infectious.
B = Acute δ-superinfection. Highly infectious early.
C = Chronic δ-superinfection. Highly infectious.
D = Resolved δ-superinfection. Immune to δ, infectious for HBV.
E = Resolved δ-coinfection. Immunity to both delta and HBV.
F = No present or past δ in an acute or chronic hepatitis B.

Table 7-11 HEV serologic markers

Test results		Diagnosis
Anti-HC	**ALT/AST**	
Positive	Increased/increased	A
Positive	Normal	B
Negative	Increased/increased	C
Negative	Normal	D

Diagnoses:
A = Active infection. Infectious.
B = Previous exposure. Immunity questionable.
C = R/O NANB hepatitis, other type(s).
D = No previous or present infection.

ing mainly the nucleolars. These patterns are more typical of certain nonhepatic autoimmune diseases. For example, the homogeneous pattern is typical in systemic lupus erythematous patients, but the patterns add little to the characterization of specific forms of autoimmune liver disease.

SMA. Antismooth muscle antibodies occur in high frequency in acute viral hepatitis, and in a wide range of acute and chronic microbial conditions and other conditions not necessarily involving the liver. In acute infections, SMAs tend to occur transiently and in relatively low titers, being predominantly of the IgM class. The highest titers (>85%) are seen in patients with untreated autoimmune chronic active hepatitis.

Table 7-12 Most frequent serum immunoglobulin patterns

Liver Disease	IgG	IgM	IgA
Autoimmune hepatitis	++*	0/+	0/+
Acute viral hepatitis (transient			
A, B)	++	++	0/+
C	0/+	0/+	0
Chronic viral hepatitis			
B, C	+	+	0
Alcoholic liver disease	+	0	++
With cirrhosis	+	+	++
PBC	+	++*	+
PSC	0/+	+	0/+
Hemachromatosis	0	0	0
Wilson's disease	+	0	0
Drug-induced hepatitis	0	0	0

Code: 0 = No increase.
+ = Increased.
++ = >2 × N.
* = Characteristic finding.

Table 7-13 Frequency and type of autoantibodies found in various hepatic diseases

Disease	ANA group	AMA group	SMA group	LAA group
AIH	60-85% [ANA(H)]	5-30% (M4)	60-85%	>85% (anti-LSP)
DIH	60-85% [ANA(H)]	30-60% (M6)	30-60%	>85% (HMA)
PBC	30-60% (*)	>85% (M2)	30-60%	>85% (HMA)
PSC	5-10% [ANA(H)]	1-5% (*)	5-10%	5-30% (anti LSP)
CH-B	5-30% (anti ds DNA)	1-5% (*)	5-30%	60-85% (anti ASGP-R)
CH-C	5-10% (?)	1-5% (*)	1-5%	30-60% (HMA)
AH-A,B(t)	30-60% (anti ds DNA)	1-5% (*)	60-85%	>85 (anti-LSP)
AH-C(t)	1-5% (?)	<1% (?)	1-5%	30-60% (HMA)
ALD	30-60% (anti ds DNA)	1-5% (*)	30-60%	30-60% (HMA/LMA)
WD	1-5% (*)	<1% (*)	1-5%	1-5% (anti-LSP)
IHC	<1% (*)	<1% (*)	<1%	?

There is considerable overlap in the percentages because these data are derived from referral-type populations and reflect approximate frequencies. Many of these autoantibody subspecificities are available only from investigative laboratories. Techniques for autoantibody screening differ among laboratories, and the clinical interpretation of the test results depends greatly on the precise method used.

Key to codes:
* = No outstanding subspecificities.
( ) = Most frequently positive auto antibody subspecificity.
dsDNA = Double standard DNA.
ASGP-R = Hepatic asialoglycoprotein receptor protein.
LSP = Liver-specific membrane lipoprotein group.
LAA = Liver autoantibodies.
LMA = Liver membrane antibodies.
HMA = Hepatocyte membrane antibodies.
ANA(H) = Antinuclear antibody: homogeneous pattern.
? = Insufficient data available.
t = Transient.
V = Widely varying, frequently reported.
DIH = Drug-induced pseudo lupus with hepatitis.
IHC = Idiopathic hemochromatosis.
WD = Wilson's disease.
ALD = Alcoholic liver disease.
AH-A,B,C = Acute viral hepatitis types A, B and C.
AIH = Autoimmune chronic active hepatitis.
CH-B = Chronic hepatitis B.
CH-C = Chronic hepatitis C.

Table 7-14 Liver disease associations with antimitochondrial antibodies

	AMA specificity
PBC	M2,* M8, M9, M4
Autoimmune CAH	M4
Drug-Induced hepatitis	M6
Healthy individual	M9

*Highly specific for PBC.

ACUTE PHASE REACTANTS COMMONLY ELEVATED IN ACTIVE LIVER DISEASE

α-1 antitrypsin
Ceruloplasm
Ferritin
Fibrinogen
Haptoglobin
Prothrombin
C-reactive protein
Complement components

AMA. Antimitochondrial antibodies (AMA) represent a broad group of autoantibodies that react with several different antigens in mitochondria. At present, nine subspecificities of AMA are recognized. Most subspecificities of AMA are associated with particular diseases though not all of them involve the liver. The M2-AMA antigen on the inner side of the mitochondrial membrane is highly specific for PBC. The M-4-AMA, outer mitochondrial membrane antigen, appears to identify cases of PBC that overlap with autoimmune chronic active hepatitis, or vice versa. Table 7-14 identifies the AMA specificities and their associated liver disorders.

Acute phase reactants. The majority of acute phase proteins (see box at right) are synthesized by the liver, but the stimuli are diverse and variable with certain notable exceptions. Although routine estimations of these proteins have little practical clinical use in the routine laboratory investigation of liver disease, their increased concentration during an acute phase response can cause diagnostic dilemmas. Only an elevated ferritin (suggesting hemochromatosis) requires more definitive diagnostic investigation in relationship to the cause of the liver disease.

Tumor markers. α-Fetoprotein (AFP) is by far the most important serologic tumor marker in liver disease. The ideal tumor marker is one that is easily and reliably detectable, specific for the histologic type, highly sensitive to identify the tumor at a treatable stage, and possessing of a serum concentration proportional to the viable tumor cell mass. To date, no such marker exists, but in primary liver cell cancer, AFP approaches the closest approximation. AFP is normally produced in fetal liver tissue and in actively replicating, regenerating hepatocytes. In clinical practice, AFP has a wide range of serum concentrations from <4 ng/ml in normal subjects to 10,000,000 ng/ml in hepatocellular-cancer patients. Table 7-15 illustrates the approximate range and frequency of AFP found in various hepatic disorders. When the most sensitive methods of AFP detection are used, serum concentrations are found to be elevated above 0-10 ng/ml in 80% of the patients with symptomatic hepatocellular carcinoma. This

Table 7-15 Distribution of α-fetoprotein levels in liver disease†

Disease	Range†	AFP levels‡ <10 ng/ml Unlikely percentage	10-500 ng/ml Suspect percentage	>500 ng/ml Characteristic percentage
HCC* without cirrhosis	$<5\text{-}1 \times 10^7$	~15	~46	~41
Cirrhosis with HCC*	$<5\text{-}1 \times 10^6$	~23	~42	~36
Extrahepatic primary cancer	$<5\text{-}1 \times 10^4$	~92	~7	~1
FHF	$<5\text{-}1 \times 10^3$	~85	~14	~1
Acute hepatitis	$<5\text{-}1 \times 10^2$	~85	~15	0
Chronic hepatitis	$<5\text{-}1 \times 10^2$	~90	~10	0
Cirrhosis without HCC*	$<5\text{-}1 \times 10^2$	~90	~9	~1
Inactive cirrhosis	$<5\text{-}1 \times 10^2$	~98	~1	~1
Alcoholic hepatitis	<5-75	~93	~7	0

*HCC = Hepatocellular carcinoma.
†Range detected by radioimmunoassay (RIA) in ng/ml.
‡These approximate figures reflect the average frequency reported from 10 studies.

frequency is affected by geographic location (high-incidence areas vs. low-incidence areas), sex (males > females), positive HBV serology (positive > negative), and age (older > younger). Clinical deterioration (i.e., formation of ascites) in patients with cirrhosis may be an indication of developing hepatocellular carcinoma. A serum AFP level >500 ng/ml is virtually diagnostic in this situation. However, values between 10 and 500 ng, require further confirmation. With hepatic tumors in a noncirrhotic liver, only levels in excess of 1,000 ng/ml should be considered strong evidence of hepatocellular carcinoma. As a screening test, AFP is not clinically or economically effective in populations at low risk of developing this tumor. However, in high-risk populations, e.g., viral hepatitis B carriers, cirrhotic patients, and patients from high endemic areas, an AFP concentration of >500 ng/dl is virtually 100% diagnostic of hepatocellular carcinoma. A value of 50 to 500 ng/dl warrants more detailed investigation by both test repetition and radiologic imaging techniques. Values between 10 and 15 ng/dl should be repeated every 3 months with ultrasonographic imaging (Figure 7-9, Decision algorithm VIII). Serial AFP measurements can be extremely useful in monitoring responses to chemotherapy, post-tumor resection, transplantation, or treatment with arterial embolization in HCC patients who are AFP positive.

Hematologic Studies

Prothrombin time. The normal prothrombin time (PT) is between 12 and 16 seconds. Test results should be reported as normal/control value and expressed as

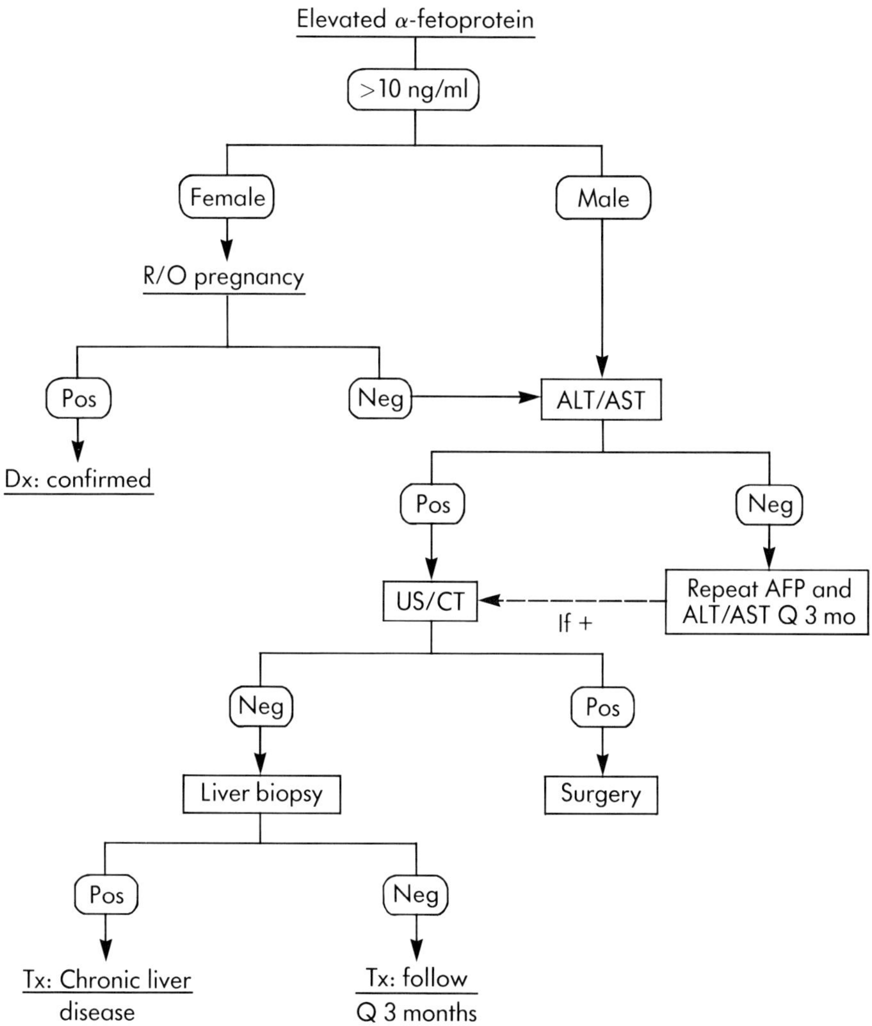

Figure 7-9
Decision algorithm VIII.

Table 7-16 The anemias of liver disease

Type of anemia	Tests							Type of liver disease
	RBC MCV	Serum Fe	TIBC	Transferritin Percentage of SAT	Ferritin	Vitamins: Folate	Vitamins: B_{12}	
Megaloblastic normochromic	>110	N	N	N	N	Decreased	N	Alcoholism with injury
		N	N	N	N/increased	Decreased	Increased	Acute injury
		Decreased	Decreased	Decreased	N	N	N	Chronic disease
Microcytic hypochromic	<80	Decreased	Increased/N	Decreased	Decreased	N	N	Chronic disease with blood loss
Hemolytic	>95	N	N	N	N/increased	N	Increased/N	Autoimmune
		N	N/decreased	N	N	N	Increased/N	Zieve's syndrome, Wilson's disease
Normochromic normocytic	80-95	Decreased	Decreased	Decreased	N	N	N	All forms of chronic chronic disease
Pancytopenia	80-95	N	N	N	N	N	Increased	Acute viral hepatitis, drug toxicity, hypersplenism
Megaloblastic hypochromic	>95	Increased	Increased	Increased	Increased	N	N	Hemochypochromic, thalassemia
		Increased	Increased	Increased	N	Decreased	N	Alcoholic injury

a ratio or as seconds prolonged (Table 7-16). Prolongations of >3 seconds or an International Normalized Ratio (INR) of >1.2 is usually considered abnormal. A prolonged PT suggests either (1) a deficiency less than 30% of normal of one of the four clotting factors; (2) a deficiency of vitamin K; (3) the presence of a specific inhibitor, e.g., warfarin anticoagulation drug; or (4) high concentrations of fibrinogen degradation products (for use of PT as a liver test, see p. 152).

In acute hepatitis a prolonged PT of >5 seconds defines a group of patients at increased risk progressing to acute FHF. PT is the best widely available prognostic indicator.

Partial thromboplastin time. The partial thromboplastin time (PTT) test indicates the integrity of the intrinsic common pathways for coagulation. Although it is frequently used with PT, this test adds little further information for patients with liver disease.

Fibrinogen and its degradation products. Disseminated intravascular coagulation (DIC) is a hemorrhagic syndrome in which any appropriate initiation of the coagulation cascade leads to widespread intravascular coagulation or consumption of the circulating chronic coagulation factors and platelets and, consequently, a fibrinolytic process. It is characterized by (1) a low platelet count, (2) damaged RBCs (schistocytes), (3) a low fibrinogen concentration, (4) a prolongation of PT and PTT, and (5) high titers of fibrinogen-degradation products. The diagnosis of DIC in liver disease is difficult because many of these abnormalities are seen for reasons other than DIC. Patients with severe chronic liver disease also have a low-grade DIC that is not clinically significant.

Anemia. Anemia and abnormalities of the RBCs are common in patients with chronic liver disease and are usually of multifactoral etiology. Table 7-16 identifies laboratory patterns seen in various chronic liver diseases and their associated RBC morphology.

Metabolic Studies

A large number of inherited disorders affect the liver either directly or indirectly. The most frequent include idiopathic hemochromatosis, Wilson's disease, α-1 antitrypsin deficiency, and the porphyrias.

Hemochromatosis. Idiopathic hemochromatosis (IHC) is a genetic disorder with an autosomal recessive mode of inheritance of the gene located on the short arm of chromosome 6. This gene has a close proximity to HLA-A loci and has inheritance patterns of HLA, antigen A-3, and other HLA allotypes, notably B7 and B14. Their clinical significance is uncertain. Standard biochemical liver tests are not very helpful in the diagnosis of IHC. The main diagnostic problem relates to the differentiation of IHC from alcoholic liver disease and secondary iron overload. Specific tests of the body's iron storage must be requested. Table 7-17 identifies typical laboratory findings in various forms of chronic disease with excessive iron concentration. Transferrin saturation is almost always >50% and often >60% in untreated IHC. False-positive rates are also high (approximately 30%). It is generally agreed that the serum concentration of ferritin, an iron-storage protein, is the best index of both hepatic and total body iron stores. RIA, or enzyme-linked immunoassay, is available. Serum ferritin concentrations of <200 ng/dl are considered normal. Most patients with IHC

Table 7-17 Laboratory finding in iron overload liver disease

Diagnosis	Tests				
	SLT	Serum Fe*	TIBC	TF % SAT	Serum ferritin†
No liver disease	WNL	10-30 (50-150)	45-70 (250-410)	20-50%	<200
Subclinical IHC	Often WNL	N/>30	N	>50%	>200-1000
Clinical IHC+	Abnormal	>30	Usually N	>60%	>500-5000
Iron overload CLD	Variable	N/>30	Usually N	N/>50	N/<50

* = mol/L.
SLT = Standard liver tests; TF% SAT = transferrin percent saturation.
WNL = Within normal limits.
Fe = Iron; TIBC = total iron binding capacity.
† = μg/l.
( ) = g/dl.
N = Normal.
+ = hepatomegaly, cardiomyopathy, pseudogout, diabetes mellitus, or increased skin pigmentation.

Table 7-18 Laboratory findings in diagnosis of Wilson's disease

Stage of disease	SLT	Serum ceruloplasmin	Serum	Copper* urine	Hepatic	D-Penicillamine challenge
Subclinical	Usually normal	<20	Variable	>1	1-4	Urine Cu > × 10
Clinical	Abnormal	<13	Variable	>2	>4-10	Urine Cu > × 20
Fulminant	Severely abnormal	<13	>30	>15	>4-10	Unknown

*Serum 10-30 μmol/L (70-150 μg/dl).
Urine 0.25-0.75 μmol/24 hr (15-45 μg/24hr).
Hepatic <1 μmol/gm dry weight.
Ceruloplasmin 13-30 μmol/L (23-43 mg/dl).

have levels >1,000 μgm/dl, but in the early stages, a patient may be in the normal range.

Wilson's disease. Wilson's disease is an inborn error of metabolism leading to abnormal deposits of copper, initially in the liver and then progressively in the kidneys, brain, eyes, and other tissue. It is essential that Wilson's disease be excluded in any young person with evidence of chronic liver disease. Wilson's disease may be asymptomatic (subclinical) or may present insidiously as CAH (clinical) or acutely as fulminant hepatitis, with a hemolytic crisis. Table 7-18 illustrates the laboratory findings in Wilson's disease at

Table 7-19 Association of adult liver disease with α-1AT phenotypes

α-1AT level*	Association				
	None	Occasional	Often	Established	Unknown
200-400	MM				
120-240		FS, SS	MZ		
80-160			SZ		MS
20-60				ZZ	Z nul

*N = 200-400 mg/dl.

its various stages. Overlapping typical laboratory findings related to copper status may be found in acute hepatic necrosis, chronic cholestasis (e.g., PBC), and Indian childhood cirrhosis.

α-1 antitrypsin deficiency. α-1 antitrypsin (α-1AT) is a protease inhibitor (Pi) that occurs normally in the serum in concentrations of 2.4 gm/dl (200 to 400 mg/dl). Deficiency of this protein is associated with lung disease (pulmonary emphysema) and liver disease. Because α-1AT is one of the acute phase reactants, serum levels may be artificially increased in response to inflammatory disease or acute or chronic liver disease, even in α-1AT–deficient subjects. Artificially low levels can occur in patients with severe hepatic necrosis or protein-losin enteropathies. Where there is doubt, the issue can be resolved by determining the phenotype of the individual and, if necessary, of family members. The association of α-1AT phenotypes, serum levels, and liver disease in adults is shown in Table 7-19.

Porphyrias. The porphyrias are a group of hereditary diseases and acquired disorders of heme metabolism that lead to abnormal production of porphyrins and other precursors of heme synthesis. Patients most frequently present with abdominal pain. Unless there is concomitant liver disease of some other etiology, standard liver tests show either a modest increase in ALT/AST activity as the main abnormality or normal liver biochemical studies. Figure 7-10 identifies the types of porphyria and the laboratory tests useful in its differential diagnosis.

DIAGNOSTIC PROCEDURES AND STRUCTURAL STUDIES OF LIVER DISEASE

Hepatic-Imaging Modalities

Several imaging modalities are available for examination and evaluation of the liver and biliary system (see box on p. 170). Some techniques (e.g., abdominal plain film) provide only estimates of liver size while others supply information regarding intrahepatic lesions and hemodynamic status of hepatobiliary vascular systems. It is important to remember that many imaging modalities, like diagnostic procedures, are heavily dependent on operator experience.

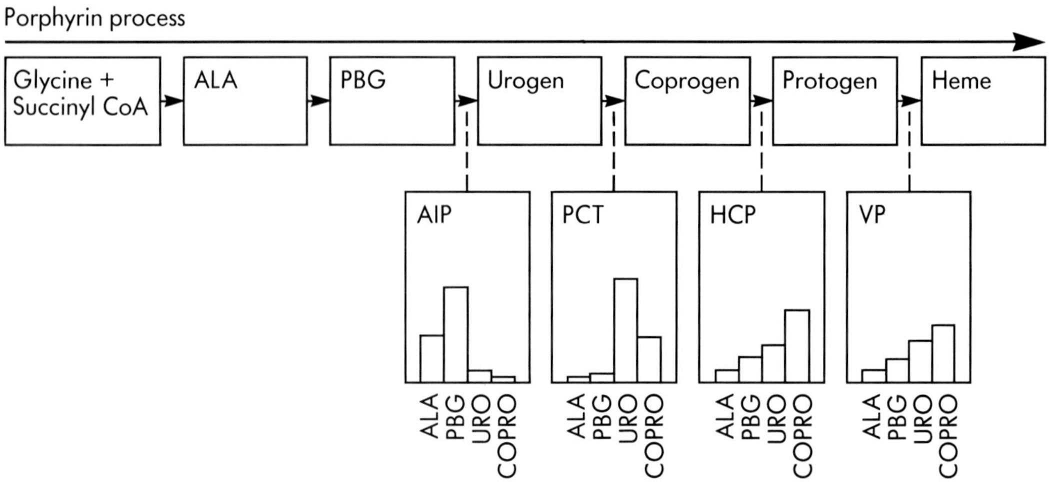

Figure 7-10
Hepatic porphyrias: urine excretion patterns of the various porphyrins and other heme precursors during heme metabolism. *AIP,* acute intermittent porphyria; *PCT,* porphyria cutanea tarda; *HCP,* hereditary coproporphyria; *VP,* variegate porphyria; *ALA,* δ-aminolevulinic acid; *Copro,* coproporphyrin; *PBG,* porphobilinogen; *URO,* uroporphyrin.

Abdominal plain film. The plain film of the abdomen can provide an estimate of liver and spleen size and can demonstrate parenchymal or biliary calcification, air in the biliary tract, cysts or abscesses, and excessive fluid in the abdomen. It is of limited usefulness in the evaluation of hepatic lesions or hemodynamic changes.

Oral cholescystogram. For many, oral cholecystogram (OCG) remains the screening procedure of choice for patients suspected of having chronic cholecystitis. It is easy to perform, requires minimal technology, has low morbidity, and is highly accurate when the gallbladder visualizes. Normal opacification of the gallbladder and an absence of filling defects virtually excludes inflammation. Demonstrations of gallstones implies the presence

HEPATIC IMAGING MODALITIES

- Plain film of the abdomen
- Oral cholecystography
- Hepatobiliary scintigraphy
- Hepatic scintigraphy
- Ultrasonography
- Computed tomography
- Magnetic resonance imaging
- Vascular angiography
- Percutaneous transhepatic cholangiography
- Endoscopic retrograde cholangiopancreatography

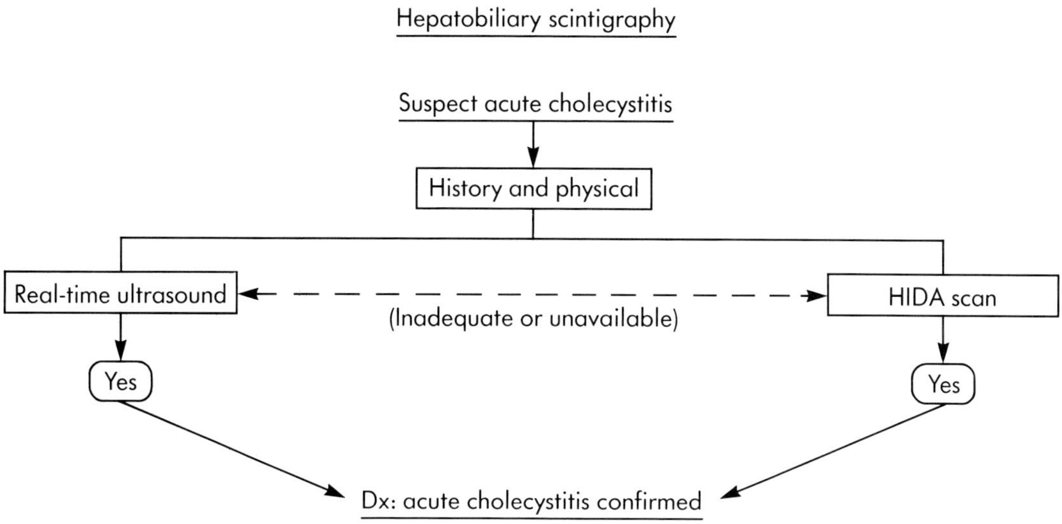

Figure 7-11
Decision algorithm IX.

of cholecystitis in the context of clinical symptoms and abnormal laboratory findings. Nonvisualization of the gallbladder is not specific with numerous causes and requires US examination. Figure 7-11, Decision algorithm IX, and Figure 7-12, Decision algorithm X, used for suspected acute and chronic cholecystitis, respectively.

Radionuclide imaging. Radionuclide imaging (scintigraphy) depends on three functional hepatic components: the RES, bile production, and hepatic blood flow. Hepatocytes account for 65% of total liver cells. Of the remaining liver cells, 10% are RE cells (Kupffer cells), and the other 25% are endothelial and Ito cells.

Hepatic scintigraphy. Hepatic scintigraphy (HS) is used widely for noninvasive evaluation of the liver. Radionuclide colloid, e.g., 99 m Tc–tagged sulfur colloid, is taken up by the RES in the liver. Liver lesions are typically nonspecific "cold" defects (no uptake) because of metastatic primary tumor, cyst, vascular lesion (e.g., hemangioma), abscess, infiltrating disease, or extensive fibrosis. All these lesions lack RES cells to take up the colloid. The sensitivity and specificity of this evaluation system is in the 0% to 85% range, but the system rarely detects lesions less than 2 cm in diameter. It is better at recognizing superficial lesions than deep central ones.

Radionuclides taken up by the hepatocyte, e.g., gallium, can characterize primary tumor or tumorlike conditions as focal, nodular hyperplasia and adenoma, but 99 m Tc–tagged RBCs allow accurate imaging of vascular lesions, e.g., hemangioma.

Radionuclide imaging is useful in determining liver and spleen size. Relative splenic, bone marrow, and lung uptake in

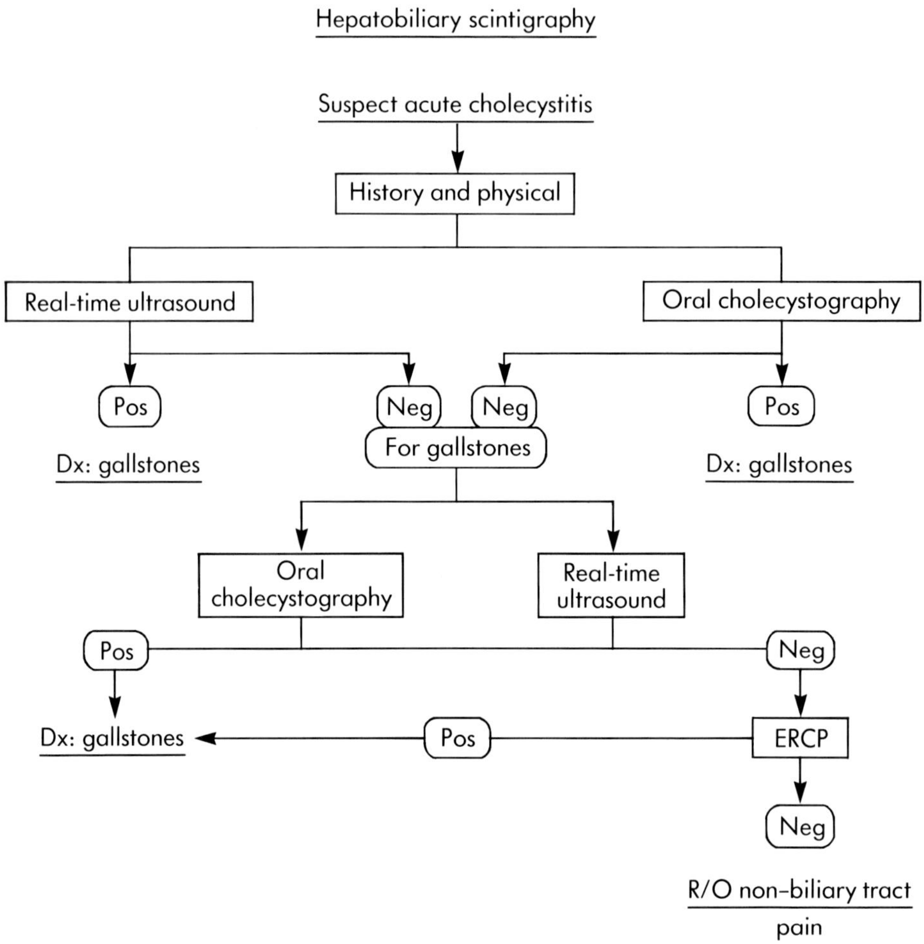

Figure 7-12
Decision algorithm X.

comparison with that of the liver is a good indicator of altered hepatic blood flow in acute disease and the degree of portal hypertension in chronic disease.

Hepatobiliary scintigraphy. The biliary transport system can be studied by immodiacetic acid (IDA), which is promptly taken up by hepatocytes and excreted unconjugated in the bile. The gallbladder and small bowel are usually visualized within 1 hour in normal individuals. The primary role of hepatobiliary scintigraphy (HBS) is the evaluation of the gallbladder and biliary duct system. Nonvisualization of the gallbladder implies an obstructed cystic duct, a hallmark of acute cholecystitis. Delayed visualization (1 to 4 hours) is typical of (1) chronic cholecystitis, presumably caused by partial cystic duct obstruction; (2) secondary fibrosis of the gallbladder wall with decreased compliance; (3) alcoholic liver injury; (4) chronic

INDICATIONS FOR HEPATOBILIARY SCINTIGRAPHY

Preoperative

- Cholescystitis
  - Acute
  - Chronic
- Cholestasis
  - Intrahepatic vs. extrahepatic
  - Acute common duct obstruction
  - Choledochal cyst
- Biliary dyskinesia
- To distinguish hepatic left lobe from spleen

Postoperative

- Postcholescystectomy syndrome
- Biliary enteric anastomosis
- Bile leak
- Patency
- Bile-flow route
- Post–liver transplant function

hepatitis; (5) parenteral hyperalimentation; (6) prolonged fasting (>24 hours); and (7) severe intercurrent disease. This delay can result in a high occurrence of positive findings not indicative of acute cholecystitis.

HBS is useful in the detection of early common bile duct obstruction before dilatation on ultrasound, postsurgical biliary leaks, evaluation of biliary-enteric anastomosis, and the functional status of liver transplants. The indications for HBS are listed in the box above.

Ultrasound. Ultrasound (US) is a totally noninvasive imaging modality that does not require radiation and that can best define cystic vs. solid structures and, more importantly, hepatic vascular flow. In experienced hands, US plays a major role in imaging of the biliary system, especially imaging related to the hepatic duct, common bile duct, cystic duct, and gallbladder. Under normal conditions the intrahepatic bile ducts cannot be completely visualized. US is very effective in evaluating dilation of intrahepatic biliary ducts and enlargement of extrahepatic ducts and in visualizing impacted gallstones within the common duct, pancreatic head tumors, primary gallbladder cancer, and biliary ductal cancers. In very experienced hands, even strictures and ampulla of Vater tumors can be identified. The accuracy of US for diagnosing cholelithiasis is approximately 95%. Exceptions to this accuracy are acute obstruction and a ball-valve type intermittent obstruction.

Stones are detected as brightly echogenic structures with associated acoustic shadowing. However, not all stones are detectable. In experienced hands, using real-time US imaging, hepatic lesions as small as 1 cm can be detected. Table 7-20 gives, in descending order, the areas in which US is most diagnostically useful and identifies complementary imaging or diagnostic procedures.

Computed tomography. Computed tomographic (CT) scanning of the liver is performed with and without the use of intravenous contrast administration. CT is very accurate as an imaging test for detecting liver masses, with a reported sensitivity of >90% for lesions 1 cm or larger. Metastasis, primary liver tumors, and benign lesions (e.g., regenerative nodules) are often indistinguishable. Contrast-enhanced CT of the liver more accurately identifies vascular lesions (e.g., hemangioma), fluid-containing masses (e.g., hematomas), and abscesses. Cirrhosis can be diagnosed using CT and distin-

Table 7-20 Ultrasound evaluation of the liver

Disorder	For detection	For diagnosis
Benign lesions		
Cysts	Very good	—
Solid lesions:		
Cavernous hemangioma	Good	+RN, CT, VA
Focal nodular hyperplasia	Good	+RN
Hepatic adenomas	Good	+RN
Primary lipomas	Good	+CT
Angiomyolipomas	Good	+CT
Abscess		
Echinococceal (hydatid) cyst	Good	+NA/B
Amebic	Good	+NA/B
Pyogenic	Fair to good	+NA/B
Fungal	Poor	+NA/B
Malignant tumor		
Hepatocellular	Very good	+NA/B
Fibrolamellar carcinoma	Good	+CT, NA/B
Metastatic	Good	+NA/B
Lymphomatous lesion	Fair	+NA/B
Leukemia	Poor	+NA/B
Hepatic disease		
Portal hypertension	Very good	+DD
Fatty liver	Good	+NA/B
Cirrhosis	Good	+NA/B
Chronic hepatitis*	Poor	+NA/B
Acute hepatitis*	Poor	+NA/B
Intrahepatic biliary lesion		
Stones	Very good	+ERCP
Stricture	Good	+ERCP, PTC
Sclerosing cholangitis	Good	+ERCP
Congenital abnormalities	Good	+ERCP
Tumor	Fair to good	+CT, surgery

Table 7-20 Ultrasound evaluation of the liver—cont'd.

Disorder	For detection	For diagnosis
Liver transplantation		
Portal/arterial vascular	Very good	+DD
Biliary complication	Very good	+CT
Fluid collection	Very good	+CT
Rejection	Poor	+CT, B

*All types—drug, viral, alcohol-induced, and metabolic.

Code:
Excellent = Most effective diagnostic method (>90%).
Very good = Other procedures add little (>80%).
Good = Should be used with other procedures to corroborate (>70%).
Fair = Varies, depending on stage of disease (50 to 70%).
Poor = Much overlap (<50%).
RN = Radionuclide.
CT = Computed tomography.
VA = Vascular angiography.
NA/B = Needle aspiration/liver biopsy.
DD = Duplex Doppler.

guished from diffuse or multifocal hepatoma, provided adequate contrast enhancement is performed (80% sensitive). Moderate to severe fatty infiltration can be identified using CT if an area of low attenuation with geographic boundaries can be identified. Contrast-enhanced, dynamic scanning of the liver is the study of choice for evaluating vascular lesions. Indications for CT imaging in hepatic disease are shown in the box at right.

Magnetic resonance imaging. Magnetic resonance imaging (MRI) differs from other techniques in that it produces images based on the response of hydrogen and other protons to a known, pulsed, radiofrequency and does not depend on tissue density. The response of these protons, which exist predominantly in body water and fat, is related to the relationship

INDICATIONS FOR COMPUTED TOMOGRAPHIC IMAGING OF THE LIVER

- Evaluation for suspected metastatic disease
- Evaluation for presence and extent of hepatocellular cancer
- Identification of cystic disease
- Detection of hepatic or perihepatic abscess
- Differentiation of obstructive vs. nonobstructive jaundice
- Clarification of anastomic variations
- Assessment of hepatic trauma
- Demonstration of altered hepatic parenchymal density (e.g., fatty liver, cirrhosis, and hemachromatosis)
- Localization and guidance of liver biopsy and PTC
- Evaluation of therapeutic response
- Detection of ascites and peritoneal tumors
- Confirmation of space-occupying lesion found on other noninvasive studies

Table 7-21 MRI proton spin-lattice relaxation times

Normal tissue	Time (msec)
Liver	140-170
Pancreas	180-200
Spleen	250-290
Blood	340-370
Bile	400-600
Pathologic conditions	
Hemochromatosis	120-150
Hepatitis	180-200
Cirrhosis	180-300
Pancreatitis	200-275
Pancreatic carcinoma	275-450
Metastases	290-450
Hepatocellular carcinoma	300-450
Cholangiocarcinoma	300-450
Hemangioma	340-370
Pus	350-500
Ascites	600-1,000
Simple cyst	800-1,000

of water to body proteins; i.e., MRI gives a measurement that varies according to body chemistry not density. This response produces two types of images: (1) using proton density as the image parameter and (2) using proton spin-lattice relaxation time, or Tl.

In the first case, a 90° radiofrequency pulse causes the protons to absorb this energy, changing their alignment relative to the applied magnetic field. When the pulse is ended, the protons relax one by one back to their original alignment, reradiating the absorbed energy that is measured and known as "proton density."

In the second case a 180° radiofrequency pulse is used. The proton spins are completely inverted, and the length of time needed for their relaxation is associated with their environment. The rate of the omitted radiation falls exponentially at a rate characteristic of the environment or lattice, of which they are part. This is known as "proton spin-lattice relaxation time", or Tl. The Tl times for normal hepatobiliary related tissue and some pathologic conditions are shown in Table 7-21.

HEPATOBILIARY MASSES IDENTIFIABLE BY VASCULAR ANGIOGRAPHY

Solid masses

- Malignant
  - Hepatocellular carcinoma
  - Metastatic carcinoma
  - Angiosarcoma
  - Miscellaneous tumor
- Benign
  - Adenoma
  - Nodular hyperplasia
  - Regenerative nodules
  - Hemangioma

Cystic masses

- Cysts
  - Solitary
  - Polycystic
  - Hydatid
- Abscesses
  - Pyogenic
  - Amebic
  - Tuberculoma
  - Gumma
- Hematoma

Vascular angiography. Selective hepatic arteriography is the most accurate means of detecting a lesion occupying hepatic space and assessing its nature. Its overall rate for diagnosis of hepatic tumor is reported to be from 74% to 97%. In addition, it also delineates vascular supply of both normal and tumor tissue which is important for hepatic resection or devascularization procedures. A list of solid and

INDICATIONS AND CONTRAINDICATIONS FOR PTC

Indications

Differentiation of intrahepatic vs. extrahepatic cholestasis
Demonstration of the site and nature of biliary obstruction
Identification of the anatomic structure of the biliary tract
Identification of a choledochoduodenal junction lesion
Study of the postcholecystectomy syndrome
Indirect diagnosis of hepatobiliary disease and a pancreatic-enteral lesion

Contraindications

Uncontrollable bleeding tendency
Continuous high fever*
Hypersensitivity to contrast medium
Extremely poor general health

*Fever caused by biliary tract obstruction requires drainage combined with PTC.

cystic liver masses demonstrable by VA are listed in the box on p. 176.

Percutaneous transhepatic cholangiography (PTC). Although the first roentgenologic visualization of the biliary tract by percutaneous puncture of the gallbladder was carried out in 1921, the technique was made safer and more effective by the development of the unsheathed Chiba needle technique (developed by Chiba University Hospital) in the late 1960s. With the use of real-time US and a puncture transducer, both the intrahepatic bile duct system and the portal vein system can be studied selectively. PTC is also effective for percutaneous drainage of and shunt placement in the biliary tract in the management of obstructive jaundice. The indications and contraindications for this procedure are listed in the box at top, left.

INDICATIONS FOR ERCP

Diagnostic endoscopy

Biliary diseases
- Visualization of ampulla of Vater
- Visualization of biliary tree
- Visualization of gallbladder
- Study of gallbladder function and sphincter of Oddi

Pancreatic diseases
- Pancreatitis
- Neoplasia
- Cyst
- Trauma

Therapeutic endoscopy

Sphincterotomy
Sphincter dilation
Nasobiliary drainage/decompression
Biliary stent placement
Dissolution of calculi
Duct stenosis dilation
Duct stone removal

Diagnostic studies

Bile analysis and culture
Cytology
Pancreatic secretion
Manometry: biliary duct and sphincter of Oddi

Endoscopic retrograde cholangiopancreatography. Endoscopic retrograde cholangiopancreatography (ERCP) is an excellent procedure for studying the biliary tract, even though the success rate in selective cannulation (85% to 90%) is a problem. ERCP is performed to investigate jaundice of obscure etiology when other imaging techniques (HBS, US, CT, etc.) fail to visualize the biliary ducts adequately and to investigate upper abdominal pain without demonstrable etiology.

ERCP also has therapeutic capabilities in hepatobiliary disease. The indications for ERCP are shown in the box on p. 177 and discussed in detail in Chapter 30.

Liver Biopsy

Diagnostic aspiration of liver tissue as a routine application began with reports on the histopathology of viral hepatitis obtained in the late 1930s using this technique and became widely used with the introduction of the Vim-Silverman and later the Menghini biopsy procedures. The liver biopsy plays a very important role in the investigation of human hepatic disease and is a necessary and often sufficient means of correct assessment of disease and response to therapy.

Needle biopsy is a safe procedure when done by an experienced operator. In trained hands the risk of complication (morbidity) is 0.3% to 0.5%, and the risk of mortality is in the range of 0.01% to 0.02%. The indications and contraindications for liver biopsy are shown in the box at right.

Either of the two percutaneous methods of liver biopsy will obtain adequate tissue in <95% of noncirrhotic individuals. In cirrhotic individuals, the core type needle (e.g., Tru-Cut) consistently obtains a contiguous adequate specimen. Suction-type needles often yield fragmented tissue (>50%).

Aspirated biopsy specimens are usually adequate (>10 mm) for assessing any diffuse hepatic condition. Fragmentation results from faulty technique. Unusual fragmentation caused by excess stability of tissue, especially from tumor or cirrhosis, can be minimized with core-type needles. Focal lesions, which were often missed by the "blind" technique, can now be accurately examined by directing the needle to

INDICATIONS AND CONTRAINDICATIONS FOR PERCUTANEOUS LIVER BIOPSY

Indications

- To diagnose suspected primary liver disease (e.g., persistent abnormal liver laboratory studies) or unexplained hepatomegaly
- To assess the course of certain liver disease (e.g., CAH or alcoholic hepatitis) and response to therapy
- To assist in the diagnoses of metabolic disease (e.g., glycogen-storage disease), multisystem disease (e.g., sarcoidosis, tuberculosis, or hemochromatosis), or pyrexia of unknown origin. (Biopsies may be cultured and stained for specific organisms.)
- To assess the effect of hepatotoxic drugs (e.g., methotrexate, in treatment of psoriasis or exposure to hepatotoxic agents)
- To confirm the presence of malignant disease
- To assist in the diagnosis and staging of lymphomas

Contraindications

- Uncooperative patient
- Abnormal clotting parameters:
  - PT >3 seconds of control
  - PTT >20 seconds of control
  - Platelet count <30,000/mm^3
  - Prolonged bleeding time (>10 min.)
- Severe anemia (hematocrit <30)
- Local infection
  - Infected pleural effusion
  - Peritonitis (Ascites should be cultured before biopsy.)
- Massive, tense ascites
- High-grade extrahepatic obstructive jaundice
- Severe uremia (BUN >50 mg/dl to 18 nmol/L)

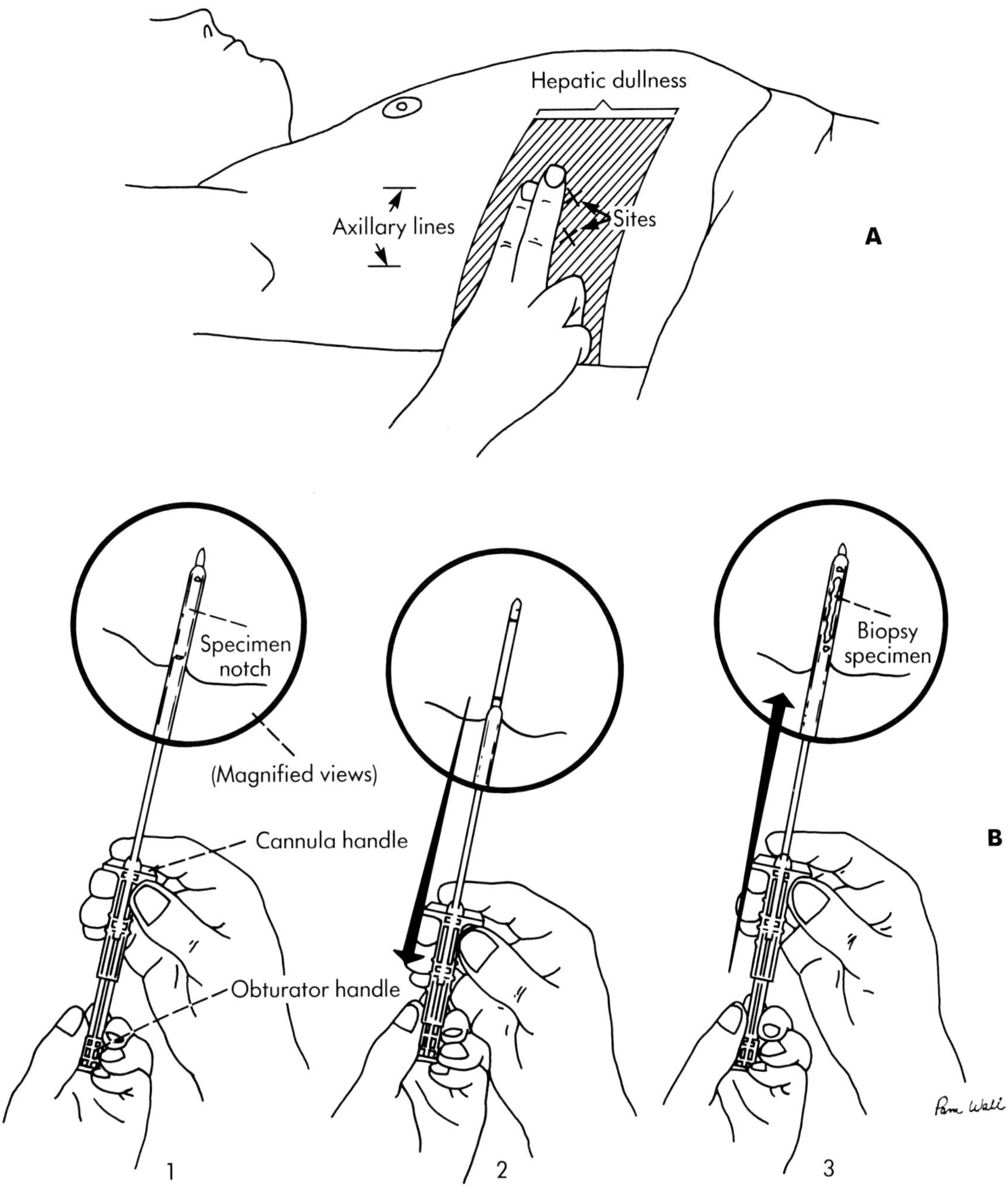

Figure 7-13
Percutaneous liver biopsy: illustration of **(A)** location and **(B)** method using "punch" type biopsy, e.g., TruCut.

particular targets revealed by imaging techniques and peritoneoscopy. Wedge biopsy at laparatomy should be supplemented by single or multiple intraoperative needle biopsies to avoid subcapsular tissue, which may not be typical of the liver as a whole.

Light microscopic examination of paraffin and specially stained plastic-prepared sections is the conventional means of examination. These stains are supplemented with increasingly sophisticated immunohistochemistry, electron microscopy, micro-chemical, and serological techniques.

Figure 7-13 provides an illustration of standard methods for percutaneous liver biopsy and procedures for punch biopsy. An excellent review of liver biopsy today is given by Dame Sheila Sherlock in the Journal of Hepatology (see Annotated Readings).

Appendix B-6 provides "normal" laboratory values in both conventional units and SI units (Systeme International d'Unités).

SUMMARY

The rapid progress of scientific methodology has through the past 25 years provided the clinician with an amazing array of tests for the more accurate diagnosis of liver disease and monitoring of patients with liver disease. In addition, the development of more sophisticated diagnostic techniques (both invasive and noninvasive) has contributed greatly to the physician's investigative technology, especially during the past decade.

However, with these technical advancements has come an overload of information that is often contradictory. This contradiction sometimes causes even the experienced hepatologist difficulty in grasping or fully understanding the complexities of interpretation of these tests and procedures.

This chapter is designed to complement the history assessment and physical evaluation of patients with liver disorders. Both routine laboratory studies and some more specialized and newer tests have been included. The chapter begins with a summary of the pathophysiologic bases of liver injury and attempts to relate the use and interpretation of these many tests and diagnostic procedures to the clinical presentation and pathogenesis of the disease. The tables and figures are designed as interpretive guides to the differential diagnoses and treatment monitoring of the more common hepatic disorders. Decision algorithms have been added to assist the clinician in performing the steps involved in differentiation and interpretation of the more frequent liver-test abnormalities. Appendices to the section include well-tested laboratory summary flow sheets that the author strongly encourages readers to use if such a practice is not already in place. All these components were structured for quick review and reference on a day-to-day working basis.

However, the reader is reminded that no test or diagnostic procedure can substitute for the cognitive skills of an attentive and perceptive clinician.

ACKNOWLEDGMENT

Appreciation to the VAMC, Louisville, Kentucky, medical illustration department, especially to Ms. Luann Rierdon for excellent photography and Mr. Hal Marquette for creative illustrations and artwork.

SUGGESTED READINGS

Alpern MB et al: Focal hepatic masses and fatty infiltration detected by enhanced dynamic CT, Radiology 158:45, 1986.

This is a prospective study of 185 patients that demonstrates the utility of contrast-enhanced dynamic CT. The authors discuss diagnostic criteria for neoplasia and fatty infiltration in the liver.

Beka S, ed: Diagnostic procedures in the evaluation of hepatic diseases: laboratory and research methods in biology and medicine, Vol 7, New York, 1983, Alan R Liss, Inc.

This multi-authored (37 world experts), in-depth comprehensive reference volume is clinically applicable and still up-to-date; the one exception is viral hepatitis serology, especially those related to hepatitis C.

Clermont RJ and Chalmers TC: The transaminase test in liver disease, Medicine 46:197-207, 1967.

A classic review of the clinical interpretation of serum transaminase values in the diagnosis of liver disorders is described.

Drane WE et al: The need for routine delayed radionuclide hepatobiliary imaging in patients with intercurrent disease, Radiology 151:763, 1985.

This is a review of HBS and US in 42 patients showing HBS to be of greater value than US in these complicated cases.

Herbert JC: Efficacy of liver scanning in malignant disease, Serum Nucl Med 14:287, 1984.

A review of scintigraphy for the evaluation of metastatic disease is presented with a a breakdown by all types.

Kaplan MM: Serum AP: another piece is added to the puzzle, Hepatology 6:526-528, 1986.

This is the most comprehensive update and analysis of the serum AP test and its interpretive application to liver disease.

Kelly DA and Tuddenbaum ECG: Hemostatic problems in liver disease, Gut 27:339-349, 1986.

An excellent review of the coagulation problems complicating chronic and acute liver disease is presented.

McFarlane IG: Autoimmunity in liver disease, Clin Sci 67:569-578, 1984.

This is one of the best reviews of and perspectives on the role of autoimmunity in a wide variety of liver diseases.

Okude K, ed: Endoscopic/cholangiographic imaging and treatment, Semin Liver Dis 2:1-85, 1982.

This issue focuses on the newer imaging techniques for visualizing the hepatobiliary system that are changing long-standing standard patterns of treatment.

Preisig R, ed: Clinical evaluation of hepatic function, Semin Liver Dis 3:265-354, 1983.

This is an excellent, clinically applicable monograph reviewing conventional liver tests and imaging techniques with regard to their role in the detection and management of liver disease.

Rothschild MA and Oratz M, eds: Hepatic imaging, Semin Liver Dis 9:1-100, 1989.

This issue describes the rapidly evolving and numerous liver-imaging procedures. It provides the clinician with practical and understandable information that allows more informed use of these techniques and gives their advantages and disadvantages.

Sawabu N and Hattori N: Serological markers in hepatocellular carcinoma. In Okudu K and Ishak KG, eds: Neoplasms of the liver, Tokyo, 1987, Springer-Verlag.

This is an authoritative, comprehensive presentation of clinically applicable markers for the detection and management of hepatic cancers.

Scharschmidt BF, et al: Approach to the patient with cholestatic jaundice, N Engl J Med 308:1515-1519, 1983.

This is an authoritative in-depth review and clinically applicable presentation of differential diagnosis of parenchymal jaundice.

Sherlock S et al: Liver biopsy today: Royal Free Hospital experience, J Hepatol 1:75-85, 1984.

An excellent review of liver-biopsy experience throughout a 23-year period is presented. The selection of patients, techniques, complications, and indications is reviewed.

APPENDIX A-1
PATIENT'S PROBLEM LIST

NAME: ____________________

SSN: _ _ _ _ _ _ _ _ _
1-9

PRIMARY DX: ____________________

____

Medical record

Problem number	Approximate date of onset _ _ / _ _ / _ _ 15-20	Active problems	Inactive/resolved problems	Date resolved _ _ / _ _ / _ _ 21-26	ICD code _ _ _ . _ _ 10-14

Study protocol: _ _ _
27-29

APPENDIX A-2
HISTORY—INITIAL VISIT (PART 1)

SSN	Date	Age	Study protocol
___ __ ____	__/__/__	___	
1-9	10-15	16-17	18-20

Chief complaint

Code: 1 = Negative/absent, 2 = Positive/present, NA = Not applicable, NE = Not examined

Symptoms		Chronologic comments/facts
21. Fatigue/malaise	_____	____________
22. Abdominal pain	_____	____________
a. Location: 1—RUQ, 2—LUQ, 3—RLQ, 4—LLQ, 5—Combination, 6—Other	_____	____________
b. Radiating to 1—Back, 2—shoulder, 3—ribs, 4—groin, 5—other	_____	____________
c. Relationship to meals: 1—worsened immediately, 2—15-60 min later, worsened 3—1-3 hrs later, 4—none	_____	____________
d. Relieved by antacids, alcohol, milk or food	_____	____________
23. Change in abdominal girth	_____	____________
24. Pruritus	_____	____________
25. Weight change	_____	____________
26. Anorexia or early satiety	_____	____________
27. Nausea	_____	____________
28. Vomiting	_____	____________
29. Hematemeses	_____	____________
30. Blood: 2—around stool, 3—mixed with stool, 4—without stool, 5—just on toilet tissue, 6—melena	_____	____________

APPENDIX A-2
HISTORY—INITIAL VISIT (PART 1)—cont'd.

Symptoms		Chronologic comments/facts
31. Stool: 1—hard, 2—soft but formed, 3—watery	_____	______________________
32. Diarrhea	_____	______________________
33. Constipation	_____	______________________
34. Fever and chills	_____	______________________
35. Epistaxis	_____	______________________
36. Impotence/abnormal menses	_____	______________________
37. Icterus	_____	______________________
38. Rash	_____	______________________
39. Paresthesia	_____	______________________
40. Dysphagia/odynophagia	_____	______________________
41. Urine color	_____	______________________
42. Pyrosis/reflex	_____	______________________
43. Joint pain	_____	______________________
44. Other	_____	______________________

APPENDIX A-3
HISTORY—INITIAL VISIT (PART 2)

SSN	Date	Age	Study protocol
_ _ _ _ _ _ _ _ _	_ _ / _ _ / _ _	_ _ _	
1-9	10-15	16-17	18-20

Code: 1 = Negative/absent, 2 = Positive/present, NA = Not applicable, NE = Not examined

Intake		**Comments/Facts**
Alcohol (in ounces of whiskey per week or equivalent: 1 oz. whiskey = 4 oz. wine = 12 oz. beer		______
45-46. a Present	____	______
47-48. b Past	____	______
49. Presently taking medications	____	______
50. Diet adequacy: 1—Poor, 2—Fair, 3—Good	____	______
51-52. Smoker, pack years (packs per day x number of years)	____	______
Past history		______
53. Hepatitis	____	______
54. Contact with jaundiced persons	____	______
55. Transfusions	____	______
56. Needle use	____	______
57. Cirrhosis	____	______
58. Oral medication	____	______
59. History of hepatotoxic chemicals/drugs	____	______
60. Delirium tremens	____	______
61. Convulsions	____	______
62. Pancreatitis	____	______
63. Ulcer disease	____	______
64. Gallbladder disease	____	______
65. Gastrointestinal disorders	____	______
66. Cancer	____	______
67. Other	____	______
68. History of anesthesia	____	______
69. Hospitalizations	____	______
70. Surgery	____	______

APPENDIX A-3
HISTORY—INITIAL VISIT (PART 2)—cont'd.

Family history		**Comments/Facts**
71. Alcoholism	_____	____________________
72. Liver Disease	_____	____________________
73. Gallbladder disease	_____	____________________
74. Gastrointestinal disease	_____	____________________
75. Central nervous system disease	_____	____________________
76. Cancer	_____	____________________
77. Cardiovascular disease	_____	____________________
78. Pulmonary disease	_____	____________________
79. Renal disease	_____	____________________
80. Blood disorders	_____	____________________
81. Other	_____	____________________

APPENDIX A-4
HEALTH ASSESSMENT SURVEY/SCREEN

Date: __ __ / __ __ / __ __
SSN: __ __ __ - __ __ - __ __ __ __
Name: ____________________
Address: ____________________
____
____

Date of birth: __ __ / __ __ / __ __
Age: __ __
Sex: __
Ethnic origin: __ __

I. Review of systems

Have you ever had any of the following medical conditions for more than 1 week? Have they recurred frequently (more than three times per year)? Have they required you to seek medical attention (see a doctor)? Check only if the answer to the question is yes.

Have you had the following?	**In the past?**	**In the past 6 months?**
System category	**Yes**	**Yes**
A. General		
1. Weight loss (>20 lbs)	____	____
2. Fever/chills	____	____
3. Night sweats	____	____
4. Dizziness	____	____
B. Endocrine system		
5. Heat/cold intolerance	____	____
6. Thyroid problems	____	____
7. Neck surgery/radiation	____	____
8. Diabetes/sugar in your blood	____	____
C. Eye		
9. Eye problems	____	____
9a. Glasses to read or to improve vision	____	____
D. Ear/nose/throat		
10. Difficulty hearing	____	____
11. Ringing in your ear	____	____
12. Frequent nosebleeds	____	____
13. Hoarseness	____	____
14. Sinusitis	____	____

APPENDIX A-4
HEALTH ASSESSMENT SURVEY/SCREEN—cont'd.

Have you had the following?	**In the past?**	**In the past 6 months?**
System category	**Yes**	**Yes**
E. Pulmonary (lung) system		
15. Breathlessness/shortness of breath	_____	_____
16. Cough/sputum production	_____	_____
17. Spitting or coughing up blood	_____	_____
18. Wheezing/asthma	_____	_____
19. Positive TB skin test	_____	_____
20. Past positive PPD test	_____	_____
21. Previous chest x-ray	_____	_____
22. Respiratory infections/pneumonia	_____	_____
23. Smoking	_____	_____
24. Environmental inhalation of toxic material	_____	_____
F. Cardiovascular (heart) system		
25. Regular exercise	_____	_____
26. Shortness of breath when lying down at night	_____	_____
27. Chest discomfort/pain	_____	_____
28. Palpitation (fast heart beat)	_____	_____
29. Fainting episodes	_____	_____
30. Edema (swelling) of feet/ankles	_____	_____
31. Phlebitis/inflamed varicose veins	_____	_____
32. Leg pains when walking	_____	_____
33. Hypertension	_____	_____
34. Rheumatic heart disease	_____	_____
35. Past heart diseases (any type)	_____	_____
36. Family history of heart disease	_____	_____
G. GI system		
37. Nausea/retching	_____	_____
38. Vomiting	_____	_____
39. Vomiting blood	_____	_____
40. Black stools	_____	_____
41. Difficulty swallowing	_____	_____
42. Indigestion	_____	_____
43. Heartburn	_____	_____
44. Abdominal pain/stomach pain	_____	_____
45. Abdominal swelling/stomach swelling	_____	_____

Continued.

APPENDIX A-4
HEALTH ASSESSMENT SURVEY/SCREEN—cont'd.

Have you had the following?	In the past?	In the past 6 months?
System category	**Yes**	**Yes**
46. Jaundice/yellow eyes	_____	_____
47. Bloody stools	_____	_____
48. Diarrhea	_____	_____
49. Constipation	_____	_____
50. Hernia	_____	_____
51. Hemorrhoids	_____	_____
52. Peptic ulcer disease	_____	_____
53. Gallbladder disease	_____	_____
54. Pancreatitis	_____	_____
55. GI/stomach surgery	_____	_____
56. Alcohol consumption	_____	_____
H. Hematopoietic system		
57. Excessive bleeding/bruising	_____	_____
58. Anemia	_____	_____
59. Paint consumption as a child	_____	_____
60. Family history of sickle cell disease	_____	_____
I. Genitourinary system		
61. Urinary frequency/urgency/dysuria	_____	_____
62. Urinary tract infection	_____	_____
63. Flank pain [pain in your side(s)]	_____	_____
64. Increased urination at night	_____	_____
65. Blood in urine	_____	_____
66. Passing of stones	_____	_____
67. Abnormality of urinary-stream flow	_____	_____
68. Any sores of penis or scrotum	_____	_____
69. Syphilis/positive serology	_____	_____
70. Male genital lesions	_____	_____
71. Pain or lumps in testes	_____	_____
72. Impotence/difficulty having sex	_____	_____
73. Family history of kidney disease	_____	_____
J. Neurologic system		
74. Headaches	_____	_____
75. Epileptic seizures	_____	_____
76. Neurologic problems	_____	_____
77. Pain or numbness in hands or feet	_____	_____
78. Weakness	_____	_____
79. Head trauma	_____	_____
80. Muscle cramps	_____	_____
81. Stroke	_____	_____
82. Sleep disorder	_____	_____

APPENDIX A-4
HEALTH ASSESSMENT SURVEY/SCREEN—cont'd.

Have you had the following?	**In the past?**	**In the past 6 months?**
System category	**Yes**	**Yes**
K. Psychiatric		
83. Previous psychiatric problems or hospitalizations	____	____
84. Difficulties in interpersonal relationships	____	____
85. Anxiety		
86. Depression	____	____
87. Loss of control/potential for violence	____	____
88. Disturbances of vegetative function	____	____
89. Substance abuse; use of nonprescribed	____	____
drugs	____	____
L. Birth control		
90. Use of birth control pills		
M. Gynecologic system	____	____
91. Pelvic pain		
92. Vaginal discharge	____	____
93. Pelvic mass/tumor	____	____
94. Abnormal vaginal bleeding	____	____
a. Bleeding after sex	____	____
b. Bleeding after menopause	____	____
c. Menopause, age: ____ years	____	____
d. Menstrual flow Interval: ____ days Duration: ____ days Amount: ____		
e. Date of last menstrual period: ____		

II. Medical, family, and social history

A. Medical history

1. Current medications

Year started	**Reason for medication**
a. 19 __ __	________________
b. 19 __ __	________________
c. 19 __ __	________________
d. 19 __ __	________________
e. 19 __ __	________________
f. 19 __ __	________________
g. 19 __ __	________________
h. 19 __ __	________________

Continued.

APPENDIX A-4
HEALTH ASSESSMENT SURVEY/SCREEN—cont'd.

II. Medical, family, and social history—cont'd.

2. Past hospitalization

Year	Reason for hospitalization
a. 19 __ __	______
b. 19 __ __	______
c. 19 __ __	______
d. 19 __ __	______
e. 19 __ __	______
f. 19 __ __	______
g. 19 __ __	______
h. 19 __ __	______

3. Immunizations (last)	Dates
3a. Childhood immunizations	__ __ / __ __ / __ __
b. Tetanus shots	__ __ / __ __ / __ __

B. Family history of chronic illness

	Yes	Body system(s) code
Father's		
4a. Grandfather	_____	_____
b. Grandmother	_____	_____
Mother's:		
4c. Grandfather	_____	_____
d. Grandmother	_____	_____
e. Father	_____	_____
f. Mother	_____	_____
g. Son(s)	_____	_____
h. Daughter(s)	_____	_____
i. Grandson(s)	_____	_____
j. Granddaughter(s)	_____	_____

Body system code

1. Anemia.
2. Bleeding problems.
3. Cancer.
4. Circulation (vein/arteries).
5. Depression.
6. Drug/alcohol.
7. Ear, nose, throat, and mouth disorders.
8. Endocrine.
9. Thyroid.
10. Diabetes (sugar).
11. Other glands.
12. Gallbladder.
13. Gynecologic.
14. Heart.
15. Intestine.
16. Liver.
17. Lung/chest.
18. Neurologic/nerve.
19. Headaches.
20. Epilepsy/seizures.

APPENDIX A-4
HEALTH ASSESSMENT SURVEY/SCREEN—cont'd.

II. Medical, family, and social history—cont'd.

C. Social history

5. Occupational history (chronologic)

Year	Type	Code
a. 19 ___ ___	____________	_____
b. 19 ___ ___	____________	_____
c. 19 ___ ___	____________	_____
d. 19 ___ ___	____________	_____
e. 19 ___ ___	____________	_____
f. 19 ___ ___	____________	_____
g. 19 ___ ___	____________	_____
h. 19 ___ ___	____________	_____

Codes for occupational categories

0. Professional.
1. Technical.
1a. Managerial.
2. Clerical.
2a. Sales.
3. Service.
4. Agricultural.
4a. Fishery, forestry, etc.
5. Processing.
6. Machine trades.
7. Benchwork.
8. Structural work.
9. Miscellaneous.

6. Hobbies

a. ______________________________
b. ______________________________
c. ______________________________
d. ______________________________
e. ______________________________

7. Nutrition

Do you regularly (almost daily) eat:	Yes	No
Breakfast	_____	_____
Lunch	_____	_____
Dinner (supper)	_____	_____
Snacks	_____	_____

8. Education

Have you completed:	Yes	No
Elementary school?	_____	_____
High school?	_____	_____
College/professional school?	_____	_____
Graduate school?	_____	_____

APPENDIX A-5
MEDICATION SUMMARY

Name: ______________________

SSN: _ _ _ _ _ _ _ _ _
1-9

Primary dx: ______________________

____

Treatment or medication	Dosage	Date started _ _/_ _/_ _ 15-20	Date stopped _ _/_ _/_ _ 21-26	Adverse drug reactions	Drug code _ _ _ _ _ 10-14

APPENDIX A-6
PHYSICAL—INITIAL VISIT

SSN	Date	Age	Study protocol
_ _ _ _ _ _ _ _ _	_ _ / _ _ / _ _	_ _ _	
1-9	10-15	16-17	18-20

Temperature __ Pulse __ Respiration __ Blood pressure __ / __ Weight __ Height __

21-24 25-27 28-29 30-35 36-38 39-40

Exams 1 = Negative, 2 = Positive

1. Jaundice _____ ____________________
2. Spiders _____ ____________________
3. Parotid swelling _____ ____________________
4. Tongue atrophy _____ ____________________
5. Oral findings _____ ____________________
6. Fetor _____ ____________________
7. Gynecomastia _____ ____________________
8. Adenopathy _____ ____________________
9. Ascites _____ ____________________
10. Abdominal collaterals _____ ____________________
11. Abdominal tenderness _____ ____________________
12. Hepatomegaly _____ ____________________
13. Splenomegaly _____ ____________________
14. Other masses _____ ____________________
15. Midline diastasis hernia _____ ____________________
16. Liver size, right lobe, MCL _____ ____________________
17. Liver size, left lobe, MSL _____ ____________________
18. Liver texture/tenderness _____ ____________________
19. Spleen size: L _____ ____________________
20. W _____ ____________________
21. BELOW LCM _____ ____________________
22. Bruits _____ ____________________
23. Bowel sounds _____ ____________________
24. Rectal masses/hemorrhoids _____ ____________________
25. Stool color: 1—brown, 2—black, 3—chalk _____ ____________________
26. Guaiac _____ ____________________
27. Sensory changes _____ ____________________
28. Deep tendon reflexes _____ ____________________
29. Flap/asterixis _____ ____________________
30. Apraxia _____ ____________________
31. Tremors _____ ____________________
32. Ankle edema _____ ____________________
33. Clubbing _____ ____________________
34. Palmar erythema _____ ____________________
35. Skin _____ ____________________
36. Dupuytren's contractures/clubbing _____ ____________________
37. Other _____ ____________________

APPENDIX A-7
FOLLOW-UP EXAMINATION

Patient name ______________ Study protocol __________ Visit # __________
Date ____ BP ____ Pulse ____ Temperature ____ Respirations ____ Weight ____ Height ____
Medications ____

1 = Negative/absent, 2 = Positive/present, ND = Not done

Subjective

1. __ Fatigue ______________
2. __ Fever ______________
3. __ Pruritus ______________
4. __ Urine color ______________
5. __ Rash ______________
6. __ Abdominal girth ______________
7. __ Paresthesia ______________
8. __ Anorexia ______________
9. __ Weight change ______________
10. __ Vomiting ______________
11. __ Nausea ______________
12. __ Hematemeses ______________
13. __ Pyrosis ______________
14. __ Constipation ______________
15. __ Diarrhea ______________
16. __ Blood/stool ______________
17. __ ABD pain ______________

Objective Head

18. __ Icterus: Eye ____ Skin ____ Oral ____
19. __ Parotid size ______________
20. __ Oral findings ______________
21. __ Fetor ______________

Chest:

22. __ Spiders ______________
23. __ Gynecomastia ______________
24. __ Lungs ______________
25. __ Heart ______________

Abdomen

26. __ Abdominal surface ______________
27. __ Collaterals ______________
28. __ Bowel sounds ______________
29. __ Bruits ______________
30. __ Liver tenderness ______________
31. __ Liver midclavicular line (MCL) ______________
32. __ Liver palpation ______________
33. __ Spleen L __________ W __________
34. __ Spleen palpation ______________
35. __ Masses ______________
36. __ Ascites ______________
37. __ Midline hernia ______________

Extremities

38. __ Palmar erythema ______________
39. __ Dupuytren's ______________
40. __ Ankle edema ______________
41. __ Clubbing ______________

Neurologic

42. __ Asterixis ______________
43. __ Tremors ______________
44. __ Sensory changes ______________
45. __ D T reflexes ______________
46. __ Gait ______________
47. __ Adenopathy ______________
48. __ Skin ______________
49. __ Others ______________

Assessment:
Plan:
Orders:

APPENDIX B-1
LABORATORY SUMMARY DATA

Name: ______________________________ SSN: ___ ___ ___ ___ ___ ___ ___ ___ ___

Date:													
Year:													
Tx:													
Day/week:													
Hematology													
Hematocrit (Hct)													
Hemoglobin (Hbg)													
RBC													
Mean corpuscular volume (MCV)													
WBC													
Polymorphonuclear													
Bands													
Lymphs													
Monocyte													
Eosinophils													
Basophils													
Reticulocyte													
Sedimentation rate													
Plate													
PT (patient/control)													
PTT (patient/control)													
Fibrin													
Chemistry													
Glucose													
BUN													
Creatine													
Na													
K													
Cl													
CO_2													
Ca													
Phosphatase													
Amylase/lipase													
Uric acid													
Cholesterol													
Triglyceride													
HDL cholesterol													
ratio													
LDL													

Continued.

APPENDIX B-1
LABORATORY SUMMARY DATA—cont'd.

Hepatic

Total bilirubin													
Direct/indirect													
AST													
ALT													
AP													
LDH													
GGTP													
Total Protein													
Albumin													
Globulin													
BA													
NH_3													

APPENDIX B-2
LABORATORY SUMMARY DATA

Name: ______________________________ SSN: ___ ___ ___ ___ ___ ___ ___ ___ ___

Date:													
Year:													
Tx:													
Day/week:													
Hepatitis serology													
HBV=deoxyribonucleic acid (HBV=DNA)													
HBeAg													
HBsAg													
Anti-HBc IgM													
Anti HBc IgG													
Anti-HBe													
Anti-HBs													
HAV													
Anti HAV IgM													
Anti-HAV IgG													
HDV-RNA													
Anti-HD IgM													
Anti-HD IgG													
HCV-RNA													
Anti-HC Ig													
Anti-HC													
HEV													
Anti-HE													
Human immunodeficiency virus (HIV)													
Autoimmune													
α=fetoprotein (AFP)													
Antimitochondrial antibody (AMA)													
Antinuclear antibody (ANA)													
Double-stranded DNA (dsDNA)													
Smooth muscle autoantibody (SMA)													
Quantitative IgG													
IgM													
IgA													
Histology													
HBsAg													
HBcAg													
HDV													
HCV													

APPENDIX B-3
LABORATORY SUMMARY DATA

Name: ______________________ SSN: ___ ___ ___ ___ ___ ___ ___ ___ ___

Date: ___ ___ ___ ___ ___ ___ ___ ___ ___ ___ ___ ___ ___

Other liver studies:

Metabolic

α1 AT
Ferritin
Ceruloplasmin
Copper
Iron

Porphyrin test

ALA
Prostaglandin B (PGB)
Uroporphyrin (URO)
Coproporphyrin (COPR)

ELECTROPHORESIS

Albumin
α=1
α=2
β
γ

Urinalysis

Specific gravity
pH
Glucose
Protein
Occult blood
Ketone
Bile
Urobilinogen
WBC
RBC
Casts
Bacteria
Sodium
Potassium

Other studies

Thyroid-stimulating hormone (TSH)

APPENDIX B-4
DIAGNOSTIC STUDIES

Name: ______________________ SSN: __ __ __ - __ __ - __ __ __ __

Date:						
Chest roentgenogram						
Abdomen roentgenogram						
Esophagogastroduodenoscopy (EGD)						
Upper GI series						
Fiberoptic sigmoidoscopy (FOS)						
Colonoscopy						
Barium enema (BE)						

APPENDIX B-5
HEPATIC DIAGNOSTIC STUDIES

Name: ______________________________ SSN: __ __ __ - __ __ - __ __ __ __

Procedures: liver

Date:						
Path #						
Liver biopsy						
Ultrasonography (US)						
Liver/spleen scan (LSS)						
CT scan						
Endoscopic retrograde cholangiopancreatography (ERCP)						
Transhepatic cholangiogram, (TPC)						
Portal manometry						
Oral cholecystography (OCG)/intravenous cholecystography (IVC)						
MRI						

APPENDIX B-6
NORMAL LABORATORY VALUES
(particularly relevant to liver disease)*

Determination	Reference range: Conventional units	Reference range: SI units
Blood chemistries		
AP	20-140 U/L; in infants and adolescents, 45-260 U/L	217-650 nmol/sec/L (<100 IU/L); up to 1.26 μmol/sec/L (<350-500 IU/L)
Aminotransferase		
(ALT serum glutamic-pyruvic transaminase [SGPT])	1-55 U/L	17-350 nmol/sec/L (<40 IU/L)
(AST, serum glutamic-oxaloacetic transaminase [SGOT])	1-50 U/L	117-450 nmol/sec/L (<40 IU/L)
Ammonia	12-55 μmol/L	400-800 μg/L
Amylase	12-55 mg/dl	86-268 IU/L
Bilirubin		
Direct	Up to 0.4 mg/dl	Up to 7 μmol/L
Total	Up to 1.2 mg/dl	Up to 20 μmol/L
Calcium	8.5-10.6 mg/dl	2.1-2.6 mmol/L
Ceruloplasmin	23-43 mg/dl	13-30 μmol/L
Chloride	95-110 meg/L	95-105 mmol/L
Cholesterol	120-220 mg/dl	3.10-5.69 mmol/L
Copper, total(s)	70-150 μg/dl	11-24 μmol/L
Copper, liver		< μmol/gmdry weight
Creatinine	0.6-1.5 mg/dl	53-133 μmol/L
Ferritin (serum)		
Iron deficiency	0-12 ng/ml 13-20 ng/ml (borderline)	0-4.8 nmol/L 5.2-8.0 nmol/L (borderline)
Iron excess	>400 ng/ml	>160 nmol/L
Folic acid†		
Normal	>3.3 ng/ml	>7.3 nmol/L
Borderline	2.5-3.2 ng/ml	5.75-7.39 nmol/L
Iron	50-150 μg/dl (higher in males)	9.0-26.9 μmol/L
Lactic dehydrogenase	45-90 U/L	750-1,500 nmol/sec/L
Magnesium	1.8-3.0 mg/dl	0.7-1.2 mmol/L
5'NT	1-11 U/L	17-183 nmol/sec/L

*Values provided in this appendix represent data compiled from several laboratories. Theses are provided for interpretation of values shown on charts or in the text. In actual clinical situations, it is essential to check the "normal" ranges of the laboratory that performed the tests.

†Age-dependent.

‡(B)=Blood; (S)=Serum.

Continued.

APPENDIX B-6
NORMAL LABORATORY VALUES—cont'd.

Determination	Reference range	
	Conventional units	**SI units**
Blood chemistries—cont'd.		
Phosphorus	2.5-4.5 mg/dl	0.8-1.5 mmol/L
Potassium	3.5-5.3 mEq/L	3.5-5 mmol/L
Protein total	6.0-8.4 gm/dl	60-84 gm/L
Albumin	3.5-5.0 gm/dl	35-50 gm/L
Globulin	2.3-3.5 gm/dl	23-35 gm/L
Sodium	135-148 mEq/L	135-148 mmol/L
Total iron-binding capacity (TIBC)	250-410 μg/dl	44.8-73.4 μmol/L
Transferrin	1.5-3.4q/L	
Percentage of saturation	25-50%	
Triglycerides	40-150 mg/dl	0.4-1.5 gm/L
Blood urea nitrogen (BUN)	8-25 mg/dl	2.9-8.9 mmol/L
Uric acid	4.0-8.5 mg/dl	89-417 μmol/L
Vitamin B	205-876 pg/ml 140-204 pg/ml (borderline)	150-674 pmol/L 102.6-149.0 pmol/L (borderline)
Zinc	0.5-1.5 mg/dl	8-23 μmol/L
Clinical immunology laboratory values		
α-Fetoprotein	0-10 ng/ml in normal adults	—
α_1-antitrypsin (B)‡	100-200 mg/dl	1-2 qm/L
Antinuclear antibodies (serum)	Negative at a 1:8 dilution	—
Anti-DNA antibodies (serum)	Negative at a 1:10 dilution	—
Autoantibodies to:		
Microsomal antigens (serum)	Negative at a 1:10 dilution	—
Smooth muscle (SMA) (serum)	Negative at a 1:20 dilution	—
Mitochondria (AMA) (serum)	Negative at a 1:20 dilution	—
Carcinoembryonic antigen (CEA)	0-2.5 ng/ml	0-2.5 μg/L
Immunoglobulins		
IgG	639-1,349 mg/dl	6-14 gm/L
IgA	70-312 mg/dl	<3.1 gm/L
IgM	86-352 mg/dl	<3.5 gm/L

‡(B)=Blood; (S)=Serum.

APPENDIX B-6
NORMAL LABORATORY VALUES—cont'd.

Determination	Reference range: Conventional units	Reference range: SI units
Hematologic values		
Complete blood count:		
Hematocrit	Male: 40%-54% Female: 37%-48%	Male: 0.40-0.54 Female: 0.37-0.48
Hemoglobin	Male: 13-18 gm/dl Female: 12-16 gm/dl	Male: 8.1-11.2 mmol/L Female: 7.4-9.9 mmol/L
Leukocytes count (total)	4300-10,000/mm	4.3-10×10^9/L
Total neutrophils	1800-7200/mm	1.8-7.2×10^9/L
Band neutrophils	100-2000/mm	0.1-2×10^9/L
Segmented neutrophils	1000-6000/mm	1-6×10^9/L
Lymphocytes	1500-4000/mm	1.5-4×10^9/L
Monocytes	200-900/mm	0.2-0.9×10^9/L
Eosinophils	0-700/mm	0-0.7×10^9/L
Basophils	0-150/mm	0-0.15×10^9/L
Mean corpuscular volume (MCV)	86-98 μm/cell	86-98 fl (μ^3)
Platelet count	150,000-350,000/mm	150-350×10^9/L
Erythrocyte count (RBC)	Male: 4.2-5.9×10^6/mm^3 Female: 3.9-5.6×10^6/mm^3	4.22-5.9×10^{12}/L 3.9-5.6×10^{12}/L
Coagulation tests		
Bleeding time	3-9.5 min	180-570 sec
Clotting time (Lee-White)	5-11 min	300-660 sec
PTT activated	25-38 sec	25-38 sec
PT	<2 sec deviation from control	<2 sec deviation from control
Urine values		
ALA	0.1-7.5 mg/24 hr	0.8-57 μmol/24 hr
Copper	15-45 μg/24 hr	0.25-0.75 μmol/24 hr
Coproporphyrin	Adults: 50-300 μg/24 hr	75-460 nmol/24 hr
Isomer ratio I:III	1:4	
	Children: <80 lb (36 kg): 0-75 μg/24 hr	0-115 nmol/24 hr
Potassium	1.4-3.5 gm/24 hr	35-90 mmol/24 hr
Porphobilinogen	<2 mg/24 hr	<9 μmol/24 hr
Sodium	1.8-12.9 gm/24 hr	80-560 mmol/24 hr
Urobilinogen	1.0 Ehrlich units (EU) (<4 mg/24 hr)	Up to 1.0 arbitrary unit
Uroporphyrin	0-26 μg/24 hr	0-31 nmol/24 hr

SECTION FOUR

Disorders

8 Liver Disease and Pregnancy

Douglas R. LaBrecque

RC. Cross, writing in the American Journal of Obstetrics and Gynecology in 1929, observed that "the liver is the largest, the most abused, the most neglected, one of the most important, and the least understood organs in the body." Although a great deal has been learned about the liver since that time, (as detailed throughout this book), many of the liver problems related to pregnancy remain mysterious. This is partly due to the fact that liver disease is relatively uncommon in pregnancy. No comprehensive prospective studies of liver disease in pregnancy are available, but the best estimates are that clinical jaundice develops in only 1 of every 1500 to 2500 pregnancies. This is clearly an underestimate of the true incidence of liver abnormalities in pregnancy, and subicteric liver disease must occur with a considerably higher frequency.

Pregnancy is generally uneventful, and most internists and hepatologists come into contact with the condition only when they or a spouse or relative becomes pregnant. Conversely, obstetricians rarely encounter liver disease and do not routinely screen pregnant women for underlying liver problems. It is only the clinically apparent, and usually the more dramatic, manifestations of liver disease that bring the pregnant patient to the attention of the hepatologist. Because each specialist has limited experience in the other's area of expertise, both obstetricians and internists/hepatologists are uncomfortable when faced with the evaluation of an otherwise healthy pregnant woman who may have liver disease. The problem is complicated by the fact that in addition to the acute and chronic liver diseases that may occur in any patient, there are several liver diseases unique to pregnancy. Poignancy surrounds the evaluation of such patients because two individuals are involved: the mother and her fetus. The pressure to reach an accurate diagnosis quickly is magnified because urgent therapeutic measures are required to treat certain liver diseases of pregnancy successfully and save the lives of both mother and child. The threat of harm to the developing fetus places limits on the techniques available for diagnostic evaluation, adding another level of complexity that requires careful cooperation between the obstetrician and internist/hepatologist.

In this chapter I will not reiterate details of the common adult liver diseases that make up the body of this book. Rather, I will review briefly the major physiologic changes in liver function that develop during pregnancy, the liver diseases that are unique to pregnantcy and the special considerations necessary to evaluate and treat other liver diseases that happen to coincide with a woman's pregnancy.

THE NORMAL PREGNANCY

The female body tolerates the tremendous demands of a normal pregnancy remarkably well. Pregnancy is a dynamic state. Significant changes in the body's metabolism and physiology occur throughout the pregnancy—right up to the time of delivery. The liver has a tremendous reserve, and overall liver function is not significantly impaired. However, the increased demand on its many functions, including protein and lipid synthesis, production of blood coagulation factors and albumin, glucose homeostasis, and clearance and detoxification of endogenous and exogenous compounds, plus a multitude of other activities, does produce some evidence of strain, particularly late in pregnancy. After these minor abnormalities are recognized as occurring during the course of a normal pregnancy, it becomes clear that any other abnormalities in liver tests indicate a preexistent liver disease or the development of a new liver disease, both of which demand prompt evaluation.

Physical Findings

Palmar erythema and spider angiomata are common findings in patients with acute and chronic liver disease (see box and Chapter 2). They are also frequently seen in pregnant women. Bean reported that spider angiomata develop in approximately two thirds of pregnant white women, appearing first in the second month of pregnancy and peaking at the time of delivery. Palmar erythema is found in a similar percentage of white women and develops at the same time. These skin changes can also be observed in non-white persons, though they are more difficult to demonstrate in dark-skinned individuals. In most women the spider angiomata and palmar erythema disappear within several months following delivery. However, in some women they will persist indefinitely. The presence of a few spider angiomata and/or palmar erythema in a multiparous woman must always be suspect as an indicator of underlying chronic liver disease.

NORMAL PHYSICAL FINDINGS IN PREGNANCY

Spider angiomata
Palmar erythema
Impalpable liver
Tachycardia

Liver size does not appear to increase during pregnancy. In the third trimester, the liver tends to be displaced superiorly and posteriorly with a consequent reduction in the area of percussion dullness, suggesting a decrease in size that is apparent but not real. Conversely, because of this shift in position, the ability to palpate the liver late in pregnancy strongly suggests underlying liver disease and requires further evaluation. Only subtle changes have been found in the histologic appearance of the liver, by both light and electron microscopy, and these changes are not considered significant. Similar changes have also been noted in women taking oral contraceptives. These findings may be related to the high circulating hormone levels achieved under these conditions.

Physiology

Dramatic changes in cardiovascular hemodynamics occur during pregnancy. Cardiac output increases 30% to 50%, with an increase in total plasma and blood volume of 40% to 50%. The majority of this excess is delivered to the placenta and the expanded splanchnic bed. Despite the significant increase in cardiac output, blood pressure actually falls because of a decrease in the mean peripheral vascular resistance. Total hepatic blood flow is unchanged, but the fraction of total blood flow received by the liver decreases from 35% to approximately 29%. Thus, the liver receives no increase in blood flow despite the increased metabolic demands on it. The decreased fractional blood flow to the liver leads to decreased efficiency in clearing compounds from the blood, which becomes more apparent as pregnancy progresses.

Laboratory Tests

The majority of liver tests are unchanged during pregnancy (Table 8-1). ALT, AST, GGTP, 5′NT, PT, and bilirubin do not change during pregnancy. AP progressively increases after the fifth week but rarely exceeds two to three times the normal level at delivery. The rise in AP is due to the increase in a heat-stable fraction of placental AP, with an occasional contribution from bone AP. These increases can be readily differentiated from liver AP by noting the normal or near-normal levels of GGTP and 5′NT when they are measured simultaneously. Cholesterol and triglyceride levels rise progressively during pregnancy, producing a striking 50% increase in serum cholesterol and a threefold rise in serum triglycerides. Blood urea nitrogen, uric acid, and serum albumin fall early in pregnancy, at least partly because of the hemodilution produced by the increased circulating blood volume, and an increase in fractional renal blood flow. Levels of serum globulins, fibrinogen, and ceruloplasmin increase progressively throughout pregnancy.

Table 8-1 Liver tests during pregnancy

Normal	Increased	Decreased
AST	AP	Albumin
ALT	LDH	γ-Globulin
GGTP	Cholesterol	
5′NT	Triglycerides	
PT	Fibrinogen	
Bilirubin	Ceruloplasmin	
	α1-Globulins	
	α2-Globulins	
	β-Globulins	
	Transferrin	

Summary

The remarkable physiologic changes that occur during pregnancy have significant effects on the liver, which may lead the uninformed physician to an incorrect diagnosis of underlying liver disease. The development of cutaneous changes, including the appearance of spider angiomata and palmar erythema, and a rise in AP can suggest the onset of liver disease. However, AP is the only standard liver test that rises during pregnancy. The absence of any other liver-test abnormalities and knowledge of the high frequency with which skin changes occur during pregnancy should reassure the worried physician and patient of the lack of underlying liver disease.

LIVER DISEASES OF PREGNANCY

Acute Fatty Liver of Pregnancy

The most dramatic liver disease of pregnancy, acute fatty liver of pregnancy, presents with the abrupt onset of rapidly progressing liver failure in a previously healthy young woman as she nears the end of the third trimester. For almost half of these women, it is their first pregnancy, and the likelihood that they are carrying twins is increased tenfold. In its most catastrophic presentation, acute fatty liver of pregnancy is heralded by the abrupt onset of persistent vomiting, hematemesis, and abdominal pain. The pain may be midepigastric or in the RUQ and right lower chest areas, or it may consist of substernal burning. Severe headaches, intense jaundice with minimal or no fever, and somnolence follow in rapid succession. If untreated, premature labor usually ensues, followed by coma, renal failure, and death 2 to 4 weeks after the onset of the disease and 3 to 4 days postpartum. The course of the disease is quite similar to that of fulminant viral hepatitis, but acute fatty liver of pregnancy is readily distinguishable in most cases by laboratory testing. The baby is usually stillborn, and until recently the mortality in mothers was quite high.

Fortunately, not all cases are quite so catastrophic. The presenting symptoms can vary, and initial reports stress high mortality rates (greater than 50%) for both mother and child. More recent series, in which the diagnosis was made early and the fetus was delivered promptly, showed mortality rates of only 15% for the mother and 36% for the infant. It has also become clear that there is a broad spectrum of severity of acute fatty liver of pregnancy. Many women appear to have mild forms of the syndrome that do not progress to severe liver failure. Thus the mortality rates in the reported series are biased in favor of severe cases, and they almost certainly overstate the morbidity and mortality of the disease. Originally thought to occur in as few as one per 1 million pregnancies, the incidence is now believed to be closer to 1 per 13,000 deliveries.

Symptoms and signs. Presenting symptoms can vary, and the disease can occur any time after the twentieth week of pregnancy, but most often between the thirty-sixth and fortieth weeks. Symptoms may be nonexistent, or they may be typical of hepatic failure. Although the disease may not become manifest until after delivery, most women are still pregnant at the time of presentation. Physical examination is not usually helpful in distinguishing acute fatty liver of pregnancy from hepatitis or other liver diseases, particularly in light of the frequent association of the cutaneous signs of liver disease with pregnancy. Almost 50% of the reported patients with acute fatty liver of pregnancy manifest evidence of eclampsia or preeclampsia, with physical signs of hypertension, edema, and agitation with hyperreflexia.

Diagnostic evaluation. Laboratory studies most often allow distinction from FHF caused by viral hepatitis. The AST and ALT are usually below three hundred and fifty international units per liter (IU/L) and rarely greater than 500 (IU/L), with the ALT lower than the AST. The AP may be elevated threefold or more, but this value must be interpreted in light of the increased placental AP. Published studies have not provided sufficient information on concurrent levels of GGTP or 5′NT to allow more clear interpretation of the increased AP values. The WBC count is frequently quite elevated, reaching levels 20 to 30 times normal. PT may also be prolonged dramatically. Thrombocytopenia is common, as is true disseminated intravascular coagulation, which frequently complicates acute fatty liver of pregnancy.

Interpretation of the coagulopathy may be difficult because of the occurrence of the hemolysis, elevated liver enzymes, and low platelet count (HELLP) syndrome in association with preeclampsia. The HELLP syndrome includes mild intravascular hemolysis, elevated liver tests, and thrombocytopenia, which may be marked (see p. 212). Hypoglycemia and hyperammonemia may also be present. Acute renal failure is a frequent complication and may require temporary renal dialysis until the liver disease dissipates.

CT scan and liver ultrasound examinations may suggest the presence of underlying fatty liver. However, definitive diagnosis can be made only through liver biopsy. As with the clinical presentation, pathologic findings also can vary greatly. Usually the liver appears shrunken and yellow during gross examination (thus the former name of the disease,) and is reduced in weight. The critical finding on light microscopy is the presence of microvesicular fatty infiltration of the zone 3 (pericentral) parenchymal cells. This infiltration may extend throughout the lobule, and there is minimal evidence of necrosis or inflammation. Microvesicular fat may be difficult to recognize on standard sections stained with hemotoxylin and eosin. If the disease is suspected, it is best to make arrangements with the pathologist ahead of time to snap freeze a portion of the biopsy for staining with oil red O, which readily demonstrates the presence of the microvesicular fat.

Therapy and outcome. As noted previously, early reports indicated a mortality as high as 85% for mother and child. More rapid recognition of the disease and initiation of intense supportive care have improved the outlook markedly. In patients with severe acute fatty liver of pregnancy, prompt delivery is thought to be critical to the survival of the mother and child. Survivors of acute fatty liver of pregnancy have no sequelae of their illness, and follow-up liver biopsies demonstrate no continuing damage or residual fibrosis.

A serious question for survivors is the risk of subsequent pregnancy. Nineteen cases have been reported in which the patient experienced an uncomplicated pregnancy and delivery following a pregnancy complicated by acute fatty liver of pregnancy. Other normal deliveries presumably have gone unreported. Conversely, no cases of recurrent acute fatty liver of pregnancy have been reported in the literature. Thus, although only limited data are available, the lack of any reported case of recurrent acute fatty liver of pregnancy suggests that the risk may be reasonable for the patient who strongly desires another child. However, any such patient should be followed very closely in a high-risk obstetrics clinic, preferably in close conjunction with care provided by a gastroenterologist/hepatologist.

Pathogenesis. Acute fatty liver of pregnancy is one of a small number of diseases that shares the common pathologic finding of microvesicular fatty infiltration. Other diseases in this category include Reye's syndrome, valproic acid–induced hepatotoxicity, tetracycline toxicity, Jamaican vomiting sickness, and systemic carnitine deficiency. Electron microscopic studies suggest that the structural abnormalities underlying these diseases are not identical although they share a similar clinical syndrome, including the abrupt onset of coma, hyperammonemia, and hypoglycemia. Abnormalities in mitochondrial function or the intermediary metabolism of fatty acids, or both, have been shown in each of these syndromes. Tetracycline localizes in the mitochondria and interferes with protein synthesis, acetate metabolism, and oxidative phosphorylation. The precise pathogenic mechanism of acute fatty liver of pregnancy has not been deciphered. However, it is a condition unique to pregnancy, and the fatty metamorphosis produced by tetracycline has occurred almost exclusively in the pregnant patient. The high degree of association between acute fatty liver of pregnancy and eclampsia/preeclampsia may also provide clues to its etiology.

Summary. Acute fatty liver of pregnancy is a disease unique to pregnancy that has potentially catastrophic consequences for mother and fetus unless the disease is diagnosed quickly and the fetus is delivered promptly. With early diagnosis, intensive supportive care, and prompt delivery, a successful outcome can be expected in more than three fourths of pregnancies. No case of recurrent acute fatty liver of pregnancy has been reported to date.

Preeclampsia and Eclampsia

The syndrome of toxemia of pregnancy, now commonly designated preeclampsia/eclampsia, is unique to pregnancy and the rare condition of hydatidiform mole. The nonobstetrician rarely comes in contact with this syndrome. However, it is not rare in the pregnant woman, developing in 7% of all pregnancies in the United States and 24% in one study of primigravidas in Scotland. It is a problem of the third trimester of pregnancy and is more common in primiparous women and those who have had multiple gestations.

Symptoms and signs. Preeclampsia is characterized by hypertension, proteinuria, and central nervous system (CNS) irritability. Because the normal blood pressure usually falls in pregnancy, a diastolic pressure as low as 80 to 90 mm Hg may represent relative hypertension. A blood pressure above 130 over 80 in the pregnant patient is automatically considered elevated, and a rise during pregnancy of 30 mm Hg systolic or 15 mm Hg diastolic is considered abnormal regardless of absolute values. The development of seizures denotes a progression of preeclampsia to the true eclampsia stage. Renal failure, coagulopathy, microangiopathic hemolytic anemia, and widespread patchy systemic necrosis of many tissues occur. Approximately 8% of all maternal deaths are secondary to eclampsia.

The liver may be involved in eclampsia or preeclampsia as part of this widespread vascular disorder. At least 10% of women with preeclampsia demonstrate hepatic involvement. The true incidence of liver disease in eclampsia is unclear, and mild cases are almost certainly missed.

HELLP syndrome. The HELLP syndrome is the most common liver manifestation of preeclampsia. It is named after its triad of characteristic laboratory findings, hemolysis, elevated liver enzymes and low platelet count. Patients with this syndrome often present with complaints of abdominal pain and only limited evidence of preeclampsia.

Diagnostic evaluation. Liver test abnormalities vary. AP generally shows only modest increases. Transaminase levels range from normal to 250 IU/L but occasionally exceed 1000 IU/L. Similarly bilirubin is most often elevated minimally but may rise to 10 mg/dl or more in severe cases.

Pathogenesis. Liver biopsy in the syndromes of eclampsia and preeclampsia shows changes similar to those found in other tissues in eclampsia. Fibrin thrombae in the hepatic sinusoids, particularly in periportal areas, with associated sinusoidal dilitation and hemorrhage in the space of Disse are characteristic. Periportal necrosis and hemorrhage, the "classic" lesion of preeclampsia-associated liver disease, was more common before early diagnosis and treatment. It has been hypothesized that preeclampsia is the result of altered or inadequate protection of the fetal-placental unit from immune attack.

Therapy and outcome. Treatment of preeclampsia/eclampsia and the HELLP syndrome consists of early delivery. The desire for early delivery must be balanced against the degree of fetal maturation and the severity of the syndrome. The time of delivery is determined by the standards of good obstetric practice. However, the mother and the fetus can deteriorate rapidly unless delivery is initiated as soon as possible.

Summary. The considerable overlap in the manifestations of acute fatty liver of pregnancy, preeclampsia/eclampsia, and the HELLP syndrome suggest a causal relationship. Some authors, including Riely, have argued strongly that these diseases are disparate representations of a broad clinical spectrum of "hepatic toxemia" unique to pregnancy.

Spontaneous Liver Rupture and Hemorrhage

Hepatic rupture represents the most severe presentation of preeclampsia-associated liver disease. It is thought to be caused by confluent hepatic necrosis caused by the vascular thrombosis induced by preeclampsia. Evidence of hepatic hematoma can be found in 1% to 2% of women with preeclampsia and minimal symptomology if it is looked for diligently by abdominal CT scan. The abrupt onset of shock and RUQ pain, usually referred to the right shoulder tip, is an obstetric and surgical emergency in a patient with preeclampsia. Typically older and multiparous, the patient requires immediate surgery if a subcapsular hematoma has ruptured. Although it confirms the presence of bleeding, the return of blood during paracentesis, provides none of the anatomic information required for surgical correction of the catastrophe. Aggressive medical support and large volumes of red cells and plasma expanders may be required until confirmation is obtained by abdominal CT scan, ultrasound, and/or angiogram. Maternal and fetal mortality exceeds 50% despite heroic efforts by physicians.

Intrahepatic Cholestasis of Pregnancy

Recurrent idiopathic intrahepatic cholestatic jaundice of pregnancy may be expected to occur in 1 out of every 2000 pregnancies and accounts for about 20% of all cases of jaundice during pregnancy. In contrast with acute fatty liver of pregnancy, it is a benign condition with no permanent effect on the mother or child. It usually appears in the third trimester, although it may begin in the second trimester. Pruritus gravidarum, a condition of severe generalized pruritus without jaundice, probably represents a forme fruste of the same syndrome.

Symptoms and signs. The major symptom of intrahepatic cholestasis of pregnancy is pruritus, which may become excruciating, followed by the onset of jaundice. A few patients will exhibit mild RUQ pain, but the presence of severe pain, fever, hepatomegaly, splenomegaly, or other signs and symptoms of liver disease, should initiate a search for other causes of jaundice. The bilirubin rises to a plateau and then persists with little fluctuation until delivery. About one third of newborns will be premature, but this occurrence appears to be a feature of the individual patient rather than of the illness, with mothers having all premature newborns or all full-term newborns. Jaundice declines rapidly in the postpartum period, with pruritus often disappearing within 2 days and jaundice disappearing in 1 to 2 weeks. However, almost 50% of patients will suffer a recurrence of the condition in one or more subsequent pregnancies. The symptoms may also develop during oral contraceptive therapy.

Diagnostic evaluation. Other than pruritus, clinically the patients are strikingly well, with no fever, nausea, vomiting, anorexia, food intolerance, or other symptoms of hepatitis. The bilirubin is typically conjugated and is less than five times normal. Bile salts can be dramatically elevated, ranging up to ten times normal. AST, ALT, and AP rarely exceed two to four times normal, although tenfold to fifteenfold elevations have occurred. Liver biopsy shows mild, focal, and irregular bile stasis, which can be missed easily. Hepatocellular necrosis and inflammatory cell reaction are absent. Thus it is a disease in which cholestasis is clinically marked (as manifested by the severe pruritus), biochemically moderate, and histologically minimal.

Pathogenesis. The pathophysiology of the condition is unclear, but intrahepatic cholestasis of pregnancy appears to be an unusual cholestatic reaction to normal physiologic processes in pregnancy. A positive family history is present in almost 50% of patients. A higher frequency of cholestasis has been reported in certain ethnic groups, including Scandinavians and Chilean Indians (1% to 6% of pregnancies in these ethnic groups vs. less than 1% in the United States and Europe). The Araucanian Indians of Chile display a 27% prevalence of this syndrome. It is rare in black women and has not been reported in Korean, Japanese, or Chinese women. An inherited sensitivity to the cholestatic effects of estrogens is further supported by the frequent recurrence of intrahepatic cholestasis with menstruation and with the ingestion of oral contraceptive pills.

Therapy and outcome. Treatment of intrahepatic cholestasis of pregnancy is symptomatic. Most patients will respond to oral cholestyramine, often requiring 16 to 20 gm/day in divided doses. Oral phenobarbital has been reported to be useful in patients unresponsive to oral cholestyramine, and hypnotics may make it easier for them to sleep. However, only delivery produces 100% successful results. With prolonged cholestasis, PT should be followed, and vitamin K should be administered if PT is prolonged because of malabsorption of dietary vitamin K. Cholestyramine therapy may exacerbate the vitamin K malabsorption. Prophylactic administration before delivery is recommended regardless of PT and may be necessary for the newborn as well. S-adenosyl-L methionine has been advocated as a possible therapy. It has been shown to reverse the cholestatic effects of estrogens in humans and animals. It significantly improved pruritus and biochemical tests in one randomized clinical trial, in which six women with intrahepatic cholestasis of pregnancy were treated with large intravenous doses of the medication. In an uncontrolled study, oral treatment with S-adenosyl-L methionine prevented the development of cholestatic abnormalities in four women treated with estrogen. Considerably more work is required before this medication can be recommended for routine use in this condition. In addition, potential risks for the fetus have not yet been determined.

Summary. Intrahepatic cholestasis of pregnancy is a benign condition related to increased sensitivity to estrogens. The laboratory abnormalities are usually mild, but the pruritus can be incapacitating. Most patients will obtain at least partial relief from cholestyramine. The condition vanishes within days of parturition but often recurs with subsequent pregnancies or oral contraceptive therapy.

Hyperemesis Gravidarum

The nausea and vomiting that occur in up to 50% of pregnancies during the first trimester can be confused with the symptoms of acute viral hepatitis when the nausea and vomiting are severe. Up to 10% of patients with hyperemesis gravidarum will develop minor bilirubin elevations. However, cholestatic markers are absent, and transaminases are usually normal, rising only threefold to fourfold in small numbers of patients. Liver biopsies should not ordinarily be necessary to distinguish hyperemesis gravidarum from viral hepatitis, though the typical histologic changes in viral hepatitis will be absent if a liver biopsy is obtained.

LIVER DISEASES DURING PREGNANCY

Any form of acute liver disease can develop during pregnancy, and many women with chronic liver disease remain fertile. The major conditions that must be considered in the differential diagnosis of the pregnant patient with liver disease are listed in Table 8-2. Diagnosis and management are the same as for the nonpregnant patient except for modifications required to avoid harm to the infant. Only the most common illnesses will be discussed in detail.

Viral Hepatitis

By far the most common cause of jaundice in pregnancy is viral hepatitis, which accounts for more than 40% of cases. A number of misconceptions have developed over the years concerning the relationship between viral hepatitis and pregnancy. These misconceptions have only recently begun to be disproved.

Incidence and susceptibility. Earlier studies suggested that pregnant women were particularly susceptible to hepatitis and that it occurred most frequently in the last trimester of pregnancy. Both of these suggestions have now been examined in careful prospective studies. These studies found that the incidence of hepatitis in pregnant women runs parallel to that of the general population. One study of an epidemic in Hamburg, Germany, found that the incidence of hepatitis among 270,000 women of childbearing age was 0.04% in pregnant women and

Table 8-2 Liver diseases in the pregnant female*

Liver Diseases of Pregnancy	
Acute Fatty Liver of Pregnancy	
Eclampsia/preeclampsia	
HELLP syndrome	
Spontaneous liver rupture	
Intrahepatic cholestasis of pregnancy	
Hyperemesis gravidarum	
Liver diseases during pregnancy	
Acute	**Chronic**
Viral hepatitis (A,B,C,D,E, CMV,HSV, EBV)†	Chronic active hepatitis Viral (B,C,D) Autoimmune
Drug hepatitis, including alcoholic	Portal hypertension, cirrhosis Alcoholic cirrhosis
Gallstones	PBC
Sepsis, pyleonephritis	PSC Wilson's disease
Hepatic tumors	Hemochromatosis
Budd-Chiari syndrome	Dubin-Johnson syndrome
Variceal bleeding	Porphyria

*This table contains the liver problems most commonly encountered by the pregnant patient (some liver diseases are unique to pregnancy ["of pregnancy"], and other diseases happen to occur in a patient who is pregnant ["during pregnancy"]). It is not meant to be encyclopedic, and it excludes those problems for which there is no clear association with pregnancy. More details can be found in the text and in the annotated readings.

†CMV = cytomegalovirus; HSV = Herpes simplex virus; EBV = Epstein-Barr virus.

0.07% in nonpregnant women of childbearing age, compared to 0.07% in the general population. Studies in Vienna, Jerusalem and Haifa, Israel, Copenhagen, and India found similar results. A number of early series suggested an increase in the incidence of hepatitis with advanced stages of pregnancy; however, these data were collected from obstetric departments that saw patients primarily in the latter stages of pregnancy. Two large, carefully conducted prospective series, which followed women from the first trimester of pregnancy, found a fundamentally identical incidence of hepatitis through all three trimesters.

Morbidity and mortality. Another misconception is that the morbidity and mortality of hepatitis are significantly increased in pregnant women. Most of these studies have originated from North Africa, the Middle East, and Asia and included patients primarily from the lowest socioeconomic groups. These patients suffered from very poor nutrition, which was exacerbated by the increased demands of pregnancy. They had virtually no prenatal or postnatal care, and only the sickest patients received care in a hospital, thereby greatly biasing the reports in favor of those with the most severe disease. In these studies, many of the patients also received parenteral tetracycline, which may have contributed to the high mortality. In addition, very few studies have characterized their patients serologically, and no definitive statements can be made concerning the true incidence and severity of the various forms of viral hepatitis in the pregnant female. Because most individuals in Third World countries acquire hepatitis A during childbirth and hepatitis B is similarly endemic, many of the deaths may have been caused by Hepatitis E (Table 8-2).

Studies originating in the United States and Europe show mortality rates for pregnant women that are similar to those of the general population but are higher in hospitals serving women with the lowest income and poorest prenatal care. Alcoholism and abuse of intravenous (IV) drugs may also have played a role in the higher observed mortality rates. The clinical course of hepatitis in the pregnant patient, including the results of liver tests and the appearance of the liver on needle biopsy, is the same as in the general population. Mortality from hepatitis depends primarily on the general health of the mother and not on the coincidental presence of pregnancy. It should be noted further that the course of viral hepatitis is not influenced by termination of the pregnancy and that the stress of surgery and anesthesia only adds to the strain on an already failing liver. One exception may be hepatitis E (epidemic non-A non-B hepatitis). Some epidemics in Third World countries have recorded a significantly higher mortality rate, approaching 20%, in pregnant women who have acute hepatitis E. The same problems of poor nutrition and limited prenatal care may have contributed to the higher mortality in these cases, as the epidemics of hepatitis E have all occurred in areas with poor public hygiene and limited public health measures.

Effects on the fetus. The effects of hepatitis on the fetus are somewhat more controversial. Some studies have found an increase in premature delivery and stillbirths when hepatitis occurs in the third trimester. There is no correlation between the duration of jaundice or the severity of the hepatitis and prematurity. The survival of the newborn depends on the infant's degree of maturity at the time of birth, so the pregnancy should be carried as long as possible while remaining consistent with good obstetric practice.

There is no convincing evidence that maternal hepatitis causes an increase in congenital malformations. Despite occasional anecdotal reports, two large prospective studies performed in New York City and Great Britain failed to demonstrate an increase in congenital malformations.

Vertical transmission of hepatitis. The major risk to the fetus is acquisition of hepatitis, primarily hepatitis B, from the mother. Evidence of vertical (maternal to fetal) transmission of hepatitis A, hepatitis C, and hepatitis D is very limited. Hepatitis A has an extremely brief viremic phase, and the fetus is at risk only if the mother has acute hepatitis A at the time of delivery. In that case, 0.5 ml of human immune serum globulin given intramuscularly (IM) is protective. The data necessary to estimate the risk of vertical transmission of hepatitis C are just now being collected. Such transmission appears to be a rare event, but if the mother has hepatitis C in the third trimester, treatment of the fetus with 0.5 ml of immune serum globulin would seem to be reasonable until more information becomes available. There are isolated reports of maternal transmission of hepatitis D, but immunoprophylaxis directed against hepatitis B should also prevent hepatitis D.

In contrast to hepatitis A, C, and D, hepatitis B is readily passed from mother to fetus; in fact, vertical transmission is probably the most frequent means of transmission worldwide. From a global perspective, hepatitis B is the commonest cause of liver disease and is second only to tobacco as a cause of cancer. Vertical transmission at or around the time of birth or horizontal transmission through close contact with virus carriers in hyperendemic areas is thought to account for up to 40% of hepatitis B transmission worldwide. Mothers who are both HBS_SAg and HB_eAg positive transmit hepatitis B to their fetuses in up to 90% of cases. Although it is rare for the fetus to develop significant clinical illness from hepatitis B, 80% to 90% of infants who acquire hepatitis B as newborns become chronic carriers. This is in stark contrast to the outcome in adults, who experience only a 10% rate of chronic hepatitis. When hepatitis B is acquired during the neonatal period, more than 50% of those who contact it will die of hepatitis B-related disease. These newborns' risk of developing hepatoma increases by 200 times. Fortunately, hepatitis B transmission can be prevented in all but 5% to 10% of newborns by administration of hyperimmune globulin (HBIG) and hepatitis B vaccine at the time of delivery. Within 12 hours of delivery (ideally while the newborn is still in the delivery room), 0.5 ml of HBIG should be injected into one of the newborn's thighs. A course of hepatitis B vaccination should be initiated by simultaneous IM injection in the other thigh, with subsequent vaccination at 1 and 6 months. Because of the high risk of hepatitis B transmission, the serious sequelae of the chronic carrier state, and the efficacy of immunoprophylactic techniques in preventing hepatitis B infection, the Centers for Disease Control in 1988 recommended screening of all pregnant women for the presence of hepatitis B virus.

Summary. The incidence of viral hepatitis and the course of the disease are similar in pregnant and nonpregnant females. An exception may be hepatitis E. There is no increased risk of congenital defects in infants born to mothers with viral hepatitis, and the occurrence of maternal hepatitis is not an indication for termination of the pregnancy. The main risk to the infant is vertical transmission of hepatitis B, with the subsequent development of chronic hepatitis B. Universal screening of pregnant women for hepatitis B should allow successful immunoprophylaxis of infants at risk of acquiring hepatitis B. Vertical transmission of hepatitis A almost never occurs, and it appears to be rare with hepatitis C and D.

Gallstones

Occurring more frequently in women than men, cholelithiasis is especially prevalent among women less than 50 years of age, though it can occur in women of all ages. It is associated with obesity and parity (but not the number of pregnancies). Pregnancy produces a number of changes in biliary physiology, including decreased contractility of the gallbladder, increased gallbladder volume, decreased chenodeoxycholate synthesis, increased cholesterol secretion into bile, decreased enterohepatic recycling of the bile salt pool, and an overall increase in the lithogenicity of the bile. Because of these remarkable changes in biliary physiology, it would seem reasonable to expect an increased incidence of acute cholecystitis and choledocolithiasis during pregnancy. In fact, gallbladder surgery is second to appendectomy as the commonest nonobstetric surgical procedure performed on pregnant women. However, acute cholecystitis requiring cholecystectomy occurs in only approximately 1 per 1000 deliveries, and gallstones cause only approximately 6% of all cases of jaundice in pregnancy. Diagnosis is most accurately made with ultrasound. This procedure creates the least risk of harm to the fetus and the mother. Surgery remains the treatment of choice for acute cholecystitis.

Cirrhosis and portal hypertension. Pregnancy is distinctly uncommon in patients whose liver disease remains active or has progressed to cirrhosis. However, as therapy and management of cases of acute and chronic liver disease continue to improve, more young women have been able to arrest the progress of their liver disease and become pregnant. The secondary amenorrhea and anovulatory cycles produced primarily by the direct effects of alcohol in patients with alcoholic liver disease and secondarily by the cirrhosis-induced alterations in estrogen metabolism in patients with nonalcoholic cirrhosis may be resolved when the underlying liver disease is stabilized. The major risk to patients with chronic liver disease and portal hypertension is bleeding. Esophageal varices may appear transiently during pregnancy, even in the normal individual, because of the increased blood volume associated with pregnancy and the shunting of venous return to the azygous system. The latter is caused by increased resistance to blood flow through the inferior vena cava caused by increasing obstruction of the cava by the enlarging uterus. Up to two thirds of women with normal pregnancies will demonstrate esophageal varices near term.

Limited studies of pregnancy occurring in cirrhotic patients have demonstrated the ability of these patients to carry a pregnancy to term. Numerous individual reports in small series have suggested an increased risk of variceal hemorrhage in pregnant women with portal hypertension. Variceal hemorrhage is a significant cause of the morbidity and mortality reported in these patients. However, no good prospective studies are available comparing the frequency of variceal hemorrhage in pregnant females with portal hypertension to the frequency in nonpregnant individuals with portal hypertension. Variceal hemorrhage occurring during one pregnancy does not indicate that such hemorrhage will occur during a subsequent pregnancy. Given the lack of controlled prospective studies, published reports are no doubt biased in favor of the occurrence of complications. Successful decompressive shunt surgery performed as emergency therapy for bleeding esophageal varices during pregnancy has been successful in a number of reported cases. Experience with obliterative variceal sclerosis in pregnant patients is more limited, and adequate data are not available to allow clear recommendations concerning its use in this setting. However, sclerotherapy would appear to be a reasonable and safe alternative to a portal decompressive shunt in the treatment of bleeding esophageal varices during pregnancy.

Summary. The coincidence of portal hypertension and pregnancy does not demand termination of the pregnancy. Meticulous care, provided in a team effort by the obstetrician and hepatologist/internist, can be expected to produce a spontaneous delivery in a majority of highly motivated patients who are aware of the potential increased risks caused by portal hypertension.

OTHER LIVER DISEASES

Pregnancies have been carried to term successfully in patients with well-compensated *PBC, Wilson's disease,* steroid-treated *autoimmune CAH, and hemochromatosis.* Therapy for these diseases needs to be continued throughout the pregnancy, though the steroid dose for CAH should be limited to less than 15 to 20 mg if possible. Penicillamine taken for Wilson's disease should be reduced to 750 to 1000 mg/day during the first two trimesters and 250 mg/day during the third trimester. Discontinuation of therapy for either of these diseases has led to severe reactivation of the underlying condition with dire consequences for the mother and fetus.

Drug hepatitis is unusual during pregnancy, probably because pregnant patients are advised to avoid drugs studiously. However, although some authors have speculated that the liver of the pregnant woman is more sensitive to drug toxicity, particularly to the phenothiazines that are often used to treat first-trimester nausea, there is no conclusive evidence to support this claim.

Reports of enlargement and/or rupture of benign *hepatic adenomas* or tumors of *focal nodular hyperplasia* have led to the recommendation that individuals with large lesions should have them surgically removed before conception.

The level of conjugated bilirubin in *Dublin-Johnson syndrome* increases during pregnancy, but in *Rotor's syndrome* it does not. Unconjugated bilirubin is unaffected in *Gilbert's syndrome.*

Budd-Chiari syndrome, caused by thrombosis of the large hepatic veins, has been reported to occur during pregnancy, especially in the immediate postpartum period. The association of Budd-Chiari syndrome with use of oral contraceptives has been well established. The etiology in both instances is thought to be related to estrogen-induced increases in clotting factors, with an associated decrease in the activity of antithrombin III.

Acute pyelonephritis was a common cause of jaundice in pregnancy before the availability of antibiotics, but it was replaced by jaundice associated with IV tetracycline therapy. *Sepsis,* or severe infection, should always be considered when direct hyperbilirubinemia develops that is disproportionate to the elevation of other liver tests, (keeping in mind the expected elevation in AP).

SUMMARY: APPROACH TO THE DIAGNOSIS OF LIVER DISEASE IN THE PREGNANT WOMAN

Several factors must be kept in mind when approaching the diagnosis of liver disease in the pregnant patient (Table 8-3):

1. Normal pregnancy produces a number of physical (e.g., spider angiomata and palmar erythema), biochemical (e.g., AP and albumin), and symptomatic (e.g., nausea and fatigue) changes that are typical of acute and chronic liver disease (see Table 8-1 and the box on p. 210).
2. Several liver diseases are unique to pregnancy. Differentiation of these diseases from liver diseases common to both pregnancy and nonpregnancy is essential because the treatment of those liver diseases peculiar to pregnancy may require early delivery of the fetus (see Table 8-2).
3. Any form of liver disease can occur in the pregnant woman. The effects of the liver disease on the mother and the fetus and the effects of the pregnancy

Table 8-3 Differential diagnosis of liver disease in pregnancy

First trimester	Second trimester	Third trimester
Normal pregnancy	Normal pregnancy	Normal pregnancy
Viral hepatitis	Viral hepatitis	Acute fatty liver of pregnancy*
Drug reactions	Gallstones	Eclampsia/Preeclampsia*
Hyperemesis gravidarum*	Cirrhosis	HELLP syndrome*
	Pyelonephritis/sepsis	Intrahepatic cholestasis of pregnancy*
		Spontaneous hepatic rupture*
		Viral hepatitis
		Gallstones
		Cirrhosis/portal hypertension
		Variceal bleeding
		Pyelonephritis/sepsis
		Dubin-Johnson syndrome
		Budd-Chiari syndrome

*Diseases unique to pregnancy.

on the severity and complications of the liver disease must be considered in determining the best course of action and the timing of treatment of the liver disease and delivery of the fetus.

4. The stage of pregnancy at which the liver disease first becomes manifest may be helpful in narrowing down the list of diagnostic possibilities (see Table 8-3). Fatty liver of pregnancy cannot be confused with viral hepatitis in the first trimester because the former occurs only in the third trimester. Similarly, eclampsia, preeclampsia, and HELLP are basically third-trimester diseases. Unfortunately, the largest number of diseases occurs in the third trimester, which is also the period of greatest liver-test abnormalities in normal pregnancy. A correct diagnosis is probably most critical in the third trimester because of the potential benefit of induced labor for both mother and fetus. The key is to identify quickly and accurately those patients who require urgent surgery (e.g., because of hepatic rupture complicating eclampsia, or acute cholecystitis) or delivery (e.g., because of acute fatty liver of pregnancy, severe eclampsia, or HELLP syndrome).
5. The care of all pregnant patients with liver disease should involve a carefully coordinated team effort between an obstetrician and a hepatologist/internist who has broad experience in the care of patients with liver disease. Decisions must always be based on the standards of good obstetric care, maximizing the opportunity for the fetus to mature fully while minimizing the risks to the mother.

SUGGESTED READINGS

Bean WB: Vascular spiders and related lesions of the skin, Springfield, Ill, 1958, Charles C. Thomas, Publisher.

This medical classic is the most comprehensive and detailed description of spider angiomata and other skin lesions as they appear in liver disease, pregnancy, and other conditions.

Beer AE: Immunology, contraception and pre-eclampsia, JAMA 262:3184, 1989 (editorial).

This is a brief discussion of the possible role of immunologic mechanisms in the pathogenesis of preeclampsia.

Centers for Disease Control: Protection against viral hepatitis: recommendations of the Immunization Practices Advisory Committee (ACIP), MMWR 39 (RR-2): 1-26, 1990.

Recommendations concerning screening of pregnant women and immunoprophylaxis of newborns are included in this detailed examination of hepatitis risks and prevention measures.

Fagan EA: Disorders of the liver, biliary system and pancreas. In de Swiet M, ed: Medical disorders in obstetric practice, Oxford, 1989, Blackwell Scientific Publishers, Ltd, 426-520.

This is a detailed, up-to-date review with comprehensive references (467) that covers every aspect of liver disease and pregnancy.

Frezza M et al: Reversal of intrahepatic cholestasis of pregnancy in women after high dose S-adenosyl-L-methionine administration, Hepatology 4:274-278, 1984.

Experimental therapy of intrahepatic cholestasis of pregnancy is described, with discussion and references on standard therapies.

Haemmerli UP and Wyss HI: Recurrent intrahepatic cholestasis of pregnancy, Medicine 46:299-321, 1967.

This is a classic review of intrahepatic cholestasis of pregnancy through 1967.

Kaplan MM: Current concepts—acute fatty liver of pregnancy, N Engl J Med 313:367-370, 1985.

An excellent summary of acute fatty liver of pregnancy and approaches to therapy is given.

Neerhof MG, Zelman W, and Sullivan T: Hepatic rupture in pregnancy, Obstet Gynecol Surv 44:407-409, 1989.

This is a brief review of a rare problem, with good references.

Riely CA et al: Acute fatty liver of pregnancy, Ann Intern Med 106:703-706, 1987.

This article discusses the spectrum of acute fatty liver of pregnancy and its possible relationship to preeclampsia and eclampsia.

Rolfes DB and Ishak KG: Liver disease in pregnancy, Histopathology 10:555-570, 1986.

This is an authoritative review of the histopathology of liver diseases unique to pregnancy.

Sheehan HC: The pathology of acute yellow atrophy and delayed chloroform poisoning, J Obstet Gynecol Brit Empire 47:49-61, 1940.

This is the original description of the "other Sheehan's syndrome"—the first reported review of patients with acute fatty liver of pregnancy.

Snyder RR and Hankins GD: Etiology and management of acute fatty liver of pregnancy, Clin Perinatol 13:813-825, 1986.

This is a detailed review of acute fatty liver of pregnancy with extensive references.

Snydman DR: Hepatitis in pregnancy, N Engl J Med 313:1398-1401, 1985.

A good discussion of the effects of hepatitis on mother and fetus is provided.

Tong MJ: Hepatitis B vaccination of neonates and children, Am J Med 87(suppl 3A):33S-35S, 1989.

This is an excellent review of hepatitis B prevention in neonates and children.

VanDyke RW: The liver in pregnancy. In Zakim D and Boyer T, eds: Hepatology—a textbook of liver disease, Philadelphia, 1990, WB Saunders Co pp. 1438-1459.

This is a detailed, up-to-date review with comprehensive references (376) that covers every aspect of liver disease and pregnancy.

VanThiel DH, ed: Seminars in Liver Disease 7:1-66, 1987.

This is an erudite, multiauthored review of the unique effects of being female on the function of the liver and the occurrence of liver disease.

9 Congenital and Inherited Disorders

David A. Gremse and *William F. Balistreri*

The developing liver is predisposed to manifest cholestasis in response to a variety of insults (the concept of "physiologic cholestasis"); therefore, significant jaundice may occur even in infants with mild liver disease. In addition, symptoms of most congenital and inherited liver disorders present in infancy. Therefore the differential diagnosis of conjugated hyperbilirubinemia in infancy differs from that in adults. There are a wide range of congenital and inherited diseases of the liver that can present with cholestasis (see box on p. 228). These conditions may exhibit similar clinical, biochemical, and histologic features, necessitating a thorough evaluation for accurate diagnosis. When evaluating an infant with liver disease, the aims should be to identify (1) diseases for which *specific treatment* is available, such as galactosemia, (2) conditions for which *surgical treatment* is required, such as biliary atresia, and (3) inherited disorders such as α-1AT deficiency or cystic fibrosis because of their implications for treatment and *genetic counseling*.

Congenital hepatic diseases can be divided broadly into extrahepatic and intrahepatic disorders (Figure 9-1). The intrahepatic diseases can be further classified as infectious, anatomic, or metabolic; the metabolic category includes defects in amino acid, lipid, or carbohydrate metabolism in addition to conditions in which the defect is uncharacterized. For those patients in whom the etiology is undefined, the term *idiopathic neonatal hepatitis* is used. The clinical findings and evaluation and management of cases of these disorders are discussed below.

INFANTILE CHOLANGIOPATHIES

Although many conditions may cause cholestasis in infants, two disorders, extrahepatic biliary atresia and idiopathic neonatal hepatitis, are responsible for 70% to 80% of cases. The term *infantile cholangiopathy* is derived from a common theory used to explain those hepatic diseases that variably produce hepatocellular or biliary tract injury in neonates. The *infantile obstructive cholangiopathy theory* is one of two pathogenic mechanisms used to explain the pathogenesis of extrahepatic biliary atresia and neonatal hepatitis; the alternative theory is the *ductal plate malformation theory*.

Embryologically the rudimentary bile duct is in the form of a cylindric ductal plate, which matures by its interchange

NEONATAL CHOLESTASIS

- I. Extrahepatic disorders
  - A. Biliary atresia
  - B. Sclerosing cholangitis
  - C. Bile duct stenosis
  - D. Anomalies of the choledochal-pancreatico-ductal junction
  - E. Spontaneous perforation of the common bile duct
  - F. Mass (neoplasia, stone)
  - G. Bile/mucous plug
- II. Intrahepatic disorders
  - A. Idiopathic
    - 1. Idiopathic neonatal hepatitis
    - 2. Intrahepatic cholestasis
      - a. Paucity of intrahepatic ducts (nonsyndromic)
      - b. Arteriohepatic dysplasia (Alagille's syndrome)
      - c. Hereditary cholestasis with lymphedema
      - d. Byler's disease
      - e. Inborn errors of bile acid metabolism
      - f. Zellweger's syndrome (and other peroxisomal disorders)
      - g. Microfilament dysfunction
      - h. Benign recurrent
  - B. Anatomic
    - 1. Congenital hepatic fibrosis or infantile polycystic disease
    - 2. Caroli's disease
  - C. Metabolic disorders
    - 1. Disorders of amino acid metabolism (e.g., tyrosinemia)
    - 2. Disorders of lipid metabolism
      - a. Wolman's disease
      - b. Niemann-Pick disease
      - c. Gaucher's disease
    - 3. Disorders of carbohydrate metabolism
      - a. Galactosemia
      - b. Fructosemia
      - c. Glycogenosis type III and type IV
    - 4. Disorders of bile acid metabolism
      - a. 3-β-hydroxysteroid dehydrogenase/isomerase
      - b. δ-D^4-3-oxosteroid 5-β-reductase
    - 5. Metabolic diseases in which the defect is uncharacterized
      - a. α-1-AT deficiency
      - b. Cystic fibrosis
      - c. Idiopathic hypopituitarism
      - d. Hypothyroidism
      - e. Neonatal hemochromatosis
      - f. Indian childhood cirrhosis
      - g. Multiple acyl-CoA dehydrogenase deficiency
      - h. Familial erythrophagocytic lymphohistiocytosis
      - i. Arginase deficiency

From Balistreri WF: Interrelationship between the infantile cholangiopathies and paucity of the intrahepatic ducts. In Balistreri WF and Stocker JT, eds: Pediatric hepatology, New York, 1990, Hemisphere Publishing Corp, pp. 1-18.

NEONATAL CHOLESTASIS—cont'd.

D. Hepatitis
   1. Infectious
      a. Cytomegalovirus
      b. Hepatitis B
      c. Rubella
      d. Reovirus type 3
      e. Herpes
      f. Varicella
      g. Coxsackie
      h. Echovirus
      i. Parvovirus B19
      j. Toxoplasmosis
      k. Syphilis
      l. Tuberculosis
      m. Listeriosis
   2. Toxic
      a. Cholestasis associated with parenteral nutrition
      b. Sepsis with endotoxemia
E. Genetic or chromosomal
   1. Trisomy E
   2. Down's syndrome
   3. Donohue's syndrome (leprechaunism)
   4. Cat's-eye syndrome
F. Miscellaneous
   1. Shock or hypoperfusion
   2. Histiocytosis X
   3. Intestinal obstruction
   4. Polysplenia syndrome
   5. Neonatal lupus erythematosis

with the ingrowing mesenchyme. The *ductal plate malformation* theory proposes that abnormal remodeling of this ductal plate results in a spectrum of hepatobiliary diseases ranging from atresia to cystic lesions. Alternatively the *infantile obstructive cholangiopathy theory* postulates that atretic disorders of the biliary tree are the result of neither agenesis nor malformation but are caused by progressive obstruction caused by inflammation. According to this theory, an inflammatory process involving primarily the biliary system could result in biliary atresia, inflammation of the hepatocytes could result in neonatal hepatitis, and inflammation of the intrahepatic bile ducts could result in bile duct paucity.

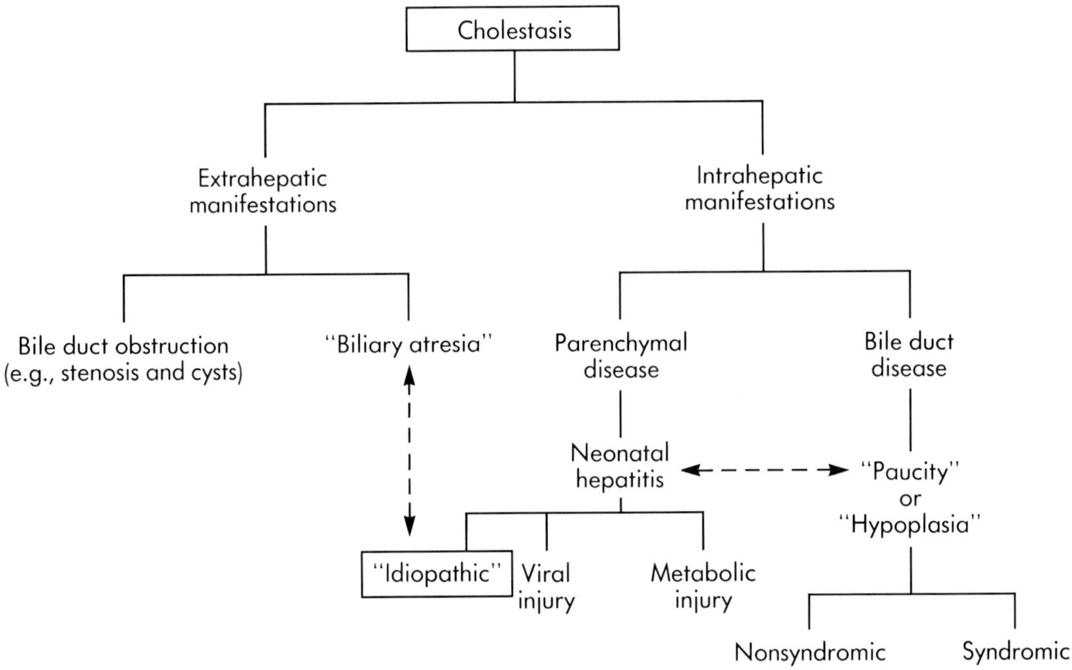

Figure 9-1
Conceptualization of neonatal cholestasis. This figure divides the causes of neonatal cholestasis based on the region of involvement in the hepatobiliary tree. The broken arrows demonstrate areas of potential overlap. For example, some patients with neonatal cholestasis may develop progressive bile duct disappearance resulting in paucity. Similarly, some patients with bile duct patency and the clinical appearance of neonatal hepatitis on initial evaluation may develop biliary atresia. (From Balistreri WF: Foreword, Seminars in Liver Disease, vol 7, No. 2, New York, 1987, Thieme Medical Publishers, Inc).

Extrahepatic Biliary Atresia

Atresia of the extrahepatic bile ducts accounts for 25% to 30% of the cases of neonatal cholestasis and occurs at a frequency of 1 in 8000 to 15,000 live births. In infancy this disorder is the most common cause of jaundice for which surgery is indicated. The etiology of this condition remains undefined. A genetic cause is unlikely based on the rarity of documented familial recurrence and reports of discordance for biliary atresia in both monozygotic and dizygotic twins.

Schweitzer and Müller have described two clinically distinct groups of patients with extrahepatic biliary atresia. The more common *perinatal* form, which occurred in 67% of the patients in their series, usually develops following a jaundice-free interval after birth. During surgical dissection of the porta hepatis, bile duct remnants are often found in these cases, and associated congenital malformations are absent. Although biliary atresia usually is not detected in premature infants or stillbirths, apparently there is a *fetal or embryonic form* of the disease, which accounts for 33% of cases in the Schweitzer and Müller series in which jaundice is present from birth. Biliary remnants in the porta hepatis are absent in these infants, and congenital malformations, including polysplenia, malrotation, ectopic pancreas, and vascular malformations, such as a preduodenal portal vein, may be present. Distinguishing the fetal forms from perinatal forms of biliary atresia may have clinical relevance because the establishment of adequate bile drainage is less likely to occur in the fetal form of the disease and cirrhosis may develop earlier. In contrast, the chances of successful biliary drainage occurring with portoenterostomy are presumably greater in the perinatal form of the disease, and the progression to cirrhosis is less rapid. Regardless of whether biliary atresia assumes the fetal or perinatal form, the disease is most often progressive. Indeed, even those patients with a "successful" portoenterostomy whose jaundice resolves and in whom bile flow is established will eventually develop cirrhosis and portal hypertension. This development implies that the condition affects both the intrahepatic and the extrahepatic bile ducts and that simply relieving the extrahepatic biliary obstruction is not sufficient to reverse the progressive intrahepatic biliary destruction.

Infants with biliary atresia are usually products of uncomplicated pregnancies and are of appropriate size for gestational age. Jaundice develops during the first week of life in the fetal form of the disease, but in the more common, postnatal form, it develops later, up to 6 weeks of age. Besides jaundice, other physical findings include an enlarged, firm liver and acholic stools. The presence of acholic stools in an infant, which indicates extrahepatic biliary obstruction, should alert the clinician to the possibility of biliary atresia, because there are relatively few clues in routine examination to distinguish biliary atresia from other forms of neonatal cholestasis. If any question remains regarding the patency of the extrahepatic biliary tree, a cholangiogram (usually intraoperative) and liver biopsy should be performed. The presence or absence of a gallbladder has been proposed as a means to discriminate neonatal hepatitis from biliary atresia, respectively, but the gallbladder (or absence thereof) may be found in both conditions. Therefore hepatobiliary ultrasonography cannot reliably distinguish between medical and surgical causes of neonatal cholestasis. Other diagnostic tests, such as assessment of duodenal fluid for bile acid content or hepatobiliary scintigraphy, may exclude biliary atresia if the bile ducts are patent but are not as specific as cholangiography and liver biopsy for diagnosis.

Because the histologic features of biliary atresia are characteristic, liver biopsy is a reliable method to distinguish biliary atresia from other conditions of conjugated hyperbilirubinemia. The most consistent histologic findings in biliary atresia are bile duct proliferation and expansion of the portal areas. Canalicular and hepatocellular bile stasis is often present. In addition, bile plugs may be seen in the portal bile ducts; this finding is specific for biliary obstruction but is present in only 40% of cases. The lobular hepatic architecture may be preserved early in the course of the disease, but some patients may have multinucleated giant cells in the hepatic parenchyma, making the differentiation from neonatal hepatitis more difficult.

The key to the initial management of biliary atresia is early diagnosis. There is a correlation between the success of hepatoportoenterostomy and the age of the patient at the time of operation. Bile flow after hepatoportoenterostomy may occur in as many as 90% of infants less than 2 months of age but in less than 20% of infants greater than 3 months of age. The type of biliary conduit used during surgery depends on the extrahepatic biliary anatomy present because correctable and noncorrectable types of biliary atresia exist. In the so-called "correctable" lesions, which make up only 10% of cases, patent proximal hepatic ducts are present, and the atretic biliary segment is distal to the porta hepatis. In infants in whom the level of obstruction is at the hepatic ducts but with a patent cystic duct and distal common bile duct, the gallbladder may be connected to the porta hepatis and may be used as the biliary conduit. If only a small segment of the bile duct is atretic with a patent remainder of the extrahepatic biliary tree, a careful evaluation should be performed to exclude conditions other than biliary atresia that can mimic biliary obstruction. "Noncorrectable" types of biliary atresia, which account for 90% of cases, have macroscopic obliteration of the *entire* extrahepatic biliary tree. A portal dissection should be performed in these patients, followed by apposition of the mucosa from a limb of jejunum to the porta hepatis.

The short-term prognosis for patients with biliary atresia depends in part on the amount of bile flow following hepatoportoenterostomy, although the ultimate outcome depends on the progression of the intrahepatic disease. It is reasonable to expect that patients in whom bile flow is established after surgery will tend to fare better than those in whom minimal bile flow occurs. Indeed, hepatoportoenterostomy will result in long-term improvement in some patients with biliary atresia; however, the majority of patients will develop progressive hepatic dysfunction leading to cirrhosis and portal hypertension. Nevertheless, surgery is often helpful in these patients as well because delaying the time at which cirrhosis occurs will allow the infant to grow to a size at which the chances for successful liver transplantation are increased. On the other hand, orthotopic liver transplantation has been recommended by some clinicians as the *primary* surgical therapy for extrahepatic biliary atresia. However, because of the documented success of hepatoportoenterostomy in some cases of extrahepatic biliary atresia combined with a shortage of suitable donors, this approach is not widely practiced.

Cholangitis is a frequent postoperative complication in patients with biliary atresia, especially in patients with good bile flow after surgery. Cholangitis usually occurs within 3 months of surgery, with 93% of cases occurring during the first year of life. Although the development of cholangitis was proposed to affect adversely the progress of patients with biliary atresia, in one series the incidence of portal hypertension in patients with biliary atresia and good postoperative bile flow was similar whether or not cholangitis occurred. This observation reinforces the concept that the limiting factor affecting the condition of patients with biliary atresia is the progression of the intrahepatic component of the disease.

The factors contributing to this progression are not yet fully elucidated.

Idiopathic Neonatal Hepatitis

The diagnosis of "idiopathic neonatal hepatitis" should be reserved for those newborns with cholestasis who exhibit the characteristic histologic features and in whom the known infectious and metabolic diseases have been excluded. This term should not be confused with hepatitis in a newborn because of an infectious agent, such as HBV or cytomegalovirus. This condition probably encompasses a heterogeneous group of disorders, and it remains the most common diagnosis for newborns with cholestasis, accounting for 35% to 40% of cases.

The heterogeneity of idiopathic neonatal hepatitis contributes to the variability of the presenting symptoms and clinical outcome in patients with this illness; however, clinical experience allows several observations to be made. Jaundice develops in all patients with the disease during the first 2 months of life and is present within the first week of life in more than half the patients. Despite the presence of cholestasis, many infants appear to be well and exhibit appropriate weight gain. In contrast, approximately one third fail to thrive and may experience a fulminant course. The most consistent finding in this condition is hepatosplenomegaly. The presence of pigmented stools in jaundiced infants with idiopathic neonatal hepatitis distinguishes them from infants with extrahepatic biliary obstruction. On the other hand, in patients with severe cholestasis the stools may be acholic and similar in appearance to those seen in cases of biliary atresia. Although hemolytic anemia is occasionally associated with idiopathic neonatal hepatitis, the presence of other extrahepatic symptoms, such as thrombocytopenia, microcephaly, hydrocephalus, or chorioretinitis, is unusual and implies an alternative diagnosis, such as congenital infection.

The diagnostic approach to the jaundiced infant is shown in Figure 9-2. Of the diagnostic tests available, liver biopsy is the most reliable means to distinguish idiopathic neonatal hepatitis from other causes of neonatal cholestasis. Histologic features of idiopathic neonatal hepatitis include (1) lobular disarray with a marked variation in hepatocellular size caused by swelling, regeneration, and individual cell necrosis; (2) a mixed inflammatory exudate of lymphocytes, eosinophils, and neutrophils; (3) extramedullary hematopoiesis; and (4) canalicular bile stasis without bile duct plugging and minimal or absent bile duct proliferation. Hepatocellular giant cell transformation, commonly seen in neonatal hepatitis, is also present in other conditions associated with neonatal cholestasis, such as biliary atresia. Thus it carries no diagnostic specificity.

There is no specific treatment for idiopathic neonatal hepatitis. Therefore management of these cases is supportive and pertains mostly to careful monitoring, maintaining adequate nutrition, and responding to the complications of cholestasis (Table 9-1). The goals of therapy should be to optimize growth, minimize discomfort, anticipate and manage complications of CLD, such as cirrhosis, and facilitate psychologic and social development.

The prognosis for patients with idiopathic neonatal hepatitis varies because of the heterogeneity of the disorder. Nevertheless, the risk of death or development of CLD is greater in familial cases than

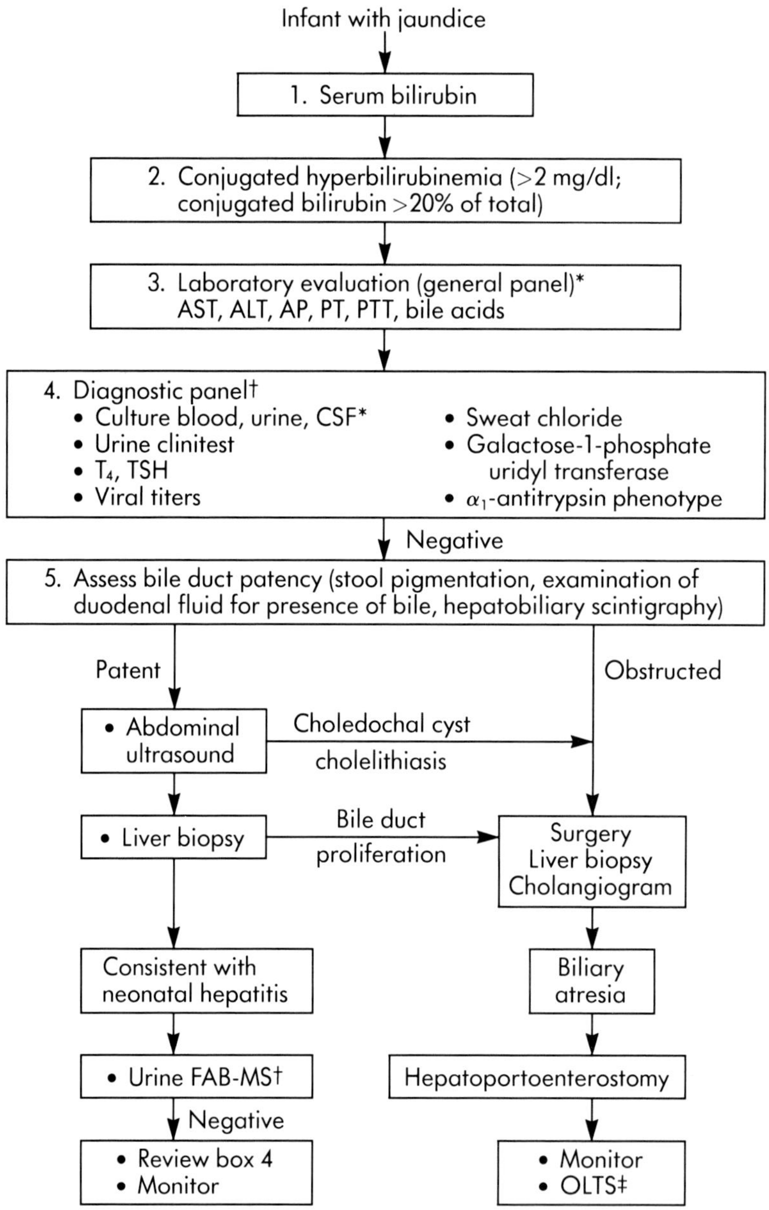

Figure 9-2
Evaluation of the cholestatic infant. This algorithm outlines the general approach to the evaluation of neonates with cholestasis. *CSF = cerebrospinal fluid; T4 = thyroxine; TSH = thyroid stimulating hormone; †FAB-MS = fast atom bombardment-mass spectrometry; ‡OLT, orthotopic liver transplantation.

Table 9-1 Management of Cases of Chronic Cholestasis

Effect	Management
Malnutrition	
Malabsorption of dietary long-chain triglycerids	Replace with formula or supplement containing medium-chain triglyceride
Poor intake (ascites, apathy)	Provide adequate protein Provide adequate calories (complex starches)
Deficiency of fat-soluble vitamins	
A (night blindness, lichenification)	Replace with 10,000-15,000 IU/day of Aquasol A
E (neuromuscular degeneration)	Replace with 50-400 IU/day as oral α-tocopherol (may require parenteral administration)
D (metabolic bone disease)	Replace with 4000-8000 IU/day vitamin D_2 or 3-5 μg/kg/day 25-hydroxycholecalciferol
K (hypoprothrombinemia)	Replace with 2.5-5.0 mg every other day as menadione
Micronutrient deficiency	Supplement with calcium, phosphate, and zinc
Deficiency of water-soluble vitamins	Supplement with double the recommended daily allowance (RDA)
Retention of biliary constituents	
Bile acids and cholesterol (pruritus/xanthomas)	Bile acid binders (cholestyramine 8-16 gm/day) Enrichment of bile acid pool (ursodeoxycholic acid ?)
Trace elements (e.g., copper)	? Avoid copper-enriched foods
Hepatotoxicity ?	? Chelating agents
Progressive liver disease	
Portal hypertension (variceal bleeding, ascites, hypersplenism)	Interim management (control bleeding, treat with sclerotherapy, restrict salt, administer diuretics)
End-stage liver disease	Transplantation

From Balistreri WF: Foreword. In Seminars in Liver Disease, vol 7, no 2, New York, 1987, Thieme Medical Publishers, Inc.

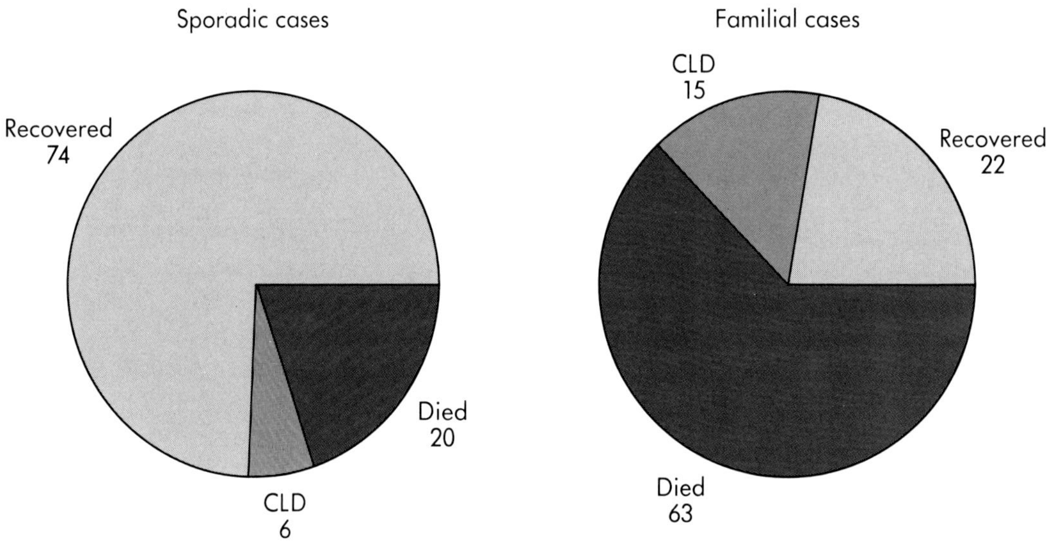

Figure 9-3
Prognosis of neonatal hepatitis. The data shown were compiled from 5 series representing 251 patients. The morbidity and mortality of chronic liver disease, shown as a percentage of the total, is greater in patients with the familial form of idiopathic neonatal hepatitis.

sporadic cases (Figure 9-3). Although one series reported a worse prognosis in infants with a peak total bilirubin greater than 15 mg/dl, no clinical or biochemical feature has consistently been found to correlate with outcome in patients with idiopathic neonatal hepatitis.

It is important to emphasize that infants with conditions diagnosed in the past as neonatal hepatitis have in recent years been diagnosed more specifically. The most commonly defined subset of idiopathic neonatal hepatitis is that of α-1AT deficiency.

A-1 Antitrypsin Deficiency

α-1AT, the predominant plasma α-1 globulin, is a hepatically synthesized protease inhibitor. A deficiency of α-1AT can cause hepatic or pulmonary disease. Phenotyping of various protease inhibitor *(Pi)* alleles is determined by electrophoretic mobility. The normal phenotype *(PiM)* is present in 95% of the U.S. population; the phenotype associated with the most severe deficiency state of α-1AT *(PiZ)* occurs in 1% of the U.S. population but is highest in Scandinavians (2.6%). In a large Swedish study that screened for *Pi* phenotype in more than 200,000 newborns, 125 individuals with *PiZZ* were identified. The hepatic complications observed in these patients included neonatal cholestasis (12%), clinical liver disease that developed later in infancy (7%), and elevations of liver enzymes without clinical symptoms (47%).

Infants with α-1AT deficiency account for 5% to 10% of cases of neonatal cholestasis. The clinical presentation and histologic features in these patients are usually indistinguishable from those of idiopathic neonatal hepatitis. Therefore the *Pi* phenotype and α-1AT concentration should be determined in all infants with cholestasis. The *Pi* phenotype should also be determined in parents of any child with α-1AT deficiency to confirm the diagnosis, and to identify asymptomatic patients with *PiZZ*. The serum α-1AT concentration, which is 10% to 15% of the normal value of 200 to 400 mg/dl in patients with *PiZZ*, also provides evidence supporting the diagnosis of α-1AT deficiency. However, because α-1AT is an acute-phase reactant, its concentration is increased with inflammation, estrogen therapy, or pregnancy and may be intermediate even in patients with *PiZZ* under those conditions. Another diagnostic test for α-1AT deficiency is periodic acid-Schiff (PAS) staining of liver biopsy tissue treated with and without diastase.

The prognosis for liver disease in patients with *PiZZ* varies. Earlier series have reported the development of cirrhosis in approximately 30% of patients who present with neonatal jaundice. However, more recent series of such patients indicate a more grave outcome, with cirrhosis developing in approximately 50% of patients, persistent liver disease without cirrhosis developing in 26% to 50% of patients, and recovery from liver disease occurring in only 0% to 20% of patients.

Currently the treatment for α-1AT deficiency is supportive, involving therapy aimed at the complications of cholestasis or cirrhosis when appropriate. Liver transplantation is indicated in patients with end-stage liver disease. After transplantation the recipient assumes the *Pi* phenotype of the donor liver.

INTRAHEPATIC CHOLESTASIS

The group of disorders causing intrahepatic cholestasis accounts for 5% to 10% of the cases of conjugated hyperbilirubinemia in infants, with an estimated frequency of 1 in 70,000 (see box on p. 228-229). Within this broad category, syndromic paucity (arteriohepatic dysplasia) is the diagnosis in approximately three fourths of the patients.

Arteriohepatic Dysplasia

Recognition of a unique constellation of clinical features (familial pulmonary arterial stenosis and neonatal liver disease) is credited to Alagille and colleagues. The phenotypic expression in patients with this syndrome varies, but the combination of features is distinctive (Table 9-2). Hepatomegaly is invariably present and is associated with cholestasis in more than 90% of patients. The other commonly associated clinical manifestations include (1) *unusual facies*, characterized by a broad forehead, hypertelorism with deeply set eyes, a long, straight nose, and an underdeveloped mandible; (2) *ocular abnormalities*, such as posterior embryotoxon, which represents incomplete iridocorneal separation; (3) *cardiovascular abnormalities*, including peripheral pulmonic stenosis (90%), ventricular septal defect, or tetralogy of Fallot; (4) *vertebral arch defects* and anterior vertebral arch fusion with butterfly vertebrae; (5) paucity of interlobular bile ducts. In the series of Alagille, 26 of 80 patients had all 5 features (complete

Table 9-2 Features of alagille syndrome (arteriohepatic dysplasia)

Major criteria	Incidence (%)
Decreased number of interlobular bile ducts/ chronic cholestasis	91
Extrahepatic anomalies	
Unusual facies	95
Vertebral arch defects	87
Cardiovascular abnormalities	70
Posterior embryotoxon	89
Associated features	
Growth retardation	50
Mental retardation	16
Renal abnormalities	68
Hypogonadism	<10
Bone disease	<10

From Balistreri WF: Interrelationship between the infantile cholangiopathies and paucity of the intrahepatic ducts. In Balistreri WF and Stocker JT, eds: Pediatric hepatology, New York, 1990, Hemisphere Publishing Corp, pp. 159-176.

syndrome), 42 patients had 4 features, and 12 had 3 features (partial syndrome). Renal abnormalities, such as tubulointerstitial nephropathy and decreased creatinine clearance, have also been reported. The associated findings of growth retardation and spermatogenic hypoplasia may represent nutrient deficiency secondary to chronic liver dysfunction.

The diagnosis may be difficult to make in early infancy because the facial features may be subtle and the bile duct paucity, which is progressive, may not be complete on the initial liver biopsy. Histologic features that may be present in infancy include ballooning of hepatocytes, giant cell transformation, and portal inflammation. Serum aminotransferase levels may be normal or elevated, but SBA, AP, cholesterol, and triglycerides are invariably elevated. The importance of differentiating intrahepatic cholestasis from extrahepatic biliary obstruction is emphasized by the report of four patients with intraoperative cholangiographic evidence of extrahepatic ductal atresia. These patients underwent hepatoportoenterostomy but were ultimately shown to have arteriohepatic dysplasia with hypoplastic but patent extrahepatic ductal systems. The prognosis became that of a patient with a hepatoportoenterostomy. Thus the difficulty in establishing an accurate diagnosis and the hazards associated with performing hepatoportoenterostomy in patients who do not have clearly defined biliary atresia warrant extreme caution and a high index of suspicion.

The prognosis for prolonged survival is good; however, patients with arteriohepatic dysplasia are at high risk for morbidity because of pruritus, xanthomas, and complications secondary to vitamin deficiency. Recurrent episodes of cholestasis, which often occur in association with upper respiratory infections, are most severe in the first 4 years of life. There were 21 (26% of patients studied) deaths in Alagille's series. Four patients died of liver complications (two each of hepatic failure and portal hypertension, and six died of cardiovascular complications. There are two reports of hepatocellular carcinoma occurring in patients with arteriohepatic dysplasia. Inheritance of this disorder appears to be autosomal dominant with variable penetrance.

Nonsyndromic Paucity of the Intrahepatic Bile Ducts

Nonsyndromic paucity is a diagnosis applied to patients whose liver biopsy shows an absence or reduced number of interlobular bile ducts but in whom none of the features of arteriohepatic dysplasia are present. These patients most likely have an eclectic group of diseases (see box below). Commonly occurring symptoms include cholestasis with hepatomegaly, pruritus, xanthomas, and hyperlipidemia. The prognoses vary because of the heterogeneous nature of this condition; however, the outcome is generally worse than that of arteriohepatic dysplasia. Alagille reported that in a series of 31 patients with nonsyndromic paucity, the diseases of 21 of the patients became manifest in the neonatal period but 10 were of a delayed onset. Seven of the patients whose diseases became manifest in the neonatal period were subsequently shown to have α-1AT deficiency. The diseases of the remaining 14 patients were of unknown etiology, as were the diseases of all 10 of those with delayed onset. In the last group of patients, any of the diseases listed in the box at left may have been present. There was a high mortality in the first 15 cases of the series; of these cases, 11 died of cirrhosis.

HEPATOBILIARY DISEASES ASSOCIATED WITH BILE DUCT PAUCITY

I. Infectious diseases
   A. Cytomegalovirus
   B. Rubella
   C. Herpes
   D. Coxsackie
II. Metabolic/ endocrine diseases
   A. α-1-AT deficiency
   B. Cystic fibrosis
   C. Inborn errors of bile acid metabolism
   D. Peroxisomal disorders
   E. Panhypopituitarism
III. Chromosomal
   A. Down's syndrome
   B. Trisomy 17, 18
IV. "Immunologic"
   A. Graft vs. host disease
   B. Disappearing bile duct syndrome (after liver transplant)
V. Toxic
VI. Idiopathic
   A. Sclerosing cholangitis
   B. Syndromic paucity (arteriohepatic dysplasia)
   C. Nonsyndromic paucity

From Balistreri WF: Interrelationship between the infantile cholangiopathies and paucity of the intrahepatic ducts. In Balistreri WF and Stocker JT, eds: Pediatric hepatology, New York, 1990, Hemisphere Publishing Corp, pp. 1-18.

Hereditary Cholestasis with Lymphedema

A Norwegian kindred with intrahepatic cholestasis and lymphedema was initially described by Aagenes and colleagues. Lower extremity lymphedema, appearing late in childhood, may be secondary to lymphatic vessel hypoplasia, according to the study. The cholestasis is enigmatic and may be related to either hepatic lymph hypoplasia or a defect in hepatic lymph flow. The cholestasis is also episodic: serum aminotransferases, AP. BA, and cholesterol are elevated during exacerbations but may be normal between episodes. Cirrhosis may develop as a late complication. The inheritance is thought to be autosomal recessive.

Byler's Syndrome

Byler's syndrome is a progressive familial intrahepatic cholestasis initially manifest as neonatal cholestasis in the majority of cases. The major clinical distinction from arteriohepatic dysplasia is the absence of nonhepatic malformations and the less frequent occurrence of bile duct paucity. The name "Byler's syndrome" is derived from the Amish kindred of Jacob Byler in whom the condition was first described; however, "Byler-like" syndromes of familial cholestasis have been reported from all parts of the world. Its inheritance appears to be autosomal recessive.

Patients with Byler's syndrome often have a positive family history of liver disease. The course of the disease may vary, and the symptoms of jaundice, pruritus, and hepatomegaly may not appear until later in the first year of life. The laboratory evaluation will document cholestasis with marked elevation in SBA levels, AP, and bilirubin. Cholesterol values may be paradoxically normal or only mildly elevated. A low GGTP may also be found in this syndrome, and it may be associated with a poor prognosis. The aminotransferase levels are only mildly elevated. Histologically, giant cell transformation and paucity of the intrahepatic bile ducts may be present initially, followed by the development of periportal fibrosis or progression to biliary cirrhosis. Complications of chronic cholestasis frequently occur with neurologic manifestations of vitamin E deficiency, rickets (caused by vitamin D deficiency), and lichenified skin (caused by vitamin A deficiency). Older patients may have Kayser-Fleischer rings caused by chronic copper overload from prolonged cholestasis. In addition, cholelithiasis, chronic pancreatitis, and hepatocellular carcinoma have been reported. The clinical course is progressive and persistent cholestasis resulting in end-stage liver disease. Currently the only known treatment is orthotopic liver transplantation, though supplementation with ursodeoxycholic acid may ameliorate some of the complications of cholestasis.

Benign Recurrent Intrahepatic Cholestasis

Benign recurrent intrahepatic cholestasis is characterized by multiple transient episodes of jaundice, which resolve spontaneously with symptom-free intervals of months to years. Additional diagnostic criteria include biochemical evidence of cholestasis, normal intrahepatic and extrahepatic bile ducts by cholangiography, and absence of other conditions known to produce cholestasis. The symptoms include intense pruritus, malaise, and lassitude. Laboratory findings include an increase of serum bilirubin and AP levels with minimal increase in aminotransferase values. The hepatic architecture is normal histologically with mild to moderate centrolobular bile stasis. The onset is usually in the second or third decade of life, though 20% of patients experience jaundice within the first year of life. Affected women may develop cholestasis during pregnancy or while taking oral contraceptives. Despite years of recurrent cholestasis, cirrhosis does not develop.

Inborn Errors of Bile Acid Metabolism

At present, in addition to the peroxisomal disorders, the known congenital defects in BA metabolism that cause cholestasis are trihydroxycoprostanic acidemia, Δ^4-3-oxosteroid 5-β-reductase deficiency, and 3-β-hydroxy-δΔ^5steroid dehydrogenase-isomerase deficiency. Infants with these conditions previously might have been considered to have familial neonatal hepatitis because the clinical course and histologic findings are nonspecific. The diag-

GENETIC DISORDERS OF PEROXISMAL NUMBER OR FUNCTION

- General impairment of numerous peroxisomal functions and reduced or undetectable peroxisome number
  - Cerebrohepatorenal (Zellweger's) syndrome
  - Infantile Refsum's disease
  - Neonatal adrenoleukodystrophy
  - Hyperpipecolic acidemia
  - Rhizomelic chrondroplasia punctata
- Generalized impairment of peroxisomal function but normal peroxisome number
  - Pseudo-Zellweger's syndrome
- Single peroxisomal enzyme defect but normal number of peroxisomes
  - X-linked adrenoleukodystrophy
  - Adult Refsum's disease
  - Acatalasemia

From Setchell KDR and Street JM: Inborn errors of bile acid synthesis, Semin Liver Dis 7:85-99, 1987.

nosis may be made by examining the urinary BA–excretion pattern with fast atom bombardment–mass spectrometry and gas chromatography–mass spectrometry. The prognosis is usually poor, but investigational treatment with BA-replacement therapy and ursodeoxycholic acid is being evaluated.

Zellweger's Syndrome

The cerebrohepatorenal (Zellweger's) syndrome was the first described entity in a group of diseases known as the peroxisomal disorders (see box above). Affected infants exhibit a high forehead with flat facies, hepatomegaly, psychomotor retardation, renal cortical cysts, and intrahepatic cholestasis. Paucity of the intrahepatic bile ducts, lobular disarray, and focal necrosis may occur. The absence of hepatic peroxisomes is associated with biochemical abnormalities, which include the accumulation of pipecolic acid and very- long-chain fatty acids. There is no known treatment, and death usually occurs within the first 6 months of life. Genetic counseling is important because prenatal diagnosis is possible through the detection of increased hexcosanoic and hexcosenoic acids in amniotic fluid and cultured amniocytes.

ANATOMIC CAUSES OF CHOLESTASIS

Infantile Polycystic Disease of the Liver and Kidney/Congenital Hepatic Fibrosis

Congenital hepatic fibrosis usually presents in late childhood with hepatomegaly, portal hypertension, and esophageal varices; however, liver function is normal. The hepatomegaly may be asymmetric, with most of the liver enlargement occurring in the left lobe. Because the pathologic lesion of congenital hepatic fibrosis may not be uniformly distributed throughout the liver, a percutaneous needle biopsy of the liver may be normal if the tissue sampled is not affected. In such patients an operative liver biopsy may be indicated. Histologically the parenchymal lobules are separated by broad bands of diffuse periportal or perilobular fibrous tissue. In addition, there are multiple "bile duct–like" structures located at the periphery of the portal area. Cystic disease of the kidney occurs in approximately 50% of cases. The renal lesion in some patients may resemble the medullary sponge kidney disease of adults. Treatment is aimed at controlling variceal hemorrhage; esophageal sclerotherapy is often effective. Because liver function is normal in this condition, patients who have recurrent variceal hemorrhage are candidates for a portocaval shunting procedure. The prognosis is generally good for children with this disease; however, renal disease, expecially *infantile* polycystic disease, is a significant mortality risk in some patients.

Caroli's Disease

Caroli's disease is a condition of saccular dilatation of the intrahepatic bile ducts with intervening areas of focal stenosis, which may involve multiple segments of the biliary system. The ectatic biliary lesions may lead to recurrent cholangitis, cholelithiasis, or abscess formation. This disorder is also associated with choledochal cysts and renal involvement. Renal cortical cysts are present in approximately 25% of patients.

Neonatal Sclerosing Cholangitis

Sclerosing cholangitis, a chronic fibrosing inflammation of the bile ducts, has been described in infants who presented with jaundice and hepatosplenomegaly during the first week of life. The diagnosis was made by ultrasonographically guided percutaneous cholecystography, which revealed decreased arborization with stenosis and focal dilatations of the intrahepatic bile ducts. Liver biopsy revealed an initial absence of interlobular bile ducts, followed by the development of biliary cirrhosis. The underlying pathophysiologic mechanism in this disorder remains undefined; however, this condition may be another entity in the spectrum of infantile obstructive cholangiopathies.

METABOLIC CAUSES OF CHOLESTASIS

Disorders of Amino Acid Metabolism

Tyrosinemia. An elevation of serum tyrosine may occur in transient neonatal tyrosinemia or acute and chronic forms of hereditary tyrosinemia. Transient neonatal tyrosinemia often occurs in premature infants and is thought to be the result of decreased tyrosine aminotransferase activity, decreased intake of ascorbic acid, or a combination of the two. This biochemical abnormality is not associated with liver disease, and tyrosine concentrations normalize with maturation.

Hereditary tyrosinemia may present in acute or chronic forms. Its inheritance is autosomal recessive, and both acute and chronic forms may occur within the same family. The acute form usually presents the first month of life with hepatosplenomegaly, jaundice, ascites, edema, and a bleeding diathesis. Hypoalbuminemia, prolonged PT, and marked hyperbilirubinemia are disproportionately abnormal, considering that the aminotransferase levels may be normal or only slightly elevated. Renal dysfunction with hyperphosphaturia, glucosuria, proteinuria, and aminoaciduria resembling Fanconi's syndrome often accompanies the liver disease. The marked elevation of serum tyrosine is accompanied by hypermethioninemia. The diagnosis can be made by analyzing the urine for elevations in nitrosonapthol, succinylacetone, succinylacetoacetone, or δ-ALA. The most common enzymatic defect is due to a deficiency of fumarylacetoacetase, though variants caused by deficiencies of 4-hydroxy-phenylpyruvic acid oxidase or 4-hydroxy-phenylpyruvic acid dioxygenase have also been reported. Prenatal diagnosis is possible by measuring succinylacetone levels in amniotic fluid or fumarylacetoacetase activity in cultured amniocytes. In the acute form, death caused by liver failure usually occurs within the first year of life. The chronic form of the disease has a more gradual onset, occurring over the first several years of life, but cirrhosis invariably develops. In addition, hepatocellular carcinoma occurs in up to one third of patients with the chronic form. Orthotopic liver transplantation has been performed successfully for infants with hepatic failure and older children with carcinoma caused by this condition.

Disorders of Lipid Metabolism

Wolman's disease. Wolman's disease is a fatal autosomal recessive condition that presents in the first year of life with steatorrhea, hepatosplenomegaly, jaundice and failure to thrive. Diffuse intracellular accumulations of triacylglycerol and cholesterol ester occur in the liver, spleen, small intestine, lymph nodes, bone marrow, and adrenal glands because of a deficiency of lysosomal acid lipase. However, the plasma lipid concentrations are usually normal. Stippled calcifications of the adrenal glands are a characteristic radiographic feature in these patients. The liver tissue is yellow grossly; microscopically, large lipid droplets are present in the hepatocytes, and cholesterol ester crystals are seen in Kupffer cells. There is no known treatment for this condition, and all reported cases have been fatal.

Cholesterol ester storage disease. Cholesterol and triglyceride accumulate in the liver and intestine in patients with cholesterol ester storage disease (CESD). Hepatomegaly, present at birth, progresses with increasing age. In contrast to Wolman's disease, hyperbetalipoproteinemia is present in CESD. The liver biopsy specimen is a brilliant yellow-orange color. Enlarged, polygonal hepatocytes with a fine lacework pattern to the cytoplasm are seen microscopically. Even though the enzymatic defect is similar to that found in Wolman's disease, patients with CESD have a normal life expectancy.

Gaucher's disease. Three forms of Gaucher's disease have been identified: *type I*, the adult or chronic nonneuropathic type; *type II*, the infantile or acute neuropathic type; and *type III*, the juvenile or subacute neuropathic type. Type I Gaucher's disease may present at any age, with symptoms that include hepatosplenomegaly, thrombocytopenia, bone pain, and yellow to brown skin pigmentation; however, neurologic symptoms are absent in this type. Type II is usually fatal during the first year of life and is characterized by hepatosplenomegaly, strabismus, spasticity, and head retroflexion. These symptoms are due to progressive neurologic dysfunction. In contrast to patients with type II, individuals with type III Gaucher's disease have neurologic symptoms but prolonged survival. The defect in all types is a deficiency of glucocerebrosidase, which produces "Gaucher cells." These cells are reticuloendothelial cells with an accumulation of glucosylceramide in the lysosomes. Histologically Gaucher cells have an eccentric nucleus and cytoplasm with the appearance of "wrinkled tissue paper." Gaucher's disease is usually suspected after examination of bone marrow. However, Gaucher cells are also found throughout the hepatic parenchyma and around the central veins.

They may even obliterate the sinusoids. The diagnosis is confirmed by WBC or fibroblast assay for glucocerebrosidase activity. Serum acid phosphatase is often elevated in Gaucher's disease, unlike other lysosomal storage diseases. Portal hypertension and ascites may occur but are rare in this condition. Treatment by replacement of purified glucocerebrosidase has been attempted, but it remains experimental.

Niemann-Pick disease. Niemann-Pick disease applies to a group of sphingolipidoses and clinically similar variants. Initially as many as five variants were suggested, but the enzymatic defect has been defined only in type A (acute neuronopathic variant) and type B (chronic variant without neurologic involvement). Deficient activity of the lysosomal enzyme sphingomyelinase is present in both types, though type B cells exhibit greater metabolism of sphingomyelin in skin fibroblasts. Patients affected with type A Niemann-Pick disease present with hepatosplenomegaly, developmental delay, and failure to thrive in infancy, with death caused by progressive neurologic dysfunction usually occurring by 4 years of age. Patients with Niemann-Pick variants may present with cholestasis, which may be confused with neonatal hepatitis. Diagnosis of the disease is suggested by the presence of lipid-laden foam cells in bone marrow or liver and sea blue histiocytes, which are best seen with Wright's stain. The cherry red spot of macular degeneration is seen in 30% of cases. There is presently no effective treatment for this condition; therefore, management of carrier families involves genetic counseling, because prenatal diagnosis is possible for types A and B.

Disorders of Carbohydrate Metabolism

Galactosemia. Galactosemia is an autosomal recessive disorder that causes hepatic and central nervous system dysfunction. It occurs in 1 in 40,000 live births. Affected infants develop vomiting, diarrhea, hepatomegaly, jaundice, and cataracts soon after exposure to lactose (or other sources of galactose) in the diet. The disorder is due to a deficiency of galactose-1-phosphate uridyl transferase, the activity of which can be assayed in erythrocytes. All infants with conjugated hyperbilirubinemia should be screened promptly after birth for this condition by testing the urine for reducing substances. However, vomiting or decreased lactose intake at the time of urine collection may result in a false negative test. Therefore if galactosemia is suspected, all sources of galactose should be eliminated from the diet until the diagnostic evaluation is complete. The prognosis is good for patients who are diagnosed and for whom treatment is instituted in infancy. Compliance with a galactose-free diet can be monitored by measuring erythrocyte galactose-1-phosphate concentrations.

Hereditary fructose intolerance. Hereditary fructose intolerance is an autosomal recessive disorder with an incidence of 1 in 20,000 live births. Unlike fructose-1,6-diphosphatase deficiency, fructose-1-phosphate aldolase deficiency causes liver disease. Vomiting, diarrhea, hypoglycemia, jaundice, and failure to thrive may occur in infants with fructose-1-phosphate aldolase deficiency after fructose is introduced into the diet. The onset usually occurs between 6 and 12 months of age, though a neonatal onset is possible in infants fed a formula containing sucrose. The diagnosis is confirmed by detection of deficient fructose-1-phosphate aldolase activity in hepatic tissue. The hepatic lesions of fatty infiltration, hepatocellular necrosis, and bile duct proliferation may be reversible after elimination of fructose from the diet. However, steatosis and growth failure may persist in patients who are noncompliant or who have hidden sources of dietary fructose, such as sorbitol.

Type III glycogen storage disease. Type III glycogen storage disease is due to deficient activity of the debrancher enzyme, amylo-1,6 glucosidase. Most commonly affected are the liver and skeletal muscle, though cardiomegaly with nonspecific electrocardiographic changes may also occur. Patients with hepatic symptoms often present in infancy with abdominal distension, marked hepatomegaly, and short stature. Biochemical abnormalities include asymptomatic fasting hypoglycemia and elevations of serum cholesterol, triglycerides, and aminotransferases. Patients with myopathy will also have elevated creatinine phosphokinase levels. Liver biopsy demonstrates enlargement of hepatocytes caused by glycogen accumulation in the nucleus and cytosol. Unlike patients with type I glycogen storage disease, patients with type III may have less fatty change, and fibrosis may be present. The diagnosis is confirmed by measuring amylo-1,6-glucosidase activity in liver or muscle. The goal of treatment should be to prevent episodes of fasting hypoglycemia by administering oral cornstarch or nocturnal nasogastric feeding. In children such treatment has been shown to decrease hepatic size, improve linear growth, and decrease serum aminotransferases. The hepatic symptoms often diminish during the second decade of life, but symptoms caused by myopathy predominate in adults.

Type IV glycogen storage disease. Type IV glycogen storage disease is due to a deficiency of α-1,4 glycan-6-glucosyl transferase (brancher enzyme), which causes a putatively toxic glycogen molecule with fewer branch points and longer chains to accumulate in liver and muscle. Affected patients develop hepatosplenomegaly and fail to thrive in infancy. In the classic form, complications of cirrhosis, such as portal hypertension with ascites and esophageal varices, usually result in death by the second year of life, though variants with less severe liver involvement have been described. In one report, preventing episodes of hypoglycemia by oral administration of cornstarch decreased hepatic size and serum aminotransferases, improved growth and muscle strength in two patients. However, liver transplantation is often required for prolonged survival. The effect of liver transplantation on the development of myopathy in this condition is unknown.

Miscellaneous Metabolic Disorders

Cystic fibrosis. Neonatal cholestasis may be a presenting symptom in 5% to 10% of patients with cystic fibrosis. Therefore sweat chloride concentration should be considered in all infants with conjugated hyperbilirubinemia. Of the reported cholestatic infants with cystic fibrosis, meconium ileus was often (in 50% to 60% of patients) an associated condition, along with hepatosplenomegaly. Conjugated bilirubin concentrations were elevated up to 15 mg/dl, and the jaundice persisted for 1 to 9 months. Histologically, liver biopsy may demonstrate inspissated bile plugs and mucus in the bile ducts. The resulting biliary obstruction can mimic extrahepatic biliary atresia.

Other than steatosis, the most common hepatic lesion in cystic fibrosis is focal biliary cirrhosis. It occurs almost exclusively in patients with cystic fibrosis. In autopsy series this lesion is seen in more than 70% of cystic fibrosis patients but is clinically apparent in only one fourth of affected individuals. The histologic features of focal biliary cirrhosis include bile duct proliferation, chronic portal inflammation, and inspissated eosinophilic material in the bile ducts. Another suggested cause of biliary obstruction in cystic fibrosis is common bile duct stricture. Surgical relief of common bile duct obstruction has been reported to reduce the severity of hepatic complications in cystic fibrosis. However, the role of such biliary surgery in patients with cystic fibrosis remains controversial. The incidence of multinodular cirrhosis is age-dependent in patients with cystic fibrosis. It occurs in 2% to 3% of all patients but in 5% of adolescents and 10% of adults over 25.

It is difficult to predict the course of liver disease in cystic fibrosis patients. The liver disease in cholestatic infants may resolve clinically. Conversely, patients with end-stage liver disease may not present with neonatal jaundice.

Neonatal hemochromatosis. Neonatal hemochromatosis can be a cause of hepatic failure in infancy. Most reported cases of this poorly understood disorder have been diagnosed at autopsy, when increased iron deposition was noted in the liver, pancreas, heart, and endocrine organs with normal iron stores in the reticuloendothelial cells. Laboratory features include hypoglycemia, hypoprothrombinemia, hypoalbuminemia, and hyperbilirubinemia. Serum aminotransferase concentrations may be elevated early in the disease process but can fall to the normal range as hepatocellular necrosis becomes more extensive. Histologically, hemosiderin deposits, diffuse fibrosis, regenerative nodules, and giant cell transformation are prominent in the liver.

Premortem diagnosis of this disorder has rarely been made in reported cases. Hyperferritinemia, which has occurred in all cases, may also be present in other causes of neonatal cholestasis. Siderosis of the minor salivary glands, which may be seen on an oral mucosal biopsy, has been proposed as a unique pathologic finding of neonatal hemochromatosis.

The prognosis for infants with neonatal hemochromatosis is poor, with most patients dying within the first 6 months of life. The iron-chelating agent deferoxamine, used in the care of adults with hemochromatosis, was ineffective in the treatment of one infant. The only patients known to have survived with this condition have undergone orthotopic liver transplantation.

Cholestasis associated with hypothyroidism. Conjugated hyperbilirubinemia may occur in association with neonatal hypothyroidism. It accounts for approximately 1% of infants with cholestasis. The jaundice may persist for longer than 2 weeks in affected infants. The precise mechanism by which hypothyroidism and cholestasis are associated is unknown, though it has been postulated that thyroid hormones play an important role in the development of hepatic excretory function. Hypothyroidism as a component of panhypopituitarism has also been reported in association with neonatal cholestasis. One specific syndrome that may also occur with conjugated hyperbilirubinemia is septo-optic dysplasia (deMorsier's syndrome), in which panhypopituitarism is combined with optic nerve hypoplasia and diabetes insipidus. Wandering nystagmus may be an early finding in these infants. The cholestasis in all of these conditions usually resolves following appropriate hormone-replacement therapy, though micronodular cirrhosis was reported in one patient 2 years of age with septo-optic dysplasia.

Indian childhood cirrhosis. Named because of its original description in Hindu children, Indian childhood cirrhosis has also been reported in Americans and Europeans. This disorder causes progressive liver injury that leads to hepatic failure and death usually by age 3. Early symptoms of Indian childhood cirrhosis are vague, such as changes in bowel movements, and unusual behavior, including irritability, behavioral changes, and reversal in the day/night cycle. On physical examination hepatomegaly is invariably present, with splenomegaly and abdominal distension developing as the disease progresses. The histologic features in the liver are micronodular cirrhosis, increased orcein-staining copper-associated protein, portal inflammation, Mallory's hyaline bodies, and the lack or paucity of regenerative activity or fatty change. The exact role copper plays in the pathogenesis of this disorder is unknown; increased dietary copper intake is thought to be responsible in the Indian variety. However, a congenital abnormality in copper metabolism has been postulated as the cause in the non-Indian variety.

Familial erythrophagocytic lymphohistiocytosis. Familial erythrophagocytic lymphohistiocytosis is an autosomal recessive condition that presents from 6 weeks to 36 months of age. Fever, wasting, and hepatosplenomegaly are found in almost all patients, but lymphadenopathy and rash are also common (occurring in 40% to 60% of patients). In one series, more than 80% of patients died within 3 months of diagnosis, with all patients dying within 2 years. Pathologic findings in this condition include a lymphohistiocytic infiltrate in the bone marrow, lymphoid tissue, brain, and liver and phagocytic activity of histiocytes against erythrocytes and other formed blood elements. A marked hyperlipidemia is also present with a disproportionate concentration of hepatic gangliosides, suggesting a pathophysiologic role for abnormal lipid metabolism. Attempts to treat familial erythrophagocytic lymphohistiocytosis with corticosteroids and cytotoxic agents have been unsuccessful.

SUMMARY

Cholestasis is often the reaction of the developing liver to a variety of toxic insults. Therefore many congenital and inherited conditions may be associated with conjugated hyperbilirubinemia. Thus it is imperative that a thorough evaluation be performed on infants with jaundice to arrive at an accurate diagnosis and to initiate appropriate therapy. If inherited diseases are discovered, it is also important to initiate genetic counseling and genetic screening where indicated.

It is not possible to detail every metabolic disorder in this rapidly expanding field. Orthotopic liver transplantation has greatly increased the survival for many children who suffer from these conditions. It is hoped that in the future, more advanced medical therapy will emerge to improve the outlook for patients who are affected by this group of diseases.

SUGGESTED READING

Alagille D et al: Syndromic paucity of interlobular bile ducts (Alagille syndrome or arteriohepatic dysplasia): review of 80 cases, J Pediatr 110:195-200, 1987.

This article includes a description of the clinical features of Alagille's syndrome and prognosis for patients with the syndrome.

Balistreri WF: Neonatal cholestasis: medical progress, J Pediatr 86:63, 1984.

An overview of the clinical scope, evaluation, and management of cholestatic infants is presented.

Balistreri WF: Neonatal cholestasis: lessons from the past; issues for the future, Semin Liver Dis 7:1-7, 1987.

The author presents a historical perspective on neonatal cholestasis and a discussion of the conceptual approach to the jaundiced infant.

Balistreri WF: Interrelationship between the infantile cholangiopathies and paucity of the intrahepatic bile ducts. In Balistreri WF and Stocker JT, eds: Pediatric hepatology, New York, 1990, Hemisphere Publishing Corp, pp. 1-18.

This paper discusses the current theories of the intrahepatic cholangiopathies and the intrahepatic cholestatic syndromes.

Balistreri WF: Liver disease associated with α_1-antitrypsin deficiency. In Balistreri WF and Stocker JT, eds: Pediatric hepatology, New York, 1990, Hemisphere Publishing Corp.

A discussion of the pathophysiology, diagnosis, and management of α-1-antitrypsin deficiency-associated liver disease in children is presented.

Danks DM et al: Prognosis of babies with neonatal hepatitis, Arch Dis Child 52:368, 1977.

This is a report on the outcome of 62 patients with this condition.

Landing BH: Consideration of the pathogenesis of neonatal hepatitis, biliary atresia and choledochal cyst: the concept of infantile obstructive cholangiopathy, Prog Pediatr Surg 6:113, 1974.

This article is an overview of the infantile obstructive cholangiopathy theory.

Markowitz J et al: Arteriohepatic dysplasia. I. Pitfalls in diagnosis and management, Hepatology 3:74, 1983.

The authors report on the tragic outcome for patients with arteriohepatic dysplasia who were erroneously diagnosed as having biliary atresia.

Riely CA: Familial intrahepatic cholestatic syndromes, Semin Liver Dis 7:119-133, 1987.

The author presents an overview of the syndromic and nonsyndromic forms of intrahepatic cholestasis.

Ryckman FC and Noseworthy J: Neonatal cholestatic conditions requiring surgical reconstruction, Semin Liver Dis 7:134-154, 1987.

A discussion of the evaluation and surgical management of patients with biliary atresia and choledochal cysts is presented.

Schweitzer P and Müller G, eds: Gallengangsatresie. Cholestase-Syndrome im Neugeborenen- und Sauglingsalter. Bibliothek für Kinderchirurgie. Stuttgart, 1984, Hippokrates.

This paper includes a discussion of the fetal and perinatal forms of extrahepatic biliary atresia.

Setchell KDR and Street JM: Inborn errors of bile acid synthesis, Semin Liver Dis 7:85-99, 1987.

The authors discuss the known inborn errors of bile acid synthesis and techniques available for evaluation and diagnosis.

10 Acquired Cholestatic Syndromes of Infancy

Robert J. Rothbaum and Jerry L. Rosenblum

In infancy, cholestasis is defined as the presence of elevated total and direct-reacting serum bilirubins. Infants have serum levels of bile acids above the usual normal range for older children and adults; this physiologic cholestasis results from immature enterohepatic circulation of bile acids and complicates interpretation of SBA measurements.

The extensive list of potential etiologies of neonatal cholestasis includes infections, metabolic diseases, anatomic abnormalities, endocrinopathies, cardiovascular disorders, drugs, and toxins. This chapter will review the most common and threatening etiologies of neonatal cholestasis.

CAUSES OF CHOLESTASIS IN INFANCY

The clinician evaluating the cholestatic infant less than 3 months of age begins with the general framework outlined in the box at left on p. 250. Many discussions focus on biliary atresia and neonatal hepatitis, but in actual practice, systemic disorders such as infection, shock, and hypoxemia are far more common. An appreciation of the association of these systemic disorders with hepatic dysfunction directs attention to the therapy for the underlying disease and avoids unnecessary evaluation and intervention in cholestatic infants.

The clinician must assess rapidly the infant with jaundice for the presence of particular diseases that require urgent and specific therapy. The infant's general appearance is an essential guide to the order of this evaluation. The infant with poor feeding, lethargy, hypothermia or hyperthermia, vomiting, and inadequate perfusion may suffer from any of the entities listed in the box at right on p. 250. Laboratory tests of hepatic synthetic function or dysfunction alone are not likely to differentiate between these entities. Most of these infants have elevated total and direct bilirubin and moderate elevation of aminotransferase levels. In addition, coagulation times may be prolonged, and serum albumin values may be low, though the pathophysiology of these abnormalities differs among disease states. Thus other examinations must be completed rapidly to reach an accurate diagnosis and begin appropriate therapy.

Certain features of history and physical examination are helpful in the rapid cate-

CAUSES OF CHOLESTASIS IN INFANCY

Common causes

Bacterial sepsis
Left-sided cardiac lesions with low output state
Hypoxemia and hypotension (shock)
Prematurity with complications of necrotizing enterocolitis or severe respiratory distress syndrome, often associated with parenteral nutrition

Unusual causes

Biliary atresia
Neonatal hepatitis
Metabolic disease (e.g., galactosemia and hereditary fructose intolerance)
α_1-antitrypsin deficiency
Cystic fibrosis
Intrahepatic paucity of bile ducts, syndromatic and nonsyndromatic
Congenital infection with virus, syphilis, and toxoplasmosis

Very rare causes

Neonatal cirrhosis with liver failure
Hereditary tyrosinemia
Chromosomal defects (e.g., Trisomy 13, 18, and 21 and Turner's syndrome)
Other anatomic lesions (e.g., spontaneous perforation of the common bile duct, and thrombosis of the hepatic veins or portal vein)
Neonatal hypopituitarism
Extremely rare cholestatic syndromes (e.g., lymphedema-associated syndromes and unusual BA synthetic defects)

ETIOLOGIES OF CHOLESTASIS THAT REQUIRE PROMPT THERAPY

Bacterial sepsis
Neonatal infection with herpes virus and other less common organisms that can be treated with specific therapy
Serious cardiac disease with poor cardiac output and hypoxemia
Galactosemia and hereditary fructose intolerance
Neonatal cirrhosis with severe coagulopathy and hypoglycemia

gorization of an individual infant to allow for the initiation of specific therapy. The infant with bacterial sepsis may have been delivered from a mother with ongoing infection after prolonged rupture of amniotic membranes. Congenital anomalies, such as obstructive uropathy, may predispose the infant to urinary tract infection and bacteremia. Premature infants may develop endotoxemia or sepsis in association with necrotizing enterocolitis. Indwelling catheters in the umbilical artery or vein may provide a portal of entry for organisms. In addition to jaundice, the septic infant may show lethargy, hypothermia or fever, irritability, pallor, and hypotonia. Leukocytosis or leukopenia, thrombocytopenia, DIC, and metabolic acidosis may occur. Cultures of blood, cerebrospinal fluid, and urine should be obtained, and parenteral-antibiotic therapy should be initiated.

The newborn suffering from congenital infection with herpes simplex virus (HSV), cytomegalovirus, rubella, syphilis, or toxoplasmosis may have had gestation complicated by a notable illness or exposure. Intrauterine growth retardation, microcephaly, marked hepatosplenomegaly, thrombocytopenic purpura, chorioretinitis, and at times fetal hydrops are common striking features. Infants with HSV infection often have multiple skin vesicles that contain the virus. Pathologic examination and cultures of the placenta may also demonstrate characteristic findings consistent with one of these infections. A rapid serologic test for syphilis in both mother and infant is essential, and penicillin therapy should be started immediately if the results are positive. Documentation of HSV infection mandates acyclovir therapy in an effort to minimize morbidity and mortality. Therapies for congenital cytomegalovirus and toxoplasmosis are currently available only as part of investigational protocols.

Severe congenital heart disease is usually evident by refractory cyanosis, congestive heart failure, or poor perfusion caused by low cardiac output. Other congenital anomalies may be present, especially with chromosomal abnormalities, such as trisomy 21, 13, or 18. Arterial blood gases, chest roentgenogram, electrocardiogram, and echocardiogram will provide essential information as to the exact anatomic defects. The type of defect dictates the specific therapy.

A history of consanguinity, early death in siblings, and early feeding of lactose or sucrose suggest the presence of metabolic disease. Galactosemic infants may have mild hemolysis, and reducing sugar usually is detectable in urine. Measurement of RBC galactose-1-phosphate uridyl transferase before any transfusion provides an exact diagnosis. After sucrose intake, infants with hereditary fructose intolerance may suffer metabolic acidosis, hypoglycemia, hypokalemia, and hypophosphatemia. These additional metabolic abnormalities can complicate management and require specific correction. The exact diagnosis of hereditary fructose intolerance requires liver biopsy for measurement of specific enzyme activities.

Neonatal cirrhosis is difficult to diagnose rapidly because the severe synthetic dysfunction may be attributed initially to other, more treatable entities, such as infection or metabolic disease. The absence of these specific diagnoses and the persistent nature of the coagulopathy, low serum albumin, and progressive jaundice indicate severe and often irreversible hepatic damage. Galactosemia, α_1-antitrypsin deficiency, erythroblastosis fetalis, Parvovirus B_{19} infection, and neonatal iron-storage disease have been reported as causes of neonatal cirrhosis. Important supportive measures include provision of continuous glucose to prevent hypoglycemia, management of ascites to prevent respiratory embarrassment, infusion of fresh frozen plasma if hemorrhage develops, and monitoring for hypoxemia, renal failure, and infection. Aggressive and intensive support is warranted to reverse the components of hepatic dysfunction that may occur with galactosemia or coincident infection and to support the infant until liver transplantation can be done.

The clinician should recall that some infants may suffer from more than one cholestatic disorder. For example, the galactosemic infant is susceptible to gram-negative bacteremia that may exacerbate the hepatic dysfunction and the seriousness of the illness. Thus ill-appearing infants with jaundice are often treated for more than one of the serious causes of cholestasis as the clinical course evolves and diagnostic testing progresses.

CHOLESTASIS ASSOCIATED WITH PARENTERAL NUTRITION

Persistent pulmonary hypertension, severe necrotizing enterocolitis, multiple congential anomalies, hypoplastic left-heart syndrome and other very complex congenital heart disease, diaphragmatic hernia, and severe respiratory distress syndrome can be fatal for newborns. Antibiotics, successful cardiac surgery, long-term IV nutrition, extracorporeal membrane oxygenation, and new methods of ventilation help many of these infants survive; however, some infants develop cholestasis during or after their period of severe illness. A small percentage of the cholestatic infants have permanent hepatic damage and cirrhosis.

These severely ill infants often require support with parenteral nutrition. Their cholestasis has been attributed to a hepatotoxic effect of the parenteral nutrition solutions. Analysis of clinical data suggests that the rate of amino acid infusion, the length of the period of fasting, the use of medications, such as diuretics or antibiotics, or the length of time of parenteral nutrition could be contributing factors to the development of cholestasis. Subsequent changes in patient care, such as early feeding, alteration of the constituents of amino acid solutions, and provision of additional medications, followed in an effort to prevent the development of cholestasis and progressive liver disease.

More recent studies demonstrate that sepsis, hypotension, and hypoxemia may be more important factors in the development of cholestasis than parenteral nutrition. Dosi and others analyzed the clinical course of a group of infants on parenteral nutrition for more than 15 days and found that infants with cholestasis had a significantly increased incidence of hypotension and severe hyaline membrane disease with hypoxia. The duration of parenteral nutrition was not a significant factor in this study. Retrospective analyses have found that the risk of cholestasis in a group of premature infants was related to shock, hemolytic disorders, multiple transfusions, and exchange transfusion. Wolf and Pohlandt concluded that proven or suspected bacterial infection with either gram-positive or gram-negative organisms was the major factor preceding cholestasis in newborns. Duration of parenteral nutrition and age at institution of enteral feeding had no discernible effect on the likelihood of jaundice. Critically ill infants treated with extracorporeal membrane oxygenation may develop marked direct hyperbilirubinemia. Extracorporeal membrane oxygenation results in extensive hemolysis that increases the amount of hemoglobin metabolized to bilirubin and therefore the load of bilirubin to be conjugated and excreted. Antecedent hypoxemia and hypotension may impair the ability of the newborn's liver to accomplish these processes.

The jaundice that occurs in association with parenteral nutrition does not require specific therapy, usually resolves within several weeks, and does not generally indicate severe permanent liver damage. Rarely an infant will develop cirrhosis, most often with persistence of refractory pulmonary, intestinal, or cardiac disease that mandates continuation of the parenteral nutrition.

The infants in the cited studies suffered from complex illnesses. Such infants are at risk of hepatic injury from multiple mechanisms. Any or all of these mechanisms may contribute to the abnormalities in hepatic function; therefore, attributing their cholestasis to a single cause, such as parenteral nutrition or other intervention, is overly simplistic.

HEPATIC HISTOPATHOLOGY

The hepatic histology of infants with fatal episodes of bacterial sepsis includes intracellular and intracanalicular bile stasis, nuclear and nucleolar enlargement in hepatocytes, and varying degrees of giant cell transformation. Extensive liver cell necrosis is not common. Bacterial endotoxin may contribute to cholestasis because it induces a selective decrease in bile salt independent bile flow secondary to inhibition of hepatocyte Na-K-ATPase activity. Endotoxemia may occur with urinary tract infection or necrotizing enterocolitis and may produce marked cholestasis even without overt bacteremia. Hepatic microabscesses may occur with bacterial contamination of an umbilical venous line or in association with bacteremia or fungemia. The hepatic damage that occurs in association with bacterial infection does not produce sufficient necrosis to result in permanent sequelae although the cholestasis may take several weeks to resolve.

Congenital infection with HSV may produce extensive hepatic necrosis and acute liver failure. Characteristic intranuclear inclusions may be seen in hepatocytes, but because hepatic disease is part of the spectrum of disseminated herpes infection, examination of other specimens, such as skin vesicles, can provide the diagnosis more rapidly, easily, and safely. Congenital syphilis may produce intralobular dissecting fibrosis with centrilobular mononuclear infiltration. Even with prompt treatment, elevated aminotransferase levels may persist for 8 weeks, though chronic liver disease is not reported. The rubella virus produces focal areas of hepatocyte necrosis, mononuclear inflammatory infiltrates of portal areas, and intralobular fibrosis. This fibrosis may be persistent. Cytomegalovirus infection results in extensive giant cell transformation and less commonly in large intranuclear inclusions with a clear halo in bile duct epithelium. Intracytoplasmic inclusions in hepatocytes rarely occur. Up to 20% of asymptomatic infants excrete cytomegalovirus in their urine by age 2 months and have no clinical manifestations of infection. Thus the isolation of cytomegalovirus in the urine of an infant with jaundice may not be related to the hepatic dysfunction but may be a coincidental finding.

The histologic findings in association with cardiac disease vary depending on the nature of the cardiac dysfunction. Acute passive congestion from right-heart failure may produce massive elevation of aminotransferase enzymes with little overt hepatocyte necrosis. With the development of aggressive medical therapy and corrective cardiac surgery, the development of "cardiac cirrhosis" has become quite rare. Low cardiac output in association with obstructive left-heart lesions or systemic venous congestion with hypoxemia are the most common settings associated with hepatic dysfunction. This dysfunction may take the form of "hepatitis," with moderate elevation of aminotransferase levels or more striking interference with synthetic functions producing hyperbilirubinemia, hypoalbuminemia, or hypoprothrombinemia. In the few available pathologic specimens, centrilobular necrosis is prominent, and the degree of necrosis correlates with the severity of the biochemical abnormalities. Hepatic damage associated with shock also takes the form of centrilobular necrosis. This zone of hepatocytes is most susceptible to hypoxemia and ischemia. Improvement of oxygenation, perfusion, and cardiac function results in simultaneous improvement in synthetic function and resolution of jaundice.

The histologic changes that occur in association with parenteral nutrition are well documented and include giant cell transformation, intracellular and intracanalicular bile stasis in the central zones of the hepatic lobule, and hepatocellular damage. Portal fibrosis also may be present. These changes are not specific, and they clearly overlap with pathologic changes that occur in sepsis, shock, and hypoxemia.

INFANTILE OBSTRUCTIVE CHOLANGIOPATHY

The infant who does not have an obvious infectious, metabolic, or circulatory cause for cholestasis may have infantile obstructive cholangiopathy. The histopathologic findings of this disorder include (1) giant cell transformation of hepatocytes (2) portal fibrosis, (3) bile duct proliferation in portal triads, and (4) bile stasis within hepatocytes, canaliculi, and bile ducts. Several authors have attempted to divide infantile obstructive cholangiopathy into the following two distinct entities based on histologic findings in the liver: (1) neonatal hepatitis, defined as giant cell transformation with intracellular and intracanalicular cholestasis, and (2) biliary atresia, indicated by bile duct proliferation with portal fibrosis. However, in clinical practice, all of the histologic findings in infantile obstructive cholangiopathy may be present to some extent in both intrahepatic cholestasis (neonatal hepatitis) and extrahepatic cholestasis (biliary atresia). Landing used the term *infantile obstructive cholangiopathy* to explain (1) the overlapping histopathologic findings in the livers and biliary systems of infants who had choledochal cysts, extrahepatic biliary atresia, or neonatal hepatitis and (2) the observation that infants initially diagnosed as having one disorder were later found to develop a second disorder. For example, infants initially diagnosed as having neonatal hepatitis later developed findings of biliary atresia. Landing stressed that infantile obstructive cholangiopathy is a *dynamic process* that may have different dominant manifestations at different times during the illness. This concept of an ongoing extrauterine inflammatory process explains why some infants who initially show bile duct proliferation in portal triads consistent with extra hepatic atresia or obstruction at age 2 months may develop sclerosis and may demonstrate disappearance of intralobular bile ducts by 9 months. Landing's hypothesis also provides an explanation for the limited ability of any diagnostic technique (e.g., liver biopsy and cholangiogram) to predict with certainty the final diagnosis or the potential outcome of interventions, such as reconstructive surgery. Thus infants who appear to have only extrahepatic biliary atresia may develop intrahepatic biliary damage that precludes the reestablishment of bile flow and leads to progressive liver disease.

Attempts to define the cause of infantile obstructive cholangiopathy center on uncovering an initial viral insult or a genetic predisposition to neonatal liver disease. Infantile obstructive cholangiopathy has been noted in reports of individual cases to be associated with cytomegalovirus, Epstein-Barr virus, and rubella infections, but such infections are not present in most infants with infantile obstructive cholangiopathy. HAV and HBV have not been found in infants with the disorder. The most recent viral candidate is reovirus type 3, but serologic and immunohistologic evidence of this infection is lacking in most infants with infantile obstructive cholangiopathy. Many infants with jaundice with α_1-antitrypsin deficiency have histopathologic findings of infantile obstructive cholangiopathy, suggesting that a hereditary abnormality in hepatocyte metabolism may be a predisposing factor. However, no such defect is found in most infants with this disorder. Extrahepatic biliary atresia may occur in association with other intraabdominal problems, such as transverse liver, intestinal malrotation, preduodenal portal vein, and polysplenia. No clear inheritance pattern has been defined for this set of anomalies. In summary, the various manifestations of infantile obstructive cholangiopathy may result from a dynamic postnatal inflammatory process, but the initial event in the process and the determinants of its course remain unknown.

Most newborns with infantile obstructive cholangiopathy present with jaundice at 2 to 4 weeks of age. Biochemical abnormalities include direct hyperbilirubinemia with elevated serum aminotransferase and AP levels. Serum albumin and PT are usually normal. Of the infants with the extrahepatic forms of infantile obstructive cholangiopathy (biliary atresia and choledochal cyst), 60% to 70% are female. These infants generally appear to be healthy and growing well except for their jaundice. Stools are persistently acholic.

The differentiation of intrahepatic forms of infantile obstructive cholangiopathy from extrahepatic forms is important in that the latter requires surgical intervention within the first few months of life to try to reestablish bile flow and prevent progressive liver damage. Exploratory laparotomy with liver biopsy and intra operative cholangiogram can provide definitive diagnosis, but they may not be necessary in infants with intrahepatic cholestasis. In the past, laparotomy was also thought to worsen the prognosis of infants with intrahepatic disorders. Therefore, much emphasis has been placed on less invasive diagnostic tests. Although the obstruction is extrahepatic in biliary atresia and choledochal cyst, ultrasound will not show generalized dilation of the extrahepatic or intrahepatic biliary tree. Often a small gallbladder and common bile duct can be identified. Hepatobiliary radionuclide scan is designed to quantitate hepatic uptake and excretion of an organic anion that follows the same route as BAs. A patent biliary tree should allow for excretion from the liver to the intestine, but poor hepatic uptake or marked intrahepatic cholestasis may interfere with excretion, creating the false impression of extrahepatic obstruction.

In evaluating the cholestatic infant, medical diagnoses must be excluded by appropriate testing (see box at left on p. 250). If the ultrasound shows choledochal cyst, then exploratory laparotomy and operative cholangiogram are mandatory to define the anatomy of the extrahepatic biliary tree and provide appropriate reconstruction. If the ultrasound fails to show a cyst, a radionuclide scan shows no excretion of radioisotope from the liver into the intestine, and no other diagnosis is evident, many clinicians proceed with laparotomy, operative liver biopsy, and cholangiogram. Other clinicians believe it is prudent to perform an initial percutaneous liver biopsy to document changes thought to be more consistent with extrahepatic atresia, e.g., bile duct proliferation in portal triads, portal fibrosis, bile plugs in interlobular ducts, and relatively little giant cell transformation. If these changes are present, laparotomy is necessary.

Because infantile obstructive cholangiopathy is a dynamic process that may progress or regress with time, findings at the time of biopsy, laparotomy, or cholangiogram may not represent the final results of the process, which will be present months later. A good example is the dilemma involving the cholangiogram that shows a patent gallbladder, cystic duct, and common bile duct, with flow into the duodenum but no proximal flow into the main hepatic duct or its right or left branches. The infant with such a condition can have progressive sclerosis of the patent extrahepatic ducts, or the inflammatory process in the hepatic ducts can regress with eventual resumption of bile flow. The former process would necessitate a Kasai procedure to establish bile flow; the latter process would not necessitate further surgery. A decision based on multiple factors, possibly including the appearance of the hepatic duct, the findings of liver biopsy, and the degree of apparent fibrosis, must be reached in the operating room. Faced with this dilemma, some surgeons leave a cholecystomy tube in place and perform repeat cholangiography over the next few weeks to judge the patency of the extrahepatic system. This situation highlights the continuing clinical problem of differentiating extrahepatic cholestasis from intrahepatic cholestasis for even the most experienced clinicians.

If an atretic gallbladder with no apparent lumen is found during laparotomy with a sclerotic extrahepatic biliary tree, then a Kasai procedure or roux-en-Y portoenterostomy, is indicated. In 50% to 60% of infants, "successful" surgery will result, as indicated by disappearance of jaundice within 3 months. Failure of jaundice to resolve and worsening of liver disease are most likely due to progression of the infantile obstructive cholangiopathy with obliteration of the intrahepatic biliary system rather than to a delay in timing of surgery or incorrect surgical technique. Biliary cirrhosis and liver failure lead to death at 18 to 24 months of age unless liver transplantation is done.

CARE OF INFANTS WITH PERSISTENT CHOLESTASIS

Most of the common causes of cholestasis in infants require no specific treatment for the jaundice other than care directed at improving an underlying disease state. For example, the infant with bacterial infection needs antibiotics, the infant with shock needs circulatory support, and the infant with hypoxemia needs oxygen and ventilatory support.

The infant with cirrhosis and liver failure needs careful monitoring of coagulation status and infusion of fresh frozen plasma if bleeding occurs. Also, sufficient glucose must be provided to prevent hypoglycemia. Ascites may be severe enough to compromise respiration, but electrolyte imbalance may develop as diuretics are given to reduce the ascites. Intensive support is warranted if a portion of the hepatic dysfunction is thought to be reversible or if liver transplantation is being considered. In other instances the

Table 10-1 Management of nutritional problems associated with persistent cholestasis

Problem	Clinical findings	Therapy
Fat maldigestion and malabsorption	Poor weight gain or slow growth	Formula containing medium chain triglyceride
Vitamin K deficiency	Prolonged PT and PTT	Water-soluble vitamin K (Synkayvite) 2.5 mg p.o./day
Vitamin D deficiency	Low serum 25-OH-vitamin D level, elevated serum AP; early: normal serum calcium, low serum phosphorus; later: low serum calcium, low serum phosphorus, rickets	Vitamin D 2000-10,000 IU/day or 25-OH-vitamin D 25-50 μg/day
Vitamin E deficiency	Early: Low serum vitamin E or low serum vitamin E to total lipids ratio; later: areflexia, ophthalmoplegia, ataxia	Vitamin E acetate p.o. up to 100 IU/kg/day; may need investigational forms of vitamin E or tocopheryl-polyethylene-glycol-succinate(Liqui-E)
Vitamin A deficiency	Low serum vitamin A	Water-miscible vitamin A (Aquasol A)

severity of the liver damage coupled with a decision not to consider transplantation may lead to a therapeutic program that provides palliation until the infant dies. Strong consideration should be given to obtaining immediate postmortem specimens of liver and skin for appropriate biochemical or genetic studies that could define an inherited cause for the liver disease.

The infant with infantile obstructive cholangiopathy may have cholestasis that persists for months to years. The cholestasis may interfere with fat digestion and absorption, necessitating special formulas and vitamin supplements to provide adequate nutrition for growth and to prevent deficiencies of fat-soluble vitamin. Table 10-1 describes the overall management of nutritional problems in infants with persistent cholestasis.

From birth to approximately 4 months, an infant multivitamin preparation may be given twice a day. Oral, water-soluble vitamin K is given once a day. At 4 to 6 months, serum concentrations of vitamin E and 25-OH-vitamin D may fall, indicating a deficiency. Additional supplements may then be added (see Table 10-1). In our experience vitamin A deficiency is unusual, and supplemental doses of vitamin A beyond those in most multivitamin preparations are not usually necessary.

SUMMARY

Infants may develop cholestasis in association with many infectious, circulatory, and metabolic illnesses. Systemic infections, marked respiratory distress, and severe cardiac dysfunction are common antecedents of direct hyperbilirubinemia. Parenteral nutrition has been blamed for cholestasis, but other illnesses often complicate the clinical presentation. By comparison, infantile obstructive cholangiopathy (biliary atresia and neonatal hepatitis) is relatively uncommon. Liver dysfunction associated with systemic disease usually improves along with the underlying illness, and extensive investigation may not be required. Persistent cholestasis may necessitate special nutritional management.

SUGGESTED READINGS

Alagille D and Odièvre M: Liver and biliary tract diseases in children, New York, 1979, John Wiley & Sons, Inc.

This book considers the various causes of liver dysfunction in a form that follows the usual clinical evaluation of a patient. Hepatic histology is well illustrated.

Bernstein J and Brown A: Sepsis and jaundice in early infancy, Pediatrics 29:873-882, 1962.

The clinical course, types of infection, and hepatic histopathology of sepsis in nine infants with hepatic dysfunction are presented in detail. Most infants had fatal gram-negative sepsis with various degrees of acute hepatic damage without extensive necrosis. Jaundice was due to intracellular and intra canalicular bile stasis.

Brown W et al: Lack of correlation between infection with reovirus 3 and extra-hepatic biliary atresia or neonatal hepatitis, J Pediatr 113:670-676, 1988.

The authors tested the serums of 35 infants with infantile obstructive cholangiopathy for a specific anti-reo-3 antibody by an immunoabsorbent assay for total antibodies and for IgM antibodies in younger infants. There was no difference in antibody titers between infants with infantile obstructive cholangiopathy and infants of similar ages with other liver diseases.

Dosi P et al: Perinatal factors underlying neonatal cholestasis, J Pediatr 106:471-474, 1985.

This case control study of 31 infants treated with parenteral nutrition for more than 15 days demonstrates that hypotension and hypoxemia with severe hyaline membrane disease were major determinants of neonatal cholestasis. Younger infants were also more likely to develop jaundice.

Felber S and Sinatra F: Systemic disorders associated with neonatal cholestasis, Semin Liver Dis 7:108-118, 1987.

This is a concise review of a multitude of disorders that present with neonatal cholestasis. By necessity the discussion of each entity is short, but 97 references provide guidance for additional reading.

Grand R, Sutphen J, and Dietz W: Pediatric nutrition: theory and practice, Stoneham, Mass, 1987, Butterworth Publishers.

This is a comprehensive text that reviews normal and abnormal nutrition in pediatrics.

Hays D et al: Diagnosis of biliary atresia: relative accuracy of percutaneous liver biopsy, open liver biopsy, and operative cholangiography, J Pediatr 71:598-607, 1967.

This careful review compares the diagnostic accuracy of percutaneous liver biopsy, open liver biopsy, and operative cholangiography in differentiating biliary atresia from neonatal hepatitis. The studies were performed in infants with jaundice at age 3 weeks to 13 weeks. The final diagnosis was determined by subsequent clinical course and autopsy findings. The study was done before the Kasai procedure was used to influence the course of biliary atresia. The results show an error rate of approximately 20% in assigning cases to biliary atresia or neonatal hepatitis, emphasizing the difficulty of an accurate diagnosis from investigations done early in the course of illness.

Landing B: Considerations of the pathogenesis of neonatal hepatitis, biliary atresia, and choledochal cyst: the concept of infantile obstructive cholangiopathy, Prog Pediatr Surg 6:113-139, 1974.

Dr. Landing presents the pathologic evidence that neonatal hepatitis, biliary atresia, and choledochal cyst are the products of a single pathologic process with different manifestations. Some of the speculations concerning the viral etiology of infantile obstructive cholangiopathy have not proven true, but the article provides an important unifying hypothesis for the understanding of this disorder.

Mace S, Borkat G, and Liebman J: Hepatic dysfunction and cardiovascular abnormalities, Am J Dis Child 139:60-65, 1985.

Sixty-five infants, children, and young adults had tests of liver synthetic function, serum aminotransferases, and serum bilirubin that were correlated with hemodynamic abnormalities in well-defined heart disease. Hypoxemia with systemic venous congestion and low cardiac output were most often associated with elevated bilirubin and serum aspartate aminotransferase levels. In addition, low cardiac output states were accompanied by prolonged PTs and hypoproteinemia.

Merritt R: Cholestasis associated with total parenteral nutrition, J Pediatr Gastroenterol Nutr 5:9-222, 1986.

Prematurity, immature metabolism of BAs, and each of the constituents of parenteral nutrition are considered in detail as possible contributing factors to the development of cholestasis. Various alterations in patient care are reviewed.

Mowat A: Liver disorders in childhood, ed 2, London, 1987, Butterworth Publishers.

This 400-page text by an experienced pediatric hepatologist reviews the entire spectrum of liver diseases in infants and children. The clinical orientation combines information from the literature with the author's extensive experience.

Rosenblum JL et al: A progressive neurologic syndrome in children with chronic liver disease, N Engl J Med 304:503-508, 1981.

The authors describe seven children with documented chronic vitamin E deficiency beginning with cholestasis in early infancy who develop a progressive neurologic syndrome that disables as the child gets older. Neuropathologic findings in two of the children who died are similar in character and location to those described in vitamin E-deficient nonhuman primates and rodents.

Schneider B et al: Cholestasis in infants supported with extacorporeal membrane oxygenation, J Pediatr 115:462-465, 1989.

The authors describe the development of marked direct hyperbilirubinemia in infants who required extracorporeal membrane oxygenation for various conditions, as well as the occurrence of extensive hemolysis and its possible contribution to the severity of the jaundice.

Wolf A and Pohlandt F: Bacterial infection: the main cause of acute cholestasis in newborn infants receiving short-term parenteral nutrition, J Pediatr Gastroenterol Nutr 8:297-303, 1989.

This retrospective and prospective study examined the clinical course of 250 infants. All of the infants with cholestasis had clinically suspected or culture-proven sepsis. About 25% of the infants with sepsis developed cholestasis. No other factors, such as birth weight, duration of parenteral nutrition, timing of initial enteral feeding, or gestational age, correlated with the development of cholestasis.

11 Infectious Disorders of Childhood

Jerry L. Rosenblum and *Robert J. Rothbaum*

VIRAL HEPATITIS

Multiphasic biochemical screening in children, in contrast to screening in adults, is not common, partly because of the large volume of blood required. Without routine serum transaminase determinations, the clinical manifestations of viral hepatitis in anicteric children may appear as a "flulike syndrome," a self-limited symptom complex caused by a host of infectious agents. Thus the clinician's ability to diagnose hepatitis depends on a high index of suspicion, which must be based on careful consideration of potential risk factors. Also, diseases of other organ systems may occasionally present with laboratory findings that mimic those of viral hepatitis. For example, simultaneous elevation of serum creatine phosphokinase activity may point to muscle as the site of organ injury, or an elevation in aminotransferase levels may reflect right-heart failure caused by a congenital anomaly of the heart valves. The clinician should be reasonably confident using data gathered from a careful history, physical examination, and appropriate biochemical studies that viral injury to the liver is likely before launching into a serologic evaluation to identify the cause of infection.

Clinical Manifestations and Epidemiology of Viral Hepatitis

Hepatitis A. The most common type of acute viral hepatitis in the pediatric age group is hepatitis A. This type of hepatitis is caused by an RNA virus (HAV) belonging to the enterovirus group of picornaviruses. Susceptibility is greatest among young children and is primarily a function of overcrowding coupled with poor hygiene. The virus is highly contagious, and infection is typically spread through fecal or oral contamination of food or water supplies. In more developed countries hepatitis A outbreaks are commonly observed in day care centers, where good hygiene, including hand-washing, can be difficult to maintain. Institutionalized individuals also constitute a high-risk population. Clinical presentation may vary with age. Estimates of the prevalence of HAV infection may be low because symptoms in children are nonspecific, being limited to vomiting, diarrhea, abdominal pain, and malaise. Less commonly, fever and myalgia may be present, and, depending on the study, jaundice occurs 2 to 5 times more often in adults than in children. As with other infections (e.g., giardiasis), some asymptomatic children excrete the infectious agent in their stool, underscoring the need for good hygienic measures. Fecal excretion of the virus is maximal during the late incubation period and early acute phase of the illness, and it persists for 2 to 3 weeks. Serum transaminase levels begin to rise about a month after exposure, peak within 1 week of the onset of clinical disease, and return to normal levels within 1 to 2 months. Fulminant hepatitis is rare, and more than 98% of pediatric patients recover fully from HAV infection. Chronic hepatitis is not a clearly recognized sequela.

Hepatitis B. HBV contains both double-stranded and single-stranded DNA and is approximately 42 nm in diameter. The surface antigen (HBsAg) is produced in large excess in hepatocytes and is released into the circulation, where it serves as a marker for the carrier state. Other markers for HBV infection include a DNA polymerase enzyme, a core antigen (HBcAg), and the e antigen (HBeAg). (The significance of each of these antigens is discussed in detail in Chapter 13.

In contrast to HAV infection, spread of HBV infection usually occurs through parenteral transmission or percutaneous or mucosal exposure to infected body fluids. Pediatric populations at risk for developing HBV infection include (1) patients exposed to blood or blood products, especially those who receive them on a regular basis (e.g., hemophiliacs and renal-dialysis patients); (2) adolescents who use parenteral drugs or engage in unsafe sexual practices, particularly with multiple partners; (3) institutionalized children and those exposed to children with violent behavior, such as biting, that may be associated with transmission; and (4) infants born to mothers who are acutely or chronically infected. Perinatal transmission is largely responsible for the high prevalence of HBV infection in southeast Asia. The high rate of infection in this region of the world is exemplified by Taiwan, where 15% to 20% of the general population are HBsAg carriers and approximately 80% of inhabitants have serologic evidence of prior HBV infection. Infants born to mothers who are HBsAg carriers or who develop acute HBV infection during the third trimester appear to have the highest risk for developing HBV infection. Infants infected with HBV usually have mild clinical disease, but about 90% of these infants become chronic HBV carriers because of an apparent immunologic tolerance to the virus. This fact alone may make hepatitis B the leading public health problem in Taiwan because HBsAg carriers are at risk throughout their lives for developing cirrhosis and hepatocellular carcinoma.

The symptoms of acute hepatitis B do not distinguish it from other causes of viral hepatitis. Occasionally the diagnosis of acute hepatitis B is suggested by systemic symptoms that are known to occur more frequently in this disorder, e.g., membranous nephropathy, joint pains or frank arthritis, or papular acrodermatitis (Gianotti syndrome). Histopathologic features of the liver in HBV infection are quite similar to features of the liver in other forms of viral hepatitis. Thus liver biopsy is not indicated in acute hepatitis, because the morphologic pattern of injury is not disease-specific. In fact, some pathologic changes observed in the first 6 months of acute viral hepatitis may mimic those observed in CAH. Therefore biopsies obtained prematurely during the acute process could lead to misdiagnosis and inappropriate therapy. About 5% to 10% of adults with acute HBV infection develop chronic hepatitis. This percentage may be slightly higher in children, and many children (and adults) who are diagnosed as having chronic hepatitis B infection have had no prior history of liver disease, indicating that acute HBV infection is frequently subclinical.

Hepatitis D. The recently described δ-agent is a 35 nm to 37 nm defective virus that is pathogenic only in association with HBV infection. This unique viral agent is composed of a ribonucleic acid genome and an associated δ-antigen that are encapsulated by the HBsAg. When HDV infection temporally coincides with HBV infection (coinfection) or follows HBV infection in the carrier (superinfection), it serves to worsen the severity and progression of the liver disease. Available data indicate that children are no exception to the serious consequences of HDV infection. Of particular concern, perinatal transmission of δ-agent has been reported in regions such as the Mediterranean basin, where the virus is endemic.

Hepatitis C. This category includes other viral agents that are transmitted either by blood transfusion, receipt of blood products, such as clotting-factor concentrates, illicit use of IV drugs, or sporadic acquisition in the community. Recently HCV has been described as the major agent responsible for post-transfusion hepatitis. Transfusion-related hepatitis usually follows an indolent course and is characterized by fluctuating serum aminotransaminase levels throughout a period of years. As in adult populations, children with hepatitis C appear to have a significant risk (greater than 50% in some series) of developing chronic liver disease (CLD). The incubation period varies, but most patients develop abnormalities in serum aminotransaminase levels 6 to 12 weeks after exposure. Without effective screening, children with underlying diseases, such as hemophilia, who require frequent administration of blood or blood products are at highest risk for developing this form of hepatitis.

Diagnosis

A careful history to search for the aforementioned risk factors is important in children with suspected hepatitis. The presence of jaundice, RUQ tenderness, or hepatomegaly can be useful findings during physical examination. After the diagnosis of viral hepatitis is suspected on clinical grounds and elevated aminotransaminase levels have been documented, the clinician is faced with choosing among a number of serologic tests. Diagnosis of acute HAV infection can be confirmed best by assaying IgM-specific antibody (anti-HAV IgM). In hepatitis B infection, HBsAg is usually detectable 1 to 3 months after exposure. The presence of a positive hepatitis B surface antigen coupled with a positive IgM antibody to HBcAg (anti-HBc-IgM), which is detectable shortly after the onset of symptoms, provides strong serologic support for the diagnosis of acute HBV infection. These three tests, combined in selected cases with anti-HDV or HCV determinations, provide a cost-effective approach to the initial evaluation of viral hepatitis. Other viruses, such as Epstein-Barr virus, cytomegalovirus, herpesvirus, varicella-zoster virus, and coxsackie B virus, can occasionally cause hepatitis as part of a systemic infection and may necessitate additional diagnostic investigation in some patients.

Management

The physician's primary responsibilities in caring for a patient with documented acute viral hepatitis are (1) to provide supportive care and promptly report documented cases to public health authorities, (2) to provide adequate follow-up to ensure that complete resolution has occurred and chronic hepatitis has not developed, and (3) to develop preventive strategies for family members and other contacts who may have been exposed to the virus. The management of acute hepatitis is nonspecific and supportive. Clear benefit from bed rest, dietary manipulation, or steroid administration has not been demonstrated. Most patients can be followed at home unless coagulopathy, encephalopathy, or persistent vomiting develop. Deepening jaundice or shrinking liver size reflect massive hepatocellular dropout and may be the harbingers of impending FHF. This latter complication occurs in 1% to 2% of all cases of acute viral hepatitis. Often, a specific cause for fulminant hepatitis cannot be found. In one series a viral cause could not be identified specifically in any of 26 pediatric cases of fulminant viral hepatitis, and the diagnosis was presumed to be acute hepatitis C. Treatable, nonviral causes of hepatic failure, such as Wilson's disease, deserve serious consideration in these instances.

Corticosteroids, the most effective drug in the treatment of autoimmune hepatitis in adults, may adversely affect the natural history of CAH associated with HBV infection. Other drugs, such as human α-interferon, have been reported to have therapeutic promise in preliminary trials in adults. In contrast, α-interferon has not been associated yet with sustained loss of viral replication in large numbers of Chinese children with chronic HBV infection.

HAV can survive on environmental objects for weeks. Public health measures to prevent the spread of HAV infection include good hygienic practices in caring for diapered infants and young children in day care settings. Screening of blood and blood products for HBsAg and surrogate testing of blood donors for hepatitis C infection with alanine aminotransferase and antibody to HBcAg have helped reduce the risk of transfusion-related hepatitis. Surrogate testing for hepatitis C infection was implemented in 1986 based on the statistical observation that the presence of an elevated serum alanine aminotransferase level or antibody to HBcAg is associated with an increased risk of transmission. A further reduction in the number of transfusion-related cases of hepatitis C is anticipated with the application of testing for antibody to HCV.

Under specified circumstances, serum immunoglobulin can be effective in modifying the clinical course of HAV infection when given before or after exposure. If administered within 2 weeks *after* exposure to hepatitis A, pooled serum immunoglobulin can induce immunity while preventing the symptoms of HAV infection. After an index case is confirmed by a positive anti-HAV IgM titer, immunoglobulin (0.02 ml/kg) should be given to all exposed children and staff in an institutional or day care setting, household contacts, and, in older patients, to sexual contacts. Unless an epidemic is apparent, casual exposure in the workplace or school does not warrant immunoglobulin administration.

Although no effective vaccines against hepatitis A or hepatitis C viruses are now available, the development of a vaccine against hepatitis B derived from plasma is a major breakthrough in immunoprophylaxis. (Detailed guidelines for preexposure or post exposure immunoprophylaxis with HBV vaccine are discussed in Chapter 13). It is essential to administer 0.5 ml

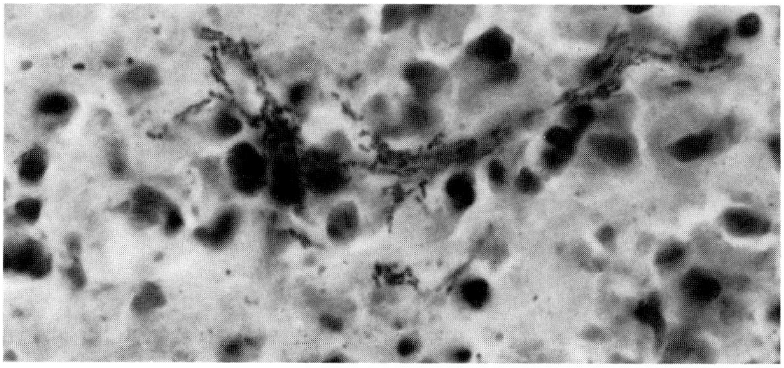

Figure 11-1
Long chains of cat-scratch bacilli (stained with Warthin-Starry stain) in collagen fibers in center of hepatic granuloma. (× 1000). (From Lenoir AA et al: Granulomatous hepatitis associated with cat-scratch disease, Lancet 1132, 1988.)

of hepatitis B immunoglobulin (HBI) IM *and* hepatitis B vaccine (0.5 ml) at birth to all infants of HBsAg-positive mothers. Vaccination (0.5 ml) should be repeated at 1 and 6 months of age. This approach has been shown to decrease the rate of chronic infection in exposed infants from about 85% to 5%. In endemic areas, such as Asia, perinatal immunization efforts are central to reducing the incidence of HBV infection and the associated high risk for developing cirrhosis and hepatocellular carcinoma.

NONVIRAL HEPATITIS (CAT-SCRATCH SYNDROME IN CHILDREN)

Apart from viruses, infectious agents causing hepatitis are uncommon in pediatrics. Parasitic, bacterial, and spirochetal infections of the liver are discussed in detail in other chapters. The cat-scratch bacillus is one organism associated with a recently recognized syndrome of granulomatous hepatitis in healthy children. In 1988 Lenoir and others reported three children who presented with a syndrome of persistent high fevers (39° C for more than 3 weeks) and findings on abdominal CT scan suggestive of a malignant or infectious process. The disorder was characterized by focal hepatic defects in two patients and periaortic and perihilar adenopathy in the third. Only one of the three patients had the usual inoculation site papule and peripheral lymphadenopathy of cat-scratch disease. At laparotomy, multiple nodules were observed on the liver surfaces of all patients. Cat-scratch bacilli were seen with the Warthin-Starry silver stain in the center of the granulomata of both the liver and lymph nodes (Figure 11-1). All three patients recovered fully without specific therapy. Thus in patients with a strong history of cat contact who present with fever and otherwise unexplained hepatic filling defects or periaortic lymphadenopathy detected by imaging studies, the diagnosis of granulomatous hepatitis should be considered. Furthermore, it may be possible to defer invasive procedures after careful consideration of treatable conditions, such as tuberculosis, fungal infection, and lymphoma. Additional studies of larger groups of patients should help determine the most appropriate course of care for individual patients.

REYE'S SYNDROME

Reye's syndrome is a rare, yet reversible metabolic encephalopathy and hepatopathy that afflicts children and adolescents. In most series the diagnosis is made with varying degrees of certainty, making reliable interpretation of the data difficult. Ideally diagnosis is based on characteristic clinical presentation and biochemical abnormalities combined with the histopathologic findings in the liver of microvesicular fat and ultrastructural parenchymal changes. Early in the course of encephalopathy, electron microscopic changes in the liver include swollen, deformed, pleomorphic mitochondria, loss of glycogen, and an increase in peroxisomes. After the first 4 to 5 days of illness, these changes resolve, and liver histology loses its diagnostic value.

Reye's syndrome classically follows an uncomplicated prodromal viral infection often with influenza B or varicella. Onset is marked by protracted vomiting, and behavioral changes may accompany or soon follow the vomiting. The child initially may be withdrawn but within 24 hours of the onset of vomiting becomes combative, often shouting obscenities in an agitated delirium. Although hepatic dysfunction is present, this encephalopathy does not represent portosystemic encephalopathy (PSE). The clinical course is unpredictable but may evolve rapidly into one of neurologic deterioration with cerebral edema and brain death over the subsequent several hours to days. Clinical findings of hepatic dysfunction are not obvious by history or physical examination, (e.g., jaundice is distinctly unusual). Serum aminotransferase levels are elevated though, with values 2 to 100 times the normal upper limit. PT is consistently prolonged and may preclude liver biopsy in some patients. Hyperammonia, although transient in some patients, can be documented in almost all cases. Hypoglycemia is a treatable if not preventable complication in young or severely affected patients.

The cause of Reye's syndrome is not known. Patients are clearly in a highly catabolic state and have extensive but potentially reversible mitochondrial enzyme dysfunction. Systematic study of pathogenesis is difficult, given the rare and sudden appearance of the disease in previously healthy children, the potential severity of the illness, and the lack of uniform diagnostic criteria. Many genetic disorders, such as mitochondrial enzyme defects and urea cycle defects, are exacerbated by acute viral illnesses and mimic many clinical aspects of Reye's syndrome. Although these diseases may provide clues to pathogenesis, they may also be misdiagnosed as Reye's syndrome, especially in children less than 3 years old, unless appropriate sophisticated diagnostic tests, which are available only in tertiary centers, are considered and performed. Encephalopathies caused by infections or toxins may also be confused with Reye's syndrome.

Between 1980 and 1982, four case-control studies demonstrated an association between Reye's syndrome and salicylate ingestion during an antecedent respiratory illness or varicella infection. Because of methodologic concerns with these studies, a Public Health Service Task Force was charged with designing a new epidemiologic study examining the relationship between Reye's syndrome and medication. This study confirmed the findings of the earlier studies but was stopped prematurely because of the marked decline in the reported incidence of this disorder in the United States. The incidence of Reye's syndrome in the United States fell to a level close to that reported in Great Britain and Australia, where paracetamol rather than aspirin is the major antipyretic/analgesic. This decline could not be explained by a fall in influenza B or varicella infection but was associated with a marked decrease in the use of aspirin and aspirin-containing substances. Despite difficulties in interpreting epidemiologic data, the avoidance of salicylates seems justified in light of our present understanding, because clear benefit from their use has never been proven and alternative antipyretics and analgesics are available.

Management of Reye's syndrome is supportive and empiric, reflecting our ignorance of the basic underlying pathogenetic mechanisms. Consideration of lumbar puncture and liver biopsy under well-controlled conditions early in the illness before increased intracranial pressure or coagulopathy develop may be useful in the diagnosis. Provision of adequate IV glucose is essential. Careful monitoring in an intensive care setting with care to avoid agitation should alert the clinician to the need for ventilatory support and to derangements in blood glucose, ammonia, liver function, serum osmolality, and fluid and electrolyte status. Maintenance of normal perfusion to the brain requires treatment of cerebral edema, usually with mannitol. Because marked increases in intracranial pressure can occur without papilledema, some experts believe that continuous monitoring of intracranial pressure is justified, despite the risks. Of the 21 patients originally described by Reye and his colleagues in 1963, 81% died. With the use of intensive management, the mortality rate in U.S. teaching institutions decreased, with three deaths occurring out of 27 patients (11%) reported with Reye's syndrome in the mid-1980s study by the Public Health Service Task Force. Patients who recover have normal hepatic histology and function but may suffer permanent neurologic sequelae. Recurrence is extremely rare and highly suggestive of an underlying metabolic disease. Similarly a familial history of this disorder or sudden infant death syndrome is rare and underscores the need to search for genetic abnormalities in such patients.

SUMMARY

Infants and children have risk factors for viral hepatitis distinct from those of adults, including repeated transfusion of blood or blood products for treatment of inherited diseases or exposure in day care settings or during parturition. The diagnosis of hepatitis A or B infection can be established using clinical findings combined with appropriate laboratory and serologic tests. Each diagnosis has its own public health implications, and careful patient follow-up is required. Future efforts must be aimed at preventing viral hepatitis and its consequences. The recently recognized syndrome of granulomatous hepatitis associated with the cat-scratch bacillus appears to be a self-limited illness and must be distinguished from malignant and other infectious processes requiring specific therapy. Reye's syndrome, which itself is not infectious but usually follows a viral illness, is a potentially fatal but reversible acute hepatopathy and encephalopathy afflicting children and adolescents.

SUGGESTED READINGS

Alagille D and Odièvre M: Liver and biliary tract diseases in children, New York, 1979, John Wiley & Sons, Inc.

This book considers the various causes of liver dysfunction in a form that follows the usual clinical evaluation of a patient. Hepatic histology is well illustrated.

American Academy of Pediatrics: Report of the committee on infectious diseases, Red Book, ed 21, 1988, Elk Grove Village, Ill, American Academy of Pediatrics.

The latest recommendations by the American Academy of Pediatrics regarding diagnosis, treatment, and control of hepatitis viruses and other infections are provided. These recommendations are updated periodically to incorporate more recent data. Risk factors and recommended immunoprophylaxis for specific situations commonly facing the clinician are presented in tabular form combined with concise discussion.

Hurwitz ES: Reye's syndrome, Epidemiol Rev 11:249-253, 1989.

This recent update summarizes the epidemiologic studies of Reye's syndrome, pointing out methodologic flaws and putting the chronology of events in historical perspective. Worldwide incidences are reviewed along with data linking Reye's syndrome with aspirin ingestion.

Lenoir A et al: Granulomatous hepatitis associated with cat-scratch disease, Lancet 1:1132-1136, 1988.

This paper describes the clinical syndrome and pathologic data of this illness in patients presenting with persistent pyrexia and hepatic filling defects. The authors make the point that cat-scratch disease should be added to the differential diagnosis of granulomatous hepatitis.

Mowat AP: Reye's syndrome: a continuing enigma, Adverse Drug Reactions and Acute Poisoning Reviews 6:211-230, 1987.

Those readers interested in learning more about the theories regarding the pathogenesis of liver injury might want to consult this review, which has 55 references and is written by an experienced pediatric hepatologist.

Psacharopoulos HT et al: Fulminant hepatic failure in childhood, Arch Dis Child 55:252-258, 1980.

This is a retrospective review of the care of 31 consecutive children seen at King's College Hospital in London from 1966 to 1977. It is one of the few larger pediatric series of FHF. Twenty-six children had presumed viral hepatitis, but no viral cause could be established. Survival (71% of children studied) correlated with the severity of the encephalopathy.

12 Liver Disease in Acquired Immune Deficiency Syndrome

Robert P. Perrillo

Patients with acquired immunodeficiency syndrome (AIDS) are predisposed to a variety of opportunistic infections and neoplasms that may involve the liver and biliary tract (see box at right). The spectrum of liver pathology associated with AIDS is due to (1) concomitant viral hepatitis, (2) AIDS-related opportunistic infections and neoplasms, (3) nonspecific biochemical and/or morphologic changes that are secondary to protein malnutrition, and (4) hepatotoxic medications. Hepatomegaly, mild elevation of aminotransferase levels, and elevation of AP levels are common findings in patients with AIDS. Jaundice may be present although significant jaundice secondary to parenchymal disease alone is rare.

HEPATOBILIARY DISORDERS ASSOCIATED WITH AIDS

Parenchymal disease

Chronic hepatitis B
Chronic hepatitis C
Mycobacterial infection (primarily *Mycobacterium avium-intracellulare)*
Cytomegalovirus infection
Lymphoma
Fungal infection: *Cryptococcus,* histoplasmosis, *Candida,* and *Coccidiodes*
Kaposi's sarcoma
Non-Hodgkin's lymphoma
Vascular lesions
 Peliosis hepatis
 Angiosarcoma
Disease induced by drugs, particularly trimethoprim-sulfamethoxazole, isoniazid, and ketoconazole)
 Others: pyrazinamide, pentamidine, and oxacillin

Biliary tract disease

Acalculus cholecystitis
Sclerosing cholangitis
Papillary stenosis
Kaposi's sarcoma
Non-Hodgkin's lymphoma

INFECTIOUS DISORDERS

Viral Hepatitis

Hepatitis B. Evidence of past or ongoing hepatitis B infection occurs in more than 90% of patients with AIDS. Approximately 10% of AIDS patients are chronic carriers of HBV. Chronic hepati-

A

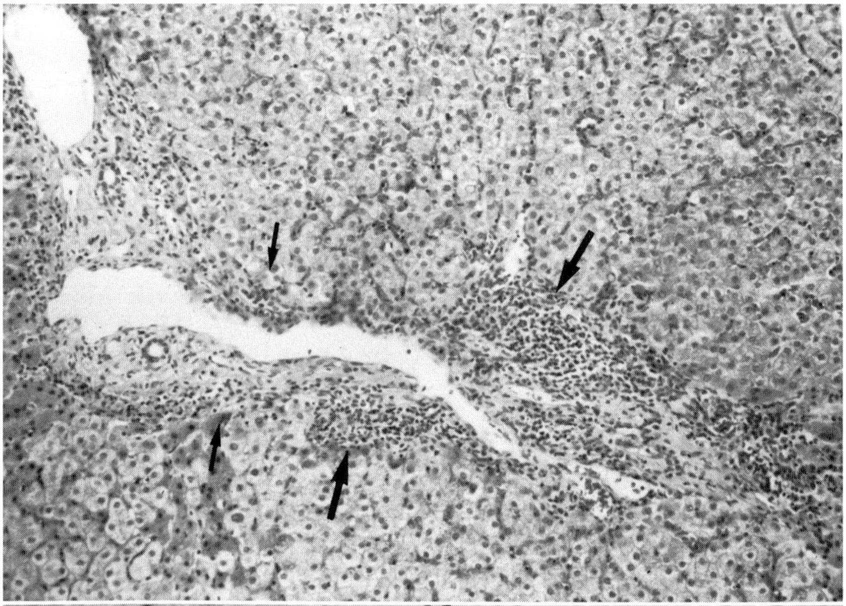

B

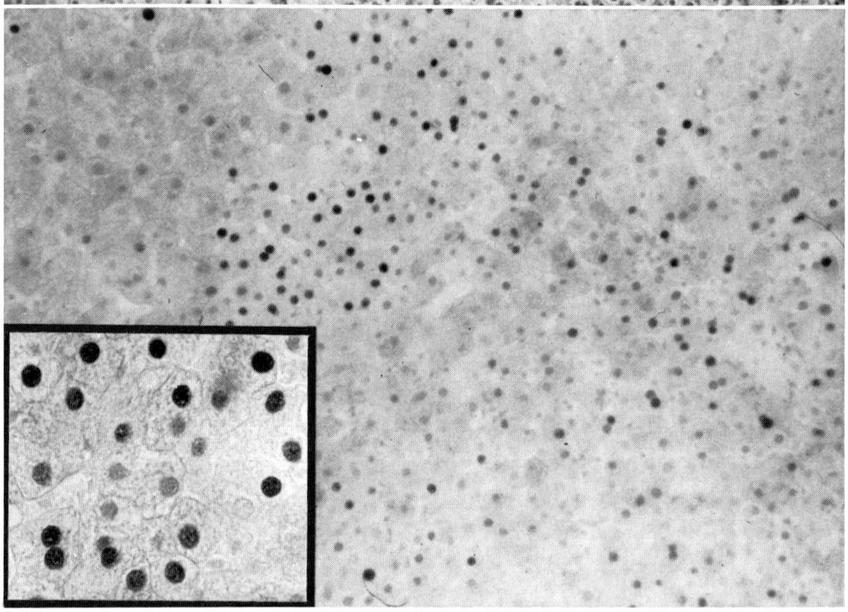

Figure 12-1
A, Liver biopsy from an asymptomatic anti-HIV-positive male homosexual illustrating minor histologic abnormality consistent with a diagnosis of chronic persistent hepatitis. Note the mild to moderate portal infiltrate *(large arrows)* with intact limiting plate *(small arrows)* (× 100). **B,** Immunoperoxidase stain for HBcAg in this patient (× 100). Note the diffuse distribution of nuclear HBcAg (inset: × 400). (From Trent-Mills C, Lee E, and Perrillo RP: Relationship between histology, aminotransferase levels, and viral replication in chronic hepatitis B, Gastroenterology 99:519, 1990.)

tis B is often typified by sparse intralobular and portal inflammatory reaction despite the presence of abundant HBcAg in liver and HBV DNA in serum. Replication of HBV tends to be potentiated in the presence of HIV infection as reflected by the increased presence of hepatocyte HBcAg and increased levels of circulating HBV DNA and DNA polymerase (Figure 12-1). Furthermore, the rate of spontaneous loss of HBeAg may be reduced, and reactivation of infection may be more common. Patients with chronic hepatitis B and concomitant HIV infection tend to have less intense histologic injury and lower aminotransferase levels when compared with a cohort of HIV-negative male homosexuals (see Figure 12-1). It is presumed that this is due to the effects of immunosuppression as reflected by lower CD4 counts in the HIV-infected group.

α-Interferon has been used to treat chronic hepatitis B in a relatively small number of HIV-infected patients. Most of these patients had not had AIDS at the time of treatment. Although a response, defined as sustained loss of HBV replication, is not precluded by the presence of a positive test for anti-HIV, at least one controlled clinical trial has indicated that HBeAg seroconversion rates are significantly lower in HIV-infected patients. Moreover, in the same study the percentage reduction of HBV-DNA was significantly less in anti-HIV-positive homosexuals when compared with the anti-HIV-negative cohort.

Hepatitis C and other forms of non-A, non-B hepatitis. In addition to hepatitis B, IV drug users with AIDS may also have chronic δ-infection and infection with hepatitis C and other forms of non-A, non-B hepatitis. Hemophiliacs may contract these viral infections through the use of clotting-factor concentrates. Concomitant infection with HIV and non-A, non-B viruses is likely to be a common association because up to 90% of IV drug users and hemophiliacs have serologic evidence of HIV infection, and non-A, non-B hepatitis has been described in greater than 50% of patients in these groups. There are data to suggest that HIV-infected patients frequently exhibit rapid histologic progression and often succumb to their liver disease. In one study, three patients with AIDS or AIDS-related complex (ARC) developed symptomatic cirrhosis within 3 years of onset of hepatitis. Such a rapid progression of liver disease was rare in 94 other patients with non-A, non-B hepatitis who did not have simultaneous HIV infection. Because non-A, non-B hepatitis is considered to be a cytopathic virus, it is possible that the immune suppression of AIDS may promote viral replication and thereby enhance liver injury. The same may hold true of δ-hepatitis virus.

Cytomegalovirus. Many patients with AIDS have persistent cytomegaloviremia. Cytomegalovirus is a major cause of dysfunction in a variety of organs. Liver involvement with cytomegalovirus has been reported to occur in 33% to 44% of AIDS cases with disseminated cytomegalovirus infection. In addition to hepatitis, patients may present with pneumonia, blinding chorioretinitis, esophagitis, colitis, meningoencephalitis, and radiculitis with polyneuropathies. Jaundice and severe liver dysfunction are very unusual with hepatic involvement. Liver biopsy often reveals intranuclear inclusion bodies within Kupffer cells, bile duct epithelium, or endothelial cells. Presence of these inclusion bodies may be demonstrated on routine hematoxylin and eosin stains or through the use of appropriate monoclonal cytomegalovirus antibodies. The intranuclear inclusions are generally quite abundant in AIDS patients but are less frequently observed in immunocompetent hosts. Most patients have demonstrable portal and periportal mononuclear cell infiltration with focal hepatocyte necrosis. Epithelioid noncaseating granulomas have rarely been reported in patients with cytomegalovirus infection. Mild increases in serum aminotransferase levels are frequently encountered; less often the AP level may be elevated. Serologic testing procedures for the virus are of limited value. Cultures of liver specimens may be useful, but may require several weeks before positive growth can be established. Patients are treated with gangciclovir.

Mycobacteriosis

Mycobacteriosis appears to be the the most frequently detected opportunistic infection involving the liver in patients with AIDS. Its presence has been noted in up to 30% of biopsy and autopsy specimens. In most instances this is due to *M. avium-intracellulare* and to a lesser extent *M. tuberculosis*. These organisms may be found on culture of liver tissue even when not detected by conventional histologic techniques. Therefore biopsies should be routinely cultured. Liver biopsy specimens are characterized by poorly formed granulomas without caseation necrosis, and acid-fast organisms are frequently evident by Ziehl-Neelsen stains. These histopathologic features are similar to those observed in lepromatous leprosy. In contrast, mycobacteria are generally not seen in the liver biopsy specimens taken from immunocompetent patients with hepatic tuberculosis, and cultures are frequently negative. Mycobacterial infection is usually a manifestation of disseminated disease, with the organism often detected in extrahepatic sites, such as the bone marrow and lymph nodes. The most typical biochemical abnormality is a disproportionately and persistently raised serum AP level. Although fever and hepatomegaly are common, jaundice is rare. Treatment is with multiple antituberculous chemotherapeutic agents, including isoniazid, rifampin, ethambutol, and pyrazinamide.

Fungal Infections

Patients with AIDS may also have a variety of fungal infections of the liver that occur as part of a disseminated process. For example, 60% of AIDS patients with disseminated cryptococcosis have hepatic involvement at autopsy. No particular clinical syndrome is associated with intrahepatic fungal disease. Liver biopsies are most often performed for unexplained fever or hepatomegaly. Budding yeast forms of cryptococcus have been described in the sinusoids. Other organisms include *Histoplasma capsulatum, Candida albicans,* and *Coccidiodes inmites*. Histologically there is generally an absence of inflammatory reaction. Granulomas may be present. Fungi are usually evident on hematoxylin and eosin sections but may be missed unless appropriate special stains (Gomori methenamine silver and PAS) are done. Mild elevations of the serum aminotransferase levels are generally observed with these disorders. Fungal abscesses may be of sufficient size to be detectable by CT scan or ultrasonography.

NEOPLASTIC DISORDERS

Kaposi's Sarcoma

Patients with AIDS are also subject to involvement of the liver with Kaposi's sarcoma. This is the most common neoplastic lesion found in patients with AIDS. Kaposi's sarcoma in AIDS patients is far more aggressive than the form that was originally recognized in elderly patients of European extraction. It occurs almost exclusively in homosexual men as opposed to IV drug users, hemophiliacs, or transfusion recipients. Widespread visceral involvement occurs almost exclusively in male homosexuals with AIDS. The tumor is often present as small focal subcapsular deposits with extension into the parenchyma through the portal tracts, suggesting lymphatic spread. Intrahepatic tumor rarely causes symptoms, but common bile duct obstruction, jaundice, and cholangitis have been reported.

Approximately one third of patients with extrahepatic Kaposi's sarcoma have liver involvement at autopsy. When present, hepatic tumors often have the appearance of purple-brown soft nodules. On histologic examination, multifocal, predominantly periportal areas of vascular endothelial cell proliferation are seen, accompanied by malignant-appearing spindle-shaped cells, extravasated RBCs, and vascular lakes. Interferon has been used to treat this condition, but therapy is only palliative.

Lymphoma

Non-Hodgkin's lymphoma also affects the liver either as a primary neoplasm or more frequently as part of widespread visceral involvement. Lymphomas in AIDS patients are unusual in several respects. First, they tend primarily to involve extranodal areas. Second, they are almost always non-Hodgkin's type and B cell or non-B, non-T cell in origin. Third, they are rapidly growing and characterized by a poor response to chemotherapy. Mean survival is about 6 months.

Fever, malaise, and weight loss are prominent complaints. Occasionally lymphoma located at the porta hepatis can cause obstructive jaundice. The most striking biochemical abnormality associated with intrahepatic lymphoma and with biliary obstruction is an elevated AP level. Large, solid, usually multifocal lesions may be noted on ultrasonography or CT scan. These procedures may be helpful in guided needle biopsy, during which two to three cores should be obtained, including a fresh sample in saline to be used for immunophenotyping. Laparoscopically guided biopsy may be helpful when percutaneous biopsy is negative or if no specific lesions are detected with the above noninvasive studies.

DRUG-INDUCED LIVER DISEASE

A wide variety of drugs used in the treatment of patients with AIDS are potentially hepatotoxic. Nevertheless, there have been few reports of adverse drug experiences in patients with AIDS, probably because of the difficulty in attributing the reaction solely to the drug. It is also possible that HIV infection may alter immune-mediated forms of drug injury. The most commonly implicated drugs are trimethoprim-sulfamethoxazole, ketoconazole, and antituberculous agents, such as isoniazid and pyrazinamide. Whereas the antituberculous medications may evoke hepatocellular injury and a selective increase in aminotransferase levels, trimethoprim-sulfamethoxazole is likely either to cause intrahepatic cholestasis or to be associated with a granulomatous reaction caused by the sulfonamide component of the drug. Ketoconazole may be associated with a hepatitis like pattern of liver injury or less commonly a pure cholestatic reaction. Abnormalities of liver tests have also been reported with pentamidine and the antifungal agent amphotericin.

BILIARY TRACT DISEASE

Acalculous Cholecystitis

This uncommon condition has been described in several series of AIDS cases. Most cases have been attributed to cytomegalovirus or cryptosporidial infection of the gallbladder, but Helicobacter (formerly Campylobacter) fetus has also been reported as cause. Most patients present with an acute or subacute illness lasting days to weeks, characterized by fever, fatigue, and RUQ pain. Liver tests are often within normal limits. Ultrasonography confirms the absence of stones and usually demonstrates a thickened gallbladder wall, often with a pericholecystic fluid collection. Air may be visualized within the wall of the gallbladder, and the gallbladder is often tender to the examiner's hand or pressure of the transducer. Most patients respond well to cholecystectomy. However, in critically ill patients, surgical cholecystostomy or percutaneous transhepatic cholecystostomy are preferred approaches. Peritonitis is absent unless perforation has occurred. At surgery the gallbladder wall is indurated and often hemorrhagic and gangrenous. Focal ulcers of the gallbladder mucosa, caused by presumed ischemic vasculitis, may be noted in cases attributed to cytomegalovirus infection. The cystic duct is usually patent. Histologically either the intranuclear inclusions of cytomegalovirus or the coccidial forms of cryptosporidia are seen within or adherent to the mucosa.

Obstructive Biliary Tract Disease

Biliary tract obstruction is being recognized with increasing frequency in AIDS. It has been reported that AIDS patients with this disorder may develop a disease similar to papillary stenosis, sclerosing cholangitis, or both. As with acalculous cholecystitis, cytomegalovirus and cryptosporidial infection of the biliary tree have been implicated, and papillary biopsy has revealed these organisms microscopically or by culture. This is generally a subacute or chronic process characterized by fever, RUQ pain, and marked elevation of the serum AP. Jaundice is rare because of the incomplete nature of the obstruction. Diarrhea is frequently observed in these patients because of concomitant infection of the GI tract.

Ductal abnormalities are usually detected on ultrasonography or CT scan. Most commonly, dilated intrahepatic and extrahepatic bile ducts are evident. Endoscopic retrograde cholangiopancreatography (ERPC) best defines the ductal irregularities in these disorders. Selective cannulation of the biliary tree typically reveals ampullary stenosis or distal common bile duct strictures with luminal irregularities producing a "beaded" appearance. Focal stricture or beading may be more prominent within the intrahepatic rather than extrahepatic ducts. Sphincterotomy and ductal decompression can be done endoscopically. A dominant stricture of the extrahepatic biliary tree may require balloon dilation or insertion of an endoscopically placed stent. If ERPC cannot be performed successfully, transhepatic cholangiography should be attempted. Balloon dilation or stent insertion can be accomplished in some patients through a transhepatic approach. Surgical sphincteroplasty is reserved for patients with papillary stenosis in whom endoscopic sphincterotomy is not possible.

MISCELLANEOUS DISORDERS

Apart from these specific disorders, a number of other hepatic histologic abnormalities may be found in patients with AIDS (see box on p. 269). In some series, hepatic macrovesicular steatosis, reflective of poor nutritional status, is the most frequent abnormality detected after liver biopsy or at postmortem examination of patients with AIDS. Hepatomegaly is commonly observed with fatty liver, and often serum AP levels are one to two times normal. Granulomas may be observed in as many as 50% of percutaneous liver biopsy specimens from patients with AIDS. These granulomas have numerous potential causes, including various opportunistic infections and drugs. However, *M. avium-intracellulare* is by far the most common infection resulting in granulomas. Portal tract lymphopenia, Kupffer cell hyperplasia, sinusoidal dilation, peliosis hepatis, and angiosarcoma have all been reported.

SUMMARY

Patients with AIDS are predisposed to a variety of opportunistic infections and neoplasms that may involve the liver and biliary tract. The liver is usually affected as part of a disseminated infectious or neoplastic process, and, in general, little morbidity extends from the liver disease itself. Clinical and histologic expression of many infectious disorders, e.g, chronic hepatitis B and mycobacterial infection, is attenuated as a result of an impaired immune response. In contrast, neoplastic diseases, particularly non-Hodgkin's lymphoma, tend to be more aggressive than usual.

SUGGESTED READINGS

Glasgow BJ et al: Clinical and pathologic findings of the liver in the acquired immune deficiency syndrome (AIDS), Am J Clin Pathol 83:582-588, 1985.

This study reviews the clinical data and hepatic histology in 42 cases of AIDS after autopsy. The infectious and neoplastic complications of AIDS did not significantly contribute to morbidity or mortality. No findings specific for AIDS were identified in the liver.

Kahn SA et al: Hepatic disorders in the acquired immune deficiency syndrome: a clinical and pathological study, Am J Gastroenterol 81:1145-1148, 1986.

Granulomas were found in 48% of percutaneous liver biopsies in 21 patients with AIDS. The most common etiology was infection with M. avium-intracellulare (seven cases).

Kavin H et al: Acalculous cholecystitis and cytomegalovirus infection in the acquired immunodeficiency syndrome, Ann Intern Med 104:53-54, 1986.

The authors report two patients with severe abdominal pain caused by acalculous cholecystitis that was associated with cytomegalovirus infection. Both cases were characterized by ulceration of the gallbladder mucosa and cytomegalovirus inclusion bodies in epithelial and endothelial cells.

Krogsgaard K et al: The influence of HTLV-III infection on the natural history of hepatitis B virus infection in male homosexual HBsAg carriers, Hepatology 7:37-41, 1987.

This is a longitudinal study of 33 male homosexuals who tested positive for HBeAg and HBV-DNA. The study demonstrates a significantly reduced rate of HBeAg seroconversion in anti-HIV positive patients when compared with anti-HIV negative persons. A single anti-HIV positive patient demonstrated reactivation of HBV infection.

Martin P et al: Rapidly progressive non-A, non-B hepatitis in patients with human immunodeficiency virus infection, Gastroenterology 97:1559-1561, 1989.

Of 97 patients with non-A, non-B hepatitis, three were found to have anti-HIV. These patients developed symptomatic cirrhosis within 3 years of the onset of hepatitis. Such a rapid progession of liver disease was observed in only 8 of 94 HIV-negative individuals. The findings suggest that HIV infection may potentiate the liver injury of chronic non-A, non-B hepatitis.

McDonald JA et al: Diminished responsiveness of male homosexual chronic hepatitis B virus carriers with HTLV-III antibodies to recombinant alpha-interferon, Hepatology 7:719- 723, 1987.

In this study, 5 of 17 anti-HIV negative homosexual men with chronic hepatitis B responded to treatment with interferon, but none of the 13 anti-HIV positive homosexuals responded to the interferon therapy. All but one of the HIV-infected homosexuals were asymptomatic. The authors postulate that the different response rates in the two groups may be due to the subclinical immunosuppressive effects of coinfection with HIV.

Perrillo RP, Regenstein FG, and Roodman ST. Chronic hepatitis B in asymptomatic homosexual men with antibody to the human immunodeficiency virus, Ann Intern Med 105:382-386, 1986.

HIV-infected male homosexuals with chronic hepatitis B had lower CD4 to CD8 ratios, less intense histologic activity, and lower aminotransferase levels when compared with HIV-negative homosexual and heterosexual persons. It is postulated that the attenuated biochemical and histologic responses reflect a diminished immune response against HBV in the HIV-infected population.

Schneiderman DJ: Hepatobiliary abnormalities of AIDS, Gastroenterol Clin North Am 17:615-630, 1988.

This is a relatively recent review of the diverse hepatobiliary complications of AIDS. The author outlines a reasonable clinical approach to evaluation and treatment of these disorders.

Schneiderman DJ, Cello JP, and Laing FC: Papillary stenosis and sclerosing cholangitis in the acquired immunodeficiency syndrome, Ann Intern Med 106:546-549, 1987.

This paper describes the clinical, biochemical, and radiologic features of eight homosexual men with AIDS who presented with stenosis of the papilla of Vater and sclerosing cholangitis. The authors conclude that most patients respond favorably to biliary decompression at the time of endoscopic papillotomy.

Trent-Mills C, Lee E, and Perrillo RP: Relationship between histology, aminotransferase levels, and viral replication in chronic hepatitis B, Gastroenterology 99:519-524, 1990.

Seventy-four untreated patients with chronic hepatitis B were examined for the degree of hepatic histologic activity, and this was compared to markers for viral replication. HIV-infected homosexual men had significantly higher levels of HBV DNA and DNA polymerase when compared to HIV-negative homosexuals. A trend was noted for higher grades of HBcAg staining in the HIV-infected population.

Ziegler JL et al: Non-Hodgkin's lymphoma in 90 homosexual men: relation to generalized lymphadenopathy and the acquired immunodeficiency syndrome, N Engl J Med 311:565-570, 1984.

This paper describes the histologic and clinical features of non-Hodgkin's lymphoma in 90 homosexual men with AIDS or ARC. Twenty-nine of these patients (32%) had AIDS when lymphoma was diagnosed. The lymphomas were histologically aggressive and poorly responsive to treatment.

13 Viral Hepatitis

Robert P. Perrillo

ACUTE VIRAL HEPATITIS

The Viruses and Their Epidemiology

Hepatitis A virus. Hepatitis A virus (HAV) is a small (27 nm), RNA-containing virus that was first identified in 1973 (Table 13-1). HAV has been propagated in cell culture and can replicate in several cell lines of human and monkey origin. HAV is not cytopathic, and the mechanisms by which it leads to cellular injury have not been defined. The RNA genome of this virus has recently been sequenced and cloned.

Hepatitis A is transmitted primarily through the fecal-oral route; thus it frequently occurs in small epidemics traced to fecal contamination of food or drinking water. The disease has a worldwide distribution and is nearly universal during childhood in developing countries because of poor sanitary conditions. Promiscuous homosexual men are at increased risk for contracting hepatitis A. Although hepatitis A is not a major health problem in the United States, approximately 200,000 cases are estimated to occur yearly. Hepatitis A has recently been recognized as a common problem in day care centers, especially where many children are in diapers. These outbreaks often result in hepatitis A cases among staff, parents, and family members. Hepatitis A rarely follows transfusion because the virus has a short viremic phase and lacks a carrier state.

Hepatitis B virus. HBV is a DNA-containing virus that belongs to a new class called the hepadnaviruses (see Table 13-1). Other members of this class include the woodchuck virus, Peking duck virus, ground squirrel virus and heron virus. The outside lipoprotein envelope of HBV, HBsAg, surrounds an inner nucleocapsid core particle with a distinct HBcAg. HBcAg is not detectable in the serum unless the complete virion is treated with detergent to remove the outer HBsAg envelope. The core also contains a double-stranded DNA with a "gap" in one of the strands and a DNA polymerase enzyme that repairs this gap region. HBeAg, a third antigen associated with the virus, is believed to represent unincorporated core polypeptide. HBeAg, HBV-DNA, and DNA polymerase are detectable in serum, and because they indicate the presence of replicating virus, they are associated with increased contagiousness. The DNA has been cloned and sequenced, and this has led to the development of second-generation recombinant hepatitis B vaccines. Various human and nonhuman cell lines

Table 13-1 The alphabet of viral hepatitis

Feature	Hepatitis A	Hepatitis B	Hepatitis C	Hepatitis D	Hepatitis E
Agent	27 nm RNA virus	42 nm DNA virus	30-60 nm RNA virus	35 nm RNA virus	32 nm virus
Envelope	No	Yes	Yes	Yes	No
Antigens	HAV Ag	HBsAg, HBcAg, HBeAg	C-100-3 (nonstructural)	HDV Ag	HEV Ag
Antibodies	Anti-HAV	Anti-HBs, anti-HBc, anti-HBe	Anti-HCV	Anti-HDV	Convalescent, immune aggregating
Genomic size	7.5 kb	3.2 kb	10 kb	1.7 kb	8.5 kb
Major routes of transmission	Fecal-oral, neonatal	Parenteral, sexual	Parenteral, sexual	Parenteral	Fecal-oral
Mortality	0.1%	1-3%	1-2%	2-20%	1-2%*
Chronicity	None	2-5%	≥50%	Yes	None
Incubation period	15-45 days	40-180 days	15-150 days	30-50 days	14-60 days
Icteric: anicteric ratio	1:1	1:2	1:4	Unknown	Unknown
Cytopathogenicity	Unlikely	No	Yes	Probably	Unknown

*Highest case fatality ratio (10%-20%) in pregnant women.

can be transfected by HBV. HBV is not cytopathic, except perhaps when the expression of the virus is greatly augmented, as occurs after liver transplantation. The damaging effects of infection are thought to result from the immune response of the host.

It has been estimated that there are more than 300 million HBV carriers throughout the world today (approximately 5% of the earth's population). Areas of high concentration include certain parts of Africa, Asia, and the Mediterranean basin. In the United States approximately 250,000 cases of acute hepatitis B occur annually, and 0.2% to 0.4% of the population are carriers of the virus.

The virus is transmitted either by parenteral exposure (e.g., needle stick or blood transfusion) or by inapparent skin or mucosal exposure (e.g., intimate or sexual contact). Anywhere from 30% to 50% of cases are not associated with an identifiable route of exposure; these cases probably result from intimate person-to-person contact. All major classes of body fluids have been shown to contain the virus with the exception of stool that is free of contamination with blood. The presence of a replicating virus in the blood, saliva, and semen of infected individuals facilitates spread by intimate contact. Infection occurs in 20% to 40% of sexual contacts of acute cases and in more than 50% of regular sexual partners of chronic carriers. Infection occurs approximately 10 times more frequently in homosexual men and IV drug users as compared with the general population.

Non-A, Non-B viruses and Hepatitis C virus. The agent responsible for most cases of post-transfusion NANB hepatitis has recently been cloned, sequenced, and designated the hepatitis C virus. The virus appears to be a small, enveloped, cytopathic RNA virus with partial genomic homology to the flavivirus group of viruses (see Table 13-1). A virus-specific polypeptide (c-100-3) has been derived in yeast and used as the antigen source in an immunoassay to detect anti-HCV. HCV is probably only one in a group of viruses (the so-called NANB viruses) that share similar clinical and epidemiological features.

NANB hepatitis is prevalent throughout the world, and the pattern of spread is primarily parenteral although sporadic cases are frequently encountered. NANB hepatitis makes up 90% to 95% of post-transfusion hepatitis cases in the world today, and more than 200,000 cases occur annually in the United States by this route. HCV appears to have a worldwide distribution, and anti-HCV is detectable in 80% to 90% of transfusion-associated cases. Anti-HCV has been detected in nearly 90% of blood donors implicated in the transmission of NANB hepatitis and in approximately 1% of healthy volunteer blood donors in the United States, making this virus the predominant if not exclusive agent involved in post-transfusion NANB hepatitis. A positive test for anti-HCV has also been observed in 60% to 80% of persons infected by IV drug use and in 50% to 60% of sporadic cases.

Patients at the highest risk for acquiring NANB hepatitis are users of illicit drugs and persons requiring multiple transfusions of blood or blood products, such as hemophiliacs and patients undergoing major surgery. Household contacts appear to be at low risk, and transmission by sexual or other intimate contact occurs less frequently than with HBV. Perinatal transmission has also been observed.

Hepatitis D virus. Hepatitis D virus (HDV) or δ-agent is a defective virus that requires coinfection with HBV to replicate. For unclear reasons this coinfection may not be necessary immediately after liver transplantation. δ-antigen contains a small RNA genome of low molecular weight and a distinct antigen that is encapsulated by HBsAg (see Table 13-1). The genome has been cloned and sequenced. Current data suggest that HDV is cytopathic.

HDV infection has a worldwide distribution, but the areas of highest concentration are the Mediterranean basin, the Middle East, and certain parts of South America. It is found infrequently in Asia, western Europe, and North America. In western nations, δ-hepatitis occurs most commonly among users of illicit drugs and among multiply transfused patients, and as many as 50% of HBV carriers in these populations may have the antibody to this agent. HDV infection is observed relatively infrequently among homosexual men, institutionalized mentally retarded persons, and hemodialysis patients.

Enterically transmitted NANB or Hepatitis E virus. An enterically transmitted form of acute viral hepatitis has recently been described that is serologically distinct from all other hepatitis viruses. The cause, termed hepatitis E virus (HEV), has been identified in stool and bile, and a viral antigen has been identified in infected liver cells by immunofluorescence (see Table 13-1). Blood-borne transmission has not been demonstrated, and a carrier state has not been observed. Preliminary studies have characterized HEV as a nonenveloped, single-stranded, RNA-containing virus. Recently the viral genome has been cloned and sequenced. HEV has been transmitted to primates but has yet to be grown in tissue culture. Epidemics in India, Pakistan, Africa, Southeast Asia, Central Asia, and Mexico appear to be related to fecal contamination of water supplies. Sporadic cases can occur in developed countries whenever travelers return from an endemic area.

Clinical/Laboratory Features of Acute Viral Hepatitis

Acute viral hepatitis is often subclinical or associated with nonspecific "flulike" symptoms (in approximately 50% of cases), and jaundice occurs in no more than 30% to 50% of cases. Patients with viral hepatitis present with similar clinical manifestations irrespective of the specific cause. The most common early symptoms are fatigue, anorexia, nausea, and a dull ache in the RUQ. Low-grade fever is often encountered. Itching is common, and many patients have typical viral symptoms, such as myalgias and arthralgias. Frank arthritis occurs but is rare. Many of the constitutional symptoms develop quickly after the jaundice develops or shortly thereafter. On physical examination the most noticeable features are icteric skin and sclerae. The liver is often enlarged and tender to palpation. The spleen is palpable in about 10% of patients.

Most patients have a relative lymphocytosis. Serum bilirubin generally does not exceed 15 to 20 mg/dl. AST and ALT levels rise 1 to 2 weeks before the onset of symptoms and begin to fall shortly after symptoms appear. Peak levels generally exceed 500 IU/L, but the degree of elevation does not necessarily parallel the severity of the disease. Aminotransferase elevations usually disappear by 8 to 12 weeks after the onset of illness.

Hepatitis A. Infection with HAV is always self-limiting, unlike infection with HBV, HCV, and HDV. The onset of hepatitis A tends to be more abrupt than the other forms of acute viral hepatitis: the fever is higher, and the duration of elevated aminotransaminase is shorter (about 1 to 3 weeks). Cholestasis, unusual with the other forms of viral hepatitis, may be a prominent feature of type A infection. Hepatitis A may be associated rarely with a syndrome of arthritis, vasculitis, and circulating cryoglobulinemia. Although life-threatening cases are rare, hepatitis A may account for as many as 25% to 30% of patients with fulminant viral hepatitis.

The first viral marker to appear is hepatitis A antigen in the stool (Figure 13-1). It appears during the incubation period, usually 7 to 10 days before the onset of symptoms of disease. The antigen generally disappears within 2 to 3 weeks after the onset of illness. Clinical relapses have occurred 30 to 90 days after the onset of the primary illness and are occasionally accompanied by more prolonged excretion of HAV in stool. Anti-HAV is the second marker to appear during infection and almost always is detectable by the

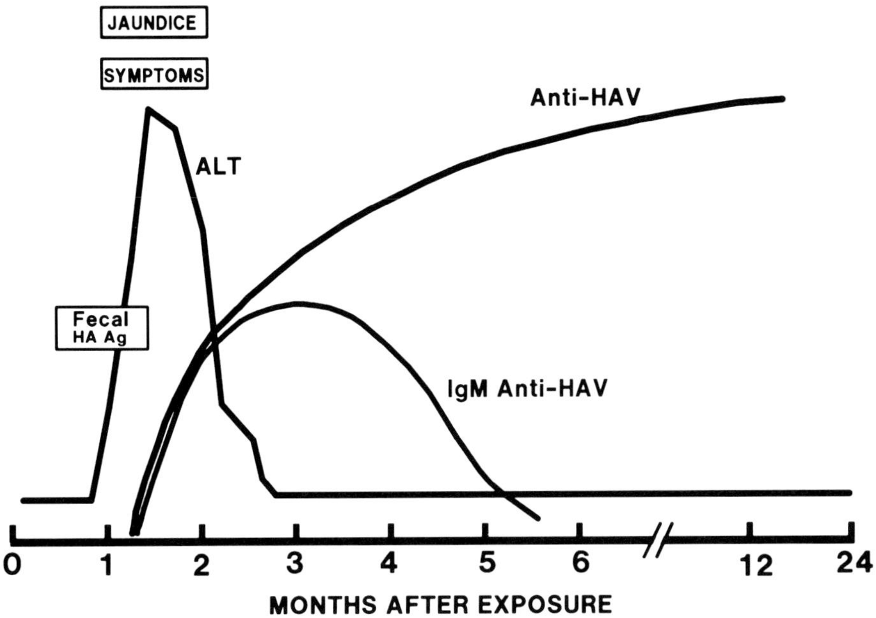

Figure 13-1
Time course of clinical, biochemical, and virologic events in typical case of acute hepatitis A.

time symptoms appear. The earliest response is composed mostly of the IgM subclass of antibody, and in this antibody usually is detectable for 3 to 6 months after the onset of illness. In approximately 5% of cases, IgM anti-HAV may be detectable for periods in excess of 6 months. Because of the usual short-lived nature of the IgM antibody, its presence in a single serum sample always implies ongoing or recent infection and serves as the most valuable test for acute hepatitis A. IgM anti-HAV is followed by IgG anti-HAV, which persists indefinitely and confers immunity against reinfection. IgG anti-HAV can be detected in 30% to 40% of the population of the United States and 90% of people living in developing countries.

Hepatitis B. The incubation period for hepatitis B varies from a few weeks to 6 months, depending in part on the size of the inoculum. A unique feature of hepatitis B is the relatively high frequency (10% to 20% of cases) of a serum sickness–like prodrome with fever, arthralgias/arthritis, and/or skin rashes, most frequently maculopapular or urticarial. This prodrome results from circulating HBsAg/ anti-hepatitis B surface (HBs) complexes that activate complement and deposit in the synovium and walls of cutaneous blood vessels. These features abate early in the illness, before the manifestations of liver disease and peak aminotransferase elevations.

In general, elevated ALT and serum HBsAg decline and disappear togeth-

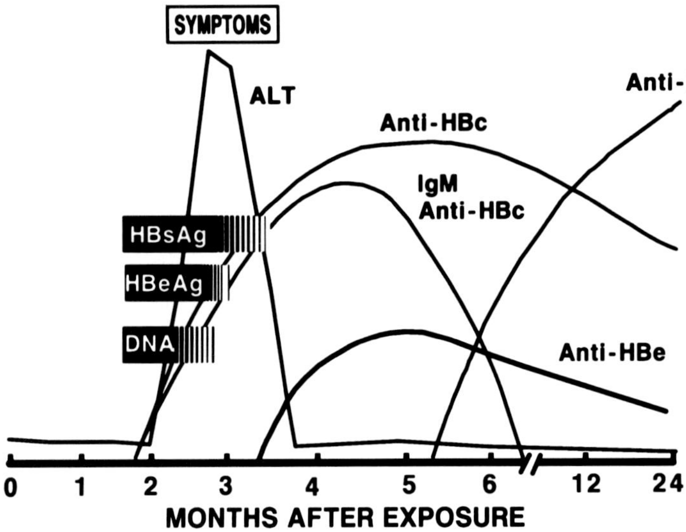

Figure 13-2
Time course of clinical, biochemical, and virologic events in typical case of acute hepatitis B. (From Kelley WN et al, eds: Textbook of internal medicine, Philadelphia, 1989, J B Lippincott Co.)

er, and in approximately 80% of cases, HBsAg disappears within 12 weeks of the onset of illness. In 5% to 10% of cases HBsAg is cleared early and is no longer detectable by the time the patient first presents to the physician. Persistence of HBsAg after 6 months implies the existence of a carrier state with only a small likelihood of recovery during the next six 6 to12 months.

In experimental studies HBeAg becomes detectable shortly after the appearance of HBsAg, but in the usual clinical situation both are detectable on presentation of the patient (Figure 13-2). The appearance of HBeAg signifies active viral replication and is usually coincident with the detection of DNA polymerase and HBV-DNA. HBeAg persists for a shorter period than does HBsAg, and persistence of HBeAg beyond 10 to 12 weeks after the onset of illness suggests that the infection is becoming chronic. The disappearance of HBeAg is followed quickly by the appearance of anti-HBe, which rarely reaches high titers and often disappears within a few months or years.

Anti-HBc appears shortly before the onset of symptoms and rises rapidly in all patients with acute hepatitis B. The initial anti-HBc response consists mainly of IgM antibody and is generally detectable for 4 to 6 months with commercially available immunoassays. Although the transient nature of IgM anti-HBc may be useful in the serodiagnosis of acute hepatitis B, approximately 10% of patients have detectable IgM anti-HBc for intervals as long as a year or more after the onset of illness. Moreover, a variable percentage of HBsAg carriers with active liver disease and evidence of viral replication express low titers of this antibody. Anti-HBc of the IgG subclass develops later and is a long-lived antibody whose titer decreases with time. In some cases, IgG anti-HBc falls to undetectable levels after many years.

Approximately 80% of patients recovering from acute hepatitis B develop anti-HBs. Anti-HBs does not usually become detectable during the acute disease but rather during convalescence. In all but a few patients, anti-HBs is not detectable in the serum until HBsAg has disappeared and recovery is complete. It is a long-lived antibody that confers immunity to reinfection although titers decrease with time and sometimes fall into the undetectable range. Of the general population 5% to 10% have anti-HBs.

Non-A, Non-B Hepatitis and Hepatitis C. The clinical features of acute NANB hepatitis do not distinguish this disease from hepatitis A or hepatitis B in any individual patient. However, in general, NANB hepatitis cases are milder, and a majority (75%) are anicteric. Of post-transfusion cases 60% to 70% have peak ALT values below 800 IU/L, but only 5% to 10% have peak levels over 2,000 IU/L. The incubation period may vary from 2 to 20 weeks, but most cases become manifest 6 to 10 weeks after exposure. Both monophasic and biphasic elevations of the aminotransferase enzymes have been observed. Many cases are asymptomatic, even when the disease progresses to chronic hepatitis or cirrhosis. The most prominent feature of NANB hepatitis is the tendency for abnormal aminotransferase levels to persist for prolonged periods in 50% to 70% of cases, reflecting the development of a carrier state and chronic hepatitis.

Before the serologic identification of HCV antibody, the diagnosis of NANB hepatitis was established solely on the basis of exclusion of other etiologic agents, including cytomegalovirus and Epstein-Barr virus. In the appropriate clinical setting, the finding of anti-HCV seroconversion confirms the diagnosis of acute hepatitis C. However, the diagnosis may be difficult to establish because the detection of anti-HCV is often delayed for 3 to 6 months after the onset of illness. In experimental studies, HCV-RNA may be detectable as early as a few days after exposure when tested by polymerase chain reaction. In these studies, HCV-RNA is detectable in serum during the early acute phase of infection, coincident with the rise in aminotransferase levels and preceding the appearance of anti-HCV (Figure 13-3).

Hepatitis D. Infection with HDV may result in either an acute or chronic illness. Acute δ-hepatitis occurs as a coprimary infection with (i.e., coinfection) hepatitis B or may be superimposed on the HBsAg carrier state (i.e., superinfection). The distinguishing feature of δ-hepatitis is its clinical severity, resulting from the cytopathic effect of the virus added to the immunologic injury induced by HBV. HDV infection accounts for an increased frequency of fulminant hepatitis among drug addicts. However, because δ-agent cannot outlive infection with HBV and more than 90% of acute HBV infections resolve, the expression of δ virus (and δ-antigen in the liver) is limited, and dual infection generally cannot be distinguished from acute hepatitis B alone. On the other hand, in HBV carriers who become superinfected with the δ-agent, the well-established HBV infection permits the active replication of δ-virus. This replication predisposes to the develop-

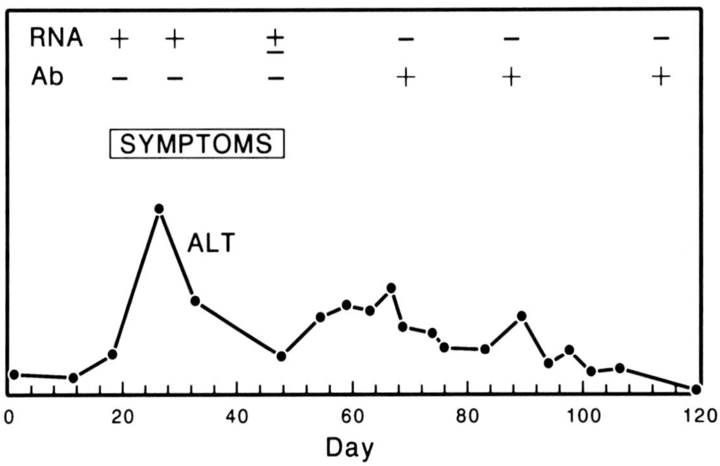

Figure 13-3
Time course of clinical, biochemical, and virologic events in typical case of acute hepatitis C. Ab refers to antibody to C-100-3 antigen.

ment of severe liver disease, which accounts for a large percentage (30% to 60%) of fulminant HBsAg-positive hepatitis in areas of high concentration. Acute δ-infection in the HBsAg carrier progresses to chronic infection in approximately 90% of cases.

Acute δ-hepatitis may be accompanied by a biphasic aminotransferase pattern, with one peak resulting from HBV-induced liver cell injury and the other resulting from the δ-agent. The serologic response to acute HDV infection as measured by currently available commercial immunoassays is often undetectable or is represented by transient appearance of IgM antibody (Figure 13-4). By methods presently confined to research laboratories, δ-antigen and HDV-RNA can be detected transiently in liver tissue and serum during acute infection.

Hepatitis E. HEV infection shares with hepatitis A a fecal-oral route of transmission, short incubation period, lack of a carrier state, and tendency to occur in large outbreaks. Nevertheless, there are also several major differences. The most striking difference between epidemics of HEV infection and hepatitis A is the case fatality rate. The overall case fatality rate has been 1% to 2%. The most severe form of the the disease occurs among pregnant women, especially those in the third trimester. The case fatality rate in this group has been 10% to 20%. During point-source epidemics, the clinical attack rate is highest among persons 15 to 39 years old. The prevalence of mild or subclinical infection is difficult to assess in the absence of specific diagnostic tests. Studies during some outbreaks have shown that for each patient with jaundice, there may be five to ten people with abnormal liver tests but no jaundice. The histologic features of this disorder are similar to those observed in other forms

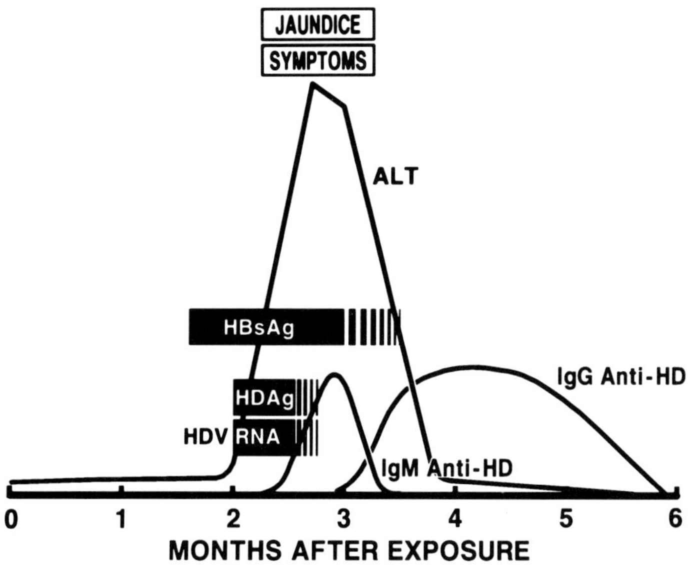

Figure 13-4
Time course of clinical, biochemical, and virologic events in typical case of acute hepatitis D.

of viral hepatitis with the exception of a greater frequency of cholestatic reaction.

Fulminant Viral Hepatitis

In less than 1% of cases, patients with viral hepatitis may lapse into coma and die within a matter of days to weeks. As conventionally defined, fulminant viral hepatitis refers to disease of less than 8 weeks in duration. All of the hepatitis viruses described previously may be associated with this condition. Mortality is extremely high (greater than 80% in most series), with the greatest chance for survival among young patients and those with hepatitis A or acetaminophen overdosage. Fulminant NANB hepatitis, halothane-induced liver failure, and drug hepatitis have been associated with the poorest prognosis. As in typical acute viral hepatitis, there is no specific treatment, and supportive care is all that can be offered. Systemic complications, such as pneumonitis, acute respiratory distress syndrome, cardiac arrhythmias, GI bleeding, pancreatitis, and renal failure are frequently encountered. The patient's fluid balance and cardiopulmonary status should be maintained, bleeding should be controlled, hypoglycemia should be corrected, and infections and other acute complications should be treated promptly. Absolute restriction of protein intake and administration of neomycin and lactulose are traditional forms of therapy, but they do not affect the outcome of disease. Cerebral edema is common, particularly among young adults, and may require therapy with mannitol and intracranial pressure monitoring. It is a leading cause of death in FHF. Dexamethasone and high-frequency ventilation have no effect on survival although the latter is associated with acute lowering of arterial CO_2 tension and intracranial pressure. H_2 receptor antagonists may reduce the frequency of GI bleeding in this setting although their use has not been evaluated extensively. Massive doses of corticosteroids have been administered to preserve liver function, but carefully controlled clinical trials have failed to support the efficacy of this treatment. Other therapies, such as exchange transfusion, porcine liver cross-perfusion, and charcoal hemoperfusion, have been tried with very limited success. Charcoal hemoperfusion was not associated with improved survival in a recent controlled clinical trial. Hyperimmune globulin has been shown to be ineffective in patients with fulminant hepatitis B. Plasmapheresis may be useful in patients with active hemorrhage and severe coagulopathy. Patients with evidence of progressive liver failure should be evaluated at centers performing liver transplantation. Those patients with grade III or greater hepatic coma should be considered for transplantation only if evidence of irreversible neurologic damage (e.g., unreactive pupils, absent brainstem reflexes, or absent cerebral activity on EEG) has not occurred. Most transplantation centers have reported survival rates in excess of 50% in patients with FHF. Mortality with transplantation is greatest for patients in prolonged grade IV coma and those with evidence of cerebral edema. Donor availability within a critical interval continues to be a problem.

The terms *late-onset hepatic failure* or *protracted hepatitis* are used by some authorities to refer to cases in which there is progressive diminution of liver function 2 to 6 months after the onset of illness. This syndrome is common among patients over 40 and may represent failure of liver cell regeneration. Such patients frequently develop ascites and renal failure, and mortality rates approach those observed with fulminant hepatitis. In selected cases liver transplantation may be an option.

Treatment of Acute Viral Hepatitis

There is no specific treatment for typical acute viral hepatitis. In approximately 10% of cases, hospitalization may be required for one or more of the following reasons: (1) uncertain diagnosis, (2) clinically severe illness with failure to maintain nutrition, progressive worsening of coagulation status, or emerging encephalopathy, and (3) unusually high patient risk, such as for elderly patients or those with serious underlying illnesses. IV feeding is necessary if the patient has persistent vomiting and cannot maintain oral intake. Alcohol and drugs that are metabolized by the liver or that are capable of producing adverse reactions, such as cholestasis (e.g., phenothiazines and oral contraceptives), should be avoided during the acute stage. The use of a bile-acid–sequestering resin, such as cholestyramine, may be indicated for the treatment of pruritus. Corticosteroid therapy has no value in acute viral hepatitis, irrespective of clinical severity. Controlled studies in severe and fulminant cases of viral hepatitis have failed to demonstrate efficacy; moreover, steroids may promote sepsis and have other adverse effects. In hepatitis B, corticosteroids have been shown to enhance viral replication, and their withdrawal may induce a flare in the illness.

Physical isolation of patients is not necessary except in cases in which patients with acute hepatitis A are incontinent or there is severe and uncontrolled bleeding in patients with hepatitis B and NANB hepatitis. Long-term isolation of patients with hepatitis A is not indicated because of the short period of fecal shedding.

Discharge from the hospital is permitted when the specific features prompting hospitalization have resolved and the patient has improved. The patient should be allowed to return to work as tolerated. Mild aminotransferase elevations and continued positive serology for HBsAg should not be considered contraindications for resumption of normal activity.

Prevention of Viral Hepatitis

Hepatitis A. Hepatitis A is preventable in more than 80% to 90% of patients exposed to HAV through prompt administration of immune globulin (i.e., within 2 weeks of exposure). Because immune globulin is inexpensive, maximally effective when given early, and virtually free of adverse effects, it is not recommended to test the recipient for anti-HAV before administration of the recommended dose (0.02 ml/kg). Immune globulin should be given to staff and clients of day care centers and institutions whenever cases of hepatitis A have been identified. For travelers to tropical and developing countries, immune globulin is recommended at a dose of 0.02 ml/kg when the travel lasts less than 3 months and at a dose of 0.06 ml/kg every 5 months for longer periods of travel. Hepatitis A vaccines are not currently available.

Hepatitis B. Hepatitis B vaccine is indicated for preexposure prophylaxis. Two recombinant yeast vaccines (10 μg and 20 μg of HBsAg protein per ml, respectively) are now available. There is overwhelming evidence that these vaccines are safe and equally immunogenic. Both preparations cost approximately $120 to $150 for a three-dose regimen (1 ml given initially and at 1 and 6 months). Plasma-derived vaccine is no longer being produced in the United States, and use is now limited to hemodialysis patients, other immunocompromised hosts, and persons with known allergy to yeast. More than 90% of healthy adults develop anti-HBs after vaccination. Sample to negative control (S/N) values in excess of 10 are generally considered to be protective. The duration of protection and the need for booster doses are not yet defined. It is essential that hepatitis B vaccine be given intramuscularly in the deltoid region because studies have indicated that injections in the gluteal region are often delivered into adipose tissue, impairing the immunogenicity of the vaccine. Preexposure prophylaxis with hepatitis B vaccine is indicated for the following high-risk groups: health care workers, clients and staff of institutions for the mentally retarded, hemodialysis patients, homosexually active men, users of illicit injectable drugs, recipients of clotting-factor concentrates and frequent blood transfusions, sexual contacts of HBV carriers, heterosexuals with multiple sexual partners, and international travelers who will reside in a country of high concentration for greater than 6 months. Universal vaccination of neonates is presently under consideration by the U.S. Public Health Service (USPHS).

HBIg (0.06 ml/kg) is recommended for postexposure prophylaxis of nonvaccinated health care personnel who have accidentally been exposed to HBsAg-positive material. Ideally, the HBIg should be given within 24 hours, and hepatitis B vaccination (1 ml delivered IM) should be initiated within 7 days of exposure. If vaccination is refused, a second, identical dose of HBIg should be administered 1 month later. In cases of heterosexual exposure to an individual with acute hepatitis B, HBIg (0.06 ml/kg) should be given within 2 weeks of exposure. It is not necessary to follow this administration of HBIg with vaccination unless the index case develops chronic infection and repeated exposures are likely. For newborns of HBsAg-carrier mothers, 0.5 ml of HBIg should be given at birth, and HBV vaccination (0.5 ml of either vaccine) should be started at the same time with repeat doses at 1 and 6 months.

Currently the USPHS recommends that all pregnant women be tested for HBsAg. Also, it has been recommended recently that school-age children become vaccinated. Prevaccination screening with anti-HBs or anti-HBc should probably be reserved for high-risk groups, such as homosexual men, multiply transfused patients, spouses of HBV carriers, clients in institutions for the mentally retarded, and household contacts of HBsAg carriers. Postvaccination screening for anti-HBs (e.g., 1 to 3 months after the booster dose) may be useful in assessing the duration of immunity, determining the relative intervals when a booster dose is necessary, and identifying nonresponders among health care workers who will require future HBIg prophylaxis for needlestick exposure.

Non-A, Non-B Hepatitis and Hepatitis C. The effectiveness of immune globulin prophylaxis has not been demonstrated consistently in NANB hepatitis. A major reduction in the incidence of posttranfusion NANB hepatitis has resulted from the use of all-volunteer blood and exclusion of patients with evidence of HIV I infection. Elevation of ALT and presence of anti-HBc in transfused blood have been shown to predispose recipients to NANB hepatitis, and screening with both tests has been adopted as a national blood-bank policy in the United States. Preliminary data indicate that screening donor blood for these surrogate markers may reduce the incidence of HCV infection by approximately 50%. It is anticipated that anti-HCV testing of donor blood further reduces the incidence of HCV-associated post-transfusion hepatitis.

Hepatitis D. There are no specific means of preventing infection with HDV. However, as δ-agent requires the presence of HBV to replicate, successful immunization against HBV also prevents infection with the δ-virus.

Hepatitis E. Limited information is available with regard to the prophylactic use of immune globulin in this disorder, and studies of the value of locally produced immune globulin are greatly needed. In humans with naturally acquired infections, higher titers of antibody are usually detected in serums collected during the acute phase of the illness rather than in serums collected during early or late convalescence. This may limit the antibody titer in conventional lots of immune globulin, and globulin derived from recently infected persons theoretically may be more protective.

CHRONIC VIRAL HEPATITIS

Clinical/Laboratory Features of Chronic Viral Hepatitis

Hepatitis A is always self-limiting and does not result in chronic liver disease. In contrast, 2% to 5% of patients with acute hepatitis B and as many as 50% to 60%

of patients with acute NANB hepatitis become chronically infected. There are approximately 1 million HBV carriers in the United States. Of this number, it is estimated that one third to one half have inflammatory changes in the liver parenchyma consistent with some form of chronic viral hepatitis. All of the morphologic variants of chronic viral hepatitis that occur with HBV infection may also be observed in association with chronic NANB infection (see Chapter 14).

Chronic viral hepatitis may be divided morphologically into chronic persistent hepatitis and chronic active hepatitis (CAH). The diagnostic distinction between the two disorders is important because their prognoses are markedly different. In chronic persistent hepatitis the inflammatory changes are limited primarily to the portal tract region, and the liver disease is seldom progressive even though inflammation and some degree of hepatocyte necrosis may be present for extended periods. In CAH, injury to hepatocytes adjacent to the portal tract is observed with focal or "piecemeal necrosis." Of greater prognostic importance, CAH may be accompanied by "bridging necrosis," in which the destruction of groups of adjacent hepatocytes interposed between portal tracts and central veins leads to collapse and disruption of hepatic architecture. Fibrosis in these regions intersects the hepatic lobule and eventually leads to cirrhosis. Thus, in contrast with chronic persistent hepatitis, CAH is a variably progressive disorder that often results in cirrhosis and possibly eventual hepatic failure.

Clinical symptoms and mild to moderate elevations of aminotransferase activity (less than three times the upper limit of normal) are generally of little value in differentiating between CAH and chronic persistent hepatitis. However, more pronounced biochemical abnormalities usually imply CAH and the presence of stigmata of advanced liver disease (e.g., portal hypertension and ascites) always indicates CAH, often with cirrhosis. Because of the similarity in clinical and laboratory features of chronic persistent hepatitis and CAH, percutaneous liver biopsy is essential for establishing the diagnosis. Sampling variations on percutaneous liver biopsy may occasionally obscure the true diagnosis. This is particularly likely with cirrhosis. When the diagnosis is in doubt, therapy should be withheld, and the patient should be observed. Repeat biopsy may sometimes be useful under these circumstances.

Patients with chronic viral hepatitis may experience a number of clinical features, including fatigue, malaise, abdominal pain, anorexia, jaundice, hepatosplenomegaly, and encephalopathy. The majority of patients who are diagnosed on the basis of abnormal liver chemistries or a positive test for HBsAg after routine evaluation (e.g., at the time of blood donation) have no symptoms or complain of only mild fatigue. For some of these patients, liver biopsy specimens may show CAH, but clinical manifestations are not seen because of the early stage of the disease. A variable percentage of such patients manifest histologic evidence of cirrhosis, reflecting the ability of chronic viral hepatitis to progress without a change in the functional status of the patient. Irrespective of the cause, only a small number of patients are critically ill when first seen by a physician.

Chronic Hepatitis B. Only 1% to 2% of HBV carriers per year lose HBsAg and develop anti-HBs; thus, many patients

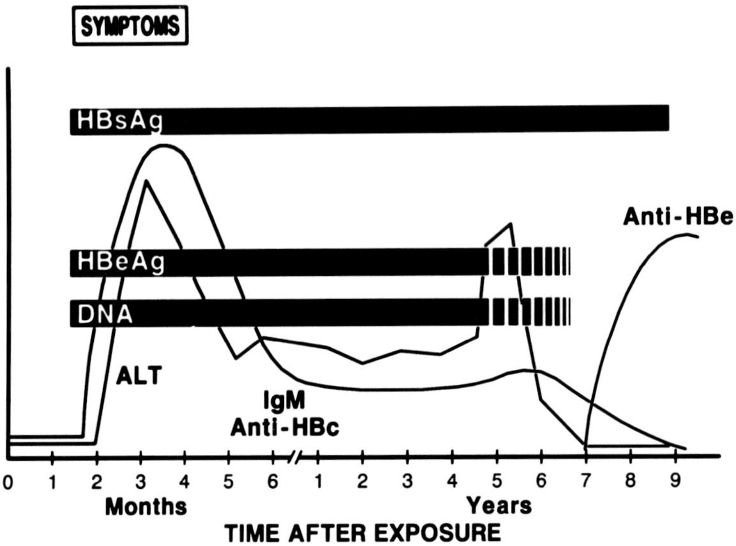

Figure 13-5
Serologic profile of chronic hepatitis B with termination of replicative phase. Note the sudden increase in ALT preceding the disappearance of HBeAg and HBV-DNA.

carry their disease indefinitely. Studies on the natural history of chronic HBV infection suggest that there are two chronologic stages of infection. In the early, "replicative" stage, HBeAg, HBV-DNA polymerase, and HBV DNA are usually demonstrated in the serum, and HBV-DNA and HBcAg are readily detectable in liver tissue. Active hepatitis with elevated serum aminotransferase levels are features of this stage. Recently a subgroup of patients has been identified in the Mediterranean countries who are chronically infected with a mutant strain of HBV that is associated with a negative test for HBeAg, a positive test for anti-HBe, detectable HBV-DNA, and severe liver disease. In time many patients become asymptomatic carriers, losing their viral-replication markers (including conversion from HBeAg to anti-HBe and loss of HBV-DNA), hepatic inflammation, and aminotransferase elevations. This second phase is referred to as the "nonreplicative phase" and is often preceded by a relatively sudden flare in the aminotransferase levels that heralds the change in course (Figure 13-5). A minority (5% to 20%) of HBeAg-positive HBV carriers undergo this transition each year. The infection may reactivate later in some of these patients, either spontaneously (particularly among homosexual men) or in association with immunosuppressive therapy. During reactivation HBV-replication markers reappear associated with biochemical and histologic deterioration. Multiple episodes may occur, contributing to histologic progression, and severe episodes have proved fatal when superimposed on ad-

Table 13-2 Defining "relapse" in chronic hepatitis B by evaluation of viral-replication markers

Situation associated with apparent worsening	Usual biochemical abnormalities	Status of HBV-DNA
Seroconversion from HBeAg to anti-HBe	Transient, preceding peak in ALT/AST	Disappears
Reactivated HBV infection	Transient or sustained rise in ALT/AST	Reappears with or without HBeAg
Superinfection with HAV, δ-virus, NANB virus	Transient or sustained rise in ALT/AST	Either no change or declining values
Hepatocellular carcinoma	Increase in AP with or without elevation of bilirubin or aminotransferase values	Usually negative with HBV-DNA integration in liver tissue

vanced CLD. The above events may be associated with worsening of symptoms and biochemical abnormalities. Thus testing for viral-replication markers, such as HBeAg and HBV-DNA, is essential in achieving a correct diagnosis (Table 13-2).

Insight into the biologic events that underlie these phases of chronic hepatitis B has come from the application of molecular-hybridization techniques. During the replicative phase most of the HBV-DNA in the liver is in the free, or "episomal" (i.e., extrachromosomal), form, whereas during the nonreplicative phase much if not all of the HBV-DNA is integrated into the host genome (i.e., intrachromosomal form). Recent studies using the polymerase chain reaction have demonstrated small amounts of circulating HBV-DNA during the "nonreplicative" phase, which disappear at the time of HBsAg seroconversion. It is not known if this HBV-DNA is integrated or episomal. Complete, infectious virions are produced when HBV-DNA is episomal, but incomplete HBsAg particles predominate when HBV-DNA is integrated. Malignant transformation (hepatoma) usually occurs several decades after the onset of infection when the HBV-DNA is integrated and the liver disease is inactive. The risk of hepatoma among Asians has been estimated to be more than 100 times greater in HBsAg carriers than in noninfected persons. For this reason HBV carriers should be screened periodically for α-fetoprotein because elevations may be expected in as many as 80% to 90% of hepatoma patients and early detection may permit resection of the tumor. Broad screening is unlikely to have a high diagnostic yield in areas of low concentration, such as the United States, where HBV infection occurs primarily in adults. Thus α-fetoprotein screening probably should be limited to HBsAg carriers over age 40 or those in whom the infection is known to have been present for more than 10 years.

Chronic Non-A, Non-B Hepatitis and chronic Hepatitis C. Awareness of NANB hepatitis as a distinct entity emerged slightly more than 15 years ago. It has become apparent that CAH and cirrhosis commonly occur in the natural his-

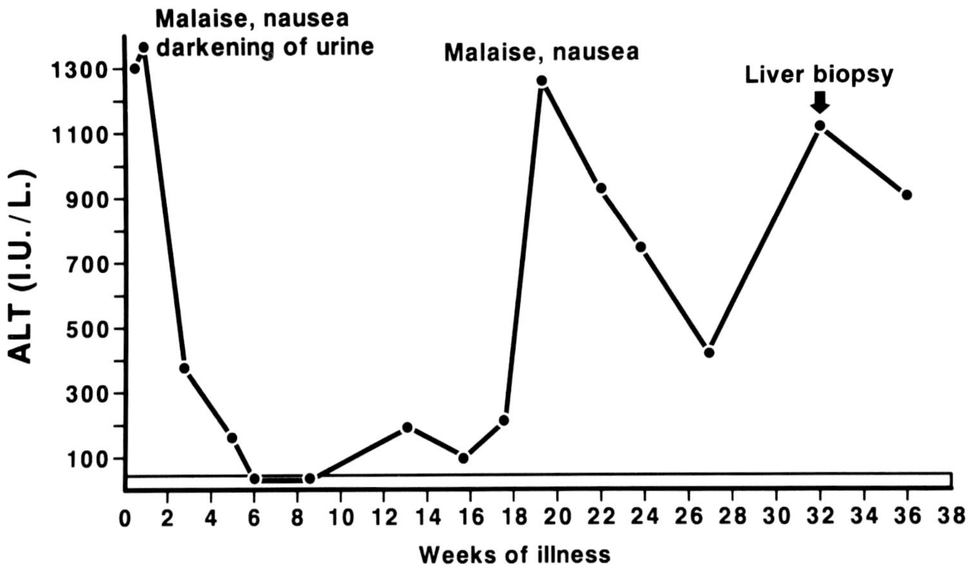

Figure 13-6
Aminotransferase fluctuations occurring in chronic hepatitis C. The liver biopsy revealed low-grade CAH. (From Kelley WN et al, eds: Textbook of internal medicine, Philadelphia, 1989, J B Lippincott Co.)

tory of NANB hepatitis. Serious liver disease (CAH, cirrhosis, or both) is found in as many as 60% of patients who undergo liver biopsy, and it has been estimated that at least 20% of patients with NANB hepatitis progress to cirrhosis during an observation period of 5 to 10 years. It is not known if the presence of cirrhosis has an effect on survival in this condition, and natural-history studies are currently underway to address this question.

Neither the amplitude of the aminotransferase elevations nor the degree of symptoms can predict the liver histology in NANB hepatitis, and progression to chronic hepatitis cannot be predicted from the clinical or biochemical severity of the acute illness. Anicteric cases are just as likely as icteric cases to be complicated by chronic infection. Irrespective of the route of exposure (e.g., transfusion vs. sporadically acquired infection), the incidence of chronicity (40% to 60%) is similar. Chronic hepatitis has not been observed after the water-borne type of "epidemic" NANB hepatitis.

During the course of NANB hepatitis, many patients have marked fluctuations in their serum aminotransferase levels, with periods of elevated enzyme levels alternating with periods of near-normal or normal levels (Figure 13-6). Evaluation of spontaneous remission or response to therapy may be difficult under these circumstances. Symptomatically, chronic NANB hepatitis may be quite mild. The majority of patients have some degree of fatigue and loss of vigor that persists after the acute episode of hepatitis. Some patients suffer from marked fatigue and weakness, with progression to liver failure and death. However, the evolution of the disease is slow, and the history of exposure to the viral agent may precede the onset of serious illness by more than 10 years. An increasing number of hepatoma cases resulting from chronic NANB hepatitis have been reported. A possible causal link between chronic hepatitis C and hepatoma was suggested recently by studies in Japan, Italy, and Spain in which 50% to 70% of HBsAg-negative hepatoma cases had detectable HCV antibody.

Chronic Hepatitis D. The clinical and laboratory features of superinfection with HDV cannot generally be distinguished from those associated with acute viral hepatitis of other causes, and this similarity can lead to a misdiagnosis of acute hepatitis B in a previously unrecognized HBsAg carrier. However, the lack of IgM anti-HBc in the serum of such a patient, should always raise the suspicion of HDV superinfection in a previously unrecognized carrier of HBsAg. Studies of both animals and humans indicate that HBV carriers with inactive HBV infection characterized by anti-HBe and integrated HBV-DNA are more likely to develop chronic δ-infection. In HBsAg carriers with active HBV-induced liver disease, HDV causes additional damage and can accelerate the course of chronic hepatitis to cirrhosis. In some cases this progression can occur in patients with an initial diagnosis of chronic persistent hepatitis. Indeed, progressive liver failure can also develop in previously healthy, asymptomatic carriers of HBsAg.

Development of chronic HDV infection is associated with a 3-year mortality rate of 15% compared with 5% in age-matched patients with HBsAg-positive, δ-negative CLD. The usual causes of death, hemorrhage from esophageal varices and hepatic coma, are similar to those of end-stage type B and NANB infections. There are no data to indicate that δ-infection predisposes to hepatocellular carcinoma.

Chronic δ-infection is diagnosed by the finding of IgM and/or IgG antibody against the virus in the serum. Unlike the weak and evanescent antibody responses seen in acute δ-hepatitis, titers of these antibodies are often persistently high in chronic infection (Figure 13-7).

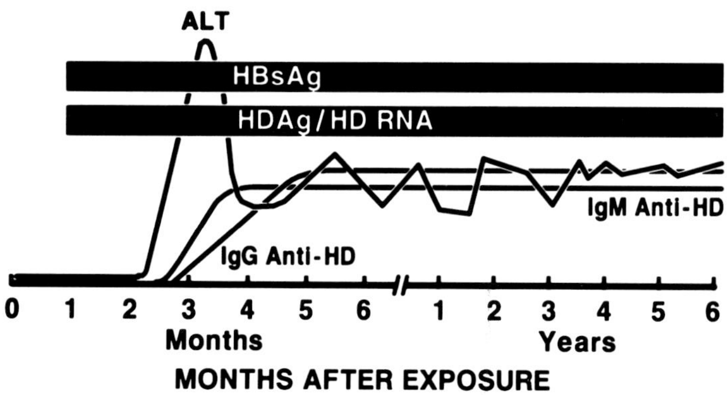

Figure 13-7
Serologic profile of HDV superinfection in a chronic HBsAg carrier with evolution to chronic δ-infection.

Differential Diagnosis of Chronic Viral Hepatitis

Chronic viral hepatitis must be distinguished from autoimmune hepatitis, drug-induced hepatitis, alcoholic liver disease, α_1-antitrypsin deficiency, hemochromatosis, PBC, sclerosing cholangitis, and Wilson's disease. In most cases the illness can be identified by history, clinical features, or biochemical and histologic findings. Chronic hepatitis B, hepatitis C, and δ-hepatitis can be diagnosed by serologic identification of the viral agents. Distinction of HCV-negative NANB hepatitis from a disorder such as autoimmune hepatitis may be difficult, particularly when there is no history of exposure to hepatitis viruses. The diagnosis of alcoholic liver disease may require liver biopsy, particularly when a history of alcoholism is not available. The finding of an AST/ALT ratio greater than 2 suggests alcoholic liver injury and is atypical for chronic viral hepatitis except possibly when active cirrhosis is present. Medications such as α-methyldopa, nitrofurantoin, dantrolene, and isoniazid can cause CAH and cirrhosis. Histologic distinction from chronic viral hepatitis may be difficult, because liver biopsy often does not reveal histologic features specific for drug toxicity. In most cases discontinuation of the offending drug results in biochemical and histologic improvement. Liver disease associated with α_1-antitrypsin deficiency can be distinguished from NANB hepatitis by the absence of α_1-globulin on protein electrophoresis and by measurement of serum α-1AT. Typical PAS-positive inclusions are seen in the liver parenchyma of these patients. Patients with hemochromatosis have elevated serum iron levels, transferrin saturation, serum ferritin in excess of 500 ng/ml, and a marked increase in liver parenchymal iron. In general the distinction between chronic viral hepatitis and chronic cholestatic syndromes is not difficult. A disproportionately high serum AP is found in the latter disorders. Visualization of the biliary tree is diagnostic in sclerosing cholangitis. Although low antimitochondrial antibody titers may be observed occasionally in chronic viral hepatitis, a strongly positive antimitochondrial antibody is virtually diagnostic of PBC. The diagnosis of Wilson's disease is supported by the findings of low serum ceruloplasmin, an elevated 24-hour urine copper, and a positive slit-lamp examination for Kayser-Fleischer rings. The liver parenchyma is marked by heavy copper deposition.

Treatment of Chronic Viral Hepatitis

Long-term corticosteroid therapy is not indicated in the management of chronic hepatitis B. Corticosteroid-associated complications frequently occur with prolonged therapy. Moreover, corticosteroids enhance viral replication and delay the disappearance of HBeAg.

A variety of antiviral and immunologically active agents have been utilized in the treatment of chronic hepatitis B. Most studies testing the use of these agents have been small, noncontrolled, nonrandomized clinical trials. The major antiviral agents under study have included the purine analogs vidarabine (and its highly soluble monophosphate ester), acycloguanosine (acyclovir), and deoxyacyclovir and various types of human interferons (α-interferon, β-interferon, and γ-interferon). Immunologic approaches have included the use of corticosteroid suppression, transfer factor, levamisole (an antihelminthic with T cell– stimulating prop-

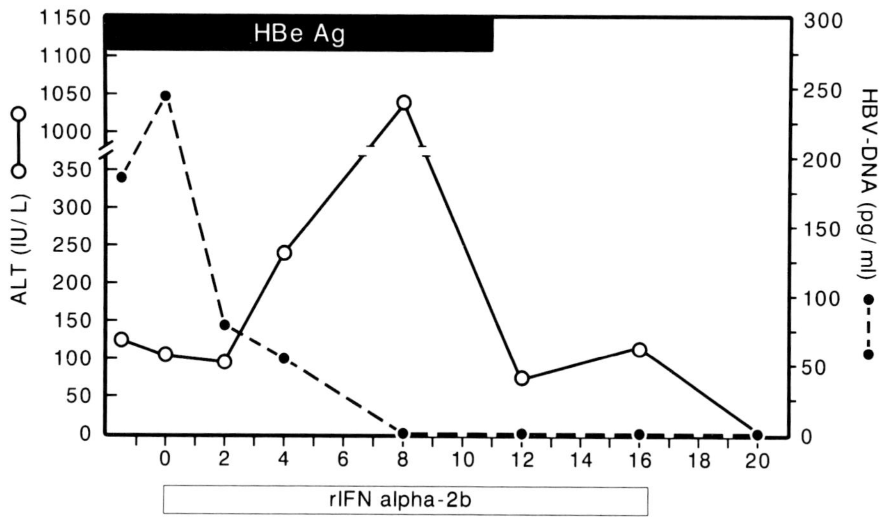

Figure 13-8
HBV-DNA and ALT curve of a patient treated with recombinant α-interferon. Note the sudden increase in ALT during the second month associated with a marked decline in HBV-DNA and clearance of HBeAg. (From Perrillo RP: Treatment of chronic hepatitis B with interferon: Experience in Western countries, Semin Liver Dis 9:240, 1989.)

erties), interferon, and short-term corticosteroids (to provide an immunologic rebound against HBV). Of these approaches, interferon has given the most promising results, perhaps because it is both antiviral and immunomodulatory. A response usually has been defined as the sustained disappearance of circulating HBeAg and HBV-DNA. Loss of these markers of viral replication has generally been associated with improvement in liver histology and a major decline in abnormal aminotransferase levels. Approximately 10% of treated patients lose HBsAg as a result of therapy. Response to interferon occurs more frequently when augmentation of aminotransferase levels, reflecting enhancement of the immune response, is observed during therapy (Figure 13-8). Studies indicate that a combination of immunostimulation (provided by steroid withdrawal) and an antiviral agent may have synergistic effects in patients with relatively mild biochemical abnormalities (i.e., ALT less than 100 U/L). Several patient characteristics are associated with a greater likelihood of a response to antiviral therapy (see box on p. 296). Baseline HBV-DNA appears to be the best independent predictor of a response to therapy in clinically stable patients.

Interferon has some activity in chronic NANB hepatitis and has recently been licensed by the Food and Drug Administration for this condition. Randomized, controlled studies have demonstrated normalization of ALT in 50% to 80% of patients who are treated with relatively low doses of interferon, e.g., 1 million to 3

FAVORABLE PROGNOSTIC INDICATORS FOR RESPONSE TO ANTIVIRAL THERAPY IN CHRONIC HEPATITIS B

Low baseline HBV-DNA level*
Short duration of hepatitis
High baseline aminotransferase level
HIV-negative status
Active disease histologically
Heterosexual lifestyle
Female gender
Anti-δ-negative
Disease acquired in adulthood†

*Best independent predictor of response to interferon therapy in anti-HIV–negative and anti-HDV–negative patients.
†Low response rates are noted in persons exposed as newborns and during early childhood (e.g., Asians).

million units three times per week. However, relapse occurs frequently after discontinuation of therapy, and additional studies are underway to determine the optimal dose and duration of therapy. Corticosteroids and acyclovir have been demonstrated to be ineffective in the management of this disorder.

δ-Hepatitis does not respond to immunosuppressive therapy. An improvement in biochemical and viral markers of disease may occur in response to interferon. Relatively high doses of interferon may be required to achieve a response. An extremely high rate of relapse has been observed after termination of therapy, even after prolonged courses (e.g., one year).

Liver transplantation is reserved for patients with advanced stages of chronic viral hepatitis. Patients presenting with variceal hemorrhage, refractory ascites, hepatic encephalopathy, worsening liver function, or deteriorating functional status should be evaluated at centers that perform hepatic transplantation. Recurrent infection of the graft invariably develops after transplantation for chronic hepatitis B. This may be associated with severe, progressive liver disease. On the other hand, recurrent NANB hepatitis, occurs relatively infrequently after transplantation.

SUMMARY

Currently, there are five known hepatitis viruses. The past decade has witnessed the discovery of two new viruses (HDV and HEV) and remarkable advances in our understanding of the genetic organization of all hepatitis viruses. Much of the current knowledge would not be possible without the ability to detect the cause in blood and other body fluids. Thus the development of immunoassays for HCV opens the way for sensitive probes for this virus and will eventually lead to greater understanding of the natural history, therapy, and prevention of this significant health problem. Major advances have recently been made in therapy for chronic viral hepatitis, with recombinant α-interferon being the first licensed treatment for chronic NANB hepatitis and hepatitis C.

SUGGESTED READINGS

ACIP: Recommendations of the Immunization Practices Advisory Committee: update on hepatitis B prevention, MMWR 36:353, 1987.

This report contains the latest recommendations for the use of hepatitis B vaccine.

Bruix J et al: Prevalence of antibodies to hepatitis C virus in Spanish patients with hepatocellular carcinoma and hepatic cirrhosis, Lancet 2:1004-1006, 1989.

The prevalence of antibodies to HCV was investigated in 96 patients with hepatocellular carcinoma, 106 patients with liver cirrhosis, and 177 persons without liver disease. Of patients with hepatocellular carcinoma, 75% had HCV antibodies, a significantly higher proportion than that observed in patients with cirrhosis (55%) or persons without liver disease (7%).

Gimson AES et al: Late onset hepatic failure: clinical, serological and histological features, Hepatology 6:288-294, 1986.

The clinical, laboratory, and histologic features of 47 patients with what is defined as late-onset hepatic failure are reviewed. Hepatic failure occurred 8 to 24 weeks after the first symptom of illness. In only four cases was a viral cause proved. In the remainder, NANB infection was likely. These patients did not respond to corticosteroids.

Gust ID and Purcell RH: Report of a workshop: waterborne non-A, non-B hepatitis, J Infect Dis 156:630-635, 1987.

This is a summary of a workshop sponsored by the National Institutes of Health (NIH). The authors describe the epidemiology, clinical and laboratory features, and transmission studies with this newly described viral agent. The article ends with important suggestions for future studies.

Hoofnagle JH: Type D (delta) hepatitis, JAMA 261:1321, 1989.

This is a current review of the advances made in our understanding of the viral structure, genomic organization, replicative cycle, clinical course, and epidemiology of this unique agent.

Hoofnagle JH and Di Bisceglie AM: Treatment of chronic type C hepatitis with alpha interferon, Semin Liver Dis 9:259-263, 1989.

The authors review the existing studies with α-interferon and conclude that future studies need to establish the correct dose and optimal duration of therapy.

Kuo G et al: An assay for circulating antibodies to a major etiologic virus of human non-A, non-B hepatitis, Science 244:362, 1989.

This report describes the pivotal series of experiments that lead to the identification of HCV and an immunoassay for its corresponding antibody.

Lemon SM: Type A viral hepatitis: new developments in an old disease, N Engl J Med 313:1059, 1985.

This is a relatively recent and lucid summary of new developments in this condition. The author reviews the physical properties and replication cycle of the virus; pathogenesis; epidemiology, clinical features, and immunization strategies.

O'Grady JG et al: Controlled trials of charcoal hemoperfusion and prognostic factors in fulminant hepatic failure, Gastroenterology 94:1186-1192, 1988.

In two controlled clinical trials, charcoal hemoperfusion was noted to be inefficacious in improving survival for FHF patients. The authors review the prognoses of patients with various forms of fulminant liver failure and find the lowest survival rate (12%) in patients with hepatitis caused by drugs, including halothane, a 20% rate in patients with NANB hepatitis, 40% in patients with hepatitis B, and the best survival (67%) in patients with acute hepatitis A.

Perrillo RP: Treatment of chronic hepatitis B with interferon: experience in western countries, Semin Liver Dis 9:240, 1989.

This is a current summary of the area with an extensive bibliography. The author explains the rationale and potential use for a short course of corticosteroids in conjunction with interferon. A treatment algorithm, based on the level of ALT and HBV-DNA, is included.

Weiner AJ, Kuo G, Bradley DW et al: Detection of hepatitis C viral sequences in non-A, non-B hepatitis, Lancet 335:1-3, 1990.

The authors describe the results of testing for HCV-RNA in naturally acquired and experimentally induced infection. Viral genome was usually detectable in serum and liver during the major peak of liver enzyme abnormalities before the appearance of circulating antibody.

14 Chronic Hepatitis

Robert P. Perrillo

The term *chronic hepatitis* refers to a group of inflammatory disorders of the liver that last for 6 or more months. Chronic hepatitis is generally classified from histologic and etiologic bases. There are several major histologic forms of chronic hepatitis: chronic persistent hepatitis, chronic lobular hepatitis, chronic active hepatitis, and cirrhosis. Chronic persistent hepatitis and chronic active hepatitis may present with similar clinical and laboratory features (Table 14-1). CAH is often associated with progressive fibrosis and may ultimately lead to cirrhosis, whereas chronic persistent hepatitis and chronic lobular hepatitis are generally thought to be benign conditions with little or no tendency for hepatic scarring. There are multiple known causes of chronic hepatitis, e.g., hepatitis virus infection, hepatoxicity caused by medications, autoimmune disease, and hereditary forms of liver disease, such as α_1-antitrypsin deficiency and Wilson's disease. This chapter presents the histologic features of the various forms of chronic hepatitis and focuses on the prototype for chronic hepatitis, chronic autoimmune hepatitis. (See elsewhere in this text for a discussion of the other disorders associated with chronic hepatitis.)

HISTOLOGIC CLASSIFICATION

Chronic Active Hepatitis

The features that characterize CAH include destruction of the limiting plate of the hepatic lobule with focal areas of liver cell necrosis, so-called "piecemeal necrosis" (Figure 14-1). The latter is best defined as the destruction of liver cells at an interface between parenchyma and connective tissue occurring in conjunction with mononuclear cell infiltration. The lobular architecture is preserved initially. A variable degree of fibrous expansion of the portal tracts is observed in this condition. The changes may be subtle, and only slight degrees of piecemeal necrosis may be evident. In such cases, it may be difficult to separate the disorder from chronic persistent hepatitis. In more active cases, there is linkage of involved portal tracts or portal tracts with central veins, so-called "bridging necrosis" (Figure 14-2). Fibrosis develops within the areas of periportal or bridging necrosis, causing architectural disruption and eventually leading to cirrhosis. Most investigators believe that bridging necrosis is the major progressive lesion in CAH that leads to cirrhosis. Further studies are needed to determine if portal-to-portal

Table 14-1 Differentiating between chronic persistent hepatitis and chronic active hepatitis

Test or clinical feature	Remark
Liver biopsy	"Brass standard"; invasive; sampling variation may be a problem
Hepatic wedge pressure	May have value; invasive
Serum bile acid levels	May have value; overlap of CPH with mild CAH
Physical examination	Splenomegaly favors diagnosis of CAH
ALT/AST	Limited value; overlap occurs frequently with low-level elevations
Serum albumin	Low levels favor CAH with cirrhosis; late manifestation
Liver scans	
CT, technetium	May reveal undetected splenomegaly; of little value otherwise
Serum bilirubin	Of little value; mild unconjugated hyperbilirubinemia may be seen with chronic persistent hepatitis
Viral markers	Worthless

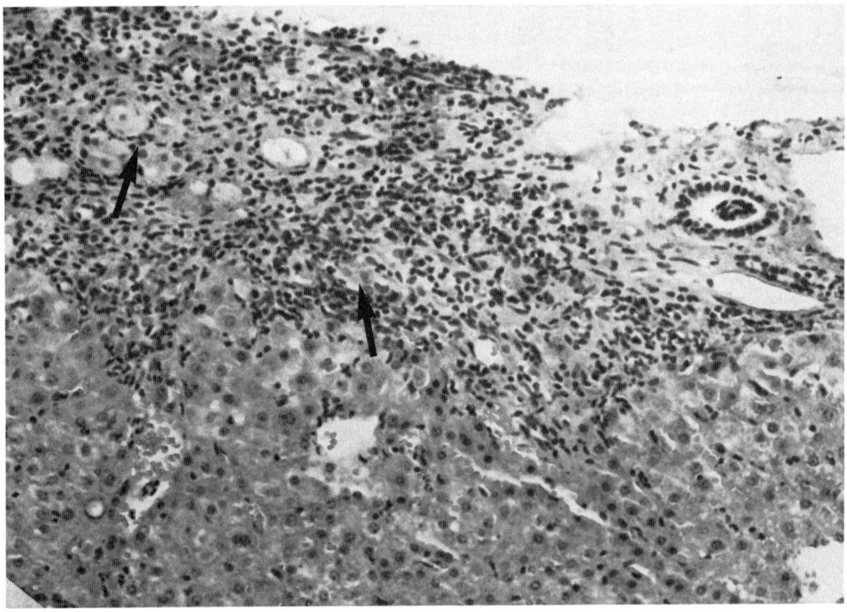

Figure 14-1
Chronic active hepatitis. The portal tract is expanded with mononuclear cells, and there is a poorly defined limiting plate with extensive piecemeal necrosis *(arrows)*.

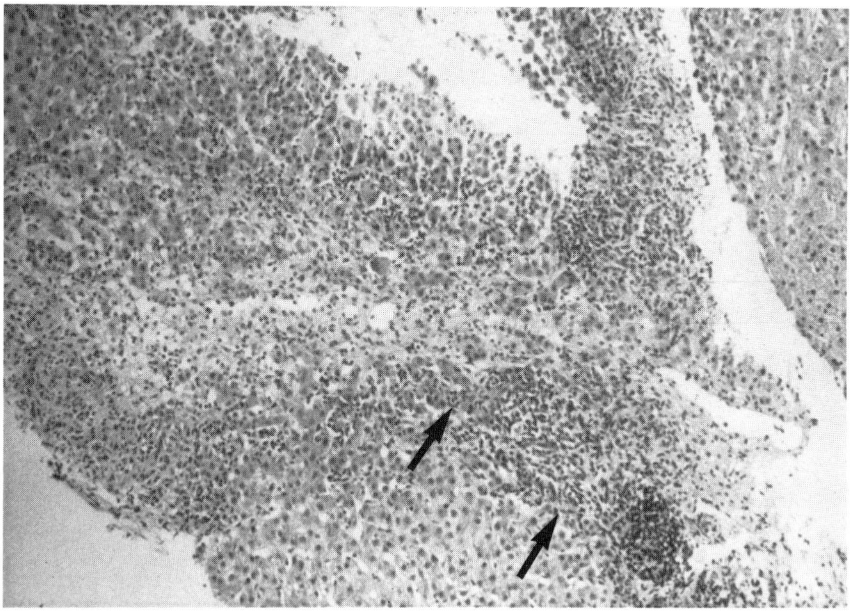

Figure 14-2
Chronic active hepatitis with bridging necrosis. There is severe inflammation in this biopsy specimen, and an area of bridging necrosis incompletely extends from the portal tract toward the central vein *(arrows)*.

bridging is a more benign finding with less predisposition to cirrhosis than is portal-to-central venous bridging. Several studies have indicated that patients with an initial lesion of piecemeal necrosis alone occasionally may progress to cirrhosis. In such cases, the evolution to cirrhosis may be relatively slow, with bridging hepatic necrosis developing as an intermediary lesion.

Chronic Persistent Hepatitis

In chronic persistent hepatitis the liver biopsy specimen shows an intact hepatic lobule with normal architecture. There is a mixed inflammatory infiltrate in the portal tracts. Generally there is sharp limitation of the infiltrate to this region, and piecemeal necrosis is absent. Occasionally, individual liver cell necrosis may occur. If this is a prominent finding or if the inflammatory infiltrate is especially dense and associated with "spillover" of the infiltrate into the surrounding parenchyma, it may be difficult to differentiate this condition from mild CAH. A benign prognosis is generally given to the patient with this condition because it is not associated with significant fibrosis and does not progress to cirrhosis or signs of portal hypertension. However, there are certain exceptions to this rule. Chronic persistent

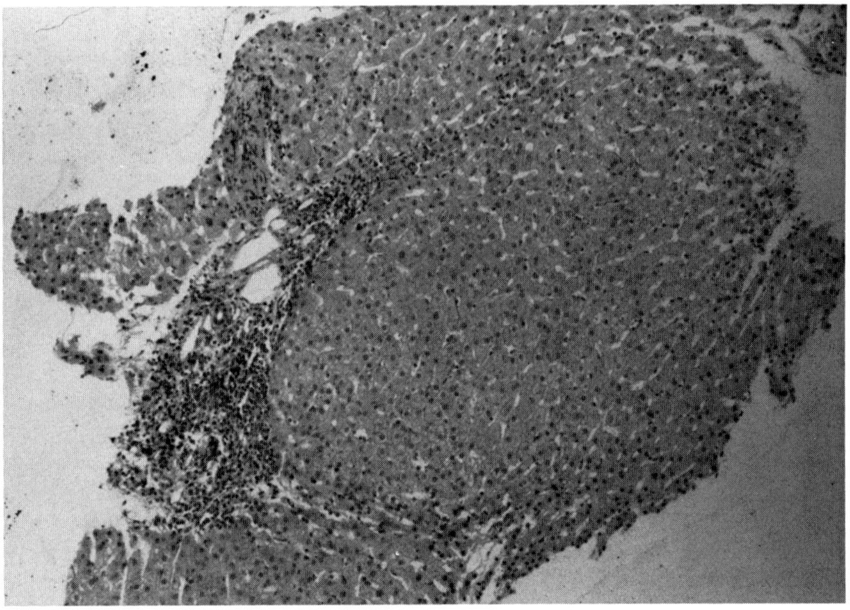

Figure 14-3
Chronic active hepatitis in remission. This is a post-treatment biopsy specimen from a patient with chronic active hepatitis B who was treated successfully with recombinant α-interferon. Note the sharp demarcation of the infiltrate in the portal tract, consistent with the findings in chronic persistent hepatitis. However, Trichrome stain revealed an increase in portal fibrosis, secondary to the CAH.

hepatitis may revert to a more serious histologic appearance, including cirrhosis, after discontinuation of immunosuppressive therapy in autoimmune hepatitis or during the natural course of chronic viral hepatitis. Progression of chronic persistent hepatitis to chronic active hepatitis has been described in chronic hepatitis B, where it occurs presumably as a result of reactivated infection. Progression of chronic persistent hepatitis to chronic active hepatitis and cirrhosis also has been documented in chronic hepatitis D and probably occurs frequently in NANB hepatitis. Chronic persistent hepatitis may be associated with increased fibrosis when it occurs during remission from chronic active hepatitis (Figure 14-3). These situations should be distinguished from instances in which an initial diagnosis of chronic persistent hepatitis is incorrectly made because of sampling variation inherent to percutaneous liver biopsy.

Chronic Lobular Hepatitis

Chronic lobular hepatitis is characterized by parenchymal necroinflammation resembling acute hepatitis but persisting for more than 6 months. It has been described most frequently in chronic hepati-

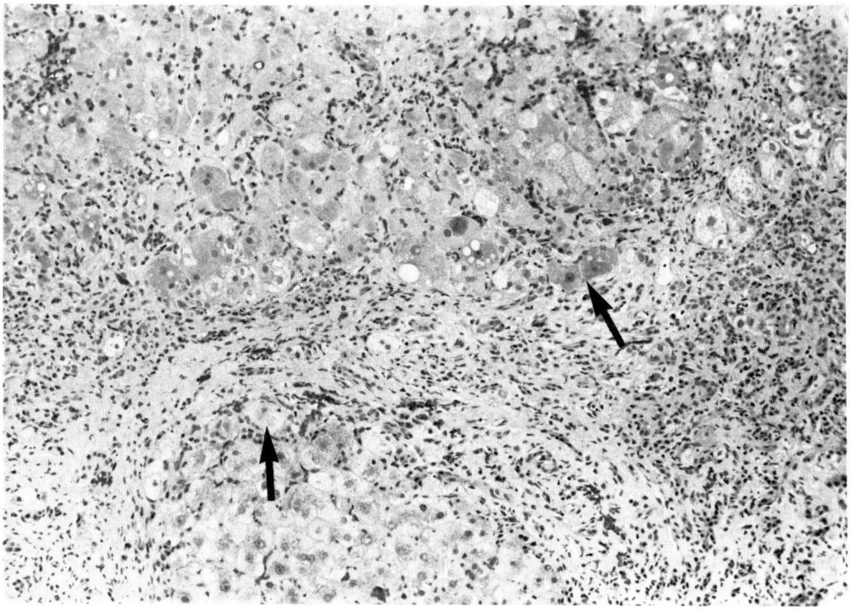

Figure 14-4
Piecemeal necrosis *(arrows)* is noted adjoining a fibrous band in this patient with well-established cirrhosis. (From Trent-Mills C, Lee E, and Perrillo RP: Relationship between histology, aminotransferase levels, and viral replication in chronic hepatitis B, Gastroenterology 99:519, 1990).

tis B and in NANB hepatitis and not in autoimmune hepatitis. Piecemeal necrosis and bridging necrosis are absent. The severity of the hepatocellular damage may vary from mild spotty necrosis and inflammation to severe injury associated with eosinophilic bodies, diffuse inflammation, and cholestasis. Chronic lobular hepatitis may last for several years with remissions and occasional relapses but without progression to cirrhosis.

Cirrhosis

Cirrhosis is the end result of CAH, usually occurring in conjunction with bridging necrosis. Cirrhosis often evolves rather insidiously and without specific clinical symptomatology. In many cases, a liver biopsy specimen demonstrates features of both cirrhosis and CAH (Figure 14-4). The regenerative nodules are surrounded by fibrous septa, and the cirrhosis is usually macronodular. The characteristic features of cirrhosis may be absent from needle biopsy specimens because the needle may be diverted from the dense fibrous septa or the needle may transect a large nodule. These possibilities led the Mayo Clinic group to propose the need for serial biopsies before excluding the diagnosis of cirrhosis. However, in clinical practice the diagnosis is supported by fragmentation of the tissue, dense fibrosis, and marked nodularity of the specimen. Laparoscopic biopsy is a more accurate means of assessment. When the necroinflammatory changes in the fibrous septa and adjoining them subside, the cirrhosis is classified as "inactive." Inactive cirrhosis may be associated with a normal 5-year survival, whereas persistence of the features of CAH superimposed on cirrhosis is likely to result in eventual liver failure.

Multilobular Necrosis

This relatively uncommon lesion implies extensive necrosis of entire hepatic lobules. Patients with this degree of histologic injury have an even less favorable prognosis than those with bridging necrosis. Cirrhosis develops early and occurs more frequently with multilobular necrosis. The liver biopsy specimen may show broad fibrotic bands in areas of extensive necrosis and collapse.

AUTOIMMUNE HEPATITIS

Definition and Pathogenesis

This condition was first diagnosed in 1951 by Kunkel and others in young females with hypergammaglobulinemia, plasma cell infiltration of the liver parenchyma, and cirrhosis. The disease was delineated further by Mackay and others in 1956 when the term *lupoid hepatitis* was coined for the subset of patients presenting with a positive ANA or lupus erythematosus (LE) cell test. Later it became clear that lupoid hepatitis was not a component syndrome of systemic LE; thus, the term *autoimmune hepatitis* was coined. Because a variety of autoantibodies occasionally may be observed with chronic liver diseases of diverse etiologies, such as drug-induced hepatitis and viral hepatitis, the diagnosis of autoimmune hepatitis remains somewhat imprecise. In the strictest sense, chronic autoimmune hepatitis may be defined as hepatitis associated with high titers of one or more circulating autoantibodies and persisting for more than 6 months. The disease occurs in patients without an identifiable metabolic abnormality or evidence of exposure to viral agents or hepatotoxins, including medications. Substantial evidence exists to suggest that aberrant immunologic mechanisms are involved in the pathogenesis of this disorder. In as many as 50% of patients with autoimmune hepatitis, other disorders with a presumed imuunologic basis are present (e.g., thyroiditis, polyarthritis, ulcerative colitis, glomerulonephritis, Coombs'-positive hemolytic anemia, and chronic fibrosing alveolitis). Additional evidence of an immunologic basis lies in finding an increased incidence of autoantibodies and autoimmune disorders in family members, elevated levels of serum immunoglobulin, the beneficial effects of corticosteroids, and the strong association of this disorder with the major histocompatibility antigens HLA-B8 and DRw3. These HLA phenotypes are observed in 70% to 80% of patients with this disorder and in approximately 25% of persons without the disorder.

Presenting Features

The clinical manifestations of autoimmune hepatitis are similar to those of chronic viral hepatitis (Table 14-2). However, unlike viral hepatitis, autoimmune hepatitis predominates in women (female/male ratio of 4:1). Patients usually present in the third to fifth decades of life; however, children and older adults can also be affected. A relatively high incidence of extrahepatic manifestations (e.g., arthritis, rash, thyroiditis, pleuropericarditis, colitis, pulmonary disease, and glomerulonephritis) may be observed at the time of presentation. Many patients

Table 14-2 Differentiating between autoimmune hepatitis and chronic viral hepatitis

Distinguishing feature	Autoimmune	Hepatitis B	Hepatitis C
Predominant sex	Female	Male	Neither
Onset	Insidious	Insidious	Insidious
Major age group	20-40	≥35	≥35*
Symptoms	Arthralgias, fatigue	Fatigue	Fatigue
Physical features	Jaundice, thyromegaly, synovitis	None	None
Key biochemical findings	Hypergammaglobulinemia	None	Fluctuating ALT/AST
Viral markers	None†	HBsAg, anti-HBc, HBeAg, HBV-DNA; immunoperoxidase stains for HBcAg, HBsAg	Anti-HCV
Autoantibodies	Common (≥1:160)	Uncommon (≤1:100)	Uncommon (≤1:100)
HLA tests	B8, Dw3	Bw15, Bw17, Bw35	None
Histology	Plasma cell predominance, microacinar transformation of hepatocytes	Ground glass cells	Sinusoidal activation, microsteatosis, prominent acidophilic degeneration

*Post-transfusion hepatitis often affects elderly patients.
†False-positive tests for anti-HCV may occur.

are currently identified at an asymptomatic stage because of the widespread application of automated blood testing. In a substantial number of these patients, the progression of disease is insidious with continued absence of symptoms on prolonged follow-up.

In asymptomatic patients the physical examination is often normal. In symptomatic patients, the most common findings include hepatomegaly (80%), jaundice (80%), and splenomegaly, spider angiomata, and palmar erythema (each in approximately 50% of patients). Signs of advanced liver disease (e.g., esophageal varices, ascites, and hepatic encephalopathy) infrequently are present when the patient first seeks medical attention.

Laboratory Features

The aminotransferase activity is often between 3 and 10 times the upper limit of normal. More striking elevations (tenfold to twentyfold) may occur, but they are unusual. Patients included in the Mayo Clinic treatment trials were identified on the basis of severe biochemical and histologic activity, and this severity of activity led to an erroneous assumption that these features were characteristic of autoimmune CAH. However, several studies subsequently indicated that the majority of patients with this disorder do not meet these critieria and are often asymptomatic with mild biochemical and histologic abnormalities. Many patients are diagnosed as having autoimmune hepatitis as a result of routine biochemical screening. Patients with autoimmune hepatitis are more likely to have elevated serum immunoglobulin levels when compared with patients with chronic viral hepatitis (see Table 14-2). Serum AP activity is elevated in approximately 80% of patients but is usually less than two times the upper limit of normal. Serum albumin levels are often decreased in the later stages of disease. In patients presenting with features of advanced liver disease, such as portal hypertension, and hepatic encephalopathy, other signs of illness, such as anemia, leukopenia, thrombocytopenia, and prolonged PT, are often present.

A variety of circulating antibodies have been identified in patients with autoimmune hepatitis. Antinuclear and anti-smooth muscle antibodies, usually in a titer greater than or equal to 1:160, remain the most clinically useful markers of this disease. Other subsets of patients who lack antinuclear and smooth muscle antibodies have been identified. Many of these individuals have detectable antibody to a liver-kidney microsomal antigen (i.e., cytochrome P-450 db1, a drug-metabolizing enzyme) or soluble liver antigen. Methods of testing for these antibodies are currently beyond the capability of most laboratories. Autoimmune hepatitis associated with antiliver/anti-kidney microsomal antibody appears to have a more aggressive course, with an acute, even fulminant, onset of hepatitis. It is characterized by more rapid evolution to cirrhosis and lower long-term survival rates. Moreover, it occurs at a younger age, often coming to appreciation in childhood. Because of the absence of the more widely performed autoantibodies, these patients might be misdiagnosed as having chronic NANB hepatitis. Further confusion may be derived from the fact that patients with autoimmune hepatitis may have false-positive tests for antibody to HCV.

On liver biopsy the features of autoimmune hepatitis may be indistinguishable from those described in chronic viral hepatitis, with the possible exception of a predominance of plasma cells infiltrating the portal tracts. Cirrhosis may be present in up to 50% of patients at the time of presentation.

Natural History

The natural history of autoimmune hepatitis is highly variable. Most studies attempting to define the natural history of this disorder are limited by failure to use uniform criteria for diagnosis, inability to exclude patients with drug-induced or viral hepatitis, predominance of seriously ill patients and those with advanced liver disease, and lack of long-term, systematic follow-up. Early studies emphasized the high mortality, with a mean survival rate of approximately 5 years in untreated patients. Patients presenting with either cirrhosis or multilobular necrosis on biopsy had the poorest prognosis. For example, in the Mayo Clinic study, approximately 80% of patients with bridging or multilobular necrosis progressed to cirrhosis during the 5-year follow-up, whereas those with piecemeal necrosis alone seemed to progress infrequently to cirrhosis (17% of patients). Spontaneous remission occurred in no more than 20% of patients. However, it is important to emphasize, that these observations were made in patients with severe disease, as reflected by pronounced clinical and laboratory manifestations. Many patients with autoimmune hepatitis have a milder form of disease, and the natural history of this form and need for treatment remain to be determined.

Management

Controlled clinical trials have demonstrated that corticosteroids alone or in combination with azathioprine are capable of inducing clinical, biochemical, and histologic remission. Therapy also appears to improve survival in patients with the more severe forms of autoimmune hepatitis at initial presentation (e.g., persons with multilobular necrosis or cirrhosis). Unfortunately, many patients, including those with CAH alone, progress insidiously to cirrhosis despite an apparent therapy-induced remission. Long-term follow-up of treated patients with histologically documented remission (i.e., with chronic persistent hepatitis) has revealed progression to cirrhosis without clinical or biochemical signs of relapse. The development of cirrhosis after treatment has not been shown to diminish survival, and complications attributable to portal hypertension have been infrequent.

Treatment with prednisone is usually initiated at dosages ranging from 20 to 60 mg per day. The dose is often tapered to a maintenance level of 10 to 20 mg per day, and therapy is continued until remission occurs. Clinical improvement and biochemical remission are noted within the first 6 to 12 months, but histologic improvement may be delayed for 18 to 36 months. Combination therapy with azathioprine, 50 mg per day, and prednisone, 10 mg per day, is associated with fewer side effects and appears to be as effective as therapy with prednisone alone. The prednisone-sparing effects of azathioprine may be particularly important for postmenopausual women (see p. 308) and patients with diabetes, hypertension, or cushingoid features. The presence of a concomitant autoimmune disorder does not appear to affect reponse to treatment, and patients with autoimmune markers have rates of response comparable to those without these markers. Alternate-day treatment with corticosteroids may improve the results of liver tests without favorably influencing the liver histology, whereas azathioprine therapy alone appears to be ineffective in controlling the disease.

Treatment is usually continued for at least 12 months. When therapy is discontinued, relapses occur in more than 50% of patients, generally within the first 6 months after the discontinuation of treatment. Patients with severe or multiple episodes of relapse generally require lifelong, low-dose maintenance therapy. Reinstitution of the original therapy usually induces remission in patients who relapse. Every effort should be made to reduce corticosteroids to the lowest dose that is able to control the symptomatic, biochemical, and histologic manifestations of disease. Control of the disorder is considered to be adequate when symptoms are no longer present, the aminotransferase values are minimally elevated (e.g., less than two times the upper limit of normal), the γ-globulin level is below 2 gm/dl, and liver histology reveals a nonspecific or chronic persistent hepatitis.

In general, symptomatic patients with laboratory and histologic evidence of active disease are most likely to benefit from therapy, whereas asymptomatic patients with mild biochemical abnormalities and minimal histologic disease (e.g., chronic persistent hepatitis or mild CAH) are least likely to benefit. Because adverse effects frequently occur during long-term corticosteroid therapy, the risk/benefit ratio for therapy needs to be evaluated individually. In many patients, particularly postmenopausal women and elderly patients, the risks of therapy (e.g., vertebral compression fracture, aseptic necrosis, and diabetes) may outweigh any potential benefits. In patients with severe liver disease that is complicated by variceal hemorrhage, refractory ascites, hepatic encephalopathy, or deteriorating functional status, liver transplantation may be necessary. Differentiation between autoimmune hepatitis and NANB hepatitis is particularly important, because the inadvertent use of interferon in patients with autoimmune hepatitis has been associated with a flare of the liver disease.

Differential Diagnosis

The clinical features of autoimmune hepatitis are similar to those of viral hepatitis (see Table 14-2). In addition, certain drugs (eg, nitrofurantoin, α-methyldopa, and isoniazid) have been implicated in production of an illness virtually indistinguishable from autoimmune hepatitis, including the presence of autoantibodies. Distinction from HCV-negative NANB hepatitis remains a clinical problem in the absence of serologic tests for the viral agent(s). However, the diagnosis of autoimmune hepatitis is more likely when circulating autoantibodies are present, serum globulins are elevated (particularly when the γ-globulin level exceeds 3.0 gm/dl), and there is no identifiable source of exposure to viral agents (e.g., blood transfusion or IV drug usage). Wilson's disease and α_1-antitrypsin deficiency need to be considered in young individuals presenting with CLD. PBC and PSC occasionally may be confused clinically and histologically with autoimmune hepatitis. The distinction between autoimmune hepatitis and PBC may be particularly difficult to make. However, the presence of high titers of antimitochondrial antibodies and markedly elevated serum levels of AP, IgM, and cholesterol favor the diagnosis of PBC.

SUMMARY

Chronic hepatitis is a spectrum of inflammatory liver disorders that includes chronic persistent hepatitis, chronic lobular hepatitis, chronic active hepatitis, and cirrhosis. Liver-function tests and tests for viral markers are of limited use in differentiating between these forms of chronic hepatitis. Although chronic persistent hepatitis and chronic lobular hepatitis are generally benign conditions that do not result in fibrosis, chronic active hepatitis often progresses to cirrhosis, particularly in cases in which bridging necrosis is a conspicuous histologic feature. There are multiple known causes, e.g., hepatitis virus infection, hepatotoxicity caused by medication, autoimmune disease, and hereditary forms of liver disease. These causes necessitate appropriate consideration because successful therapy relies on identification of the specific cause.

SUGGESTED READINGS

Chadwick RG et al: Chronic persistent hepatitis: hepatitis B virus markers and histological follow up, Gut 20:372-377, 1979.

This study describes the progression of chronic persistent hepatitis to chronic active hepatitis in chronic hepatitis B. This report antedates the recognition of reactivation of chronic hepatitis B.

Combes B: The initial morphologic lesion in chronic hepatitis: important or unimportant? Hepatology 6:518-522, 1986.

A concise, well-referenced review of the prognostic importance of the liver biopsy in CAH is presented. Emphasis is given to the different outcomes of piecemeal necrosis alone and when bridging necrosis is observed.

Czaja AJ et al: Corticosteroid-treated chronic active hepatitis in remission: uncertain prognosis of chronic persistent hepatitis, N Engl J Med 304:5-9, 1981.

The authors describe the insidious progression to cirrhosis without clinical or laboratory manifestations of relapse in patients with treatment-induced chronic persistent hepatitis.

Czaja AJ: Natural history, clinical features, and treatment of autoimmune hepatitis, Semin Liver Dis 4:1-12, 1984.

This is a concise summary of the Mayo Clinic study of autoimmune hepatitis.

Davis GL, Czaja AJ, and Ludwig J: Development and prognosis of histologic cirrhosis in corticosteroid-treated hepatitis B surface antigen-negative chronic active hepatitis, Gastroenterology 87:1222, 1984.

This article describes the frequent development of cirrhosis if remission is not achieved within the first few years of therapy. Thereafter, cirrhosis develops infrequently and does not appear to influence survival.

Hodges JR, Millward-Sadler GH, and Wright R: Chronic active hepatitis: the spectrum of disease, Lancet 1:550-552, 1982.

Alcohol (26%) and hepatitis B (20%) are described in this article as the commonest causes of chronic active hepatitis. The study included 14 patients with autoimmune hepatitis, of whom only four (14%) presented with AST levels in excess of five times the upper limit of normal. The patients ranged in age from 41 to 80, with a mean age of 62.

Koretz RL et al: Chronic active hepatitis: Who meets treatment criteria? Dig Dis Sci 25:695-699, 1980.

This report describes the relative infrequency with which patients with histologically proven CAH meet the criteria for the Mayo Clinic treatment trials. Most patients in this study did not meet biochemical criteria independent of presumed etiology.

Lebovics E et al: Autoimmune chronic active hepatitis in postmenopausal women. Dig Dis Sci 30:824-828, 1985.

In this study, steroid therapy was associated with limited benefit and substantial toxicity (e.g., glaucoma, diabetes mellitus, and pathologic fracture) in postmenopausal women with autoimmune CAH.

Liaw YF et al: Chronic lobular hepatitis: a clinicopathological and prognostic study, Hepatology 2:258-262, 1982.

A large series of patients with this disorder are described from a clinical, laboratory, and histologic standpoint. No evidence of cirrhosis was observed in a follow-up period of at least 4.5 years.

MacFarlane IG et al: Hepatitis C virus antibodies in chronic active hepatitis: pathogenetic factor or false-positive result? Lancet 1:754-757, 1990.

This study describes a high prevalence of positive reactions for antibody to hepatitis C (65%) in patients with active autoimmune hepatitis and a low prevalence (5%) when the disease is in remission. The antibody readings correlated with serum globulin and IgG levels, suggesting that the results represent false-positive reactions.

Maddrey WC: Subdivisions of idiopathic autoimmune chronic active hepatitis, Hepatology 7:1372-1375, 1987.

In this concise, well-referenced review, patients with autoimmune chronic hepatitis are divided into three groups, based on the presence of antibodies to actin, liver/kidney microsomes, and soluble liver antigen, respectively.

15 Uncommon and Exotic Viral Infections of the Liver

Cheree Trent Mills *and* ***Robert P. Perrillo***

VIRUSES THAT AFFECT THE LIVER AS PART OF A SYSTEMIC ILLNESS

Three viruses affect the liver as part of a systemic illness: cytomegalovirus, Epstein-Barr virus, and herpes simplex virus (Table 15-1).

Cytomegalovirus

Infection with cytomegalovirus is common and occurs worldwide. The virus has a DNA genome and is classified as a herpesvirus. Major routes of transmission are perinatal exposure, person-to-person contact, and blood transfusions. Most primary infections with cytomegalovirus are asymptomatic although hepatitis, an infectious mononucleosis-like illness, and Guillain-Barré syndrome have been reported. After primary infection the virus is not eradicated, and it remains latent with the potential for future reactivation.

Infection in newborns. In approximately 5% of infected newborns, cytomegalovirus infection is manifested by hepatosplenomegaly, jaundice, thrombocytopenic purpura, microcephaly, chorioretinitis, and hemolytic anemia. Serum aminotransferase levels may be increased moderately, and hyperbilirubinemia may occur. The clinical course usually consists of mild to moderate hepatitis with recovery during the first year of life.

Infection in adults. Postperfusion syndrome occurs in patients after open-heart surgery or other procedures requiring transfusions of large volumes of blood from multiple donors. Patients become febrile and lethargic and develop splenomegaly, anemia, and atypical mononuclear cells in the peripheral blood 3 to 6 weeks after transfusion. Occurrence of the syndrome is not prevented by the presence of preexisting cytomegalovirus antibodies. Patients with preexisting antibodies may demonstrate an increase in their antibody titer and are considered to have reactivated infection.

Most primary cytomegalovirus infections are asymptomatic in nonimmunocompromised hosts although mild abnormalities of AP and aminotransferase levels may be present. Liver morphology is varied with a mononuclear infiltrate in the sinusoids and portal tracts, occasional bile stasis, focal areas of liver cell necrosis, and, in general, minimal disturbance of

Table 15-1 Viruses that affect the liver as part of a systemic illness

	Route of transmission	Risk group	Characteristic liver pathology	Diagnosis	Treatment
Cytomegalovirus	Perinatal Sexual activity Blood transfusion	Immunosuppressed patients Newborns Organ transplants	Intranuclear inclusion bodies Mononuclear infiltration of sinusoids, focal necrosis	Isolation of virus Four-fold rise in IgG antibody De novo appearance of IgM antibody	Ganciclovir
Epstein-Barr virus	Transfer of saliva Blood transfusion	College and military populations	Portal and sinusoidal infiltration with mixed infiltrate, focal necrosis	Heterophile-antibodies	Supportive
Herpes simplex virus	Direct contact with infected secretions Congenital	Sexually promiscuous (prostitutes) Immunosuppressed patients Pregnant women	Multinucleated hepatocytes Eosinophilic intranuclear inclusions	Viral isolation Demonstration of viral antigens in infected cells	Vidarabine (Ara-A) Acyclovir

the lobular architecture. In approximately 20% of patients, cytomegalovirus nuclear inclusion bodies can be seen in hepatocytes, vascular endothelium, and biliary epithelium (Figure 15-1). Inclusion bodies tend to be more abundant in immunosuppressed patients.

Cytomegalovirus infection may be accompanied by a mononucleosis-like illness. This infection is most common in young adults and older children. It is characterized by fever lasting 3 to 6 weeks, fatigue, anorexia, nausea, and vomiting. Examination of peripheral blood reveals relative and absolute lymphocytosis with atypical mononuclear cells. In contrast to the Epstein-Barr virus–associated syndrome, the heterophile test is negative, and exudative pharyngitis and lymphadenopathy are absent.

Cytomegalovirus infection is a major health problem in immunocompromised patients. Unlike the situation with otherwise healthy hosts, both primary and recurrent cytomegalovirus infections are more likely to be associated with clinically evident illness in immunocompromised patients (e.g., bone marrow–trans-

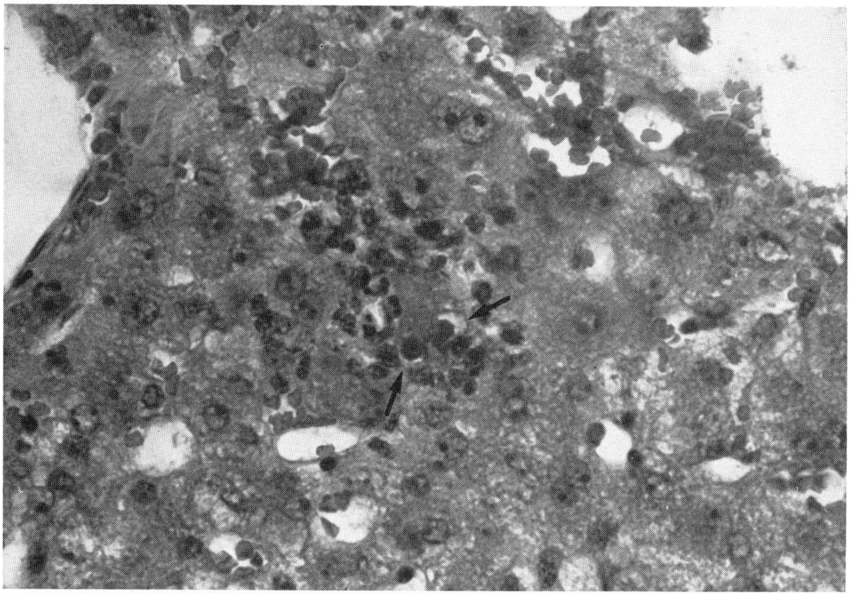

Figure 15-1
Two intranuclear inclusions *(arrows)* in an immunosuppressed patient with cytomegalovirus hepatitis. (Courtesy of Dr. Elizabeth Brunt.)

plant patients or heart-transplant patients). Viral excretion may persist for prolonged periods, and dissemination of the virus to multiple organs, including the liver and lungs, is common. Patients may present with jaundice and marked elevation in liver tests.

Cytomegalovirus infection is diagnosed through recovery of the virus from urine, saliva, or other body fluids. Isolation of the virus from blood correlates best with the presence of disseminated infection. The presence of IgM antibody to cytomegalovirus in the serum can be helpful in the diagnosis of cytomegalovirus infection and is more apt to be positive in primary infections vs. reactivated infections.

Serious cytomegalovirus infection is treated with ganciclovir. The major side effect of this guanine analog is its bone marrow toxicity.

Epstein-Barr Virus

Infection with Epstein-Barr virus is very common, and as many as 90% of patients of lower socioeconomic status have serologic evidence of past exposure. As with the other herpesviruses, Epstein-Barr virus appears to establish a lifelong latent infection after primary infection. During childhood, infections are usually asymptomatic. The infectious mononucleosis syndrome associated with this virus is usually a disease of young adults and is characterized by severe exudative pharyngitis, lymphadenopathy, relative and absolute lymphocytosis, atypical mononuclear cells, and a positive heterophile test. Severe disease occurs in elderly persons in

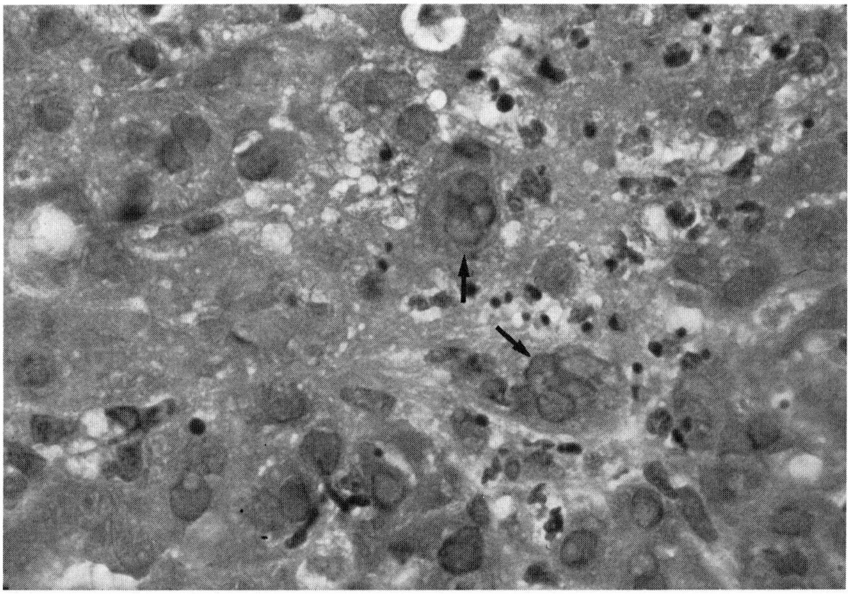

Figure 15-2
Multinucleated syncytial cells *(arrows)* adjacent to an area of hepatocyte necrosis in a patient with herpes simplex hepatitis. (From Regenstein F and Perrillo RP: Uncommon forms of viral hepatitis. In Gitnick G, ed: Modern concepts of acute and chronic hepatitis, New York, 1989, Plenum Publishing Corp, p. 148.)

rare instances. Infection is transmitted most commonly through the saliva. Transmission through blood transfusions and hemodialysis have also been reported.

Hepatic involvement with Epstein-Barr virus frequently is associated with mild elevation of aminotransaminase levels. Elevation of serum bilirubin has been noted in 37% of patients in one series, with frank jaundice occurring in 4% to 17% of cases. Fulminant hepatic failure and severe abnormalities of synthetic function rarely occur.

On liver biopsy the primary features include portal and sinusoidal lobular infiltration with lymphocytes, plasma cells, and monocytes (Figure 15-2). In the majority of cases, the lobular architecture remains intact, in contrast to the appearance of classical viral hepatitis. There is no specific therapy for Epstein-Barr virus infection.

Herpes Simplex Virus

Herpes simplex virus (HSV) is one of the most common viruses infecting humans. It is a large DNA virus. There are two major serotypes: HSV-1 and HSV-2. HSV-1 is transmitted primarily by contact with oral secretions, and HSV-2 is transmitted primarily by contact with genital secretions.

Congenital infection may be characterized by jaundice, hepatosplenomegaly, bleeding diathesis, and abnormalities of the skin and central nervous system. Liver

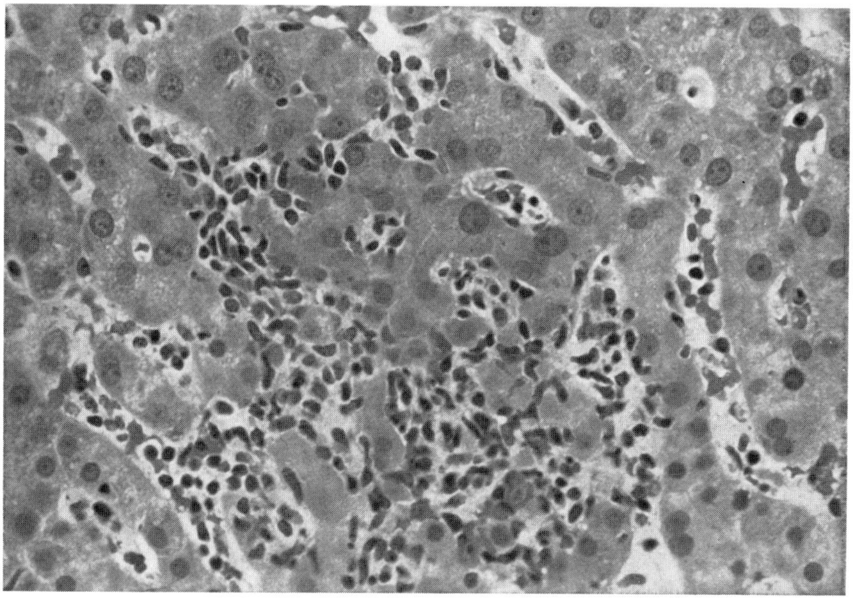

Figure 15-3
Sinusoidal infiltration with atypical lymphocytes in an immunosuppressed patient infected with Epstein-Barr virus. (Courtesy of Dr. Elizabeth Brunt.)

involvement in herpes simplex infections generally occurs in the setting of disseminated infection, as seen in newborns, immunocompromised hosts, and pregnant women. Severe hepatic necrosis may occur when herpes simplex infections involve the liver. Marked serum aminotransferase elevations, icterus, and death caused by hepatic failure have been reported. Uncommonly, immunocompetent persons may present with a febrile disorder with mild to moderate hepatomegaly and abrupt elevation of bilirubin, aminotransferase levels, and serum AP.

Laboratory diagnosis of HSV infection includes (1) detection of the virus in blood and ulcerated lesions by monoclonal antibody staining, (2) isolation of the virus in tissue culture, and (3) detection of the virus in blood and infected tissues by electron microscopy. Liver biopsy reveals multiple hemorrhagic foci, diffuse hepatocellular necrosis with sparse inflammatory reaction, multinucleated hepatocytes and eosinophilic intranuclear inclusions, so-called Cowdry's type A inclusions (Figure 15-3).

Although vidarabine (Ara-A) and acyclovir can be effective against HSV, acyclovir is much less toxic and is the preferred agent. IV and oral acyclovir are effective for reactivation of HSV in serum-positive immunocompromised patients.

Several other common human viruses (rubella, rubeola, mumps, *Coxsackie B,* and varicella-zoster) can cause minor alterations in the results of liver tests. These changes are very uncommon, and jaundice is rare.

EXOTIC VIRAL INFECTIONS THAT AFFECT PRIMARILY THE LIVER

Yellow Fever

Yellow fever is very uncommon in the United States, with the last reported cases occurring more than 40 years ago. Outbreaks can be found in Central America, South America, and Central Africa, where it is transmitted by mosquitoes.

The onset of the disease is abrupt with a short incubation period (3 to 6 days) with fever, headaches, nausea, and dizziness. In severe cases jaundice may be present with high aminotransferase levels and a mortality rate of 20%. Jaundice is a poor prognostic sign; death often occurs within 3 to 4 days. Histology reveals extensive acidophilic necrosis, which may be particularly prominent in the midzonal area.

Diagnosis is made by various serologic methods, which include plaque-reduction neutralization tests and measurement of hemagglutination or complement-fixing antibodies in paired serum. Treatment is supportive.

Rift Valley Fever

Rift Valley fever (enzootic hepatitis) is a viral infection that is borne by arthropods. It primarily affects sheep and cattle. The disease is endemic to certain areas in Africa. Transmission of the virus to humans occurs primarily through inhalation or percutaneously during handling of sick or dead animals.

In most cases the disease in humans is usually asymptomatic or associated with mild symptoms of a viral illness. Clinical features of the disease include a transient febrile course with severe headaches and myalgia occurring 3 to 7 days after exposure. Liver injury occurs with all grades of the disease. However, jaundice is rare and indicates a poor prognosis.

Liver tissue reflects a wide spectrum of injury, varying from focal to submassive or massive necrosis. Acidophilic bodies and intranuclear inclusions are frequently seen.

Lassa fever, Junin, and Machupo Viruses

These viruses are from a group known as arenaviruses, which are endemic to Africa and certain areas of South America. The clinical course is similar in all three viral infections. After a short incubation period (6 to 20 days), there is the insidious onset of fever, malaise, weakness, and myalgia. Death is usually a result of vascular collapse often accompanied by increased vascular permeability. RUQ pain and hepatic tenderness may be present with an increased aminotransferase level. Hepatic failure is a rare occurrence.

Histology of the liver reveals widespread acidophilic or coagulative necrosis, which may involve as many as 50% of hepatocytes. Diagnosis requires isolation of the virus from the blood or other body fluids or complement fixation antibody assays. Treatment is supportive. Recently, oral or IV ribavirin, a broad spectrum antiviral agent, has been applied successfully to the treatment of infection with Lassa fever virus.

Ebola Virus

The Ebola virus, isolated in northern Zaire and southern Sudan, is associated with viral hemorrhagic fever. Clinical features include the sudden onset of fever, malaise, headache, myalgia, nausea, vomiting, and watery diarrhea. During the second week of the illness, results of liver tests may be elevated. Jaundice is seen in approximately 5% of patients with fatal disease. Disseminated intravascular coagulation is a major feature of the disease.

The most prominent hepatic histologic feature is focal necrosis of hepatocytes primarily affecting the periportal and midzonal areas. The specific diagnosis depends on direct isolation of the virus or evidence of antibody development between paired serum samples. Treatment with plasma containing Ebola virus–specific antibodies has been attempted, but its efficacy is still under investigation.

Marburg Virus

Marburg virus is an RNA virus that causes an acute febrile illness. This disorder was described in 1967 after an epidemic occurred in laboratory workers who were exposed to infected tissues from imported African green monkeys. Clinically and histologically this disease is almost identical to Ebola virus. Multiple drugs have been administered to treat this condition, but they have failed to demonstrate any influence on the course of the disease.

SUMMARY

Infections with cytomegalovirus, HSV, and Epstein-Barr virus are common, but serious hepatic disease is not. Serious disease tends to occur in immunosuppressed patients. Medical therapy is available for some of these conditions. Little is known about the pathologic course of many of the so-called exotic viruses, but infection with these agents is likely to be more common than believed.

SUGGESTED READINGS

Corey L and Spear PG: Infections with herpes simplex viruses, N Engl J Med 314: 686-691, 749-757, 1986.

This is an extensive review of all aspects of infection with HSVs.

Griffiths PD: Cytomegalovirus and the liver, Semin Liver Dis 4:307-313, 1984.

This paper discusses the natural history, diagnostic methods, liver involvement, and epidemiology of this infection.

Howard CR et al: Exotic viruses and the liver, Semin Liver Dis 4: 361-374, 1984.

This is a detailed review of the clinical, laboratory, and histologic features of exotic viruses of the liver.

Regenstein FG and Perrillo RP: Uncommon forms of viral hepatitis. In Gitnick G, ed: Modern concepts of acute and chronic hepatitis, New York, 1989, Plenum Publishing Corp.

This is a concise yet authoritative discussion of uncommon forms of viral hepatitis that is primarily designed for the practicing physician. The authors discuss the clnical and laboratory aspects of infection with cytomegalovirus, herpesvirus, and Epstein-Barr virus.

Tandon BN and Acharya SK: Viral diseases involving the liver, Baillieres Clin Gastroenterol 1:211-230, 1987.

This is a clearly written and extensively referenced paper on viral diseases that involve the liver, including widespread agents that affect the liver as part of a systemic illness and unusual agents that affect the liver as the primary target organ.

White NJ and Juel-Jensen BE: Infectious mononucleosis hepatitis, Semin Liver Dis 4:306, 1984.

The authors discuss the usual and uncommon clinical forms of this infection.

16 Bacterial and Spirochetal Infection

Cheree Trent Mills** and **Robert P. Perrillo

SPIROCHETAL INFECTION

Syphilis

Congenital syphilis. Treponema pallidum infects the liver through the placenta, often leading to severe infections of the fetus with high fetal mortality. Infants who survive frequently exhibit hepatosplenomegaly with hyperbilirubinemia, although frank jaundice is believed to be rare. Liver involvement is just one manifestation of the evidence of syphilitic involvement, and infants often exhibit other stigmata of congenital infection, such as osteochondritis, periostitis, skin lesions, and a positive serology test.

The initial lesion of congenital syphilis is diffuse hepatitis. In fatal cases the liver shows a fine diffuse fibrosis extending from the portal triads into the lobules. In survivors of this acute phase, gummas (focal lesions with central necrosis) may be present. Electron microscopy has been used to identify treponema organisms in the liver.

Secondary syphilis. Although liver involvement in the congenital and tertiary stages of syphilis has been well described, liver involvement in the early and secondary stages of the disease is less well known. In recent series the incidence of hepatitis in secondary syphilis has varied from 1% to 10% of all patients.

The histologic appearances of the liver vary: a necrotic type of lesion around the central vein, miliary interascinar granulomas, and occasionally cholestatic changes. A variable amount of cell infiltration with minimal damage to the normal liver architecture is often observed. Spirochetes are rarely detected in the liver biopsy. With prompt treatment the inflammatory lesions of the liver are not thought to produce any long-term sequelae. It is not known whether delayed treatment leads to an increased incidence of cirrhosis.

The main biochemical abnormality appears to be a disproportionate increase in the level of AP with levels as high as 10 times the normal level despite the absence of jaundice. Appropriate therapy for the primary disease leads to prompt resolution of the liver involvement.

Tertiary syphilis. Gummas are the predominant histologic lesion of the tertiary stage of syphilis. They may vary in size from microscopic to large nodules. They can be single or multiple and irregular in distribution. As gummas undergo central caseation necrosis, they become encapsulated and eventually undergo fibrosis, with scar formation and lobulation producing a lesion known as *hepar lobatum*. Although this lesion may resemble cirrhosis, the normal architecture is preserved. Hepatic gummas usually are asymptomatic and discovered incidentally. They may be confused with metastatic malignancy. In cases of extensive scarring, signs of portal hypertension may be apparent. Diagnosis of syphilitic hepatitis may be difficult at this stage because a positive serology may be inconclusive. In these cases liver biopsy of an accessible nodule may prove helpful.

Relapsing Fever *(Borrelia recurrentis)*

Relapsing fever is caused by a spirochete *(Borrelia recurrentis)* that is most often transmitted by a louse. It is found throughout the world, may occur in epidemic fashion, and was particularly prevalent after both world wars. Hepatic infection frequently is accompanied by hepatomegaly and is typified by midzonal lesions in the hepatic lobule containing scattered foci of necrosis and hemorrhage. Spirochetes can be identified in the vessels and sinusoids of the liver. Treatment is with tetracycline, erythromycin, or penicillin.

Lyme Disease *(Borrelia burgdorferi)*

Lyme disease is a multisystemic disorder caused by a tick-borne spirochete, *Borrelia burgdorferi*. The disease is characterized by malaise, fever, headache, lymphadenopathy, paresthesias, myalgia, stiff neck, and a characteristic rash, erythema chronicum migrans. In one study, abnormal liver tests were found in 19% of 314 patients with early Lyme disease. Patients also had symptoms suggestive of hepatitis with nausea, vomiting, RUQ pain, hepatomegaly, and weight loss. These findings were present within days to weeks after the onset of the disease. It is postulated that the spirochete disseminates throughout the skin, blood, and other organs, such as the liver, during this early period.

Diagnosis can be made by serologic testing. Successful treatment has been described with tetracycline, erythromycin, or penicillin.

Leptospirosis

More than 170 serotypes of leptospira have been found to cause disease. The infection usually is transmitted to humans by direct contact with the urine of infected rats or infected tissue of domestic animals. In the United States several occupational groups have been identified to be at increased risk, including sewer and dock workers, veterinarians, farmers, and slaughter-house workers. The infection may be asymptomatic or associated with shock, jaundice, and azotemia in severe cases. The most common clinical features are nonspecific and include headache, nausea, vomiting, and myalgias. Liver disease can be seen in approximately 50% of patients. Jaundice is rare, but when it is present, it usually occurs in the early stage of the illness (i.e., on the fourth to seventh day). It is a sign of a poor prognosis.

Results of liver tests are nonspecifically elevated. Liver biopsy reveals focal necrosis, periportal infiltration with leukocytes, and centrizonal bile thrombi if severe jaundice is present.

Diagnosis can be made clinically in patients with typical features of the disease. However, for confirmation the organisms must be isolated from blood in the early phase of the disease or from the urine later in the illness. A rise in hemagglutination antibody titer may also be used to confirm the diagnosis. Benzyl penicillin may be effective if given during the first 4 days of the illness.

RICKETTSIAL DISEASES

Rocky Mountain Spotted Fever (Rickettsia rickettsii)

Rocky Mountain spotted fever is a disease caused by the tick-borne organism *Rickettsia rickettsii*. The clinical picture most commonly described is an acute prostrating illness with fever, headache, malaise, and generalized myalgia. A rash usually appears on the lower extremities on the second or third day of the illness. In severe cases there may be extensive vascular damage with purpura and central nervous system damage. Jaundice is rare except in fatal cases.

The most prominent finding from liver biopsy is inflammation of the portal triads. This inflammation is characterized by a predominance of large mononuclear cells and polymorphonuclear leukocytes. Other findings include portal vasculitis, ductal cholestasis, and sinusoidal erythrophagocytosis.

Diagnosis is made by the complement-fixation test, or Weil-Felix agglutination reaction. The organism may be demonstrated in liver tissue by immunofluorescence microscopy. Specific therapy is most effective when initiated during the early stages of the disease. Chloramphenicol and tetracycline have been shown to be effective.

Q Fever *(Coxiella burnetii)*

Q fever is caused by the rickettsial agent *Coxiella burnetii,* which is transmitted by an arthropod vector. It is normally a self-limited disease with predominant respira-

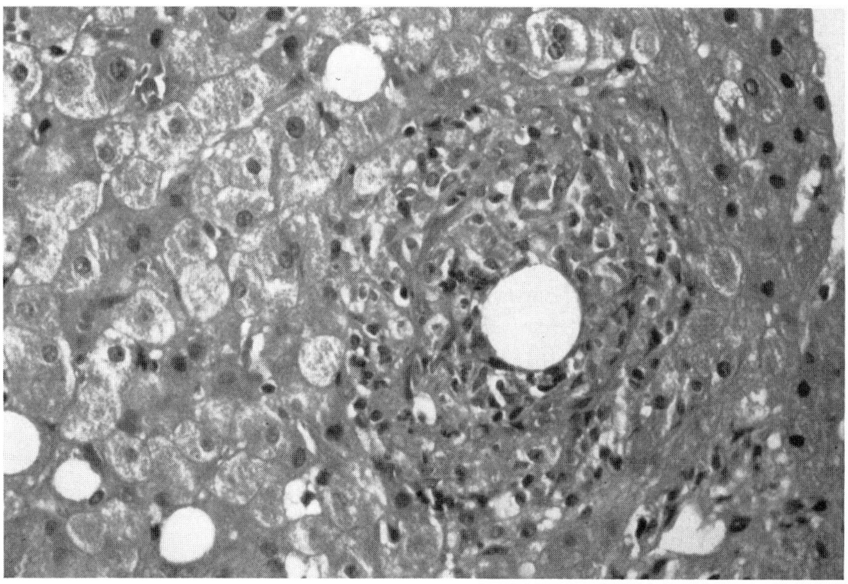

Figure 16-1
Fibrin-ring granuloma typical of Q fever hepatitis. Such granulomas are seen rarely in other disorders. (From Ishak KG. From Hepatic Pathology course conducted by Armed Forces Institute of Pathology, August, 1989, Washington, DC.)

tory symptoms. The frequency of liver involvement in Q fever is unknown. Patients usually present with symptoms and signs suggestive of viral hepatitis. The typical histologic findings include focal hepatocellular necrosis with infiltration of round cells and eosinophils. Granulomas with fibrin rings that have clear centers may be present, and in severe cases liver cell necrosis may be observed (Figure 16-1). Hepatic involvement may not appear until the second or third week of the illness.

Diagnosis is confirmed by demonstrating a rise in the complement-fixing antibodies to *C. burnetii* 2 to 3 weeks after the onset of the disease. Tetracycline and chloramphenicol are effective in the treatment of patients with this disorder.

BACTERIAL INFECTIONS OF THE LIVER

Jaundice of Bacterial Infections

Jaundice may complicate many systemic infections although other factors, such as transfusion-related hepatitis, anesthetic liver damage, and surgery, may cause additional liver impairment and obscure the role of infection. The most common laboratory abnormalities are conjugated hyperbilirubinemia with normal or minimal elevation of AP and aminotransferase levels. Cholestatic reactions to gram-negative infection may be secondary to the effects of circulating bacterial endotoxin, but the pathogenesis of hepatic dysfunction in other cases is not understood.

Gram-Negative Infections

Brucellosis. Brucellosis is caused by a small gram-negative coccobacillus transmitted to humans through direct contact with the products of infectious abortions in cattle or sheep or indirectly through contaminated milk or milk products. The incubation period varies from 1 week to several months. Clinically the onset of the illness may be either insidious or acute, characterized by fever, generalized weakness, headache, night sweats, backache, or arthralgias. Hepatosplenomegaly occurs in approximately 50% to 60% of patients, but jaundice is rare.

Biopsy studies have shown that hepatic granulomas occur frequently in active cases of brucellosis. Additional histologic findings include portal inflammation and fibrosis and necrosis of parenchymal cells. Abscesses of the liver are common complications of late or chronic brucellosis.

The diagnosis of brucellosis can be confirmed by either positive blood or positive bone marrow cultures or rising agglutination titers. Tetracycline in combination with an aminoglycoside or co-trimoxazole are effective treatments.

Melioidosis. Melioidosis is caused by a gram-negative bacillus, *Pseudomonas pseudomallei,* found in the soil and water of Southeast and Southwest Asia. The incubation period varies from a few days to several weeks although a latent subclinical infection may persist for years. Hepatosplenomegaly unaccompanied by jaundice can be found with the septicemic form of the disease. Granulomas or small hepatic abscesses may also be found. A mortality rate of greater than 50% has been reported with the septicemic form of the disease.

The diagnosis can be established by either serology or culture. Treatment depends on the form of the disease. Asymptomatic persons with positive serology generally do not require treatment. Antibiotics should be chosen according to the results of sensitivity testing.

Tularemia. Tularemia is caused by a gram-negative coccobacillus, *Francisella* *tularensis.* Elevation of liver enzymes can be found in more than 50% of reported cases, but liver damage generally is mild, and overt hepatitis is rare, being reported in less than 1% of cases. With dissemination of the organism, hepatomegaly, jaundice, abscesses, peritonitis, and ascites have been reported.

During the first 2 weeks of the disease, areas of focal necrosis infiltrated with mononuclear cells may be apparent. In later stages granulomas with areas of central necrosis may predominate. Tularemia is often diagnosed clinically because culture of the organism may be difficult. Streptomycin is the drug of choice for treatment.

Bartonellosis. Bartonellosis is caused by a small, gram-negative coccobacillus, *Bartonella bacilliformis.* The disease is concentrated in areas of Peru, Ecuador, and Colombia. After an incubation period of 2 to 4 weeks, an acute febrile illness occurs. During this phase hemolytic anemia, profound jaundice, generalized lymphadenopathy, and hepatosplenomegaly with associated splenic infarction and centrilobular necrosis may occur. Death can occur in up to 40% of cases and is caused by either acute hemolysis or overwhelming septicemia. Tetracycline and chloramphenicol are effective treatments.

Plague. The causative agent in plague is *Yersinia pestis,* a gram-negative coccobacillus. Plague has three major forms: bubonic, pneumonic, and septicemic. The bubonic stage is not characterized by liver involvement. With septicemia, hepatomegaly with multifocal necrosis, hepatic granulomas, or abscess formation may be found. Effective antibiotics include streptomycin, tetracycline, and chloramphenicol.

Salmonella. Two forms of hepatitis have been reported to be associated with *Salmonella* infection: an epidemic form associated with concurrent viral hepatitis A and a sporadic form caused by the toxic effects of *Salmonella.* In areas of crowding and poor sanitation, both types of hepatitis have been reported. Chloramphenicol is the antibiotic of choice in systemic infections.

Typhoid fever. Typhoid fever is caused most commonly by *S. typhi.* It occurs worldwide although it is most prevalent in the Indian subcontinent, Africa, and Central America. During the course of the disease, most of the tissues and organs are vulnerable to bacterial colonization. Greater than 50% of patients will show moderately elevated liver enzymes and hepatomegaly during the early phase of the disease. Severe hepatitis and jaundice occur infrequently. The hepatomegaly is associated with focal areas of parenchymal necrosis and portal inflammation. Chloramphenicol is the drug of choice for treatment.

Legionnaires' disease. Laboratory evidence of abnormal liver tests is common but appears to be related to the acute illness. It disappears with resolution of the disease.

Gonococcus and Chlamydia. Abnormalities of liver tests have been demonstrated in as many as 50% of patients with gonococcal bacteremia. Toxic hepatitis and jaundice have been described in association with fatal gonococcal endocarditis. Areas of focal necrosis and polymorphonuclear infiltration in the liver are observed in these cases.

Perihepatitis (Fitz-Hugh—Curtis syndrome) is a syndrome predominately affecting young women that is caused by *Neisseria gonorrhoeae* and *Chlamydia trachomatis.* It is characterized by the progression of cervical, local urethral, or pelvic infection to the acute onset of severe

RUQ pain with fever, leukocytosis, and abdominal tenderness. Transient jaundice and elevated liver tests may be present, but their causes are unknown. Cholecystography may reveal a nonfunctioning gallbladder, which results from adhesions between the liver capsule and the diaphragm. Elevated liver tests generally return to normal within a month of appropriate antimicrobial therapy.

Escherichia coli. *Escherichia coli* bacteremia commonly causes jaundice in children but rarely causes it in adults. Death is usually the result of overwhelming sepsis although hepatic insufficiency may be present. The liver may demonstrate bile stasis, focal hepatocellular necrosis, evidence of regenerative activity, giant cell transformation of the parenchyma, and mild inflammation of the portal triads.

Gram-Positive Infections

Pneumococcus. Patients with pneumococcal pneumonia may exhibit abnormal liver tests. The severity and extent of the pneumonia or the presence of bacteremia does not appear to play a critical role. Jaundice of pneumococcal pneumonia typically occurs on the fifth or sixth day of the illness and is usually associated with bilirubinuria. Liver abnormalities demonstrated in tests are rarely severe and resolve quickly as the pneumonia subsides. Pathologic changes in the liver include basophilic degeneration of the hepatocytes, evidence of active hepatocellular regeneration with frequent mitotic figures, and leukocytic infiltration of the portal triads.

Streptococcus. Two types of hepatic lesions have been described in association with streptococcal infections. The first is typified by centrilobular hepatocellular necrosis with an acute polymorphonuclear reaction of the portal triads that is thought to be secondary to a circulating toxin. The second consists of scattered areas of acute, nonsuppurative hepatocellular necrosis thought to be the direct result of invasion of the liver parenchyma by streptococcal organisms.

A rare syndrome characterized by prolonged chills and fever, bacteremia, weight loss, and anemia has been attributed to infection of the intrahepatic biliary radicles by *Streptococcus viridans*. Jaundice and hepatomegaly generally are not present, and ascites and splenomegaly occur only in rare cases.

MYCOBACTERIA

Tuberculosis

Alterations in liver tests can be seen in a large number of patients with active tuberculosis. Patients with extensive granulomatous involvement may exhibit marked elevations in the serum AP. Jaundice and increased bilirubin levels are rare but have been noted in patients with tuberculous cholangitis, tuberculomas, or miliary tuberculosis of the liver.

Leprosy

Hepatosplenomegaly has been demonstrated in 30% to 40% of advanced cases of leprosy. Impaired liver function is rare, and granulomas are the predominant histologic finding.

Atypical Mycobacteria

In patients with AIDS disseminated infections with atypical mycobacteria are often associated with abnormal liver tests and granulomatous infiltration (see Chapter 12).

PYOGENIC LIVER ABSCESS

Pyogenic liver abscesses are often the result of direct extension from contiguous infection of the biliary tract. They occur in association with ascending cholangitis, cholecystitis, or obstructive neoplasm. Fever, chills, malaise, anorexia, and abdominal pain are usually the most frequent symptoms. The clinical presentation varies according to the patient's age. For example, in infants and young children hepatic abscesses often result from umbilical infection or septicemia in an immunocompromised host. The most common organism in this setting is *Staphylococcus aureus,* but streptococcal and gram-negative enteric organisms occur frequently also. Hepatic abscesses may follow penetrating injuries to the abdomen in older children and adults. In elderly persons the disease onset may be insidious and may present as a fever of unknown origin without localizing complaints. The most common cause in persons in this age group is biliary tract infection, with gallstone disease and obstructive malignancies of the biliary tract the most common predisposing factors.

The organisms recovered from pyogenic liver abscesses vary greatly. The most common isolates are gram-negative aerobes, anaerobic gram-negative bacilli, and microaerophilic streptococci. In many series *E. coli* has been the most commonly isolated organism. Other species that commonly have been isolated include *Streptococcus faecalis* (enterococcus), anaerobic streptococci (e.g., *Peptococcus* and *Peptostreptococcus*), and the microaerophilic organism *S. milleri*. Approximately 50% of pyogenic abscesses are found to be caused by anaerobic organisms or a mixture of aerobic and anaerobic flora.

Routine laboratory tests generally show nonspecific abnormalities with an increased WBC and elevation of the serum AP. Blood cultures are positive in approximately 50% of cases and may reveal a single organism when polymicrobial infection has been demonstrated in the abscess cavity. Therefore culture of the abscess itself frequently is clinically useful.

Ultrasound is very useful in distinguishing a solid mass from a fluid-filled cavity, such as an abscess. CT scan can also be useful in localization of an abscess. Treatment includes percutaneous aspiration and appropriate antibiotic coverage. Usually the largest of multiple abcesses is drained, with the smaller ones resolving with antibiotic treatment. Aspirated pus should be cultured, and antibiotic sensitivities should be determined. Even with appropriate treatment, mortality remains high, particularly in patients with multiple abscesses. In some series, mortality rates have exceeded 50%.

SUMMARY

Many common and uncommon pathogens may infect the liver. The identification of these organisms often depends on appropriate culture techniques or serologic tests. Pyogenic abscess of the liver often appears in an insidious fashion in the elderly and continues to have an appreciable mortality.

SUGGESTED READINGS

Herzog C: Bacterial infections involving the liver, Baillieres Clin Gastroenterol 1:231-250,1987.

This is a concise but well-referenced discussion of many of the more serious bacterial infections of the liver.

Holmes KK et al: Disseminated gonococcal infection, Ann Intern Med 74:979-993, 1971.

The authors describe their own experience with 34 patients and review the literature. Abnormal liver tests were found in 15 episodes of disseminated gonococcal infection occurring in 14 patients.

McDonald MI et al: Single and multiple pyogenic liver abscesses: natural history, diagnosis and treatment, with emphasis on percutaneous drainage, Medicine 63:291-302, 1984.

This is a recent review based on a 15-year experience. This review contains an excellent description of the different clinical and laboratory features in 33 patients with single abscesses and 22 patients with multiple abscesses.

Rubin R and Swartz MN: Hepatic abscess: changes in clinical, bacteriologic, and therapeutic aspects, Am J Med 57:601-610, 1974.

Fifty-three cases of hepatic abscess are described. The authors emphasize the varied clinical presentations in different age groups.

Steere AC et al: The early clinical manifestations of Lyme disease, Ann Intern Med 99:76-82, 1983.

This study describes the liver manifestations of early Lyme disease based on a large series of patients. Of patients in the study, 10% had symptoms of hepatitis, and approximately 20% had abnormal aminotransferase levels.

Veeravahu M: Diagnosis of liver involvement in early syphilis. a critical review, Arch Intern Med 145:132-134, 1985.

This is a relatively recent review of an often neglected topic. The authors describe the variability in clinical, laboratory, and histologic features and suggest that some of the previously reported cases may have been caused by concomitant infection with the hepatitis viruses.

17 Parasitic Diseases of the Liver

Cheree Trent Mills and *Robert P. Perrillo*

PARASITIC LIVER DISEASE

Protozoan Infections

Amebiasis. Amebiasis is caused by the protozoan *Entamoeba histolytica* (Figure 17-1). Amebic abscess of the liver occurs in less than 10% of patients with the intestinal form of the disease. Abscesses may present either as an acute inflammatory process with fever and a tender, enlarged liver or more insidiously with wasting, anorexia, and hepatomegaly, suggesting a malignant process. RUQ tenderness is found in 50% to 60% of patients. Jaundice occurs in less than 10% of patients and is more likely in the presence of multiple or large abscesses that cause compression of the biliary tree. The most common location for an amebic abscess, occurring in more than 80% of cases, is the right lobe of the liver. The majority of these abscesses are single, and they often extend to the dome of the liver.

Laboratory findings may include marked anemia, leukocytosis, and mild increases in serum aminotransferase values. Serum AP levels are usually increased to two to three times the upper limit of normal, and a mild increase in the serum bilirubin is observed in approximately 20% of cases.

Various serologic tests are available. Counter immunoelectrophoresis provides a rapid screening method. Indirect hemagglutination testing is the most frequently used test and is positive in more than 90% of cases. The hemagglutination test is considered positive if circulating antibodies are present in a dilution titer of 1:128 or greater. Enzyme-linked immunosorbent assay (ELISA) may be useful for serum diagnosis although false negatives have been observed early in the course of the disease. In the presence of a visible abscess on ultrasound, it is rare for the serology to remain negative for greater than 1 week.

CT scan and ultrasound may be used for localization of the abscess, but the former may be more sensitive in revealing small abscesses. Metronidazole is effective in the treatment of an uncomplicated abscess and is the drug of choice. The dosage is 750 mg three times a day for 10 days. Alternative agents with greater toxicity include a combination of dehydroemetine followed in turn by chloroquine phosphate and iodoquinol or emetine followed by chloroquine and iodoquinol. Aspiration is seldom needed unless complications, such as a tense abscess or an

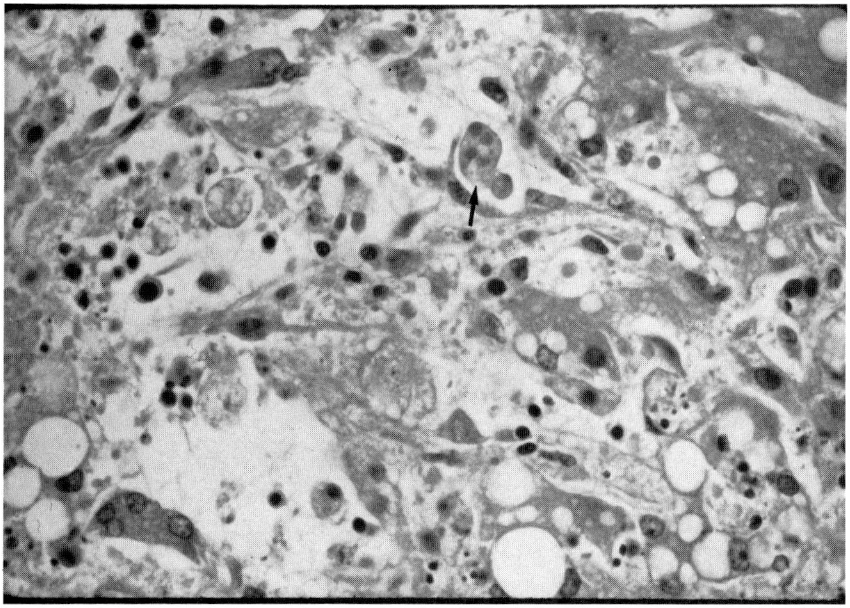

Figure 17-1
E. histolytica (arrow) in an area of liver cell necrosis. The dark inclusions within the organism are ingested erythrocytes. (From Ishak KG. From Hepatic Pathology course conducted by Armed Forces Institute of Pathology, August, 1989, Washington, DC.)

expanding lesion unresponsive to therapy, are observed. Failure to aspirate such lesions may result occasionally in rupture into the chest cavity or mediastinum, including the pericardial sac.

Malaria. Malaria is caused by four species of obligate intracellular parasites belonging to the genus *Plasmodium*. Sporozoites inoculated with the saliva of an infected female mosquito invade hepatocytes and multiply intensively. The hepatocytes rupture and release forms that quickly infect circulating RBCs. Only the intraerythrocytic stages of the organism are responsible for symptoms. Because of reticuloendothelial hyperplasia, the liver and the spleen are almost always enlarged. The striking feature histologically is the congestion of the sinusoids and centrilobular veins with parasitized red cells. Kupffer cells are hypertrophied and contain parasites. Malarial pigment is present in Kupffer cells in more than 80% of cases. In addition, hemosiderin may be found in Kupffer cells and hepatocytes. The most common abnormalities of liver tests are elevations of the aminotransferase enzymes. Patients may have mild jaundice, and serum bilirubin rarely exceeds 5 mg/dl. Coagulation abnormalities, hypoalbuminemia, and hypoglycemia have been reported.

Because of the development of many drug-resistant forms of malaria, treatment is becoming more difficult. However, the drug of choice for treatment of most uncomplicated malaria remains chloroquine phosphate, given in a dose of 25 mg/kg with an initial dose of 10 mg/kg. Chloroquine-resistant malaria is treated with quinine sulfate. Liver tests usually return to normal with successful treatment.

Toxoplasma. Hepatic infection with toxoplasma is rare. There are three clinical forms of the disease: (1) a long prodrome with lymphadenopathy followed by clinically apparent hepatitis, (2) primary hepatic involvement without lymphadenopathy, and (3) granulomatous infiltration associated with lymphadenopathy. Patients may recover spontaneously. The drugs of choice are pyrimethamine (25 mg/day) plus trisulfapyrimidine, (2 to 6 gm/day), both given for 3 to 4 weeks.

Kala azar. Visceral leishmaniasis (kala azar) is caused by *Leishmania donovani* and is characterized by varying degrees of hepatosplenomegaly, fever, weight loss, anemia, and other non specific systemic changes. Diagnosis is usually established by the demonstration of leishmanial organisms in either the bone marrow or the liver. The drug of choice for visceral leishmaniasis is sodium stibogluconate (20 mg/kg/day [maximum 800 mg/day]) for 3 weeks.

Helminthic Infections

Schistosomiasis. Of the three major species of schistosomes that infect humans, two are known to cause liver disease: *Schistosoma mansoni* and *S. japonicum*. The parasite has an intermediate phase of its life cycle in snails, but humans are the definitive hosts. More than 500 million people live in endemic areas, and schistosomal liver disease affects more than 200 million people, making it one of the most common liver diseases in the world. In the Western hemisphere, schistosomiasis is limited to areas with a large population of immigrants from endemic areas in Asia. *S. mansoni* is the only type known to be endemic in the Western hemisphere. It accounts for the majority of hepatosplenic cases of the disease.

Granulomas are the hallmark of schistosome infection, and, unlike those caused by other disease processes, the granulomas of schistosomiasis are directly responsible for most of the clinicopathologic features of the disease (see below).

The clinical features of schistosomal infection vary from totally asymptomatic cases to multiple sequelae of the chronic fibroobstructive form of the disease. During the early stages of all three forms of schistosome infection, a dermatitis caused by cercarial penetration of the skin (swimmer's itch) is often present. As the worms mature and eggs are produced, a serum-sicknesslike syndrome appears that is characterized by fever, malaise, eosinophilia, lymphadenopathy, and hepatosplenomegaly. This syndrome usually is associated with heavy infestation.

Severe illness is seen in a small percentage of patients with chronic infestation and is generally caused by ova that are lodged in the intestines and liver. Ova trapped in the liver cause granuloma formation and fibrosis with subsequent heptomegaly and portal hypertension. The liver tests usually remain within normal limits in uncomplicated cases. Presinusoidal blockage within the portal venous system can lead to portosystemic collaterals with resultant esophageal varices. Often the first evidence of schistosome infestation is hematemesis and melena. Hepatic coma is a rare occurrence, and the usual cause of death is exsanguination.

The diagnosis of schistosomal infestation can be made by finding ova in human stool or urine and by finding granulomas in biopsy specimens from the rectum or urinary bladder. Hepatic schisto-

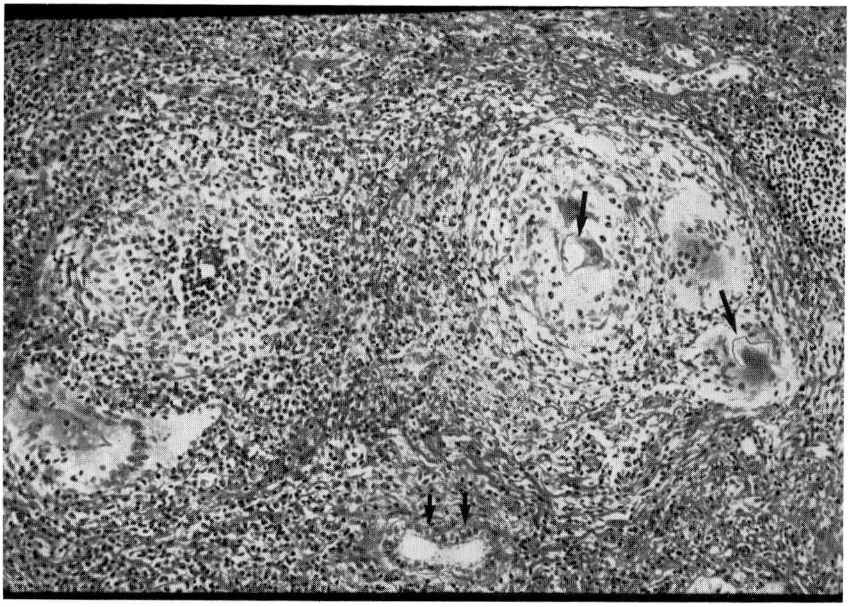

Figure 17-2
Florid portal reaction typical of schistosomiasis. Large arrows indicate oval remnants within a mixed inflammatory infiltrate. Small arrows identify a normal-appearing bile duct. (From Ishak KG. From Hepatic Pathology course conducted by Armed Forces Institute of Pathology, August, 1989, Washington, DC.)

somal infestation is easy to define when a hepatic granuloma is identified that contains ova or their remnants, although in the chronic stages ova may not be present (Figure 17-2). A large number of serum immunologic methods for diagnosis have been utilized, but none appears to be reliable.

The severity of the liver disease associated with schistosomal infection is directly related to the worm burden. Thus the goal of therapy is to decrease markedly the number of organisms. Praziquantel (20mg/kg three times a day for one day) is the drug of choice for treating all forms of schistosomiasis although the susceptibility of the different species varies. This therapy is contraindicated in patients with portosystemic collaterals because of the risk of increased neurotoxicity and central nervous system disease. An alternative agent may be a single dose of oxamniquine (15mg/kg). Bleeding esophageal varices have been treated by several methods, including portosystemic shunts, splenectomy, propranolol, and injection sclerotherapy. The distal splenorenal shunt has been advocated as the shunt of choice.

Visceral larva migrans. *Toxocara canis* is a common ascarid (roundworm) of dogs and cats and is the most frequent cause of visceral larva migrans. The most common route of infection is ingestion of soil containing larvae or embryonated ova. A less common route of infection is close contact with nursing puppies and, in particular, hand-to-mouth contact. Clinical illness is most frequent in young children. There are two forms of clinical presentation, the ocular and visceral, each with its own unique clinical and laboratory manifestations. Associated findings of visceral *T. canis* infection are hepatomegaly, splenomegaly lymphadenopathy, recurrent pneumonia, eosinophilia, and hypergammaglobulinemia. The earliest lesions in the liver are eosinophilic abscesses that subsequently develop into granulomas.

Results of stool examination may be negative because larvae may invade and reside in human tissue for long periods. Definitive diagnosis may be made by demonstration of larvae in tissues by using direct microscopy and serum fluorescent antibody testing. An ELISA using a larva-specific antigen is the serologic diagnostic method of choice. A variety of drugs have been used to treat visceral larva migrans. Of these drugs thiabendazole (25 mg/kg twice a day for 5 days) and diethylcarbamazine (2 mg/kg three times a day for 7 to 10 days) are the drugs of choice.

Ascariasis. Infestation of the human GI tract by *Ascaris lumbricoides* occurs worldwide. The adult worm lives in the lumen of the small bowel, and in the Far Eastern countries it is common for the parasite to migrate to the biliary tree. Adult worms may invade the common bile duct through the ampulla of Vater; the worm's secretions may cause spasm of the sphincter of Oddi. This in turn may lead to biliary obstruction with possible ascending cholangitis and hepatic-abscess formation. Residual dead worms and foreign material may destroy the biliary tract epithelium, causing fibrosis. Biliary calculi may complicate the course of the disease. Pancreatitis and common bile duct perforation also have been described.

T-tube cholangiography, ERCP, and operative cholangiography can demonstrate the worms that typically appear as a long-filling defect in the opacified bile duct. Surgery, with drainage and evacuation of all worms, is necessary for the treatment of hepatic abscesses. Obstruction of the biliary tree has been treated by ERCP with endoscopic sphincterotomy and mechanical extraction. In uncomplicated biliary ascariasis, pyrantel pamoate given as a single dose of 11 mg/kg appears to be the treatment of choice.

Fasciola hepatica. *Fasciola hepatica* is an unsegmented flatworm of the class Trematoda that resides in the biliary tree. Humans usually are infected by eating wild watercress or chewing grass on which metacercaria are encysted. Clinically an association of upper abdominal pain, fever, and marked eosinophilia with or without laboratory evidence of cholestasis should raise the possibility of infection with *F. hepatica*. On gross pathologic examination the infected liver appears to be covered by grayish white hard nodules that most likely represent sites of previous invasion of the liver capsule by immature migrating liver flukes. The diagnosis usually is made by finding ova in the feces or duodenal aspirate. Diagnosis may be facilitated by a variety of serologic test methods, including the complement-fixation test and indirect hemagglutination assay.

Bithionol (30 to 50 mg/kg on alternate days for 10 to 15 doses) has been shown to be effective for both relief of the clinical manifestations and eradication of the organism. Other reported complications of *F. hepatica* infection include chronic biliary tract disease in the form of portal tract fibrosis, portal hypertension, and cholelithiasis.

Clonorchiasis. Humans are infected with *Clonorchis* by eating undercooked fresh-water fish that are infested with the metacercariae of the flukes. The disease is widespread in the Far East, primarily in Japan, Korea, China, and Vietnam. Flukes ascend the biliary tree from the duodenum and may persist for decades. Infected persons may be asymptomatic, but they often present with clinical features of cholangitis, liver abscess, or lithiasis. Chronic cholangitis may lead to a severe inflammatory reaction with subsequent development of portal fibrosis. Jaundice caused by obstruction by either the flukes themselves or accompanying stone disease may occur. Relief of obstruction can be obtained through insertion of an endoprosthesis, or through surgical or percutaneous drainage.

Lingulata serata (tongue worm). Tongue worm is a common name for an endoparasite belonging to the class Pentastomidia that is prevalent in Africa, Central and South America, Asia, and parts of Europe. Several species are known to infect humans. Granulomas are found in the walls of the intestine, mesenteric lymph nodes, peritoneum, lungs, liver and spleen. It is not unusual for healed granulomas to be discovered incidentally during surgery or autopsy.

Echinococcosis. This is a disorder with worldwide distribution. Humans become infected by accidental ingestion of eggs passed in the feces of dogs and other carnivores. Four species of the organism are pathogenic for humans. *Echinococcus granulosus* and *E. multilocularis* account for most of the infections. Herbivores, such as sheep and cows, serve as intermediate hosts in *E. granulosus* infections. In this disorder onchospheres (embryos) reach the liver from the duodenum, and larval development produces a fluid-filled cyst. When the primary cyst ruptures, secondary cysts may form. The cyst grow slowly (1 to 5 cm per year) and are well tolerated until they become large enough to cause pain or hepatic dysfunction by virtue of compression of normal structures. Large cysts can obstruct blood and bile flow, causing portal hypertension and jaundice, respectively. The rupture of a cyst with sudden release of fluid has been associated with allergic reactions and even anaphylactoid shock. Unlike *E. granulosus, E. multilocularis* is not curable by surgery because of the multicystic and more invasive properties of the organism.

SUMMARY

Although relatively uncommon in the Western world, hepatic disorders caused by parasites, such as schistosomiasis and ascariasis, are important globally and affect many millions of individuals. Amebic abscess continues to be seen in the United States, particularly in the southwestern part of the country. These infections are readily treatable in the early phase of illness, but chronic infection can lead to life-threatening complications.

SUGGESTED READINGS

Barnes PF et al: A comparison of amebic and pyogenic abscess of the liver, Medicine 66:472-483, 1987.

This is a series of 96 cases of amebic abscess and 46 cases of pyogenic abscess. The authors emphasize clinical and laboratory features that are useful in distinguishing these disorders.

Chan CW and Lam SK: Diseases caused by liver flukes and cholangiocarcinoma, Baillieres Clin Gastroenterol 1:297-318, 1987.

This report describes the epidemiology, pathology, complications, and therapy of Clonorchis and Fasciola infections. Special emphasis is given to the associated finding of cholangiocarcinoma.

Degremont A: Parasitic diseases of the liver, Baillieres Clin Gastroenterol 1:251-271, 1987.

This is a concise and informative review of hepatic parasitic disorders.

Knight R: Hepatic amebiasis, Semin Liver Dis 4: 277-292, 1984.

This is an extensive review of this disorder, including an excellent discussion of the presenting features of complicated liver abscess.

Uflacker R et al: Parasitic and mycotic causes of biliary obstruction, Gastrointest Radiol 7:173-179, 1982.

This article focuses on the radiologic presentation of Clonorchiasis, Ascariasis, Echinococcosis, and Candidiasis of the biliary tract. Biliary tract manipulation with a balloon catheter and endoprosthesis is presented as an option for management.

Warren KS: The kinetics of hepatosplenic schistosomiasis, Semin Liver Dis 4:293-300, 1984.

This paper describes the dynamic interactions occurring among the worm burden, egg output, extent of host inflammatory response, and extent of fibrosis that determine the major clinical features of the disease.

18 Drug Hepatitis

Fredric G. Regenstein

Drug-related hepatic dysfunction represents a common problem in adult medicine, with approximately 4% to 5% of all adverse drug reactions reported to the Food and Drug Administration involving cases of suspected drug-induced hepatic disease. The availability of an increasing number of medications coupled with the frequent use of automated liver chemistry profiles and greater physician awareness has led to the perception that the prevalence of drug-induced liver disease is increasing. Although many cases of hepatotoxicity are mild and of little clinical consequence, severe and sometimes fatal cases of hepatic dysfunction can occur. A number of the agents discussed in this chapter are well-known hepatotoxins, and when prescribing these agents, most physicians are alert for signs of hepatic dysfunction. However, many of these agents are not generally recognized as being hepatotoxic, and severe toxicity can develop if the early signs of liver dysfunction are ignored. An additional danger exists during the administration of newly released medications not previously identified as hepatotoxic. Often it is not until after drug approval and subsequent administration to large numbers of patients that an agent's hepatotoxic potential becomes apparent. Thus clinicians need to maintain a high index of suspicion for drug-induced disease when evaluating patients with unexplained liver dysfunction. Serious drug-induced liver disease will remain a frequent problem in the United States as our population ages and the number of people taking both prescription and nonprescription drugs continues to increase.

CLINICAL FEATURES OF DRUG-INDUCED HEPATOTOXICITY

Drug-induced hepatic injury is classified most often according to the pattern of hepatic injury. Cholestatic injury is characterized by the predominant elevation of bilirubin and AP with only mild to moderate elevations of the aminotransferases. In symptomatic individuals jaundice and pruritus are the characteristic features. Of the agents associated with cholestatic injury, Zimmerman has subdivided them into those causing canalicular cholestasis and those causing hepatocanalicular cholestasis. In canalicular cholestasis the serum AP level is normal or slightly elevated, but in hepatocanalicular cholestasis, AP levels are typically elevated greater than threefold. Morphologically, canalicular jaundice is associated with little or no liver injury or portal inflammation. In contrast, hepatocanalicular jaundice is associated with significant portal inflammation and slight hepatocyte injury.

Hepatocellular injury is typified by aminotransferase elevations of varying degrees. Clinically, drug-induced hepatocellular injury resembles viral hepatitis, and the spectrum of disease severity ranges from mild anicteric cases to fulminant hepatic failure (FHF). Severe hepatocellular injury may be associated with jaundice, fever, anorexia, nausea, vomiting, and abdominal discomfort. Fatality rates often exceed 10%. In some centers, more than 60% of FHF cases are drug-induced.

Mixed hepatocellular injury refers to cases of liver damage exhibiting features of both cholestasis and hepatocellular necrosis. Individuals with mixed injury frequently have jaundice and manifest marked aminotransferase elevations (greater than tenfold) in association with moderate elevations of AP (greater than threefold).

Steatosis is another morphologic form of liver injury caused by a number of different drugs. Two distinct patterns of steatosis occur. Macrovesicular fatty infiltration is the more common form and consists of large fat globules occupying most of the cytoplasm, displacing the cell nucleus to the periphery. Patients with macrovesicular steatosis usually have mild liver injury and are asymptomatic; an occasional patient may complain of vague upper abdominal pain. The results of physical examination are usually normal, but hepatomegaly and hepatic tenderness may be present. If abnormal, aminotransferase and AP values are mildly elevated. Microvesicular steatosis is characterized by small droplets of fat scattered throughout the cytoplasm. Liver damage caused by agents producing microvesicular fatty infiltration may be severe, and in these cases moderate to severe abnormalities of liver tests may be present in conjunction with hepatic encephalopathy, hyperammonemia, and hypoglycemia.

Drugs have also been implicated in a variety of vascular abnormalities and tumors involving the liver. Budd-Chiari syndrome, hepatic venoocclusive disease, peliosis hepatitis, hepatic sinusoidal dilation, hepatic adenoma, and hepatocellular carcinoma have all been associated with drug ingestion.

MECHANISMS OF HEPATIC INJURY

Hepatotoxic medications are subdivided into intrinsic (predictable) toxins and idiosyncratic (nonpredictable) toxins. Intrinsic hepatotoxins typically cause a dose-dependent liver injury in a high percentage of exposed individuals. Idiosyncratic toxins cause dose-independent hepatic injury that occurs only in susceptible hosts. When compared with intrinsic toxins, idiosyncratic reactions tend to occur infrequently and after a somewhat longer exposure interval. In some cases idiosyncratic hepatotoxicity is mediated through a hypersensitivity reaction. In other situations it may be related to genetic or environmentally determined differences in drug metabolism or detoxification. Many drugs appear to exert injury through a combination of both intrinsic and idiosyncratic toxicity. Often these agents will manifest dose-dependent toxicity at the high doses used in experimental systems and idiosyncratic toxicity at the doses used in clinical practice. Although this system of classification undoubtedly represents an oversimplification of hepatotoxicity, it provides a framework for understanding the complexity of drug-induced liver disease. The hepatotoxicity of specific drugs is described in the remainder of this chapter.

ANESTHETIC AGENTS

Halothane

Halothane generally is considered to be an idiosyncratic hepatotoxic agent. Over the past three decades, there has been considerable controversy regarding the frequency and significance of halothane as an hepatotoxin. Currently, little controversy exists about halothane's hepatotoxicity, but it remains a rare cause of liver injury in the United States, where administration of halothane has been supplanted largely by other agents. In Europe halothane hepatotoxicity remains a frequent problem; in fact, it is the second most common cause of drug-induced hepatic failure. Liver damage is believed to occur as a consequence of halothane metabolism and biotransformation to metabolic intermediates (Figure 18-1). These intermediates bind to cellular proteins, leading to the production of neoantigens, which may then trigger an immune-mediated hepatotoxicity in susceptible patients. Alternatively the metabolites may lead to direct hepatocellular damage through lipid peroxidation. Mild, asymptomatic elevations of aminotransferase levels may occur in as many as 25% of patients exposed to halothane. Severe liver injury develops in approximately 0.01% to 0.07% of exposed persons. The relationship between the frequently occurring mild abnormalities and the rare episodes of severe hepatic dysfunction remains obscure. However, the frequently

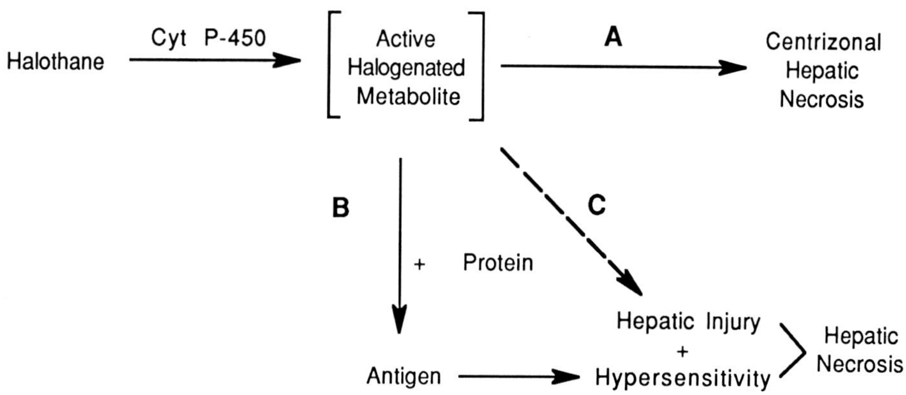

Figure 18-1
Proposed mechanisms for hepatic injury induced by halothane. **A,** Presumptive mechanism for injury caused by metabolic idiosyncrasy. **B,** Mechanism for hypersensitivity induced injury. **C,** Combined effects of intrinsic toxicity and hypersensitivity producing hepatic injury. (From Zimmerman HJ: Hepatotoxicity: anesthetic agents, New York, 1978, Appleton-Century-Crofts, p. 387.)

encountered mild liver dysfunction may be secondary to the direct hepatocellular toxicity of the metabolic intermediates, but the idiosyncratic severe hepatitis probably is due to immune-mediated injury.

Halothane-associated liver injury is less common in children and in persons receiving the agent for the first time. Factors that may predispose to halothane hepatotoxicity include obesity, female sex, and multiple halothane exposures, especially if the interval between exposures is less than 3 months. Typically the initial manifestation is an unexplained postoperative fever occurring within the first 7 to 14 days after anesthesia. In moderate to severe cases this is followed by the development of jaundice, anorexia, nausea, myalgias, and hepatomegaly. Patients previously exposed to halothane may develop fever and jaundice earlier after surgery. However, laboratory values vary, with moderate to marked elevations of bilirubin and aminotransferase levels being typical. Coagulation abnormalities are present in severe cases. Eosinophilia may be present in up to 60% of cases, and autoantibodies may be present in up to 29% of cases. Hepatic histology characteristically reveals evidence of centrizonal necrosis and less inflammatory activity than is usually seen with viral hepatitis. An inflammatory infiltrate associated with eosinophils is occasionally present. In most series case fatality rates exceed 50%. Patients with mild cases (bilirubin less than 5 mg/dl) usually recover without sequelae. Individuals with fulminant disease and those with severe biochemical abnormalities (e.g., bilirubin greater than 20 mg/dl and PT greater than 20 seconds) should be evaluated at centers performing hepatic transplantation. Corticosteroids are of no proven value, and, aside from transplantation, no specific therapy is available. Avoidance of halothane in patients with a history of unexplained postoperative liver dysfunction or fever and in patients undergoing repetitive procedures under anesthesia may reduce the frequency of significant halothane hepatotoxicity.

Methoxyflurane, Enflurane, and Isoflurane

After the introduction of methoxyflurane in 1960 and enflurane in 1963, reports appeared implicating methoxyflurane, enflurane, and isoflurane in cases of hepatic injury. The clinical, biochemical, and histopathologic similarities among cases related to ingestion of methoxyflurane, enflurane, and halothane are indicative of a similar mechanism of action. With all of these agents, injury appears to be idiosyncratic, with hypersensitivity phenomena present in some cases. Risk factors identified from cases of hepatitis induced by halothane, methoxyflurane, and enflurane are similar and include female sex, obesity, and previous exposure. Histologically the agents are associated with centrizonal necrosis, with case fatality rates approximately 50% for halothane and methoxyflurane and approximately 20% for enflurane. With haloalkane hepatotoxicity, there appears to be a relationship between the degree of biotransformation and the potential for liver damage. Methoxyflurane and halothane both undergo extensive biotransformation and are more often associated with hepatotoxicity than enflurane and isoflurane, which undergo minimal biodegradation. Estimates of hepatotoxicity range from 1 to 7 per 10,000 patients receiving halothane to less than 1 per 1 million in patients receiving enflurane. Isoflurane-induced hepatotoxicity appears to be even less frequent.

ANTICONVULSANTS

Phenytoin

Phenytoin therapy is associated with predictable rises in γ-glutamyltransferase activity and is associated occasionally with asymptomatic, mild elevations of AP and aminotransferase levels. On rare occasions phenytoin may be associated with an idiosyncratic syndrome characterized by fever, skin rash, lymphadenopathy, leukocytosis (with lymphocytosis or eosinophilia), and severe hepatic injury. The syndrome typically begins 1 to 6 weeks after initiation of therapy, and the case fatality rate may be as high as 50% in patients presenting with jaundice. The pattern of injury is usually mixed, with most cases sharing hepatocellular and cholestatic features. Liver test abnormalities are quite variable, but in most cases aminotransferase values are elevated greater than tenfold and AP values are elevated less than threefold. Hepatic histologic changes resemble acute viral hepatitis and consist primarily of hepatocellular necrosis. Massive necrosis typically is present in fatal cases. Rare cases of individuals with predominantly cholestatic injury have also been reported. Injury is believed to occur on the basis of reactions involving metabolically active intermediates that cannot be detoxified in susceptible individuals. Arene oxides, the putative toxic intermediates, covalently bind to cellular components, leading to either direct injury or altered proteins (haptens), which incite immunologically mediated hepatocyte injury (Figure 18-2).

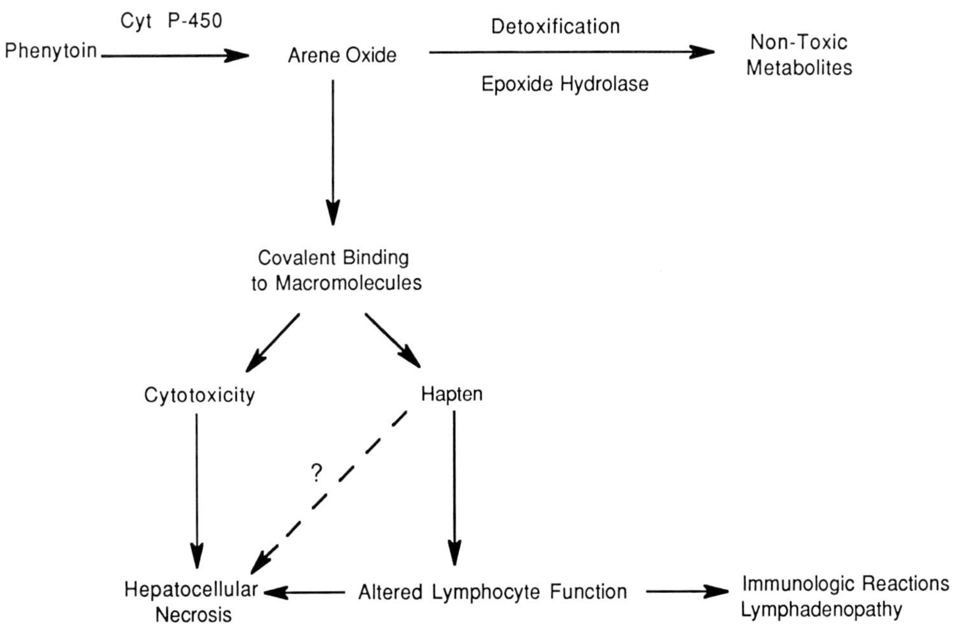

Figure 18-2
Phenytoin metabolism and the role of arene oxide metabolites in the pathogenesis of hepatotoxicity and secondary immune phenomena. (From Spielberg SP et al: Predisposition to phenytoin hepatotoxicity assessed in vitro, N Engl J Med 305:726, 1981.)

Routine monitoring of liver tests is not indicated for patients receiving phenytoin. Early recognition of potential phenytoin toxicity and prompt drug discontinuation is required if the patient develops unexplained fever, skin rash, or lymphadenopathy. Corticosteroids frequently are administered in patients with hepatocellular injury; however, the value of corticosteroids in treating hepatocellular injury has not been established clearly.

Valproic Acid

Mild asymptomatic elevations of aminotransferase levels occur frequently with administration of valproic acid. Often the elevations are transient and reach peak values 10 to 12 weeks after therapy is started. In rare cases an apparent idiosyncratic form of severe hepatocellular injury may occur. These cases are typically preceded by a prodrome of lethargy, anorexia, nausea, facial edema, and a change in seizure pattern. Severe hepatitis appears to occur within the first 6 months of therapy and is more frequent in children than adults. Aminotransferase values elevated less than tenfold, bilirubin levels less than 10 mg/dl, and prolonged PT in association with hypofibrinogenemia and thrombocytopenia are typical. Hepatic coma, hypoglycemia, hyperammonemia, and renal failure are often present in fatal cases. Hepatic histology reveals microvesicular steatosis with varying degrees of necrosis, which is often centrizonal. Hepatic injury is believed to be mediated by the accumulation of toxic metabolites in susceptible hosts. Patients with self-limited toxicity either develop alternative metabolic detoxification pathways or in some fashion become less susceptible to the putative toxic intermediates . Concomitant administration of agents known to stimulate enzymes of the cytochrome P450 system may potentiate valproic acid toxicity. Avoiding severe toxicity is critical because no specific treatment is available. Patients starting therapy with valproic acid should have liver tests monitored periodically. Medication should be discontinued in those patients developing greater than threefold increases of aminotransferase levels.

Carbamazepine

Carbamazepine is a rare cause of idiosyncratic hepatic injury. Most reported cases have described a cholestatic injury with morphologic evidence of granulomatous inflammation. In some cases AP levels have remained elevated for several months after the medication was discontinued. No specific therapy is available, and therapy is supportive.

ANALGESIC AND ANTIINFLAMMATORY AGENTS

Acetaminophen

Acetaminophen is an intrinsic hepatotoxin that leads to predictable hepatocellular injury in all patients who ingest sufficient amounts, generally greater than 10 gm/day. In patients with a history of heavy alcohol consumption, toxicity can occur with the ingestion of as little as 3 to 4 gm/day. Acetaminophen is the most common cause of drug-induced hepatic failure in the United States and Europe. Toxicity is mediated by metabolic intermediates of acetaminophen produced during biotransformation by the cytochrome P450 system. These intermediates are normally detoxified by conjugation with glutathione. When glutathione stores are depleted, the toxic intermediates are free to bind covalently to cellular proteins and macromolecules, resulting in cellular necrosis and death. Increased activity of the cytochrome P450 system and depletion of glutathione stores by chronic alcohol ingestion most likely account for the increased toxicity of acetaminophen in these patients. Symptoms of nausea and vomiting are usually present within the first few hours after ingestion. These symptoms resolve, and a "window" period occurs, during which the patient appears to be clinically well. Over the next 24 to 48 hours, patients ingesting sufficient quantities develop biochemical evidence of hepatocellular necrosis associated with anorexia, nausea, vomiting, and jaundice. Moderate to extreme elevations of aminotransferase values are seen in association with hyperbilirubinemia and disturbances of coagulation. Renal dysfunction secondary to acute tubular necrosis may also be present. Histologically centrizonal necrosis with little associated inflammation occurs. Mortality rates up to 25% have been reported in untreated patients.

N-acetylcysteine is an effective antidote for acetaminophen poisoning when given within the first 12 hours of ingestion. The efficacy of this agent diminishes thereafter but may still have a beneficial effect for up to 24 hours after ingestion. N-acetylcysteine acts by increasing glutathione stores and enhancing drug metabolism through the nontoxic sulfation pathway. Effective management of acetaminophen toxicity requires treatment as soon as possible after the exposure. Determination of serum acetaminophen levels, correlation of peak levels with the time of ingestion, and estimation of the serum elimination half-time are all employed to determine which patients are at risk for developing hepatotoxicity. Serum levels below 150 mg/L at 4 hours after ingestion or below 50 mg/L at 12 hours after ingestion are unlikely to be associated with hepatotoxicity. A calculated serum elimination half-time greater than 4 hours is associated with the development of hepatotoxicity, and a half-time greater than 12 hours is associated with encephalopathy. In suspected cases therapy should be initiated while plasma acetaminophen levels are measured. Patients who are determined not to be at risk can have treatment stopped, and those at risk can complete a full course of therapy. The current treatment schedule recommends the oral administration of N-acetylcysteine at an initial dose of 140 mg/kg, followed every 4 hours by 70 mg/kg for a total of 18 doses. An IV preparation consisting of 300 mg/kg administered over a 20-hour period is available in Canada and Europe. After patients develop significant hepatotoxicity, supportive care is provided. Patients developing stage 3 encephalopathy and those with a prolongation of PT greater than 20 seconds should be transferred to hepatic transplant centers for care and possible transplantation.

Salicylates

Aspirin and the nonacetylated salicylates appear to be intrinsic hepatotoxins, producing hepatic injury that is dose-related. Host factors may play an important role because hepatotoxicity is seen primarily in patients with juvenile rheumatoid arthritis, systemic lupus erythematosus, and rheumatic fever. As many as 50% of patients with serum salicylate levels greater than 25 mg/dl develop aminotransferase elevations. Jaundice occurs rarely, and the toxicity is reversible after aspirin is discontinued. In rare patients with aspirin-related hepatocellular injury, aminotransferase values may be elevated tenfold to

Table 18-1 Nonsteroidal antiinflammatory agents

Benoxaprofen*	Diclofenac†	Diflunisal
Fenoprofen	Flurbiprofen	Ibuprofen
Indomethacin†	Ketoprofen	Meclofenamate
Naproxen	Phenylbutazone†	Piroxicam†
Pirprofen†	Sulindac	Suprofen
Tolmetin		

*Agent withdrawn secondary to cases of fatal hepatotoxicity.
†Agent implicated in fatal cases of hepatotoxicity.

fortyfold and may be associated with changes on liver biopsy specimens of focal hepatitis and necrosis. Aspirin ingestion also has been associated with the development of Reye's syndrome in children. Recent reductions in the incidence of childhood Reye's syndrome have coincided with the reductions in aspirin usage in children.

Nonsteroidal Antiinflammatory Agents

Aminotransferase elevations in patients receiving nonsteroidal antiinflammatory agents (NSAIDs) are common and occur in up to 15% of patients. Drug toxicity may be mediated by both a direct hepatotoxic effect and a hypersensitivity reaction. Most often the abnormalities are mild or transient; however, in some cases moderate degrees of hepatic dysfunction associated with jaundice, anorexia, nausea, and vomiting may occur. Fatal cases of FHF have been reported with several of these agents (Table 18-1). One agent, benoxaprofen, was withdrawn from the market shortly after its release secondary to numerous case reports of severe hepatotoxicity. Onset of liver dysfunction usually occurs during the first 12 weeks of therapy, but delayed toxicity may also occur. Hepatic injury may resemble viral hepatitis, but in some cases prominent cholestasis or granulomatous inflammation may occur. Patients developing aminotransferase elevations while taking NSAIDs need to be followed carefully. The agent should be discontinued for patients developing elevations greater than threefold. In most cases hepatotoxicity is reversible after the NSAID is stopped. Chronic NSAID ingestion has been associated with the development of chronic hepatitis that improves with drug discontinuation.

Gold

Several cases of cholestatic injury related to chrysotherapy have been reported in patients with rheumatoid arthritis. Onset of jaundice usually occurs early in the course of therapy and often is associated with eosinophilia. Rash, proteinuria, and lymphadenopathy may also be present. Prognosis is generally good, with complete recovery within 3 months.

D-Penicillamine

D-Penicillamine has been associated with a variety of systemic toxicities. Significant hepatotoxicity appears to be rare, but isolated cases of cholestatic jaundice have been attributed to this agent.

ANTIMICROBIAL AGENTS

Antituberculous Agents

Isoniazid. Isoniazid remains the most widely prescribed antituberculous drug in use today. Although it was introduced in the early 1950s, it was not recognized as a potential cause of serious hepatotoxicity until the early 1970s. Mild, asymptomatic elevations of aminotransferase levels occur in 10% to 20% of treated patients, usually within the initial 2 to 3 months of therapy. These elevations are typically transient, and the aminotransferase levels are elevated less than threefold. In approximately 1% of treated patients, overt hepatitis develops. Symptomatic hepatitis is age-dependent; it rarely is seen in patients under 20 years of age, but it occurs in approximately 2% of patients age 50 to 64 and in almost 5% of patients more than 65 years old. In patients developing serious hepatotoxicity, about 15% develop jaundice within 4 weeks of the initiation of treatment, 50% within 8 weeks, and the remaining 35% within 6 months. The clinical features in patients developing symptomatic hepatitis are similar to those in acute viral hepatitis. Malaise, anorexia, nausea, vomiting, and abdominal discomfort are often present before the onset of jaundice. Moderate to marked elevations of aminotransferase occur in association with varying degrees of bilirubin elevation. As with other forms of hepatocellular injury, PT is prolonged in severe cases. Histologic changes resemble acute viral hepatitis, with the presence of bridging necrosis, submassive necrosis, and massive necrosis in the severe cases. In patients developing jaundice, the case fatality rate is approximately 10%. Patients over age 50 and those who continue to receive the agent despite development of symptoms are at increased risk for severe disease. Infrequent cases of chronic hepatitis evolving to fibrosis and cirrhosis have also been reported.

Isoniazid is believed to exert a direct hepatotoxic effect through metabolic intermediates formed in the liver during drug biotransformation. In some patients, there also may be a superimposed hypersensitivity-mediated reaction. The suggestion that toxicity was more common in individuals who rapidly received acetylate isoniazid has not been confirmed by subsequent studies. In experimental systems, agents that stimulate the P450 mixed function oxidase system potentiate isoniazid toxicity. Rifampin-induced stimulation of isoniazid metabolism may be responsible for the observation that isoniazid plus rifampin leads to hepatic injury more often than administration of either agent alone. Early recognition and prompt discontinuation of isoniazid is necessary to prevent additional hepatic damage. Most fatal cases have occurred in patients who continued isoniazid despite developing signs and symptoms of icteric hepatitis. Treatment is supportive, and corticosteroid administration is not indicated. Routine monitoring of liver biochemistries is of limited value in predicting severe toxicity because of the frequent occurrence of mild aminotransferase elevations. Patients developing symptoms of a viral illness should have liver-function tests checked. Those patients developing aminotransferase values elevated greater than three to five times should have their isoniazid discontinued.

Rifampin. Critical evaluation of rifampin toxicity has been hampered by its frequent coadministration with isoniazid and other agents. Approximately 20% of patients receiving isoniazid plus rifampin develop aminotransferase elevations. In most cases the elevations are minimal, but, in approximately 5% of cases, they are increased greater than fivefold. Alcoholics and patients with preexisting hepatic or biliary tract disease may be predisposed to developing liver injury. Patients developing jaundice or greater than threefold to fivefold elevations of aminotransferase should stop both isoniazid and rifampin. After aminotransferase levels have returned to normal, isoniazid, alone or in combination with other antituberculous agents, can be carefully restarted.

Paraaminosalicylic acid, ethionamide, and pyrazinamide. Hypersensitivity reactions to paraaminosalicylic acid (PAS) are associated with evidence of hepatic injury in approximately 25% of cases. The hepatotoxicity occurs as part of a generalized syndrome associated with fever, rash, and lymphadenopathy. PAS causes a mixed hepatocellular injury, with features of both hepatocellular and cholestatic injury. Ethionamide causes elevated liver biochemistries in approximately 5% of treated patients. Symptomatic hepatitis with jaundice occurs less often. Most cases are mild and resolve with drug discontinuation. Pyrazinamide rarely has been associated with hepatitis.

Antibacterial Agents

Erythromycin. Erythromycin estolate is responsible for an apparent idiosyncratic reaction leading to cholestatic injury with hepatocanalicular features. Until recently, erythromycin estolate was believed to be the only derivative of erythromycin associated with hepatotoxicity. Reports have now appeared implicating erythromycin lactobionate, stearate, and ethylsuccinate in cases of liver injury. Symptoms generally develop within 1 to 3 weeks after initiation of therapy. In cases of reexposure, symptoms may appear within 1 to 2 days. Generally, anorexia, nausea, vomiting, and abdominal pain precede the onset of jaundice. Eosinophilia associated with moderate to marked elevations of AP and mild to moderate abnormalities of aminotransferase levels are characteristic. Cholestasis associated with a mononuclear portal infiltrate and eosinophils is seen on biopsy specimen. Although erythromycin toxicity usually is believed to be a hypersensitivity-mediated reaction, there is experimental evidence for erythromycin's having direct hepatotoxic effects; thus the relative contribution of these effects to the pathogenesis of erythromycin-induced injury in humans remains unclear. Hepatic dysfunction is readily reversible on discontinuation of erythromycin.

Tetracycline. Tetracycline hepatotoxicity previously had been reported most often in patients receiving large doses of IV-administered drug. The scarcity of this syndrome in recent years appears to be due to the infrequent use of IV tetracycline. In patients developing hepatic injury, the illness develops within 10 days of drug administration and is associated with anorexia, nausea, vomiting, and abdominal pain. The course is usually progressive, with subsequent development of jaundice, renal failure, and encephalopathy. Aminotransferase levels and serum bilirubin are elevated mildly to moderately, and PTs usually are prolonged. Hypoglycemia and pancreatitis are also frequently present. Liver biopsy characteristically reveals microvesicular steatosis. Pregnancy and renal insufficiency appear to increase the susceptibility to tetracycline-induced hepatic damage. Although tetracycline appears to possess intrinsic hepatotoxicity, the precise mechanism of toxicity remains unclear.

Sulfonamides. Sulfonamides may be associated with clinically apparent hepatotoxicity in up to 0.6% of recipients. Hepatotoxicity has been reported with all of the currently available sulfonamide agents (i.e., sulfanilamide, sulfamethizole, sulfamethoxazole, sulfisoxazole, sulfadoxine, and sulfasalazine), including agents administered intravaginally. In patients developing symptoms, fever, rash, anorexia, nausea, and vomiting usually occur within 2 weeks of the start of therapy. Typically both aminotransferases and AP are elevated, consistent with a mixed-hepatocellular injury. Eosinophils and granulomas may be present on a liver biopsy specimen, and in severe cases massive or submassive necrosis may be present. Cases of chronic hepatitis can occur after prolonged or repeated administration of these agents. Most clinically significant cases of hepatotoxicity are idiosyncratic and occur as part of a generalized hypersensitivity reaction. Hepatotoxicity in patients receiving sulfa drugs in combination with other agents (i.e., pyrimethamine-sulfadoxine and trimethoprim-sulfamethoxazole) is most often related to the sulfa derivative. AIDS patients appear to be more susceptible to trimethoprim-sulfamethoxazole–induced abnormalities in liver tests. Recovery usually follows drug withdrawal; however, fatalities occur that are secondary to massive hepatic necrosis or hepatotoxicity associated with severe dermatologic disorders (i.e., Stevens-Johnson syndrome). Corticosteroids are often administered to patients with severe hypersensitivity reactions without clear evidence of any benefit. Treatment is primarily supportive.

Nitrofurantoin. Nitrofurantoin has been associated with both acute and chronic liver disease. Acute nitrofurantoin hepatotoxicity typically is associated with fever, rash, arthralgias, and eosinophilia. The nature of liver injury is variable, with hepatocellular pattern being the most common. An entity resembling autoimmune chronic active hepatitis can develop in patients receiving prolonged treatment. In these individuals, features of autoimmune disease, including autoantibodies, hyperglobulinemia, and hypoalbuminemia are typically present. The precise mechanism of drug-induced injury is unclear although in most cases an immune-mediated, idiosyncratic reaction appears responsible. Corticosteroids may ameliorate the hypersensitivity-related features and hasten biochemical resolution, but generally treatment is supportive. If nitrofurantoin is not discontinued, cirrhosis and death from progressive hepatic failure can occur. Cross-sensitization to furazolidone, a closely related nitrofuran, has been reported.

Penicillins. Almost all reported cases of hepatocellular injury with these agents have involved semisynthetic penicillins. Oxacillin and dicloxacillin have been implicated in cases of cholestatic liver injury and in cases of anicteric hepatocellular injury. Rapid improvement usually occurs when either the offending agent is discontinued or another penicillin is substituted. Rare cases of hepatotoxicity have been reported with ampicillin, amoxicillin, amoxicillin-clavulanate, carbenicillin, and nafcillin. In some cases toxicity may occur as part of a generalized hypersensitivity phenomenon. In other cases a direct toxic effect of either the penicillin or a metabolite may be responsible.

Cephalosporins. Mild, reversible abnormalities of liver biochemistries can occur with virtually all of the currently available cephalosporins. Clinically significant toxicity is extremely rare. Ceftriaxone is unique in that it may lead to the deposition of biliary sludge in up to 43% of treated patients. Occasionally symptoms mimicking acute cholecystitis may develop, and some patients have been subjected to cholecystectomy. Symptoms and gallbladder sludge usually resolve after treatment has been discontinued.

Aztreonam, imipenem-cilastatin, and fluoroquinolones. Mild abnormalities of liver biochemistries have been reported with all of these agents. Clinically significant toxicity seems to be rare.

Antifungal Agents

Ketoconazole and fluconazole. Asymptomatic elevations of aminotransferases occur in approximately 5% to 10% of patients receiving ketoconazole; symptomatic liver injury occurs in approximately 1 per 15,000 patients receiving the drug. Most patients develop symptoms within 8 weeks of the start of therapy. The pattern of liver injury is usually hepatocellular, but some patients exhibit cholestatic or mixed hepatocellular-cholestatic features. Liver injury caused by ketoconazole appears to be idiosyncratic, but the actual mechanism is unknown. Women and patients over age 40 appear to be more susceptible to hepatic injury by this agent. Recovery after drug discontinuation appears to be the rule; however, fatal cases have been reported. In some cases, biochemical resolution may be delayed for up to 6 months. Routine monitoring of liver biochemistries during therapy has been recommended. More importantly ketoconazole should be stopped in patients developing jaundice or symptoms of viral hepatitis. Fluconazole has also been associated with abnormal liver biochemistries. Two fatal cases of hepatitis occurred in patients receiving fluconazole; however, these patients were also receiving a number of other potentially hepatotoxic medications. Patients taking fluconazole who develop abnormal liver biochemistries need to be followed closely. The medication should be discontinued in those developing progressive liver test abnormalities.

Griseofulvin and amphotericin B. Griseofulvin is a predictable hepatotoxin and carcinogen in mice, but it appears to be of less importance as a human toxin. Griseofulvin-associated cholestasis has been described, but significant hepatotoxicity in humans is rare. Amphotericin B has been associated with liver biochemistry abnormalities but not significant hepatotoxicity. A dosage reduction results in normalization of liver tests in most cases.

Antiviral Agents

Acyclovir, ganciclovir, interferon, and zidovudine. These agents rarely are associated with clinically significant hepatic dysfunction. Implication of these agents as hepatotoxins is confounded by the frequent coexistence of numerous medical problems, including systemic infections involving the liver. In rare cases zidovudine may cause a mixed hepatocellular-cholestatic reaction in patients with AIDS. Recombinant α-interferon administration has been associated with mild increases in aminotransferase levels when the drug has been administered to patients without underlying liver disease. Patients receiving interferon for chronic hepatitis B often develop moderate to marked aminotransferase elevations 8 to 12 weeks after initiation of treatment.

Antiprotozoal Agents

Quinine has been associated with a hypersensitivity type of hepatic injury in rare cases. Pyrimethamine-sulfadoxine has been associated with fatal cases of hepatic necrosis in patients with hypersensitivity reactions to sulfa agents (vide supra). Amodiaquine, a 4-aminoquinolone, can lead to rare cases of idiosyncratic hepatic injury ranging from asymptomatic cholestasis or anicteric elevations of aminotransferase to severe icteric hepatitis associated with hepatic encephalopathy and coagulopathy. Patients continuing therapy after the onset of symptoms develop the most severe illness. Resolution of jaundice may be delayed for up to 6 months, and other biochemical tests may remain abnormal for more than 2 years. Parenterally administered pentamidine causes abnormal liver chemistries in approximately 8% of patients. Severe hepatotoxicity appears to be rare.

CARDIOVASCULAR AGENTS

Antianginal and Dysrhythmic Agents

Perhexiline maleate has never been approved in the United States, but it has been used in Europe for the treatment of angina. This agent has been associated with elevated aminotransferase levels in up to 50% of treated patients. Jaundice can develop, and signs of portal hypertension can occur. Liver biopsy specimens reveal changes very similar to those seen with alcoholic hepatitis, including Mallory bodies and sinusoidal fibrosis.

Amiodarone is a potent antidysrhythmic agent capable of causing multisystem toxicity. The spectrum of amiodarone hepatotoxicity ranges from asymptomatic aminotransferase elevations to a rapidly progressive, fulminant form of hepatitis. Abnormal aminotransferase levels are common and occur in 20% to 40% of treated patients. These elevations are usually less than fourfold, although in patients presenting with acute hepatitis, elevations greater than tenfold can occur. Histologic changes resemble alcoholic hepatitis and include macrovesicular steatosis, focal necrosis, presence of Mallory bodies, centrizonal fibrosis, and cirrhosis. The presence of multilamellar, lysosomal inclusions resembling those seen with the primary phospholipidoses are an ultrastructural feature of amiodarone exposure and do not appear to correlate with drug toxicity. Hepatic disease can progress despite drug withdrawal; this progression probably relates to the high concentration and slow elimination of amiodarone and its principal metabolite, desethylamiodarone, from the liver. Amiodarone usually is discontinued in patients with significant hepatotoxicity. However, with life-threatening dysrhythmias and no therapeutic alternatives, treatment may need to be continued.

Quinidine has been associated with a hypersensitivity type of hepatitis in approximately 2% of treated patients. Mild to moderate elevations of aminotransferase and AP with normal to mild elevations of bilirubin are typical. Fever is the most common clinical feature, but thrombocytopenia and rash also may be present. Hepatotoxicity characteristically appears within 1 month of the start of therapy. A variety of findings have been reported on liver biopsy, including granulomas, diffuse hepatitis with eosinophils, and centrizonal necrosis. Hepatic injury resolves with quinidine withdrawal, and liver biochemistries usually return to normal within 3 weeks of drug withdrawal.

Procainamide, disopyramide, tocainide, encainide, flecainide, mexiletine, and propafenone have all been associated with rare cases of hepatotoxicity, ranging from asymptomatic elevations of liver biochemistries to overt hepatocellular or cholestatic injury. In many of the case reports, the hepatic injury may have been related to other causes (e.g., congestive heart failure and hypotension) or coincidentally administered medications. For patients developing signs or symptoms of hepatotoxicity while on any of these agents, therapy should be withdrawn, or the patient should be observed closely. Therapy should be withdrawn if evidence of progressive injury develops.

Antihypertensive and Diuretic Agents

Methyldopa has been associated with a symptomatic acute hepatocellular injury indistinguishable from acute viral hepatitis. This syndrome is rare, and its incidence is likely to decrease in the future as methyldopa is prescribed less frequently. Asymptomatic, often transient, elevations of aminotransferase occur in approximately 5% of treated patients. Chronic active hepatitis and chronic hepatitis progressing to cirrhosis also have been documented with this agent. Some patients with methyldopa-induced liver injury develop an illness resembling typical autoimmune CAH. Patients with symptomatic disease usually present with evidence of hepatocellular injury. Death from submassive necrosis can occur if therapy is continued. Liver injury probably is mediated by a combination of both immunologic mechanisms and direct hepatotoxicity of drug intermediates produced during methyldopa metabolism. In patients with acute hepatitis, resolution of disease occurs rapidly after drug discontinuation. Resolution occurs more slowly in patients with chronic hepatitis. In rare patients with the syndrome of methyldopa-induced, autoimmune chronic hepatitis, the disease may progress despite drug withdrawal.

Ticrynafen was released in the United States in 1979 and withdrawn several months later after multiple reports of hepatotoxicity. Acute hepatitis, chronic hepatitis, and cirrhosis were associated with this agent, and death occurred in approximately 7% of cases. Many patients developed high titer antibodies against liver and kidney microsomes (anti-LKM).

A number of currently available diuretics and antihypertensive medications have been associated with hepatotoxicity (Table 18-2). The incidence of toxicity with these agents is extremely low, and in some cases the association with liver toxicity may be coincidental.

Anticoagulant and thrombolytic agents. Anticoagulant and thrombolytic agents are rare causes of significant hepatotoxicity. Of greater importance is the occasional case report of hepatic hemorrhage, usually into a cyst or hepatic tumor, in patients receiving these agents. Heparin is frequently associated with minor elevations of aminotransferase levels. This phenomenon appears to be dose-dependent and not associated with clinically significant liver dysfunction. Approximately 20% of patients spontaneously normalize their biochemistries despite continued treatment. Warfarin and dicumarol appear to be virtually free of significant hepatotoxicity. Streptokinase has been associated with rare reports of hepatic dysfunction.

Antineoplastic and Immunosuppressive Agents

The anticancer drugs are inherently toxic; thus, not surprisingly, a large number of these agents cause liver injury. Unfortunately, evaluation of hepatotoxicity in patients receiving these agents is often complicated by the underlying illness, frequent coadministration of multiple medications, and the presence of coexisting conditions or disorders. Furthermore, these agents are most often administered

Table 18-2 Antihypertensives and diuretics: frequency and nature of injury caused by selected agents

Agent	Frequency*	Nature of injury
Ethacrynic acid	VR	Hepatocellular
Furosemide	VR	Cholestatic ± hepatocanalicular
Spironolactone	VR	Hepatocellular
Thiazide	VR	Cholestatic ± hepatocanalicular
Hydralazine	VR	Hepatocellular and granulomatous
Captopril	R	Cholestatic ± hepatocanalicular
Diltiazem	VR	Granulomatous
Nifedipine	VR	Hepatocellular
Verapamil	VR	Hepatocellular
Acebutolol	VR	Hepatocellular and mixed hepatocellular
Metoprolol	VR	Hepatocellular
Labetalol	R	Hepatocellular

*VR = very rare (few case reports available); R = rare

on an intermittent schedule, which may lead to an underestimation of the true hepatotoxic potential.

Alkylating agents. The nitrosoureas (carmustine, lomustine, and semustine) have been associated with hepatocellular injury and elevations of liver chemistries in up to 25% of patients receiving therapeutic doses. These changes are usually reversible with drug withdrawal. Fatal cases of liver failure have been observed in patients receiving extremely high doses of carmustine for refractory tumors. Mechlorethamine, triethylenethiophosphoramide, cyclophosphamide, busulfan, dacarbazine, chlorambucil, and mitomycin infrequently are associated with hepatotoxicity. Most case reports of hepatotoxicity caused by cyclophosphamide have been in patients with collagen vascular disease and not malignancy. Streptozotocin has been reported to cause reversible elevations of liver chemistries in 15% to 67% of patients. Alkylating agents may lead to venoocclusive disease of the liver, particularly when used at higher than conventional doses or when used in conjunction with radiation for patients undergoing bone marrow transplantation.

Antimetabolites

Azathioprine, mercaptopurine, and thioguanine. Evaluation of reports implicating azathioprine have been complicated by the frequent inability to exclude other potential causes of hepatic dysfunction. Both azathioprine and its metabolite, mercaptopurine, are associated with hepatic injury; however, azathioprine leads to hepatotoxicity less often than mercaptopurine. Both agents cause either a cholestatic or a mixed pattern of hepatocellular injury. Fibrosis may also be a feature of azathioprine-related liver disease. Clinically apparent injury can develop at any time but most often within the first 2 months of treatment. This is usually manifested by mild to moderate elevations of aminotransferase, AP, and bilirubin. These agents appear to be directly hepatotoxic, and the toxicity is dose dependent. After drug withdrawal cholestasis improves, and elevated liver chemistries return to normal. Whether fibrosis improves is unclear. Azathioprine has also been associated with venoocclusive disease, peliosis hepatitis, and sinusoidal dilatation in patients receiving long-term treatment after renal transplantation. Thioguanine administered in combination with other agents has been implicated in cases of hepatic venoocclusive disease.

Methotrexate. Methotrexate has been in clinical use since 1955, but it was not recognized as a significant hepatotoxin until the early 1970s. Methotrexate is now widely employed in the treatment of certain malignancies and of nonmalignant disorders, such as psoriasis and rheumatoid arthritis. Most of the currently available information about methotrexate hepatotoxicity was derived from studies conducted in patients with psoriasis. Methotrexate appears to be a predictable hepatotoxin that leads to the insidious development of hepatic fibrosis and cirrhosis. In rare cases, chronic use has been associated with overt liver failure and need for liver transplantation. The mechanism of liver injury remains unknown. Mild to moderate elevations of aminotransferase levels are common in patients receiving high-dose methotrexate followed by calcium leucovorin rescue. These abnormalities are transient and not associated with permanent structural liver damage. Patients receiving chronic methotrexate who develop liver toxicity are usually asymptomatic, with aminotransferase and AP levels being normal to mildly elevated. In rare cases, patients may present with signs of portal hypertension or liver failure. Liver biopsies characteristically reveal evidence of macrovesicular steatosis, focal necrosis, nonspecific portal and periportal inflammation, and fibrosis with or without cirrhosis. Hepatotoxicity occurs more often in patients receiving methotrexate daily than in those receiving weekly treatment. Other factors associated with an increased risk of methotrexate hepatic toxicity include past or present heavy alcohol ingestion, preexisting liver disease, obesity, renal dysfunction, and cumulative doses greater than 1.5 gm. No correlation exists between abnormalities of liver tests and hepatic histology; thus liver biopsy remains the standard for evaluating patients receiving methotrexate. Although some authorities believe that liver disease occurs less often in patients with rheumatoid arthritis, this may be a function of the lower cumulative doses of methotrexate administered to these patients. Until more information becomes available, all patients receiving chronic methotrexate should be followed as outlined below.

A pretherapy liver biopsy is required in patients known or suspected of having any of the risk factors for hepatotoxicity. Patients at low risk for toxicity may forgo the pretherapy biopsy but should have a biopsy performed after 3 to 4 months of therapy if long-term treatment is anticipated. Liver tests should be monitored monthly for 3 months then repeated at intervals of 3 to 4 months. Patients developing greater than threefold elevations of aminotransferase should have the methotrexate withheld until chemistries return to normal. Elevations persisting beyond 2 months should be evaluated with liver biopsy. Patients with normal routine liver chemistries should undergo liver biopsy after receiving a cumulative dose of 1.5 gm. In patients with normal or mildly abnormal biopsy specimens, repeat biopsies are recommended at 1.5 gm intervals. Patients with evidence of increased fibrosis on the biopsy specimen need to be followed more closely and should have biopsies repeated at 6 month intervals.

5-Fluorouracil, floxuridine, and cytosine arabinoside. 5-Fluorouracil alone rarely has been associated with hepatotoxicity. In combination chemotherapy, regimens containing 5-FU have been associated with frequent, asymptomatic, and reversible elevations of liver biochemistries. The 5-FU derivative floxuridine has been associated with significant hepatotoxicity when administered through the hepatic artery for treatment of hepatic metastases. Abnormalities of aminotransferase levels, bilirubin, and AP occur frequently, usually within 2 to 4 weeks of the start of infusion therapy. Liver chemistries return to normal in most patients within 2 to 3 months after discontinuation of therapy. Approximately 15% of patients develop a cholestatic syndrome associated with cholangiographic evidence of diffuse or localized biliary strictures. Strictures most often involve the common hepatic duct bifurcation, but isolated intrahepatic and extrahepatic bile duct strictures may occur in association with abnormalities of the gallbladder and cystic duct. The mechanism of injury remains speculative but appears to be a direct toxic effect of the high concentrations of floxuridine delivered to the liver and biliary tract. In some cases ischemia related to the surgical dissection required to place the infusion catheter may contribute to injury. Individual differences in rates of hepatic drug extraction and degradation are believed to be responsible for the differing susceptibilities to this agent. Histologic abnormalities include steatosis, acute and chronic inflammation in the lobule and portal area, bile duct proliferation, periportal fibrosis, and cirrhosis. Patients receiving floxuridine should have liver tests monitored periodically during treatment. Those patients developing jaundice or a greater than threefold elevation of aminotransferase levels should have treatment discontinued until tests return to near normal. Infusion with corticosteroids has been attempted without any clear evidence of benefit. Patients with symptomatic cholestasis that does not improve with cessation of infusion therapy and is associated with cholangiographic evidence of a dominant stricture occasionally may benefit from endoscopic biliary drainage or stent placement. Percutaneous drainage procedures seem to be especially hazardous in these patients and should be avoided.

Cytosine arabinoside leads to transient abnormalities of liver chemistries in up to 46% of patients. The abnormalities often resolve despite continued therapy, and in almost all cases the biochemistries return to normal after cytosine arabinoside is discontinued. Venoocclusive disease has been reported in patients receiving cytosine arabinoside alone or in combination with radiation or other chemotherapeutic agents.

Miscellaneous agents

Asparaginase, flutamide, and mithramycin. Transient elevations of aminotransferase, AP, and bilirubin are frequent in patients receiving L-asparaginase for acute lymphocytic leukemia. Associated with these modest elevations of liver chemistries are disproportionate decreases in levels of plasma coagulation factors, lipoproteins, albumin, haptoglobin, transferrin, and β-globulins. Although most cases are mild and reversible after L-asparaginase is discontinued, occasional cases of severe coagulopathy and fatal hepatic failure have been reported. Toxicity is believed to occur as a consequence of treatment-induced asparagine deficiency and is accompanied by morphologic changes of hepatic steatosis. Hypersensitivity to L-asparaginase or impurities present in the enzyme solution may account for some of the hepatotoxic reactions. Although the biochemical abnormalities usually resolve within two weeks of discontinuation of therapy, fatty infiltration may persist for several months.

Mithramycin is a predictable hepatotoxin causing hepatocellular injury and necrosis in most patients treated with a tumoricidal dose. Dosages used in the treatment of hypercalcemia infrequently are associated with significant toxicity.

Flutamide, an antiandrogen, has been associated with jaundice and at least one fatal case of hepatic failure during clinical trials. Hepatotoxicity may be mediated through a hypersensitivity reaction.

Anthracyclines, bleomycin, etoposide, and vinca alkaloids. These agents rarely cause significant hepatic injury. Slight elevations of aminotransferase and AP have been reported with doxorubicin, daunorubicin, and mitoxantrone, and hepatic steatosis may be seen in patients treated with bleomycin. Hepatotoxicity has been reported when these drugs are used in combination with other agents.

Cyclosporine. Mild to moderate increases of bilirubin and aminotransferase occur in as many as 30% of renal transplant patients treated with high doses of cyclosporine. These biochemical abnormalities are reversible after the dosage is reduced.

Endocrine Agents

Antithyroid drugs. Hepatotoxicity with these agents is rare and appears to be idiosyncratic. Carbimazole and methimazole have both been associated with cholestatic liver injury, and propylthiouracil has been implicated in cases of acute and chronic hepatitis. Liver injury related to ingestion of carbimazole and methimazole is self-limited and reversible; however, biochemical resolution can take several months. Propylthiouracil usually is associated with hepatocellular injury, and fatal cases with massive or submassive necrosis can occur. Propylthiouracil also has been demonstrated to cause CAH that resolves with drug withdrawal. Autoantibodies may be present in patients with chronic hepatitis caused by propylthiouracil.

Lipid-lowering agents. The recent interest in cholesterol reduction has led to more patients being treated for hyperlipidemia and an increased awareness of the potential toxicity of lipid-lowering agents. Nicotinic acid occasionally is associated with hepatotoxicity and is currently one of the most common causes of drug-induced hepatic injury seen in clinical practice. The availability of niacin without prescription and the frequent use of sustained-release preparations also have contributed to the recent increase in the number of drug-induced hepatotoxicity cases. Hepatotoxicity most often occurs in patients receiving in excess of 3 gm per day of crystalline niacin and in patients taking sustained-release niacin, even at lower doses. The onset of toxicity is usually insidious and characterized by the development of malaise, anorexia, and nausea. Jaundice and pruritus may be present in some cases. The pattern of injury is usually hepatocanalicular cholestasis, but hepatocellular injury also may occur. In most cases the hepatic damage is reversible after niacin is discontinued. Symptoms disappear rapidly, and liver chemistries usually return to normal within 1 month. Nicotinic acid appears to be a dose-dependent, direct hepatotoxin, but the mechanism of injury remains to be determined. At least two cases of fulminant hepatic failure (FHF), one requiring liver transplantation, have been reported.

The hydroxy-methylglutaryl-coenzyme reductase inhibitors lovastatin and simvastatin have been associated with an apparently idiosyncratic form of hepatocellular injury. Transient minimal elevations of aminotransferase are common in hyperlipidemic patients and most likely are unrelated to drug therapy. However, in approximately 1% to 2% of treated patients, moderate to marked sustained elevations of aminotransferase occur. These abnormalities develop 3 to 15 months after the start of therapy and are characteristically asymptomatic. Liver chemistries usually return to normal within 4 weeks of discontinuation of therapy. Patients receiving concomitant therapy with other medications may be at an increased risk for hepatotoxicity with these agents. Until further information about the safety and long-term effects of these medications is available, it is recommended that patients receiving lovastatin and simvastatin have liver chemistries performed at intervals of 4 to 8 weeks for the first year of treatment and at intervals of 2 to 3 months after that. Some patients with toxicity to lovastatin have been retreated successfully with simvastatin.

Oral hypoglycemic agents. The sulfonylureas occasionally are associated with hepatotoxicity, and all of the currently available agents, chlorpropramide, tolbutamide, tolazamide, acetohexamide, glyburide, and glipizide, have been associated with hepatic injury. Several older derivatives from this class of drugs were abandoned because of problems with frequent hepatotoxicity. The pattern of toxicity with these agents is usually cholestatic. However, hepatocellular and mixed hepatocellular-cholestatic reactions have been reported. Onset of hepatotoxicity usually occurs within 1 to 2 months after the start of therapy, but in some patients the onset of injury may be delayed. Symptoms may precede or coincide with the development of jaundice. Symptoms usually include anorexia, fatigue, nausea, and pruritus. Rash and fever occur infrequently. Liver biopsy findings vary but most often demonstrate some degree of cholestasis. Eosinophils, granulomas, and evidence of cholangitis may be identified, but in long-standing cases bile duct proliferation and fibrosis can be present. The mechanism for injury is unknown, with some cases appearing to be hypersensitivity related and others seemingly caused by direct hepatotoxicity. In most cases toxicity is completely reversible after treatment is withdrawn. Rare cases of progressive, fatal liver injury have been reported. In the event of suspected hepatotoxicity, oral hypoglycemic therapy should be discontinued. Substitution with another sulfonylurea is not recommended.

Estrogenic and contraceptive steroids. Estrogens have a predictable dose-dependent effect on hepatic excretory function but are rarely associated with clinically significant hepatic dysfunction. On rare occasions women taking oral contraceptives develop jaundice and pruritus during the first few months of therapy. Systemic symptoms are usually mild or absent, and liver chemistries reveal mild to moderate direct hyperbilirubinemia with normal to slight elevations of AP and aminotransferase. Hepatic histology shows intrahepatic cholestasis with little or no associated inflammation. Signs and symptoms of cholestasis resolve rapidly when medication is discontinued. Approximately 50% of women taking oral contraceptives who develop a cholestatic reaction have a history of cholestasis of pregnancy. In addition, patients with unsuspected underlying liver disease may develop overt liver dysfunction during therapy. After estrogens are withdrawn, there is usually a rapid resolution of cholestasis. Incomplete resolution of liver biochemistries may be indicative of underlying liver disease unmasked by contraceptive therapy. Estrogens are believed to exert their effect on plasma membrane fluidity, leading to impaired transport across membranes and ultimately to decreased uptake and transport of bile acids and organic anions into bile. Estrogens and oral contraceptive steroids also have been associated with the development of cholesterol gallstones, hepatic sinusoidal dilatation, Budd-Chiari syndrome, hepatic adenomas, hepatocellular carcinoma, and focal nodular hyperplasia.

Androgenic steroids. Administration of androgenic steroids containing an alkyl group in the C-17 position can lead to the development of clinically significant cholestasis; testosterone, containing a C-17 hydroxyl group, does not. Although only a small percentage of treated patients develop a cholestatic reaction, the effect appears to be dose dependent, and patients with underlying liver disorders appear to be more susceptible to development of jaundice. Persons with cholestasis are usually asymptomatic, but pruritus, malaise, anorexia, and nausea may be present. Jaundice and mild hepatomegaly are the most common physical findings. Liver chemistries are remarkable for moderate to marked bilirubin elevation with minimal elevation of aminotransferase and AP. Liver biopsies typically reveal intrahepatic cholestasis with little or no associated inflammation or necrosis. Although the precise details are unknown, anabolic steroids are believed to act through mechanisms similar to those of estrogenic steroids. The cholestatic reaction is reversible, but in patients with deep jaundice biochemical recovery may take several months. Androgenic steroids have been associated with the development of hepatic sinusoidal dilatation and peliosis hepatitis. Cases of hepatocellular carcinoma also have been reported in patients receiving long-term treatment with androgens. The contribution of these agents to the development of hepatocellular carcinoma and the process of carcinogenesis remains to be determined.

GI Agents

Histamine-2 antagonists. Both cimetidine and ranitidine have been associated with infrequent reports of idiosyncratic hepatotoxicity. In most cases, asymptomatic mild elevations of aminotransferase are noted, and often these abnormalities resolve during continued therapy. On very rare occasions overt symptomatic hepatitis with jaundice can develop in patients receiving these agents. Cases of hepatocellular, cholestatic, and mixed hepatocellular-cholestatic injury have been reported with both cimetidine and ranitidine, but ranitidine may be associated more often with hepatocellular injury. In particular, patients receiving high doses of parenteral ranitidine appear more likely to exhibit reversible elevations of aminotransferase. Hepatotoxicity usually develops within the first 6 weeks of therapy, but isolated cases with latent periods of up to 7 months have been reported. Focal necrosis, cholestasis, and a mixed portal inflammatory infiltrate may be seen on the liver biopsy specimen. Symptoms and biochemical abnormalities resolve rapidly with drug withdrawal. Mild elevations of aminotransferase have occurred with nizatidine and famotidine; however, clinically significant hepatitis has not been reported to date. Cross reactivity among cimetidine, ranitidine, nizatidine, and famotidine has not been reported.

Chenodiol and ursodiol. Chenodiol leads to dose-dependent, mild elevations of aminotransferase in approximately 30% of patients. These abnormalities usually develop during the first few months of therapy and are often transient. More significant elevations (i.e., greater than threefold) occur in less than 3% of treated patients. Histologic findings associated with these abnormalities are often difficult to interpret because (1) many patients receiving chenodiol have liver biopsy abnormalities before treatment and (2) the coexistence of choledocholithiasis in some patients is often associated with biopsy abnormalities. The mechanism of hepatotoxicity is believed to be due to the production and accumulation of the hepatotoxic bile acid lithocholate in susceptible patients. Patients taking chenodiol who develop abnormal liver chemistries should be followed monthly. Therapy should be discontinued in those with greater than threefold elevations of aminotransferase. The biochemical abnormalities are completely reversible after therapy is discontinued. Ursodiol appears to be virtually free of hepatotoxicity.

Miscellaneous agents. Treatment with octreotide, a synthetic somatostatin analog, may predispose to development of cholelithiasis. Abnormal liver tests may occur rarely.

Psychoactive Medications

Major tranquilizers. Approximately 1% of patients receiving chlorpromazine develop cholestatic jaundice within 5 weeks of the start of therapy. Subclinical liver dysfunction occurs more frequently and is believed to be due to the direct effects of chlorpromazine and its metabolites on biliary secretion. Patients developing significant hepatic injury frequently present with anorexia, nausea, vomiting, fever, and abdominal pain. Pruritus may precede or follow the onset of icterus. AP and cholesterol may be elevated markedly, although aminotransferase levels are mildly to moderately elevated. Aminotransferase values elevated greater than tenfold are rare. Eosinophilia occurs in up to 80% of patients. Liver biopsies reveal intracellular and canalicular cholestasis, focal areas of necrosis, Kupffer cell hyperplasia, and a predominantly mononuclear portal inflammatory infiltrate. In some cases large numbers of eosinophils may be present in the portal spaces and sinusoids, and in approximately 20% of cases there is evidence of an acute cholangiolitis. Clinical and biopsy findings frequently simulate biliary obstruction; thus hepatic imaging procedures are usually required to exclude obstruction. Experimentally, chlorpromazine and its metabolites appear to have direct effects on hepatic function, as manifested by their ability to form insoluble complexes with bile salts, alter membrane fluidity, decrease bile salt uptake and secretion, and inhibit membrane Na=K ATPase activity. These effects are believed to be responsible for the subclinical cholestasis that occurs in many treated patients. The syndrome of symptomatic, cholestatic jaundice induced by chlorpromazine is believed to be caused by an unpredictable hypersensitivity reaction to either chlorpromazine or a metabolite. Hepatic dysfunction usually is reversible but may take months to resolve. In rare cases, a progressive cholestatic syndrome resembling primary biliary cirrhosis (PBC) has been reported. Aside from discontinuing chlorpromazine, management is supportive. Although documented cross reactivity with other phenothiazines appears to be extremely rare, all phenothiazine derivatives should be avoided until biochemical recovery is complete.

Other phenothiazines also may be associated with the development of cholestasis, with promethazine, perphenazine, and prochlorperazine causing hepatotoxicity less often than chlorpromazine does. Thiothixene can lead to mild, transient elevations of aminotransferase, and haloperidol and molindone rarely may cause significant hepatic dysfunction.

Antidepressants and anxiolytics. The tricyclic antidepressants have been associated with infrequent cases of hepatotoxicity. Both cholestatic and hepatocellular injury can occur, and there may be cross hepatotoxicity between tricyclic antidepressant agents. The monoamine oxidase inhibitors phenelzine, isocarboxazid, and tranylcypromine are potentially hepatotoxic and lead to hepatocellular injury in less than 1% of treated patients. These reactions usually are reversible, but progressive liver injury and cases of fatal liver failure have been reported. Although rare, significant liver toxicity may also occur with some of the following new antidepressant medications (unrelated to either the tricyclic or monoamine oxidase inhibitor antidepressants):

Tetracycline
- Maprotiline

Serotonin-uptake inhibitors
- Trazodone
- Fluoxetine

Aminoketone
- Bupropion

Extremely rare cases of hepatotoxicity have been reported with benzodiazepine agents. Cholestatic injury appears to be occurring more frequently than hepatocellular injury.

Antiparkinsonism agents. Carbidopa-levodopa, selegiline, and pergolide may cause slight elevations of liver tests.

Miscellaneous Agents

Allopurinol. Allopurinol rarely leads to hepatic injury associated with hypersensitivity features. Most patients present within 5 weeks of the start of therapy and have fever and a rash. The injury is usually hepatocellular with moderate to marked elevations of aminotransferase and moderate hyperbilirubinemia. Biopsies may reveal evidence of centrizonal, focal, or massive necrosis, along with the frequent presence of hepatic granulomas and tissue eosinophilia. The toxicity is often reversible with drug withdrawal, but deaths caused by hepatic failure or complications of the systemic hypersensitivity reaction can occur. Corticosteroids may be effective if administered early in the course of the illness.

Retinoids. The hepatotoxicity resulting from excessive doses of vitamin A has been well documented. The hepatotoxic potential of the therapeutic derivatives of retinoic acid, isotretinoin, and etretinate have not been characterized as well. Therapy with these agents has been reported to cause frequent elevations of aminotransferase. In most cases the elevations are mild and rapidly return to normal with drug discontinuation. Symptomatic icteric hepatitis can develop if treatment is continued, and several fatal cases of hepatotoxicity caused by etretinate have been reported. Patients receiving these agents should have liver chemistries checked before instituting treatment and again periodically during therapy. Patients developing hyperbilirubinemia or greater than threefold elevations of aminotransferase should be withdrawn from treatment.

Disulfiram. Severe hepatotoxicity appears to be a rare complication of disulfiram therapy. The injury is hepatocellular, and the mechanism is believed to be an idiosyncratic hypersensitivity reaction. Toxicity generally begins within 8 weeks of the start of therapy and is associated with signs and symptoms of acute hepatitis with moderate to marked aminotransferase and bilirubin elevations. With discontinuation of disulfiram, symptoms and liver chemistries generally return to normal within 12 weeks. Fatal hepatic failure can result if medication is continued after evidence of liver toxicity develops.

SUMMARY

Drug-induced hepatotoxicity represents an entire spectrum, ranging from mild subclinical hepatic dysfunction to FHF or cirrhosis. Establishing the diagnosis of drug-related hepatotoxicity can be difficult, but it should always be considered when a patient taking medication develops liver disease in the absence of any risk factors for viral hepatitis. When hepatotoxicity is suspected, proper management requires that the offending medication(s) be discontinued as soon as possible. Therapy is primarily supportive after the implicated medication is withdrawn. Corticosteroids may be useful in patients with severe hypersensitivity reactions, and hepatic transplantation can be life saving for the patient with FHF or unremitting liver injury. In cases involving recently released medications or reactions not previously described with older medications, reports should be filed with both the Food and Drug Administration and the drug's manufacturer. The procedure of voluntary reporting by physicians is critical for the management and recognition of drug-induced liver injury, and this process remains a vital link in the network tracking drug hepatotoxicity.

SUGGESTED READING

Black M: Acetaminophen hepatotoxicity, Gastroenterology 78:382, 1980.

This is a comprehensive overview of the pharmacology, epidemiology, clinical features, and treatment of acetaminophen-related liver disease.

Gilbert SC et al: Methotrexate-induced cirrhosis requiring liver transplantation in three patients with psoriasis: a word of caution in light of the expanding use of this "steroid-sparing" agent, Arch Intern Med 150:889, 1990.

Three cases of methotrexate-induced cirrhosis requiring orthotopic liver transplantation are presented to emphasize the importance of adherence to published criteria for patient selection, monitoring of cumulative drug doses, and the performance of serial liver biopsies.

Gordin FM et al: Adverse reactions to trimethoprim-sulfamethoxazole in patients with the acquired immunodeficiency syndrome, Ann Intern Med 100:495, 1984.

Of 35 patients with AIDS, 20% developed signs of hepatitis (an elevation in ALT or AP levels equal to or greater than twofold), including four with severe reactions.

Henkin Y, Johnson KC, and Segrest JP: Rechallenge with crystalline niacin after drug-induced hepatitis from sustained-release niacin, JAMA 264:241, 1990.

Based on their series of cases, the authors present evidence that sustained-release niacin is more hepatotoxic than crystalline niacin.

Lewis JH et al: Amiodarone hepatotoxicity: Prevalence and clinicopathologic correlations among 104 patients, Hepatology 9:679, 1989.

Asymptomatic elevation of aminotransferase levels was detected in one fourth of patients, and symptomatic hepatocellular injury developed in 3% of patients.

Kaplowitz N et al: Drug-induced hepatotoxicity, Ann Intern Med 104:826, 1986.

The authors present a fine review of the patterns and mechanisms of drug toxicity that includes an excellent discussion of drug-induced cholestasis.

Kopanoff DE, Snider DE, and Caras GJ: Isoniazid-related hepatitis: a U.S. Public Health Service cooperative surveillance study, Amer Rev Respir Dis 117:991, 1978.

This is a landmark study evaluating the factors associated with the development of isoniazid-related hepatotoxicity in more than 13,000 individuals receiving prophylactic therapy.

Neuberger J and Kena JG: Halothane hepatitis: a model of immune mediated drug hepatotoxicity, Medical Science 72:263, 1987.

This is a good summary of halothane hepatitis and the immune mechanisms that play a role in the development of hepatotoxicity.

Roenigk HH et al: Methotrexate in psoriasis: revised guidelines, J Am Acad Dermatol 19:145, 1988.

Up-to-date recommendations for methotrexate usage and follow-up are provided in this report.

Schaad UB, Krucko JW, and Tschaeppeler H: Reversible ceftriaxone-associated biliary pseudolithiasis in children, Lancet 2:1411, 1988.

Sixteen of 37 children being treated for serious infections developed biliary concretions. The pathophysiology is unknown but may be related to the high biliary excretion of ceftriaxone.

Seeff LB et al: Acetaminophen hepatotoxicity in alcoholics: a therapeutic misadventure, Ann Intern Med 104:399, 1986.

This is an important report warning clinicians about the significant problem of acetaminophen toxicity in alcoholics.

Stricker BHC et al: Hepatic injury associated with the use of nitrofurans: a clinicopathological study of 52 reported cases, Hepatology 8:599-606, 1988.

This is an excellent clinical description of nitrofurantoin-associated liver injury based on a series of 50 cases.

Zimmerman HJ: Hepatotoxicity, New York, 1978, Appleton-Century-Crofts.

Although somewhat dated, this textbook remains a good reference source for questions about hepatotoxicity.

Zimmerman HJ: Hepatotoxic effects of oncotherapeutic agents. In Popper H and Schaffner F, eds: Progress in liver diseases, vol 8, Orlando, 1986, Grune & Stratton.

A brief general overview of hepatotoxicity is given, followed by a thorough discussion of the toxicities of various chemotherapy agents.

19 Environmental and Industrial Hepatotoxins

Fredric G. Regenstein

Potentially hazardous materials are ubiquitous in our environment, yet there is relatively little available information on the hepatotoxicity of most of the thousands of different chemical agents in widespread use. Much of the current literature on chemical hepatotoxicity has been derived from case reports involving accidental or deliberate ingestions, and relatively little is based on carefully controlled laboratory or clinical studies. Thus a large percentage of the available information is of limited value when applied to the most frequently encountered environmental and occupational exposures. Of the more than 500,000 chemicals available in the United States, only 2800 have been classified as hazardous substances by the Occupational Safety and Health Administration. This does not imply that the remaining agents are safe, only that they have been incompletely or inadequately studied. Aside from the staggering number of agents to study, research into chemical hepatotoxicity is complicated by the complexities of environmental, drug/chemical and chemical/chemical interactions, and the enormous diversity of host responses to these toxins. Furthermore, accurate assessments of the incidence of chemical-associated liver toxicity are often hindered by the frequent coexistence of other potential causes of hepatic dysfunction (e.g., viral, alcohol, and drug).

HEPATOTOXICITY OF FOODS, FOOD ADDITIVES, AND FOOD CONTAMINANTS (see box on p. 360)

Mycotoxins

Toxic mushrooms usually are ingested accidentally by amateur mushroom hunters in their search for tasty or hallucinogenic wild mushrooms. Members belonging to the genus *Amanita* are responsible for 95% of the fatal cases of mushroom poisoning occurring in the United States and Europe. *Amanita phalloides* is the mushroom most often implicated in these exposures. *A. phalloides* produces a series of toxins, several of which are among the most lethal toxins known to exist. Ingestion leads to the development of a GI illness, generally 6 to 18 hours after the exposure. Symptoms include nausea, vomiting, abdominal pain, diarrhea, and dehydration. In many patients abatement of the GI symptoms is followed by a 24 to

> **HEPATOTOXINS PRESENT IN FOODS, FOOD ADDITIVES, AND FOOD CONTAMINANTS**
>
> **Hepatotoxins in foods**
>
> Toxic mushrooms
> Pyrrolizidine alkaloids
> Cycasin
> Hypoglycin A
> Safrole derivatives
>
> **Hepatotoxins in food additives**
>
> Nitrites
> Nitrosamines
>
> **Hepatotoxins in food contaminants**
>
> Aflatoxins
> Organic contaminants
>   Hexachlorobenzene
>   Methylenedianiline
>   Paraquat
>   Polychlorinated biphenyls
> Toxic rapeseed oil

36-hour period of apparent improvement. Liver dysfunction becomes manifest during this interval. As the liver dysfunction progresses, patients develop jaundice, coagulopathy, hypoglycemia, encephalopathy, seizures, and renal failure. Mortality is highest in children. In fatal cases hepatic histology typically reveals evidence of steatosis and centrilobular necrosis. In nonfatal cases, sinusoidal congestion and spotty necrosis may be all that is present. The diagnosis usually can be made on clinical grounds for a patient presenting with a history of wild-mushroom ingestion.

General management principles established for other toxins are applicable to cases of *A. phalloides* ingestion. In patients seen early, vomiting should be induced or gastric lavage should be performed. Because the toxins are excreted in bile and reabsorbed in the enterohepatic circulation, continuous duodenal drainage combined with charcoal administration may reduce the amount of toxin exposure. Early charcoal hemoperfusion may also lower toxin levels and reduce overall injury. Good supportive care should be provided with careful attention to fluid status, electrolyte abnormalities, and glucose levels. Although no controlled studies have been done, administration of antibiotics, corticosteroids, thioctic acid, and cytochrome *c* have been recommended by some authors. Patients developing severe coagulopathies and patients progressing to stage 3 hepatic coma should be considered for hepatic transplantation.

Pyrrolizidine Alkaloids

Pyrrolizidine alkaloids are present in more than 200 species of plants and are responsible for hepatotoxicity occurring in humans and animals. These alkaloids are distributed widely in nature and have been associated with outbreaks of human poisoning in Jamaica, Africa, and Asia. Cases in the United States usually have involved patients ingesting herbal preparations containing these alkaloids. Pyrrolizidine compounds cause a toxic injury to hepatic veins, resulting in venoocclusive disease. After exposure, patients may develop acute, subacute, or chronic venoocclusive disease. Patients with acute venoocclusive disease typically present with abdominal pain, hepatomegaly, fluid retention, and ascites. Laboratory studies usually reveal mild to moderate elevations of aminotransferase and bilirubin. The ascitic fluid protein content is almost always high. Liver biopsies show evidence of centrilobular congestion, hemorrhage, necrosis, and subintimal thickening of the terminal hepatic venules. In severe cases the central vein lumen may be obliterated. The outcome after acute venoocclusive disease varies. Most patients recover completely although some patients develop a fatal progressive disease and other patients develop subacute or chronic venoocclusive disease. Subacute venoocclusive disease is characterized by hepatosplenomegaly, ascites, and bouts of abdominal pain. Chronic venoocclusive disease leads to cirrhosis that on a liver biopsy specimen resembles the nonportal central fibrosis findings encountered with Budd-Chiari syndrome. Management is supportive and usually consists of managing ascites and the other complications of portal hypertension.

Aflatoxins

Aflatoxins are a group of toxins produced by the fungus *Aspergillus flavus*. These toxins are among the most potent known carcinogens and are present in a variety of foods contaminated with the fungus. A warm, moist environment enhances organism growth and toxin production, and the most frequently contaminated foods include nuts, corn, grain, and soybeans. Acute liver injury has been reported in animals and humans exposed to large doses of aflatoxins. In humans both FHF and an illness resembling Reye's syndrome have been seen. Chronic liver disease has been identified in animals exposed to aflatoxins, but its role in the pathogenesis of human cirrhosis remains unclear. The strong epidemiologic association between aflatoxins and human liver cancer suggests that these toxins are significant hepatocarcinogens in humans.

Organic Compound Contaminants

A number of organic agents can be identified as contaminants in our food supply. Some of these agents occur predictably as a consequence of attempts to control pests or weeds, but other agents may be present because of accidental contamination. Among the organochlorine pesticides and herbicides, many have been shown to be hepatotoxic in animals. Reports of acute hepatotoxicity in humans are extremely rare, and almost all cases involve individuals ingesting extremely large amounts of the implicated chemical toxin.

An epidemic caused by the ingestion of cooking oil contaminated with polychlorinated biphenyls was reported from Japan in 1968. The high levels of exposure to polychlorinated biphenyls in this outbreak resulted in the development of acute hepatocellular injury associated with chloracne, facial edema, conjunctivitis, and peripheral neuropathy. Some of the surviving patients eventually developed cirrhosis and hepatocellular carcinoma.

An outbreak of hepatocellular injury in Epping, England, caused by the ingestion of bread made from flour contaminated with methylenedianiline has also been reported. In the patients with "Epping jaundice," cholestatic hepatitis typically developed 3 to 5 days after the exposure and was associated with fever and abdominal pain. In a small number of patients, jaundice persisted for several months. Subsequent reports have described a toxic hepatitis in workers occupationally exposed to methylenedianiline through inhalation. In Turkey more than 3000 patients developed severe liver disease associated with porphyria cutanea tarda after the ingestion of wheat contaminated with hexachlorobenzene. The hexachlorobenzene was sprayed on the wheat as a fungicide, and it led to severe liver damage with a 10% mortality rate.

A massive outbreak of illness linked to food contamination occurred in Spain in 1981 when approximately 100,000 people consumed contaminated rapeseed oil. A multisystem (toxic-epidemic syndrome) illness developed in many of the exposed persons, and more than 18,000 persons sought medical attention. Although liver test abnormalities were common (24%), symptomatic hepatic disease occurred in less than 10% of affected persons. A single death caused by fulminant Budd-Chiari syndrome was reported from a group of more than 800 patients seen at one center. Abnormal liver tests persisted in some of the affected patients, and biopsy specimens from these individuals revealed a variety of abnormalities, including steatosis, cirrhosis, venoocclusive disease, and nodular regenerative hyperplasia.

Other Toxins

Cycasin, hypoglycin A, and safrole are naturally occurring hepatotoxins rarely implicated in cases involving humans. Cycasin, isolated from the cycad nut, appears to be hepatotoxic and hepatocarcinogenic in experimental systems and in humans. Hypoglycin A causes an illness resembling Reye's syndrome in people ingesting poorly ripened or undercooked fruit from the *Blighia surpida* tree. Safrole and related compounds derived from oil of sassafras have been shown to be both hepatotoxic and hepatocarcinogenic when administered in large doses to animals.

Nitrites are frequently added to food products as preservatives and have been shown to combine with amines present in food to form potentially carcinogenic nitrosamine compounds. Although not responsible for outbreaks of hepatic disease in humans, nitrosamine compounds have been associated with significant hepatotoxicity in livestock.

TOXICITY OF INDUSTRIAL AND ENVIRONMENTAL CHEMICALS

Inorganic Toxins

The box below lists the inorganic agents most clearly associated with toxicity in humans. Most of the available information on toxicity of the listed agents has been derived form large-dose exposures occurring as a consequence of accidental or deliberate ingestion. The effects of chronic low-dose exposure to these agents have been studied less carefully.

Arsenic toxicity, now primarily of historical interest only, can lead to acute or chronic liver injury. Acute hepatotoxicity occurs after ingestion of a large dose and is generally preceded by neurologic and GI toxicity, often with vascular collapse. Liver biopsy evidence of steatosis, necrosis, and cholestasis are generally present.

MOST IMPORTANT INORGANIC AGENTS ASSOCIATED WITH ENVIRONMENTAL OR INDUSTRIAL HEPATOTOXICITY

- Arsenic
- Beryllium
- Cadmium
- Copper
- Iron
- Phosphorus
- Thallium
- Thorium dioxide

In surviving patients, a prolonged cholestatic syndrome may occur. Chronic exposure has been reported to cause steatosis, cirrhosis, noncirrhotic portal hypertension, and hepatic neoplasms (i.e., angiosarcoma and hepatocellular carcinoma).

Phosphorus is regarded as a prototype toxin causing direct hepatocyte damage. Poisoning with phosphorus results in massive fat deposition in the liver and varying degrees of hepatic necrosis. GI, neurologic, and cardiovascular signs usually predominate during the early period after exposure. Patients surviving the early events develop evidence of hepatic and renal failure. Mortality is high, with case fatality rates in excess of 50%.

Copper and iron may be associated with hepatotoxicity, usually when ingested in a suicide attempt or accidentally. Both agents cause a similar illness, consisting of an early phase, in which GI and cardiovascular symptoms are prominent, followed in 1 to 2 days by evidence of hepatocellular injury. With copper intoxication, hemolysis and acute tubular necrosis are often present. Hepatic histology demonstrates centrizonal necrosis and cholestasis with cases of copper toxicity and periportal necrosis with steatosis in cases of iron toxicity.

Cadmium and thallium have been demonstrated to be hepatotoxic in animals but are rarely significant in human exposures. Beryllium causes a granulomatous reaction in the liver resembling sarcoidosis. The primary clinical manifestations of beryllium exposure occur in the lung. Thorium dioxide, once widely used as a radiographic contrast agent, has been associated with the development of hepatic angiosarcoma 20 or more years after an exposure.

Organic Toxins

Aliphatic hydrocarbons. The haloaliphatic agents are all potentially hepatotoxic. Exposure to the most potent hepatotoxins within this group of chemicals (e.g., tetrachloroethane, carbon tetrachloride, 1,1,2-trichloroethane, and chloroform) leads to combined steatosis and hepatocellular necrosis. Exposure to the least toxic agents (e.g., trichloroethylene, methyl chloride, and 1,1,1-trichloroethane) results in mild steatosis or minimal hepatic damage. These agents have been used primarily as industrial solvents, thus most of the reported toxicity has occurred in industrial exposures. Substitution of solvents with less hepatotoxic potential has decreased the prevalence of industrial hepatotoxicity. However, reports of toxicity involving occupational exposure to the less toxic agents have appeared (see the box on p. 364).

Carbon tetrachloride is probably the most extensively studied hepatotoxin, and it serves as a model for hepatotoxicity caused by the other haloalkanes. In past years carbon tetrachloride was used widely as a cleaner and solvent. The mechanism of hepatic injury induced by carbon tetrachloride is complex and involves several different processes. Steatosis develops very soon after exposure and appears to result from impaired transport of triglycerides out of hepatocytes. Hepatic necrosis follows but appears to be independent of the development of steatosis. Necrosis is believed to occur through two separate mechanisms. The initial phase of hepatocyte necrosis is caused by the direct solvent effect of carbon tetrachloride on hepatocyte membranes. Subsequent hepatic necrosis is thought to be mediated by free radicals and lipid peroxides produced during the metabolism of

ORGANIC AGENTS ASSOCIATED WITH OCCUPATIONAL HEPATOTOXICITY IN HUMANS

Aliphatic compounds

Halogenated compounds
- Carbon tetrachloride
- Tetrachloroethane
- Tetrachloroethylene
- Trichloroethylene
- 1,1,1-Trichloroethane
- Vinyl chloride

Nonhalogenated compounds
- Dimethylformamide

Aromatic compounds

Halogenated compounds
- Polychlorinated biphenyls
- Hexachlorobenzene

Nitroaromatic compounds

2,4,5-Trinitrotoluene (TNT)

Nitroparaffins

2-Nitropropane

carbon tetrachloride by the cytochrome P450 system. Carbon tetrachloride poisoning can occur through either inhalation or ingestion. The earliest symptoms of intoxication, dizziness, visual disturbances, confusion, and somnolence are due to the anesthetic properties of carbon tetrachloride. These symptoms are soon followed by GI symptoms and within 1 to 2 days by evidence of liver and renal dysfunction. Hepatic steatosis and centrilobular necrosis are the primary findings on the liver biopsy; however, significant histologic abnormalities may be present in many organs. Management is primarily supportive, but early administration of N-acetylcysteine may reduce the severity of the hepatorenal damage. Chronic exposure has been demonstrated to cause cirrhosis in animals but not in humans.

Vinyl chloride monomer is used in the manufacture of polyvinyl chloride. Exposure to vinyl chloride has been associated with the development of angiosarcoma and noncirrhotic portal hypertension caused by perisinusoidal fibrosis. In chemical workers exposed to vinyl chloride, focal hyperplasia of hepatocytes and sinusoidal cells has been identified as an early histologic abnormality and may precede the development of angiosarcoma. The occurrence of angiosarcoma in chemical workers appears to have decreased in conjunction with federal regulations reducing workplace exposure.

Dimethylformamide, a widely used industrial solvent, recently was implicated in an outbreak of hepatotoxicity in a fabric-coating plant. Overall, 76% of workers with direct solvent contact were found to have aminotransferase elevations, which in most cases returned to normal with cessation of exposure. Of the subjects seeking long-term follow-up, approximately 30% had persistent unexplained aminotransferase elevations.

Aromatic hydrocarbons. The halogenated aromatic compounds represent an important cause of environmental and occupational liver disease. Polychlorinated biphenyls (PCBs) have been associated with both acute and chronic liver disease in animals and humans following high-level oral exposure. These agents also have been shown to be significant carcinogens in animals. Government regulations, such as the banning of the manufacture and sale of devices containing PCBs in 1976, have reduced the occupational and environmental risks of exposure. Despite these occupational improvements, low levels of PCBs are frequently found in soil and water samples. However, even these low levels are of great concern, given that long-term exposure to PCBs may lead to the development of hepatocellular carcinoma, other cancers, and possibly chronic liver disease (see box on p. 364).

Nitroaromatic and nitroaliphatic compounds. Trinitrotoluene (TNT) was an important cause of occupational liver damage among munitions workers during both World War I and World War II. Acute, subacute, or chronic liver disease could be seen following exposure. The illness developed several months after the initial exposure, and the hepatic dysfunction was typically preceded by an interval in which constitutional symptoms predominated. Some patients then developed rapidly progressive hepatic failure, but other patients manifested a more protracted illness associated with the development of portal hypertension. Cirrhosis was reported to occur in some of the surviving patients. Extrahepatic manifestations were common (e.g., methemoglobinemia, skin lesion, and aplastic anemia) and indicative of heavy occupational exposure. Improvements in occupational safety have virtually eliminated this syndrome.

The nitroparaffins, nitromethane, nitroethane, and nitropropane, are hepatotoxic in experimental animals but rarely in humans. Several cases of FHF have been reported in workers exposed to 2-nitropropane.

SUMMARY

The classic syndromes of acute chemical hepatotoxicity have been described well and usually occur in settings in which the reactions are recognized easily. The relationship between a chronic liver disease and chronic low-level exposure to an industrial or environmental toxin is far more difficult to establish. Relatively little is known about these types of interactions, and much additional research needs to be conducted in this area. The major challenge to hepatologists and occupational medicine specialists throughout the coming years is to identify some of these agents and to remove as many as possible from the environment and workplace.

SUGGESTED READINGS

Hodgson MJ, Heyl AE, and Van Thiel DH: Liver disease associated with exposure to 1,1,1-trichloroethane, Arch Intern Med 149:1793-8, 1989.

This is an initial report documenting the potential hepatotoxicity of occupational exposure to 1,1,1-trichloroethane. The liver function test abnormalities described were mild to moderate. Two patients had advanced cirrhosis, and one was being evaluated for possible hepatic transplantation.

Kopelman H, Scheuer PJ, and Williams R: The liver lesion in Epping jaundice, Q J Med 35:553-64, 1966.

This is a detailed review of the clinical and pathologic features in seven patients who developed hepatic injury (Epping jaundice) caused by methylenedianiline.

McGill DB and Motto JD: An industrial outbreak of toxic hepatitis due to methylenedianiline. N Engl J Med 291:278-82, 1974.

This is a review of 12 cases of hepatotoxicity occurring in patients with an occupational exposure to methylenedianiline. All patients recovered completely when the exposure was discontinued.

Olson KR et al: *Amanita phalloides*-type mushroom poisoning, West J Med 137:282-9, 1982.

This review includes a description of 10 cases (3 fatal) of A. phalloides poisoning in Northern California. This report provides basic information about the diagnosis and treatment of the poisoning and speculation about why there were so many cases that particular year.

Redlich CA et al: Liver disease associated with occupational exposure to the solvent dimethylformamide, Ann Intern Med 108: 680-6, 1988.

A description of a recently detected occupational outbreak of toxic liver disease caused by dimethylformamide is reported. This study was particularly interesting because of the high prevalence of unsuspected liver chemistry abnormalities in the exposed patients.

Ridker PM et al: Hepatic venoocclusive disease associated with the consumption of pyrrolizidine-containing dietary supplements, Gastroenterology 88:1050-4, 1985.

This is a case report from the United States describing a middle-age woman with venoocclusive disease treated with a portosystemic shunt.

Ruprah M, Mant TGK and Flanagan RJ: Acute carbon tetrachloride poisoning in 19 patients: implications for diagnosis and treatment, Lancet 1:1027-9, 1985.

This is a description of 19 patients with acute carbon tetrachloride poisoning. The 13 treated with N-acetylcysteine fared better than those not receiving this therapy.

Solis-Herruzo JA et al: Hepatic injury in the toxic epidemic syndrome caused by the ingestion of adulterated cooking oil (Spain, 1981), Hepatology 4:131-9, 1981.

This is an evaluation of the hepatic manifestations occurring in 842 patients with toxic epidemic syndrome evaluated at a single medical facility.

Tamburro CH: Relationship of vinyl monomers and liver cancers: angiosarcoma and hepatocellular carcinoma, Semin Liver Dis 4:158-69, 1984.

A thorough review of the clinical and toxicologic aspects of vinyl chloride exposure is presented with a special emphasis on its role as a carcinogen.

20 Granulomatous Disease of the Liver

Cheree Trent Mills and *Robert P. Perrillo*

Granulomas of the liver are relatively common, being found in 3% to 10% of liver biopsy specimens. The finding of granulomas often presents the physician with a diagnostic challenge because of the multitude of associated infectious and noninfectious causes (see box on p. 368).

DEFINITION

A granuloma is defined as a nodular, reactive lesion composed of epithelioid cells surrounded by large fibroblasts and lymphocytes (Figure 20-1). The epithelioid cells are transformed macrophages that bear a resemblance to epithelial cells. Caseation necrosis and fibrinoid necrosis are occasionally present. Granulomas tend to be discrete and do not usually disturb the normal hepatic architecture.

The formation of granulomas is a nonspecific immunologic response to a large variety of stimuli. The designation "granulomatous hepatitis" has been used synonymously to describe hepatic granulomas. This is a misnomer in that actual hepatocellular dysfunction and significant elevation of aminotransferase levels rarely occur.

ETIOLOGY

In 5% to 36% of cases the cause remains unknown. In a series of more than 6,000 liver biopsy specimens, Klatskin found granulomas in 10%. Generalized granulomatous disease was present in 56% of patients, 31% had underlying hepatic disease, and 13% had miscellaneous disorders that appeared to be neither hepatic nor granulomatous in nature. Sarcoidosis and tuberculosis accounted for 90% of the cases with generalized granulomatous disease.

CLINICAL ASPECTS

Granulomas of the liver may be encountered in patients of any age, race, or sex. Patients may be asymptomatic, or they may complain of nonspecific symptoms, such as weight loss, malaise, anorexia, or unexplained fever. The clinical history occasionally provides valuable diagnostic clues. For example, marked weight loss

CAUSES OF HEPATIC GRANULOMAS

Infectious diseases

- Bacterial
  - Tuberculosis
  - Atypical mycobacteriosis
  - BCG immunotherapy
  - Leprosy
  - Brucellosis
  - Tularemia
  - Granuloma inguinale
  - Melioidosis
  - Listeriosis
  - Nocardiosis
  - Whipple's disease
  - Typhoid fever
  - Paratyphoid B
- Fungal
  - Histoplasmosis
  - Coccidioidomycosis
  - Cryptococcosis
  - Actinomycosis
  - Blastomycosis
  - Aspergillosis
  - Nocardiosis
  - Candidiasis
- Viral
  - Cytomegalovirus
  - Epstein-Barr (infectious mononucleosis)
  - Viral hepatitis
  - Influenza B
  - Lymphogranuloma venereum
- Parasitic
  - Schistosomiasis
  - Ascaris
  - Toxocara
  - Malaria
  - Strongyloidiasis
  - Amebiasis
  - Visceral larva migrans

Hepatobiliary disease

- Biliary obstruction
- Primary biliary cirrhosis
- Laënnec's cirrhosis
- Postnecrotic cirrhosis
- Chronic active hepatitis
- Jejunoileal bypass

Drugs

- Sulfonamides
- Diazepam
- Phenytoin
- Halothane
- Allopurinol
- Phenylbutazone
- Hydrochlorothiazide
- Chlorpropamide
- Methyldopa
- Quinidine
- Clofibrate

Miscellaneous

- Sarcoidosis
- Wegener's granulomatosis
- Hodgkin's disease
- Crohn's disease
- Foreign bodies (starch, talc, and silica)
- Celiac disease

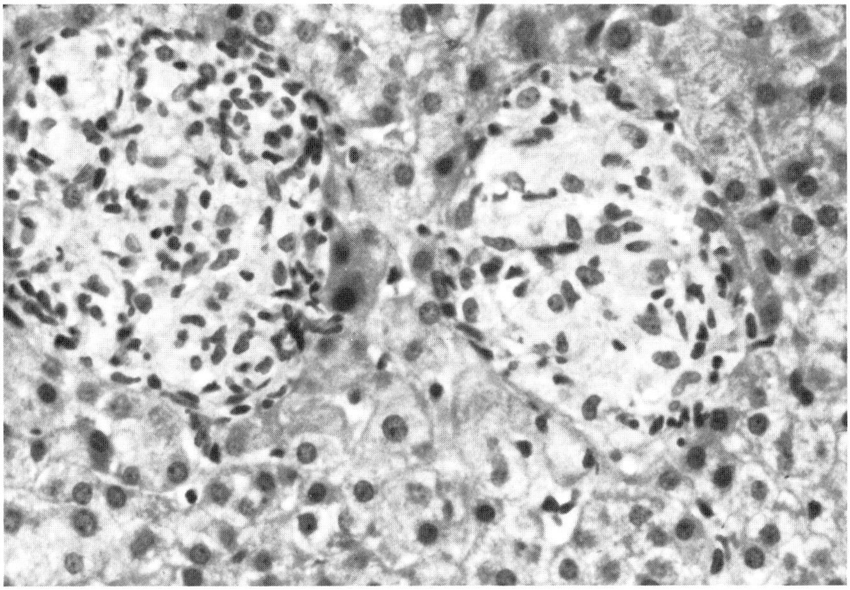

Figure 20-1
Typical appearance of noncaseating granulomas in the liver. Patient had *M. avium intracellulare* infection complicating AIDS. (From Ishak KG. From Hepatic Pathology course conducted by Armed Forces Institute of Pathology, August, 1989, Washington, DC.)

might suggest a diagnosis of tuberculosis or neoplasm. Dyspnea on exertion might suggest a diagnosis of sarcoidosis. Headaches and myalgias may lead to consideration of a diagnosis of arteritis; travel to the Middle East or Africa may raise the possibility of schistosomiasis. Physical examination is rarely helpful although pyrexia, lymphadenopathy, hepatosplenomegaly, or skin lesions may be present. Laboratory abnormalities are usually nonspecific but may include an elevated sedimentation rate, hypergammaglobulinemia, increased AP, and mildly elevated aminotransferases levels.

There is no uniform clinical pattern of illness that accompanies hepatic granulomas. However, there are several suggested indications for liver biopsy that may lead to this diagnosis: (1) hepatosplenomegaly of unknown cause, (2) abnormal liver tests, (3) unexplained jaundice, and (4) fever of unknown origin.

Serial sections of liver biopsy material may enhance the rate of detection of granulomas, and demonstration of specific organisms by appropriate culture techniques of sputum, blood, urine, gastric washings, or various tissues, including liver and lymph node, may be helpful in establishing a diagnosis. There are a few specific situations in which the pathologist might be provided with specific diagnostic clues. Extensive caseation necrosis with acid-fast bacilli are diagnostic of tuberculosis but are seen only in a small percentage of cases. Schistosomiasis ova or *Toxocara* larvae may be seen within granulomas. Granulomas surrounding or involving damaged bile ducts may suggest a diagnosis of PBC.

INFECTIOUS CAUSES OF GRANULOMAS

In the past, tuberculosis was among the most frequent causes of granulomatous liver disease and was reported in 10% to 53% of cases. Primary acute tuberculosis often involves the liver. Miliary tuberculosis can also involve the liver either by dissemination from a primary complex or from a chronic pulmonary focus. Certain clinical findings are suggestive of tuberculosis: fever of unknown origin associated with chills, anemia, meningeal involvement, weight loss, and duration of symptoms of less than 6 months. Physical examination and liver tests usually offer no additional information in differentiating tuberculosis from other causes of infectious granulomas. Skin test reactivity to PPD may be absent. A positive skin test should not be considered definitive for tuberculosis because this occasionally may be observed in patients with other causes, including sarcoidosis.

Although caseating granulomas are said to be the histologic hallmark in tuberculosis, this finding is often missing. Acid-fast bacilli are identified in fewer than one third of cases, and culture is positive only in up to 10% of cases.

Although hepatic granulomas have been considered a characterisitic finding in patients with brucellosis, this occurs in 20% of cases or fewer. *Brucella melitensis* is one of the most common causes of granulomatous hepatitis in the Mediterranean countries. Hepatic lesions also have been described with *B. abortus* and *B. suis*. In *B. suis* infection, caseation necrosis may occur with subsequent calcification. The lesions rarely progress to cirrhosis although there may be widespread hepatic involvement. Hepatomegaly may be the only finding on physical examination. Diagnosis is substantiated by an appropriate clinical history and isolation of the organism from sites, such as blood, lungs, kidneys, bone marrow, or lymph nodes, that may have a higher yield than culture from liver biopsy tissue.

Histoplasmosis is the most frequent fungal cause of hepatic granulomas in the United States. The spleen and liver are the most common sites of dissemination. Histologically the lesions of histoplasmosis are identical to those of sarcoidosis. Serologic tests and skin testing are generally low-yield procedures in establishing a diagnosis, and cultures of blood, bone marrow, or liver tissue are more frequently useful.

Hepatic granulomas have been noted in other disseminated fungal infections, such as coccidioidomycosis, blastomycosis, and candidiasis. Granulomas are a characteristic finding in hepatic schistosomiasis (see Chapter 17). The granulomas in this condition may contain schistosomal ova or their remnants. Infection with *C. burnetti* produces granulomas with a characteristic fibrinoid material in either a ring-like configuration or broken rod–shaped strands. Although highly suggestive of Q fever, similar findings also have been reported in Hodgkin's disease.

NON-INFECTIOUS CAUSES OF HEPATIC GRANULOMAS

Sarcoidosis is a disease of unknown cause characterized by widespread granulomatous involvement of various organs. In 50% to 65% of cases, liver biopsy reveals the presence of granulomas. Autopsy studies have demonstrated granulomas in 75% of cases. In many recent series sarcoidosis is the most commonly asociated disorder, occurring in 30% to 50% of cases.

Symptoms of liver disease are frequently absent, and hepatic insufficiency is rare. Features that support a diagnosis of sarcoidosis are (1) noncaseating granulomas, (2) granulomatous infiltration of at least one other tissue, e.g., skin, lymph node, lung, or eye, and (3) failure to identify other causes by appropriate cultures of sputum and gastric washings, special stains for acid-fast organisms and fungi, or skin testing. Other features that may suggest this diagnosis include a relatively long duration of symptoms, evidence of intrathoracic disease, and response to steroid treatment.

Laboratory findings generally include increased AP levels with a normal serum bilirubin. Serum angiotensin-converting enzyme may be increased but should be interpreted cautiously because elevated levels also have been found in cases of PBC, silicosis, asbestosis, and leprosy, among other disorders.

Sarcoid granulomas are usually discrete, round follicles up to 2 mm in diameter. The lesions are located predominantly around portal tracts but also may be present in midcentral and midzonal areas. Although true caseation necrosis does not occur, a central area of eosinophilic necrosis and ductular debris may be present. The reticulin framework is maintained, unlike in tuberculous granulomas. Although the histologic appearance may suggest sarcoidosis, this appearance is not diagnostic when taken alone and must be interpreted in conjunction with clinical and laboratory findings.

Primary Biliary Cirrhosis

In the early stages of PBC, granulomas may appear in association with damaged interlobular bile ducts. Histologically this lesion may be indistinguishable from sarcoidosis. The diagnosis can be established in the majority of cases by the combination of compatible histology, clinical history, and the presence of antimitochondrial antibodies.

Drug Reactions

Drug reactions may cause hepatic granulomas. Most of these reactions are thought to be hypersensitivity reactions with eosinophils present in the granulomas.

Criteria that may be useful in determining evidence for drug-induced granulomas include clear temporal relationship between the use of the drug and onset of the adverse reaction; clinical, biochemical, and histologic improvement after withdrawal of the drug; and exclusion of other causes.

Hepatic granulomas have been noted in various multisystemic diseases, e.g., collagen vascular diseases, such as Wegener's granulomatosis and temporal arteritis. In the latter disorder granulomas appear in the perivascular tissue and walls of medium-sized arteries.

Hepatic granulomas also have been reported in association with malignancies, such as lymphomas and intraabdominal solid tumors. Whipple's disease has been associated with granulomas with bacillary inclusions in the liver. Hepatic granulomas also have been associated with celiac disease and have been described following jejunoileal bypass surgery.

SUMMARY

Hepatic granulomas are relatively common. There are numerous potential causes, and it is important to determine the cause whenever possible because of the implications for treatment.

SUGGESTED READINGS

Guckian JC and Perry JE: Granulomatous hepatitis: an analysis of 63 cases and review of the literature, Ann Intern Med 65:1081-1100, 1966.

Of the patients in this study, 53% had underlying tuberculosis. The authors discuss clinical, histopathologic, and laboratory data that are helpful in establishing this diagnosis.

Harrington PT et al: Granulomatous hepatitis, Rev Infect Dis 4:638-655, 1982.

This is a thorough and relatively recent review of the area. This paper emphasizes the diagnostic evaluation and controversial management of undiagnosed cases.

Irani SK and Dobbins WO: Hepatic granulomas: a review of 73 patients from one hospital and survey of the literature, J Clin Gastroenterol 1:131-143, 1979.

The authors describe their experience with the clinical and laboratory associations in 73 patients with hepatic granulomas.

Ishak KG and Zimmerman HJ: Drug-induced and toxic granulomatous hepatitis, Baillieres Clin Gastroenterol 2:463-480, 1988.

This is a recent and extensive review of more than 50 drugs and miscellaneous hepatotoxins that have been implicated in the production of hepatic granulomas.

Klatskin G: Hepatic granulomata: problems in interpretation, Ann N Y Acad Sci:427-432, 1976.

The authors review their experience with 565 cases of biopsy-documented hepatic granulomas. The study emphasizes the heterogeneity of the causes of this disorder.

Klatskin G and Yesner R: Hepatic manifestations of sarcoidosis and other granulomatous diseases: a study based on histological examination of tissue obtained by needle biopsy of the liver, Yale J Biol Med 23:207-248, 1950.

This is one of the earliest and best descriptions of the histologic appearance of granulomas associated with sarcoidosis, tuberculosis, and other miscellaneous conditions. It is based on a series of 650 needle biopsies of the liver.

Maddrey WC et al: Sarcoidosis and chronic hepatic disease: a clinical and pathologic study of 20 patients, Medicine 49:375-395, 1970.

This is a frequently cited paper that discusses the clinical and pathological spectrum of patients with hepatic sarcoidosis. Corticosteroids are shown to be helpful only in the early phases of the disease.

21 Cystic Diseases of the Liver

Michele Woodley

CONGENITAL CYSTIC DISEASES

The biliary system develops in two parts. The intrahepatic and extrahepatic ducts form separately. They join at the interlobular ducts in the portal septa to form the complete biliary system. Cystic diseases of the liver (see box) are thought to result from faulty development of the intrahepatic ductal system. (Cysts of the bile ducts are discussed in Chapter 30.) At 4 weeks' gestation, hepatic parenchyma can be found encircling areas of mesenchyme and the portal vein. At 6 weeks' gestation the hepatocytes that are in direct contact with the mesenchyme are transformed into bile duct cells. A second layer of hepatocytes undergoes similar transformation, forming two rows of bile duct cells with a slitlike lumen between them encircling the portal vein and its surrounding mesenchymal connective tissue. This is known as the ductal plate and occurs at 9 weeks' gestation. Duplication of the ductal plate and formation of a larger lumen occur in certain areas, resulting in a "beaded necklace" appearance. These tubular structures are incorporated into the connective tissue surrounding the portal vein and become individual bile ducts. The ductal plate appears near the hilum first. At birth the smallest branches of the portal vein do not have fully developed bile ducts.

During fetal development many more bile ducts are formed than are needed. The excess ducts usually involute. Those that fail to do so form cysts. Microscopic cysts are called microhammartomas. Cysts greater than 10 cm can also develop, as seen in adult polycystic disease. Some cystic liver diseases result from a malformation of the ductal plate and not merely from a failure of involution. Ductal plate malformation is seen in congenital hepatic fibrosis, infantile polycystic disease, and some forms of Caroli's disease.

CYSTIC DISEASES OF THE LIVER

Congenital	Acquired
Microhammartomas	Inflammatory
Congenital hepatic fibrosis	Traumatic
Polycystic disease	Neoplastic
Infantile	Benign
Adult	Malignant
Caroli's disease	Metastatic
Choledochal cysts	
Solitary cysts	

Fibropolycystic Diseases

Fibropolycystic diseases of the liver consist of an overlapping family of disorders, i.e., a single patient can manifest several of the disorders. This overlapping makes strict classification of these diseases impractical. Although the following sections discuss these disorders separately, the reader should remember that they often occur together (Table 21-1).

Table 21-1 also lists those cystic diseases associated with an increased risk of malignancy. Cholangiocarcinoma is the most common associated malignancy and occurs in disorders in which the cyst epithelium is in contact with bile for prolonged periods. This occurs in congenital hepatic fibrosis, Caroli's disease, and choledochal cysts. A few cases of cholangiocarcinoma have been associated with microhammartomas and adult polycystic disease.

Microhammartomas. In 1918 von Meyenberg described clusters of small bile ducts in and near portal tracts. These clusters became known as von Meyenberg complexes, or microhammartomas. These dilated bile ductules, ranging in size from 0.1 cm to 0.3 cm, are lined by cuboidal epithelium. They represent the excess intrahepatic ducts that failed to involute. They are surrounded by a fibrous tissue stroma and can contain inspissated bile. On gross examination they appear as focal white nodular lesions in the subcapsular area of the liver. They communicate with each other and with normal bile ducts. When the surrounding fibrous tissue predominates, the disease is indistinguishable from congenital hepatic fibrosis. In some patients the cysts enlarge with time, resulting in adult polycystic disease. Microhammartomas have been found in patients with medullary sponge kidney.

Diagnosis is usually incidental at autopsy because the disease is without symptoms or laboratory abnormalities. The incidence in routine autopsies is 0.79%. Rarely they are diffuse and can be diagnosed by arteriography, which reveals stretching of the arteries and early venous filling. There have been two reported cases of cholangiocarcinoma in patients with microhammartomas. No treatment is needed for microhammartomas unless they are associated with other diseases.

Polycystic diseases. There are three types of polycystic liver diseases: childhood, adult, and Caroli's. The childhood and adult forms have multiple hepatic cysts and renal abnormalities but are otherwise unrelated. Caroli's disease is discussed in Chapter 9.

Infantile polycystic disease is a rare autosomal recessive disorder. There are four groups: perinatal, neonatal, infantile, and juvenile. The kidneys have cystic dilations of the distal and collecting tubules and are grossly cystic. In the liver there is ductal plate malformation, and the cysts are not seen on gross examination. Microscopically the portal tracts have fibrosis and an increased number of bile ducts, leading some authors to consider this a form of congenital hepatic fibrosis. The liver parenchyma is normal, as are the renal glomeruli, calyces, and ureters.

The most severely affected are stillborn. The perinatal group has minimal hepatic fibrosis but severe renal involvement, with more than 90% of the tubules affected. These infants present at birth with huge bilateral renal masses. They usually die within 6 weeks from respira-

Table 21-1 Characteristics of cystic diseases of the liver

	Micro-hammar-toma	Congenital hepatic fibrosis	Infantile polycystic disease	Adult polycystic disease	Caroli's disease	Choledochal cyst	Solitary cyst
Inheritance	—	Autosomal recessive	Autosomal recessive	Autosomal dominant	Autosomal recessive/ sporadic	—	—
Age	All ages	3-10 years	Birth-5 years	40-50 years	20-35 years	13 years	40-50 years
Male to female ratio	1:1	—	1:1	1:4	3:1		1:4
Cyst lining	Cuboidal	—	—	Cuboidal or columnar	Cuboidal	Variable	Columnar/ squamous
Liver enzymes	Normal	Mild ↑ AP	Normal	Normal	Cholestatic or normal	Cholestatic or normal	Normal
Symptoms	None	PHT	PHT, renal failure	Abdominal pain	Abdominal pain, cholangitis	Pain, jaundice, pancreatitis	Abdominal fullness
Diagnosis	Autopsy, liver bx	Liver bx	Liver bx, intra-venous pyelo-gram	Ultrasound, CT scan	Ultrasound, cholangiogram	Ultrasound, CT scan, cholangiogram	Ultrasound
Associated diseases	CHF, Caroli's	Renal tubules	Renal, CHF	Renal, Berry aneurysm, microhammar-tomas	CHF renal	Caroli's	—
Cholangio-carcinoma	(see p. 374)	1%	No	(see p. 377)	7%	4%	No
Treatment	None	Shunt, bile acid therapy	Renal transplant, liver transplant	Liver transplant, unroofing	Biliary stents, bile acid therapy, liver transplant	Excision, sphinc-terotomy	Excision, unroofing if symptoms exist

PHT = portal hypertension; CHF = congenital hepatic fibrosis; liver bx = liver biopsy.

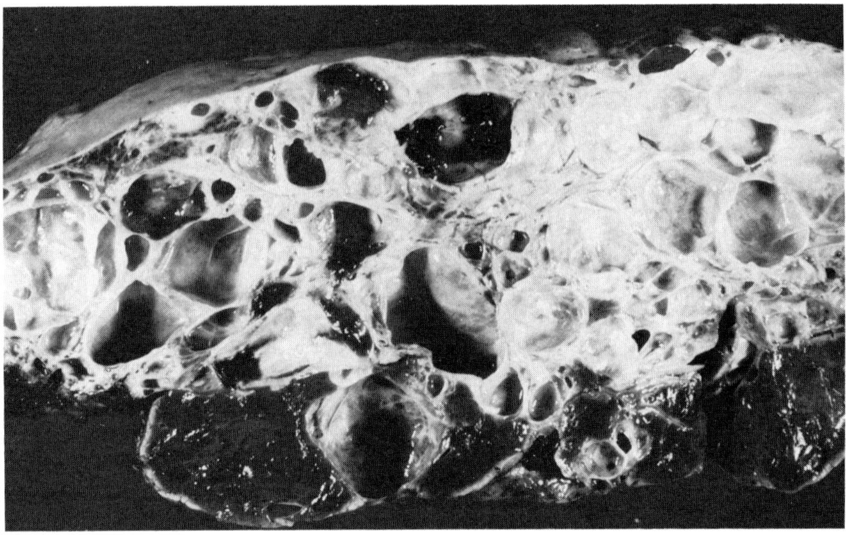

Figure 21-1
Gross specimen from a patient with adult polycystic disease who underwent liver transplantation. Note the variable size of the cysts. (Courtesy of Dr. Elizabeth Brunt.)

tory or renal failure. At the other end of the spectrum is the juvenile form. These children present between the ages of 1 and 5 years with portal hypertension and hepatomegaly. In contrast to the perinatal group, less than 10% of the renal tubules of the juvenile group are affected, but the group has severe hepatic fibrosis. The neonatal and infantile forms lie between these two extremes.

Diagnosis of the perinatal or neonatal forms is made by nephrotomograms and excretory urograms in the appropriate clinical setting. Unfortunately the diagnosis is often made at autopsy. In those who present after the age of 3 months, hepatomegaly usually is evident, along with enlarged kidneys. These children should undergo a liver biopsy in addition to the evaluation described above.

Treatment depends on the age of presentation. Neonatal disease is primarily renal. These patients require treatment for their severe hypertension, congestive heart failure, and progressive renal failure. A renal transplant or dialysis is often necessary. The juvenile group suffers primarily from liver disease and portal hypertension. Treatment includes a portosystemic shunt or liver transplantation.

Adult polycystic disease is an autosomal dominant disorder in which the liver is diffusely involved with large cysts (Figure 21-1). Occasionally it is focal. The cysts arise from gradual dilation of von Meyenberg complexes and range in size from less than 1 cm to greater than 10 cm. Cysts larger than 10 cm probably result from rupture of septa between cysts. The cysts are of bile duct origin and are lined by cuboidal epithelium, which secretes fluid resembling the bile salt independent fraction of bile. Most cysts do not communicate directly with the rest of the biliary system, so any biliary fluid within the cyst is due to rupture of a bile duct into the cyst. The hepatic parenchyma is normal. The aminotransaminase levels are normal, but mild elevations of AP and indirect bilirubin have been noted. Adult polycystic disease has been seen in conjunction with congenital hepatic fibrosis.

Adult polycystic liver disease and adult polycystic kidney disease probably result from the same developmental abnormality. The two are often found together. Of patients with renal cysts, 15% to 75% have hepatic cysts, and 50% of patients with hepatic cysts have renal cysts. Of patients with hepatic cysts, 5% have cysts in other organs, e.g., spleen, lung, pancreas, and seminal vesicles, and 10% to 36% have berry aneurysms.

Polycystic liver disease is found in 0.5% of routine autopsies. The frequency of this disorder increases with age in those who have polycystic kidneys. Only 11% of patients age 20 to 29 with polycystic kidneys have hepatic cysts, 77% of patients over 60 have them.

Polycystic liver disease is slightly more common in females. Females account for 80% of symptomatic cases and are more likely to have massive cysts. Most females present after age 40 with vague complaints of epigastric pain or abdominal distension. Rupture of a cyst or hemorrhage into it can cause severe abdominal pain. Massive hepatomegaly is often evident on physical examination, but liver size can be normal in localized disease.

The diagnosis is made by ultrasound or CT scan (Figure 21-2). When the disease is focal, the differential diagnosis includes hydatid cysts, solitary cysts, and metastases. If there are concomitant polycystic kidneys, the disorder is almost certainly polycystic liver disease.

Complications occur in fewer than 5% of cases and include hemorrhage into a cyst and infection or rupture of the cyst. Rarely, large cysts can obstruct the biliary tree, leading to jaundice. A few cases of cholangiocarcinoma have been reported. Prognosis classically has been determined by the extent of renal disease. Since the advent of dialysis and renal transplantation, patients are surviving longer. Liver complications account for up to 10% of all deaths.

Treatment is needed only for those with incapacitating symptoms. Infected cysts require external drainage and/or antibiotics. For cysts that do not contain bile, several options exist. If only a few cysts are responsible for symptoms, aspiration can be attempted under ultrasound or CT guidance, but the fluid often reaccumulates. Ethanol has been used as a sclerosant after fluid aspiration. There are also several surgical options. Unroofing larger cysts is effective in controlling symptoms. In patients with diffuse disease, fenestration of deeper cysts in addition to unroofing larger cysts has been advocated, but a recent study reports a higher morbidity and mortality in patients undergoing fenestration. Simultaneous hepatic and renal transplantation has been performed successfully.

Solitary Cysts

Solitary cysts are found in 0.1% to 0.3% of autopsy specimens. They can be congenital or acquired. Congenital cysts are more common in women and are diagnosed between age 50 and 70. Acquired

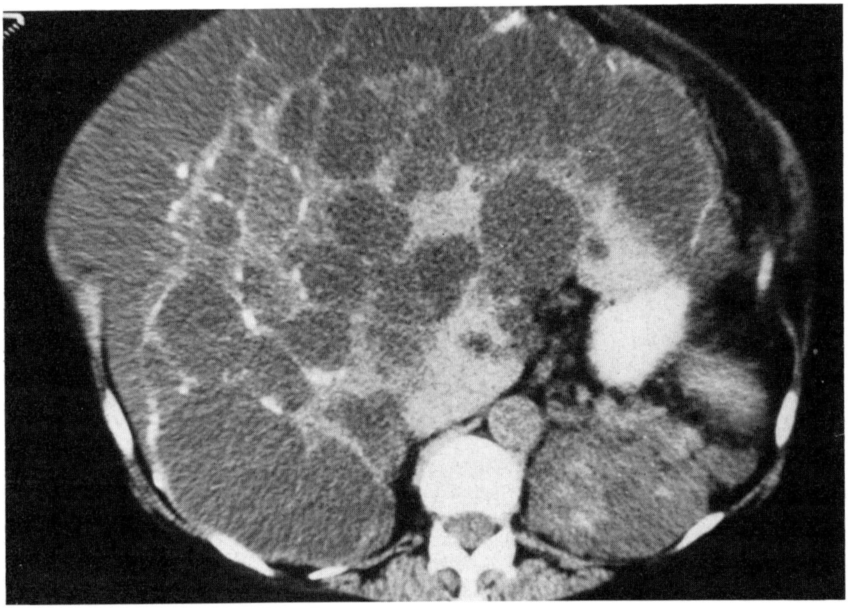

Figure 21-2
Abdominal CT scan of the same patient shown in Figure 21-1. Note the diffuse location of the cysts and their variable size. (Courtesy of Dr. Elizabeth Brunt.)

cysts are more common in men and are diagnosed between age 40 and 50.

Congenital cysts grow slowly, and their cause is unknown. They usually are found in the right lobe of the liver and are not associated with cysts in other organs. However, some solitary cysts are multiloculated and resemble focal polycystic disease. This finding should prompt a search for cysts in other organs. An intravenous pyelogram and a detailed family history are needed.

The fibrous sheath of the cyst contains bile ducts and blood vessels. It is lined by cuboidal, columnar, or squamous epithelium. Only one third of solitary cysts produce symptoms. They are often an incidental finding at surgery. In such cases they should not be removed unless pedunculated and easily resected. An asymptomatic solitary cyst can be observed for growth or signs of malignancy using ultrasonography.

Symptomatic cysts are large, with a mean size of 15 cm. Nearly 50% have neighboring smaller cysts. Symptoms include a palpable mass, RUQ or epigastric pain, and hepatomegaly. Liver enzymes are normal unless there is infection or malignancy. When large and strategically located, solitary cysts can cause jaundice and portal hypertension. Severe abdominal pain occurs with hemorrhage into the cyst or torsion of a pedunculated cyst. Fever and chills suggest hemorrhage or infection.

Diagnosis of a solitary cyst is by ultrasound, CT scan, or liver scan. Calcification is rare. If the cyst is large and the patient is symptomatic, a sample of the fluid should be sent for culture and cytology. Hydatid cysts are an exception because cyst contents can be under pressure, and aspiration can lead to peritoneal seeding.

The fluid in a solitary cyst is clear unless hemorrhage into the cyst or rupture of a bile duct has occurred. If the fluid is clear, simple excision can be performed. Aspiration is associated with fluid reaccumulation. Sclerosis with 95% ethanol is a nonsurgical alternative. Massive cysts are treated by unroofing a large portion of the cyst and allowing it to drain into the peritoneum. If this is done, a large sample of the cyst wall should be sent for frozen section to exclude malignancy. If the fluid is biliary, a cholangiogram is needed to assess communication with the biliary tree. If there is a communication, a roux-en-Y anastomosis can be performed. Alternatively, wide unroofing and oversewing of biliary radicles has been advocated. Purulent fluid requires antibiotics and/or external drainage.

Complications include infection, hemorrhage, and torsion of pedunculated cysts. Carcinoma is rare in a solitary cyst, but benign tumors have been found.

ACQUIRED CYSTIC DISEASES

There are numerous causes for acquired hepatic cysts. The cysts may be single or multiple, and determining the specific cause of a cyst can be difficult. Ultrasound and CT scan are the initial radiologic tests used. Occasionally a small cyst is seen in the periphery of the liver on ultrasound or CT scan performed for an unrelated reason. These cysts may result from focal obstruction of hepatic lymphatics. Some cysts may be microhammartomas. An asymptomatic patient with a superficial simple cyst several millimeters in size needs no further therapeutic or diagnostic procedures.

Many malignant and benign cystic liver lesions have similar imaging characteristics. A simple cyst is roughly spherical without a capsule. Separations, thick or irregular walls, papillary projections, or calcium require further investigation. Calcium is found in hydatid cysts, tumors, and lymphangiomas but is very rare in a simple cyst. Septae are found in hydatid cysts, tumors, and inflammatory cysts. Amebic abscesses classically have a halo of low-density tissue surrounding the abscess when viewed by CT scan. Other abscesses frequently have air-fluid levels.

Although a CT scan is helpful in evaluating renal cysts, hepatic cysts are evaluated better through ultrasound. Ultrasound is better at distinguishing nodules, septations, and fluid levels. If there is any question regarding the nature of the cyst, aspiration of the fluid and appropriate biochemical, microbiologic, and cytologic studies should be done.

Traumatic Cysts

Trauma is an uncommon cause of hepatic cysts in part because of the protection the rib cage affords. Traumatic cysts are usually in the right lobe of the liver and are often symptomatic. Symptoms include abdominal pain and distention, which can be dated to shortly after the occurrence of severe trauma to the abdomen. The cysts are most likely secondary to intrahepatic hemorrhage and contain old blood and bile. Treatment of traumatic cysts consists of drainage.

Tumors

Cystic liver tumors are much more likely to be metastatic than primary. Any metastasis can develop central necrosis or cystic degeneration and be radiographically identical to a cystic tumor. Ovarian, gastric, and small cell carcinomas, cholangiocarcinomas, choriocarcinomas, hepatic adenomas, and certain sarcomas are associated with cystic metastases.

Cystadenomas and cystadenocarcinomas are primary cystic liver tumors. They are developmental in origin. Cystadenomas occur throughout the biliary tree. Cystadenocarcinomas arise from cystadenomas but are confined to the intrahepatic biliary system. Both range in size from 1 cm to 15 cm and are lined by cuboidal or columnar biliary epithelium. Ulcerations and focal malignant change can occur.

The symptoms are identical to those seen with nonmalignant cysts, namely RUQ pain, increased abdominal girth, and occasionally a palpable mass. Because their imaging characteristics are also similar to those of nonmalignant cysts, a high index of suspicion is needed. Often a slight increase in transaminase levels is the only clue. Nearly three fourths occur in women, usually over age 40.

Ultrasound studies may reveal septations, mural nodules, or calcification, all of which are rare in simple cysts. Treatment is by surgical excision because cystadenomas rarely recur. If carcinoma is present in the excised cyst, surgery usually is also curative. Metastases are rare.

SUMMARY

Cystic diseases of the liver include a variety of congenital and acquired disorders. Some of these disorders are associated with an increased risk of malignancy, and these patients should be followed closely. With the advent of liver transplantation, many of the congenital diseases can be cured.

SUGGESTED READINGS

Blyth H and Ockenden B: Polycystic disease of kidneys and liver presenting in childhood, J Med Genet 8:257-284, 1971.

An extensive review of polycystic disease of the liver and kidney is provided.

Chung EB: Multiple bile duct hammartomas, Cancer 26:787, 1970.

The author reviews microhammartomas and their frequency in routine autopsy specimens.

Everson GT et al: Polycystic liver disease: quantitation of parenchymal and cyst volumes from computed tomography images and clinical correlates of hepatic cysts, Hepatology 8:1627-1634, 1988.

This article discusses hepatic parenchymal volume in polycystic disease and why patients rarely develop liver failure.

Grunfield JP et al: Liver changes and complications in adult polycystic kidney disease, Adv Nephrol 14:1-20, 1985.

This article reviews the morbidity and mortality of polycystic disease and how they have changed since the advent of hemodialysis and renal transplantation.

Honda N, Cobb C, and Lechago J: Bile duct carcinoma associated with multiple von Meyenberg complexes in the liver, Hum Pathol 17:1287-1290, 1986.

This article describes a case of bile duct carcinoma in a patient with microhammartomas and reviews the literature on this subject.

Litwin DE et al: Nonparasitic cysts of the liver, Ann Surg 205:45-48, 1987.

This article reviews the surgical options in 22 patients with liver cysts. Nearly half of the cysts are solitary. The article contains a flow chart reviewing the results of different surgical procedures.

Milutinovic J et al: Autosomal dominant polycystic kidney disease with liver and pancreatic involvement in early childhood, Am J Kidney Dis 13:340-344, 1989.

This article describes the clinical and pathologic findings in children with adult polycystic kidney disease and its relationship to polycystic liver disease.

Philips RL: The radiology of cystic liver tumors, Australas Radiol 33:66-68, 1988.

This article clearly describes the radiologic features of liver cysts.

Summerfield JA et al: Hepatobiliary fibropolycystic diseases, J Hepatol 2:141-156, 1986.

This is a recent review of polycystic liver disease.

Turnage RH et al: Therapeutic dilemmas in patients with symptomatic polycystic liver disease, Am Surg 54:365-372, 1988.

This article reviews the cases of nine patients with polycystic liver disease who underwent various surgical procedures. The risks, benefits, and complications of surgery are discussed.

Van Eycken P et al: The developement of the intrahepatic bile ducts in man: a keratin immunohistochemical study, Hepatology 8:1586-1595, 1988.

This article gives a clear and comprehensive review of bile duct formation.

22 Liver Dysfunction Secondary to Anesthesia and Surgery

Fredric G. Regenstein

EFFECTS OF ANESTHETIC AGENTS AND SURGERY ON THE LIVER

Agents administered during general anesthesia have a variety of effects on hepatic function and blood flow. All anesthetic agents reduce hepatic blood flow, with the inhalational agents causing the greatest reductions. Of the inhalational agents, halothane appears to have the most profound effects, causing a greater decrease in hepatic blood flow and hepatic oxygen content and greater impairment of hepatic excretory function than either enflurane or isoflurane. The IV anesthetic agents, ketamine, etomidate, and althesin, also can reduce hepatic blood flow by increasing vascular resistance in the mesenteric and hepatic arterial vasculature. Because laparotomy alone results in a decrease in hepatic blood flow, the effects of surgery and anesthesia are additive.

POSTOPERATIVE HEPATIC DYSFUNCTION

Patients developing postoperative hepatic dysfunction can be subdivided into three groups. The first group consists of patients with no preexisting liver disease who develop hepatic dysfunction after their surgery. Included within this category would be patients with anesthesia or drug-induced liver disease and patients with ischemic and post-transfusion hepatitis. The second group consists of patients not suspected of having liver dysfunction who are found to have liver disease either at the time of surgery or during the postoperative period. The last group consists of patients known to have liver disease before surgery. This group includes the entire spectrum of patients with liver disease, ranging from those with asymptomatic, chronic hepatitis to patients with end-stage cirrhosis, portal hypertension, and hepatic encephalopathy.

Patients without Preexisting Liver Disease

Early postoperative liver dysfunction. In patients without preexisting liver disease, postoperative hepatic dysfunction can occur immediately after surgery, or it can be delayed for several weeks. The box on p. 384 lists the most frequent causes of early postoperative liver dys-

FREQUENT CAUSES OF EARLY POSTOPERATIVE LIVER DYSFUNCTION

- Increased bilirubin production
  - Transfusions
  - Hemoglobin reabsorption from the operative field
  - Hemolysis
- Ischemic hepatitis
  - Hypotension
  - Passive congestion
  - Surgical injury to hepatic blood supply
- Sepsis
- Benign postoperative intrahepatic cholestasis
- Drug-induced hepatitis
  - Inhalational anesthetics
  - Other drugs
- Biliary tract disease
  - Surgical injury to bile duct
    - Biliary stricture
    - Bile leak
  - Choledocholithiasis
  - Acalculous cholecystitis
- Postoperative pancreatitis
- Graft vs. host disease

function. In most cases early hepatic dysfunction occurs as a consequence of increased bilirubin production. Transient hyperbilirubinemia may occur in up to 20% of patients undergoing major surgery, with as many as 3.7% of patients developing clinically significant jaundice. Individuals receiving large amounts of blood develop a slight increase in indirect bilirubin as the transfused RBCs are destroyed prematurely and the bilirubin is delivered to the liver for excretion. Resorption of hematomas and retained blood in body cavities leads to hyperbilirubinemia by the same mechanism. Coexisting alterations in hepatocyte metabolism may impair bilirubin excretion further. The mechanisms responsible for the postsurgical impairment in hepatic excretory function are incompletely understood.

Perioperative hypotension, especially when associated with massive transfusion, congestive heart failure, sepsis, or respiratory failure, frequently leads to postoperative hepatic dysfunction. Profound hyperbilirubinemia associated with marked increases in aminotransferase typically is present in these patients. The aminotransferase elevations are transient and return to near normal within several days of correction of the hypotension. In these patients hyperbilirubinemia, with or without AP elevation, may persist for weeks after surgery. This cholestatic syndrome has been designated *benign postoperative intrahepatic cholestasis.* Although the liver dysfunction in these patients is almost never life-threatening, patients with this syndrome have high mortality because of the multitude of associated medical problems. The mechanism responsible for the intrahepatic cholestatic reaction in these patients remains obscure. Recovery may be delayed further by the coincidental administration of total parenteral nutrition. After the associated medical problems have improved or resolved, hepatic excretory function gradually returns to normal.

Drugs administered perioperatively also can lead to hepatic dysfunction. Halothane has been the most extensively studied; however, other inhalational agents also have been implicated (see Chapter 18, Drug Hepatitis). In patients developing unexplained postoperative hepatic dysfunction, all potentially hepatotoxic medications should be discontinued.

Most often this involves careful chart review to see if any of the most frequently implicated agents have been administered. Particular attention should be directed to the antiemetics, antibiotics, antihypertensives, and the type of anesthesia administered. In the event that certain medications cannot be discontinued, alternative agents with less hepatotoxic potential should be substituted.

Surgery involving the liver or biliary tract may be complicated by retained bile duct stones or a bile duct injury resulting in biliary obstruction or a bile leak. In both situations hyperbilirubinemia associated with variable elevations of aminotransferase and AP is present. The diagnosis can be confirmed with hepatic imaging procedures. Postoperative pancreatitis, with or without biliary obstruction, and acalculous cholecystitis may also result in hepatic dysfunction after surgery. Graft vs. host disease may be associated with either early-onset or late-onset hepatic dysfunction.

Late-onset postoperative hepatic dysfunction. Post-transfusion and drug-induced hepatitis are the most common causes of hepatic dysfunction occurring more than 3 weeks after surgery. Post-transfusion hepatitis typically presents 6 to 8 weeks after transfusion. The presentation can vary from asymptomatic patients with mild elevations of aminotransferase to patients with deep jaundice and early signs of hepatic encephalopathy. Abnormalities of liver tests also may be identified in approximately 1% of non-transfused patients. The cause of liver dysfunction may not be apparent in many of these patients. Some patients may have hepatic dysfunction related to drugs or alcohol, and other patients may have preexisting liver or biliary tract disease that was not recognized before surgery. Patients receiving prolonged total parenteral nutrition also may present more than 3 weeks after surgery with evidence of cholestatic hepatic dysfunction.

Evaluation of the patient presenting with delayed-onset hepatic dysfunction requires careful review of the patient history. The hospital record should be reviewed to determine the presence of any evidence of liver dysfunction before surgery, the exact nature of the operative procedure, the presence of any intraoperative or postoperative complications, the amount of blood products received, and a complete list of all medications. Patients with suspected biliary tract disease should undergo hepatic imaging, and patients thought to have hepatitis should have serologic tests performed for hepatitis A, B, and C and cytomegalovirus. Most cases of acute post-transfusion hepatitis C will be negative for the hepatitis C virus antibody when tested early in their course, thus the diagnosis remains one of exclusion. Medications should be discontinued or substituted in those patients thought to have drug-induced disease.

Patients with Unrecognized Preexisting Liver Disease

Most patients with preexisting liver disease are identified preoperatively by history, physical examination, or laboratory evaluation. In occasional circumstances occult liver disease is identified either at the time of surgery or in the postoperative period. These patients usually tolerate anesthesia and surgery without difficulty. After most surgical procedures, liver tests are normal or only slightly impaired. In patients undergoing hepatic resection or major surgical procedures, more profound disturbances of liver function may occur as a consequence of hepatic oxygen deprivation. Patients with underlying liver disease may develop hepatic ischemia as a result of their inability to increase hepatic artery blood flow in response to the reductions in portal venous blood supply induced by anesthesia and laparotomy. Hyperbilirubinemia and moderate to marked aminotransferase elevations are typically present in these patients, but most patients recover without sequelae. In occasional cases severe cholestasis and progressive liver failure can occur.

Patients with Recognized Preexisting Liver Disease

Well-compensated liver disease. For the majority of patients with well-compensated liver disease, the risks of anesthesia and surgery are small. This group includes patients with a variety of liver disorders, including chronic hepatitis, early sclerosing cholangitis and PBC, hepatic neoplasms, and cirrhosis. Preoperatively these patients are well nourished and minimally symptomatic and they show no evidence of ascites or hepatic encephalopathy. Laboratory evaluation reveals normal or nearly normal values for serum albumin, bilirubin, and PT. Minor surgical procedures can be performed in this population with complication rates comparable to those occurring in normal patients. In patients undergoing major abdominal, thoracic, or emergency procedures, the complication rates are higher than for comparable operations performed on patients without liver disease.

After surgery and anesthesia these patients may develop transient deterioration of liver tests, but they rarely develop significant problems unless the surgery involves hepatic resection or is complicated by massive transfusion or hypotension. Edema and ascites may occur after surgery, but most often this can be readily managed with careful attention to fluid balance and administration of diuretics.

Moderate and advanced liver disease. Surgery in patients with severe or moderately severe liver disease is fraught with danger and is associated with markedly increased morbidity and mortality. Increased blood loss, impaired wound healing, increased susceptibility to infections, alterations of drug metabolism, and inability to tolerate the reduction in hepatic blood flow induced by anesthesia and surgery all contribute to the higher risk in these patients. Hepatic failure, bleeding, and sepsis are the most common causes of postoperative death in these patients.

The Child's classification, although intended as an estimate of hepatic reserve for patients undergoing portosystemic shunt surgery, also can be applied to estimate the operative risk of cirrhotic patients undergoing other types of surgery. Child's class A patients are well compensated and at a relatively low risk for postoperative complications. Child's class B and class C patients are heterogeneous and vary widely in their ability to tolerate surgery. A variety of factors, in addition to the Child's classification, have been analyzed to evaluate an individual's ability to tolerate surgery. The variables that appear to have some predictive value include PT, PTT, hepatic histology, and aminopyrine breath test results. A PT or PTT greater than 2 seconds prolonged, active alcoholic hepatitis on liver biopsy, and an aminopyrine breath test less than 2.3% all appear to correlate with an increased operative mortality. Also, patients requiring emergency operations and those with a large operative blood loss (greater than 1000 ml) are at high risk.

Improvements in hepatic-imaging techniques nearly have eliminated the need to perform exploratory surgery to diagnose obstructive jaundice. In past decades patients with jaundice caused by hepatocellular dysfunction occasionally were subjected to operative exploration, often with disastrous consequences. Patients undergoing laparotomy with jaundice caused by either acute viral hepatitis or acute alcoholic hepatitis are at a very high risk and should have surgery cancelled or postponed if possible.

Despite advances in surgical technique, critical care, and anesthesia, laparotomy in patients with advanced liver disease can be associated with mortality rates exceeding 80%. Thus, in patients requiring surgery, as much attention needs to be directed to the patient's underlying liver disease as to the problem necessitating the surgical procedure. A careful preoperative assessment is mandatory and should include consultations among surgery, anesthesiology, and hepatology or gastroenterology. Patients with suspected biliary tract obstruction should undergo direct cholangiography, because endoscopic management of choledocholithiasis or biliary tract obstruction in cirrhotic patients is preferable to laparotomy and common bile duct exploration. Stabilization of the patient and avoidance of an emergency procedure should be attempted if possible. Patients whose surgery could be performed on an elective basis should be allowed extra time to optimize their status. Elective operations should be avoided in patients with acute hepatitis and in patients with chronic hepatitis during a relapse or episode of decompensation. Individuals with nutritional deficiencies should receive supplemental alimentation for a period before surgery. In particular, vitamin deficiencies and electrolyte abnormalities should be corrected before surgery. Patients with coagulopathies need preoperative fresh-frozen plasma. In selected cases plasmapheresis before surgery may be beneficial in patients with severe coagulopathies. Vasopressin administration intraoperatively may reduce operative blood loss, and a Swan-Ganz catheter during the perioperative period is helpful in managing fluid status.

SUMMARY

Elective surgical procedures and general anesthesia usually are tolerated well by patients with compensated chronic liver disease. However, in patients with decompensated acute or chronic liver disease, surgical morbidity and mortality are dramatically higher. If possible, emergency surgery should be avoided, and these patients should be managed medically until their condition is stable enough for an elective procedure to be performed. Before any planned surgery, patients at high risk should be evaluated by an experienced surgeon, and any subsequent decision regarding surgery should be made after consultation with a hepatologist.

SUGGESTED READINGS

Aranha GV, Sontag SJ and Greenlee HB: Cholecystectomy in cirrhotic patients: a formidable operation, Am J Surg 143: 55-60, 1982.

This report issues a warning to surgeons about the hazards of cholecystectomy in cirrhotic patients. Mortality rates in compensated cirrhotic patients were eight to nine times greater than in controls, and in patients with decompensated cirrhosis, the mortality rate exceeded 80%!

Doberneck RC, Sterling WA, and Allison DC: Morbidity and mortality after operation in nonbleeding cirrhotic patients, Am J Surg 146:306-309, 1983.

A description of the operative outcome in a group of 102 cirrhotic patients undergoing a variety of surgical procedures is presented. The overall mortality rate was 19.6%, increasing to 66.7% in those patients with multiple risk factors.

Gill RA et al: Aminopyrine breath test predicts surgical risk for patients with liver disease, Ann Surg 198:701-704, 1983.

This is a relatively small study demonstrating the value of the aminopyrine breath test in predicting operative mortality in patients with liver disease. An aminopyrine breath test less than 2.3% was associated with an extremely high mortality, but almost all patients with an aminopyrine breath test greater than 2.3% survived.

Harville DD and Summerskill HJS: Surgery in acute hepatitis: causes and effects, JAMA 184:257-261, 1963.

This is an article of historical significance describing the outcome of surgery in a group of 42 patients with viral hepatitis and 16 patients with drug-induced hepatitis who were operated on to exclude extrahepatic obstruction.

Mikkelsen WP, Turrill FL, and Kern WH: Acute hyaline necrosis of the liver: a surgical trap, Am J Surg 116:266-272, 1968.

A stern warning to physicians and surgeons about the dangers of operating on patients with severe alcoholic hepatitis is given. Four of 10 patients undergoing exploratory laparotomy died, and 15 of 18 patients undergoing emergency shunt procedures died.

Schmid M et al: Benign postoperative intrahepatic cholestasis, N Engl J Med 272-545-550, 1965.

This is a seminal article on the entity of postoperative cholestasis. "Benign" probably should be dropped from the description, given the 50% mortality rate.

Sirinek KR et al: Improving survival in patients with cirrhosis undergoing major abdominal operations, Arch Surg 122:271-273, 1987.

This report is not as pessimistic as the previous studies. With careful attention to preoperative preparation and good intraoperative management, the mortality rate in cirrhotic patients can be reduced to 8%.

23 Benign and Malignant Neoplasms of the Liver

Swan N. Thung and *Michael A. Gerber*

Hepatocellular carcinoma (HCC) is the most common visceral cancer in the world. It has a very high incidence (as high as 40% of all cancers) in regions with large populations such as sub-Saharan Africa, Southeast Asia, China, and Japan. In some of these countries, the annual death rate from HCC is higher than 100 per 100,000 population. In the Western world, cancer metastases from other organs represent the most common neoplasms in the liver. HCC is rare in North and South America, northern and central Europe, and Australia where it represents only about 0.5% to 2% of all cancers with annual death rates of 3 to 7 per 100,000 population. During the last 25 years, the frequency of this tumor has decreased in some parts of the world, such as South Africa, but increased in others, such as Japan. Throughout the world, HCC occurs in high incidence areas at a younger age than in low incidence areas. Thus the average age of Africans with HCC is below 40 years, whereas it is higher than 50 years in Americans. In addition to geography, race, and increasing age, male sex represents a risk factor for HCC (see box at right). The tumor is 2 to 4 times more frequent in men than in women. Cirrhosis of almost any cause is an important risk factor for HCC. About 75% of cases are associated with cirrhosis. The cirrhosis is usually macronodular, as in patients

MAJOR RISK FACTORS FOR DEVELOPMENT OF LIVER TUMORS IN HUMANS

- Geographical location, race
- Male sex, increasing age
- Viral infections: hepatitis B virus, hepatitis C virus
- Chemicals and drugs: alcohol, aflatoxins, anabolic steroids, oral contraceptive steroids
- Cirrhosis
- Congenital liver diseases: glycogen storage disease type I, hemochromatosis, α_1-antitrypsin deficiency, tyrosinemia, Caroli's disease, membranous obstruction of inferior vena cava, Wilson's disease, porphyria
- Radiation
  - Internal: Thorotrast
  - External: x radiation

with chronic viral hepatitis, and is characterized by large regenerating parenchymal nodules. In alcoholic patients with micronodular cirrhosis, HCC may emerge when large nodules develop after prolonged abstinence from alcohol. The so-called precursor lesions of HCC, i.e., adenomatous hyperplasia or nodule-in-nodule and dysplastic hepatocytes, are frequently seen in association with HCC. It should be emphasized that HCC may also develop in the absence of cirrhosis, as in fibrotic or histologically normal liver.

HEPADNAVIRUS CHARACTERISTICS

Enveloped spherical viruses containing partially double-stranded circular DNA

Hepatotropic

Encode 4 proteins: surface antigen, core antigen, DNA polymerase (reverse transcriptase), and X antigen

Natural hosts: man, Eastern woodchuck, Beechey ground squirrel, Peking duck, and others

Cause acute and chronic liver diseases: acute hepatitis, chronic hepatitis, cirrhosis, hepatocellular carcinoma, or asymptomatic carriers

ETIOLOGY

The risk factors listed above indicate that the cause of HCC is multi-factorial. It is one of the few human tumors where a direct relationship to viral infection has been clearly established, but other carcinogenic factors are probably also involved. Worldwide, most HCCs are associated with chronic infection by hepatitis B virus (HBV). Multiple lines of evidence indicate that HBV is causally related to HCC. First, there is a strong parallelism between the frequency of HBV carrier rates and the incidence of HCC in different countries. Large prospective studies, as in Taiwan, demonstrated that the relative risk of HBsAg-positive Taiwanese males developing HCC is at least 200 times greater than that of HBsAg-negative males. Second, HCC is often clustered among closely related relatives, presumably because of intra familial spread of HBV. In these families, HBV is transmitted perinatally or in early childhood and results in the development of a chronic HBV carrier state. The lag time between the initial HBV infection and the discovery of HCC is usually 20 years or longer, but HBV-associated HCC has been discovered in children as young as 5 years. Third, many studies demonstrated that the prevalence of serum HBsAg in HCC patients is significantly higher than that in control patients. Fourth, as is discussed later, HBV DNA has been detected in virtually all liver tumors of HBsAg-positive patients. In addition, patients without evidence of current HBV infection may carry HBV DNA in their livers or tumors. This includes patients who presumably have recovered from HBV infection and have anti-HBc or anti-HBs, or both, in their serum as well as patients without any serologic markers of HBV infection. Fifth, in addition to HBV DNA, HBsAg and less commonly HBcAg are frequently detected by immunohistochemical methods in the tumor bearing liver and less prominently in the tumor cells. Several tumor cell lines have been established from patients with HBV-associated HCC that secrete HBsAg into the culture media. Sixth, HBV belongs to the family of hepadnaviruses, i.e., DNA viruses that infect the liver of various animals including the Eastern woodchuck, Beechey ground squirrel, and Peking duck. If chronically infected, these animals frequently develop HCC. Virtually 100% of woodchucks infected at birth by the woodchuck hepatitis virus and kept in captivity on a carcinogen-free diet develop HCC by the time they are 3 years old. This represents direct evidence that the woodchuck hepatitis virus and presumably the other hepadnaviruses, including HBV, are oncogenic.

There is no evidence that hepatitis A virus or hepatitis D virus infections are associated with the development of HCC. Recent work, however, has linked hepatitis C virus (HCV) to liver cancer. Many patients with HCC have antibodies to HCV in their serum. HCV is the most frequent cause of posttransfusion hepatitis and often leads to chronic infection and cirrhosis. In Japan, the incidence of HBV-negative HCC is rising while the frequency of HBV-associated HCC remains constant. Many of these cases may be related to infection by HCV, but much more work needs to be done to determine the role of HCV in the development of HCC.

Chemical hepatocarcinogens, well studied in animal models, appear to play a minor role in human HCCs. Mycotoxins, particularly aflatoxin B_1, produced by the common fungi *Aspergillus flavus* and *Aspergillus parasiticus,* have long been incriminated, primarily in hot humid climates in sub-Saharan Africa and Southeast Asia. The degree of exposure to dietary aflatoxin, as in fungus-contaminated grain, parallels the frequency of HCC in these areas. Quantitative data indicate a dose-response relationship between aflatoxin ingestion and HCC. Other chemicals that cause liver tumors in animals and are commonly ingested in food stuffs include other mycotoxins, plant-derived carcinogens such as cycasin and saffrole, nitrosamines, chlorinated hydrocarbons, organochlorine pesticides, arsenic, and the radioactive dye Thorotrast. The pathogenetic relationship between alcohol abuse and HCC is not established, but the epidemiologic evidence is convincing in countries where the carrier rate of HBV is low. Some drugs, particularly anabolic steroids and less convincingly oral contraceptives, have been linked to the development of HCC. Many chronic liver diseases have been associated with an increased incidence of HCC. These include congenital liver diseases such as hemochromatosis, α_1-antitrypsin deficiency, tyrosinemia, Caroli's disease, membranous obstruction of the inferior vena cava and, rarely, Wilson's disease, autoimmune chronic active hepatitis, and primary biliary cirrhosis. In these conditions, it is not known whether the underlying disease or the cirrhotic state with the associated necroinflammatory and regenerative processes are involved in the oncogenic process.

MECHANISM OF HEPATOCARCINOGENESIS

Carcinogenesis represents a multistep process involving initiation, promotion, and progression (Figure 23-1). The first step is often alteration of DNA by binding of a reactive chemical to DNA such as the aflatoxin-derived epoxide, or insertion of viral DNA into the host cell DNA. The viral DNA integrations may be associated with general chromosomal defects

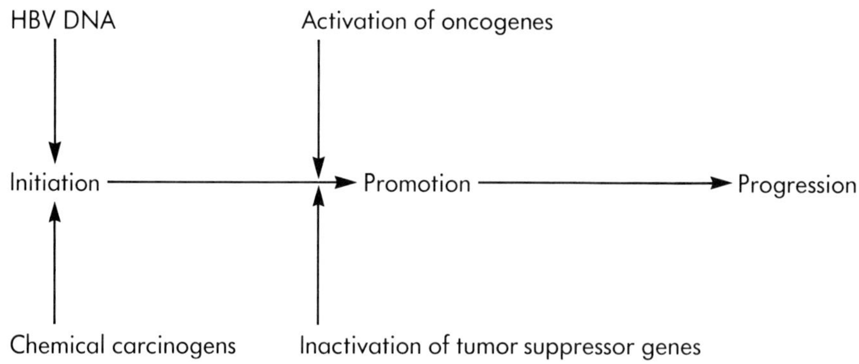

Figure 23-1
Mechanism of hepatocarcinogenesis.

such as deletions, transpositions, or translocations, or with specific effects caused by the viral DNA such as a viral oncogene, *cis*-or *trans*-activation of a proto-oncogene, or inactivation of a tumor suppressor gene. With respect to HBV, it is not known which of these mechanisms leads to malignant transformation of hepatocytes. It is clear, however, that the HCC cells have noticeable karyotypic changes (i.e., changes in chromosomal structure and number as described above and on p. 391). In addition, there are multiple random integrations of HBV DNA into the tumor cell chromosomes, and the viral DNA itself is "scrambled" with many deletions, duplications, and rearrangements. Although it appears that viral DNA integration represents a necessary event in HBV-associated hepatocarcinogenesis, it may not be sufficient and other factors, i.e., co-carcinogens, may be needed for malignant transformation. Furthermore, other etiologic factors of HCC may involve different mechanisms of carcinogenesis.

PATHOLOGY

Metastases to the Liver

Metastases are by far the most common malignant neoplasms in the liver. Usually they are not solitary but multiple irregular nodules of varying sizes scattered throughout both hepatic lobes. Areas of necrosis are often present in the center of the nodules. Occasional tumors spread diffusely through the sinusoids rather than forming distinct nodules and may not be grossly visible. The surrounding liver is usually not cirrhotic. Microscopically, metastases often resemble the primary tumor. Lung, breast, colon, and pancreas are the most common primary sites of hepatic metastases, but malignant tumors from almost any site can metastasize to the liver. Metastatic tumor has to be differentiated from intrahepatic cholangiocarcinoma and from hepatocellular carcinoma. It may be difficult when the tumor is poorly differentiated (Table 23-1).

Hepatocellular Carcinoma

HCC may exist as a solitary well-defined mass, as multiple nodules, or diffusely in-

Table 23-1 Abbreviated classification of primary liver tumors

	Benign	Malignant
Epithelial	Hepatocellular adenoma Bile duct adenoma Bile duct cystadenoma Intrahepatic biliary papillomatosis Focal nodular hyperplasia Diffuse nodular hyperplasia	Hepatocellular carcinoma Bile duct carcinoma (cholangiocarcinoma) Bile duct cystadenocarcinoma Hepatoblastoma Mixed hepatocellular and cholangiocarcinoma Carcinoid
Mesenchymal	Hemangioma Infantile hemangioendothelioma Lipoma Others	Hemangiosarcoma Epithelioid hemangioendothelioma Lymphoma Others

filtrating the liver without clear borders. The tumor is usually soft and yellow-brown in color. The liver bearing a hepatocellular carcinoma is frequently cirrhotic (Figure 23-2). Portal vein invasion is often present. Using the new imaging techniques, one can detect small hepatocellular carcinomas (1 to 3 cm in diameter). These small tumors may or may not be surrounded by a fibrous capsule.

Cellular characteristics of HCC. The most important criterion in the histologic diagnosis is the similarity between the HCC cells and normal hepatocytes (Figure 23-3). In a well-differentiated HCC, the tumor cells have eosinophilic cytoplasm with round uniform nuclei. The tumor cells, like hepatocytes may contain abundant glycogen, fat, Mallory's hyalin, or other inclusions, or produce bile. The increase in glycogen content gives the tumor cells a clear-cell appearance. Poorly differentiated tumor cells have more pleomorphic nuclei and less eosinophilic cytoplasm. Giant cells can be seen in HCC. These giant cells may have a large oval nucleus, a single multilobed nucleus, or many small nuclei ranging in number from 4 to 100 or more. Despite the size and bizarre appearance, these giant cells have many features of hepatocytes, such as eosinophilia of the cytoplasm and prominent nucleoli. Histologically, it is often difficult to differentiate HCC from hypernephroma or adrenocortical tumor.

Tissue patterns of HCC. The basic growth pattern of HCC is trabecular without significant sclerosis. The tumor cells grow in cords of variable thickness separated by prominent sinusoids lined by endothelial cells. Bile canaliculi that are formed between tumor cells may be dilated into glandlike spaces and may contain bile. In this pseudoglandular or pseudoacinar HCC, the basic trabecular growth pattern often remains. The content of glandlike spaces may be fat-laden macrophages, fibrinous exudate, cellular debris, or colloid-like material. Compact or solid HCC is seen when the sinusoids

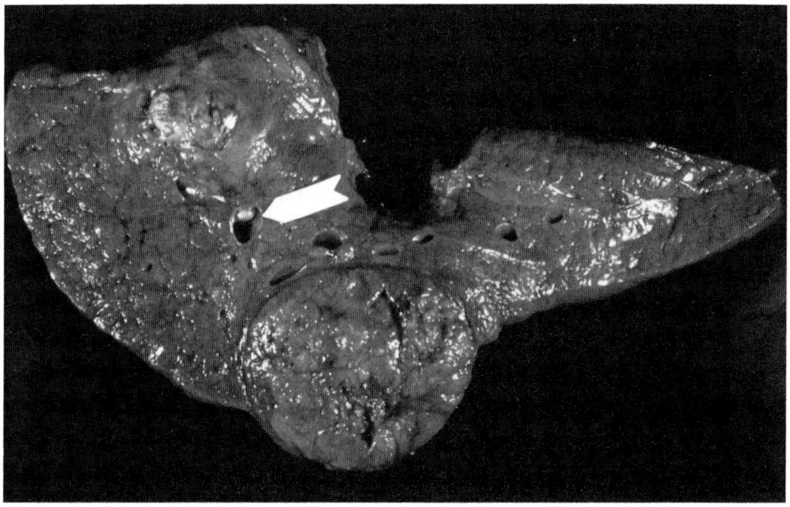

Figure 23-2
Cirrhotic liver showing large subcapsular hepatocellular carcinoma with intrahepatic metastases. *Arrow,* Tumor in a large vessel.

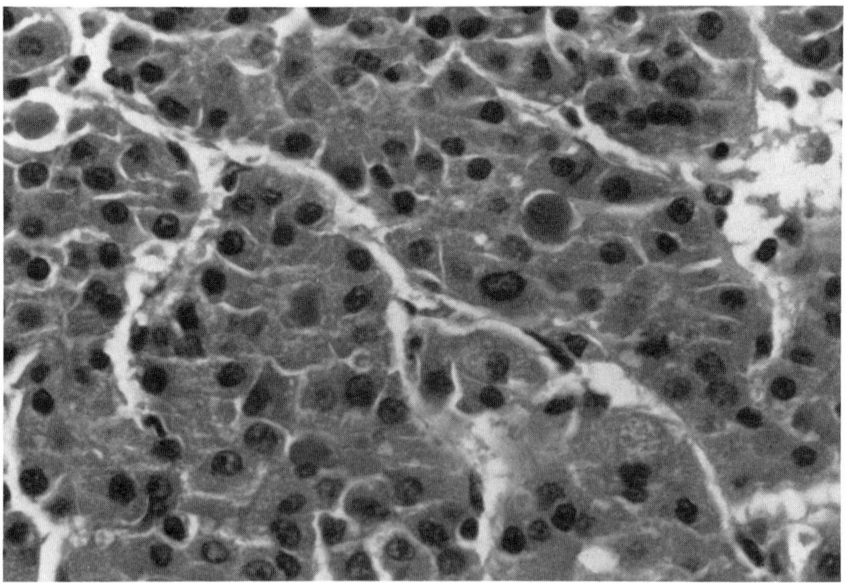

Figure 23-3
Hepatocellular carcinoma demonstrating resemblance of tumor cells to hepatocytes with bile formation.

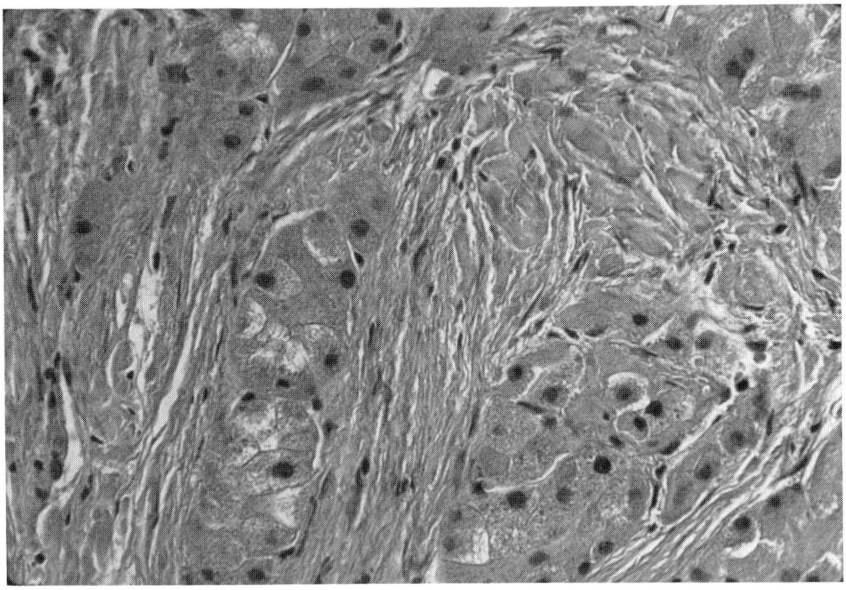

Figure 23-4
Fibrolamellar hepatocellular carcinoma showing large eosinophilic tumor cells surrounded by lamellar bands of fibrous tissue.

between the trabeculae become inconspicuous because of compression by tumor cells. When the neoplastic cells are cytologically well differentiated, distinction from nonmalignant liver may be difficult on a needle biopsy specimen.

Fibrolamellar carcinoma. The variant of HCC called "fibrolamellar carcinoma" occurs in younger patients (20 to 40 years of age) and is usually not associated with cirrhosis. It has highly characteristic histologic features. The tumor cells have deeply eosinophilic cytoplasm. They are separated by fibrous bands arranged in a lamellar fashion, hence the name "fibrolamellar carcinoma" (Figure 23-4). The cells often contain pale-staining inclusions or hyalin globules.

Sclerosing hepatocellular carcinoma. A fibrous stroma is found in tumors associated with hypercalcemia and hypophosphatemia. Some of these tumors may be of bile duct origin.

Combined hepatocholangiocarcinoma. HCC with areas of ductal or glandular changes is fairly common and should not be referred to as "combined." The tumor must contain unequivocal elements of both hepatocellular and cholangiocellular carcinoma.

"Minute" or encapsulated HCC. Minute HCC is seen in Southeast Asia and particularly in Japan. It is a small (less than 5 cm), slowly growing tumor with a thick fibrous capsule, well-differentiated trabecular pattern, lack of vascular invasion, and a high rate of cure by hepatectomy.

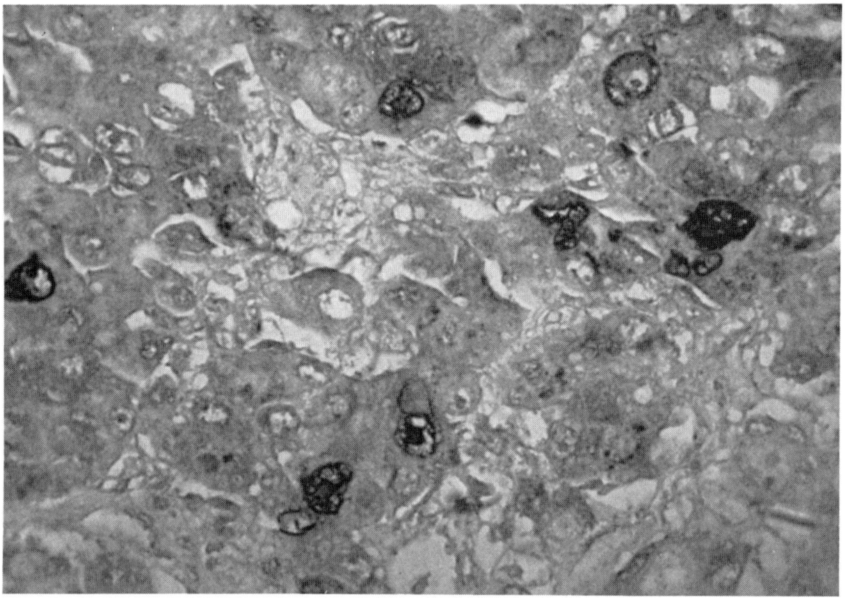

Figure 23-5
Immunoperoxidase staining of hepatocellular carcinoma for α-fetoprotein. The brown reaction product in tumor cells indicates the presence of tumor antigen.

Cholangiocarcinoma

Cholangiocarcinoma is a malignant tumor of extrahepatic or intrahepatic biliary epithelium. It is rare in the Western world, but endemic in the Orient where it is related to chronic parasitization of the biliary passages by the liver fluke, *Clonorchis sinensis*. It is usually a large, solitary, ill-defined, gray-white, firm mass. The surrounding liver often shows cholestasis without cirrhosis. Hilar cholangiocarcinoma, however, may cause secondary biliary cirrhosis.

Histologically, the degree of differentiation varies from well-formed glandular structures with mucus secretion to solid cords of anaplastic tumor cells. Abundant fibrous stroma is characteristically present. The appearance is similar to adenocarcinoma elsewhere in the gastrointestinal tract, gallbladder and pancreas. Unless dysplastic or in situ carcinomatous changes are seen in nearby bile ducts, the differentiation of a primary intrahepatic bile duct carcinoma from metastatic adenocarcinoma is difficult and often impossible. When the tumor is poorly differentiated, the differentiation between cholangiocarcinoma and HCC may also be a problem. The main distinguishing features are the amount of fibrosis that is greater in cholangiocarcinoma, the presence of cirrhosis in HCC, α-fetoprotein (Figure 23-5) and α_1-antitrypsin production in HCC, and the demonstration of different molecular weight cytokeratin

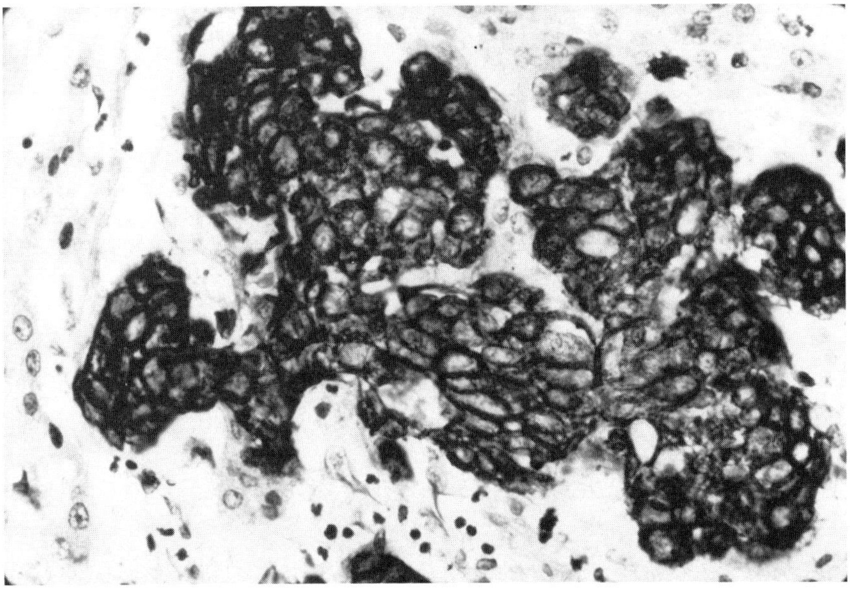

Figure 23-6
Immunohistochemical staining for high molecular weight cytokeratin. This cytokeratin is found in cholangiocarcinoma but not in hepatocellular carcinoma.

polypeptides in cholangiocarcinoma vs. HCC by immunohistochemical staining (Figure 23-6).

Hepatoblastoma

The malignant tumor hepatoblastoma occurs primarily in infants and children and has been associated with polyposis coli. It has to be differentiated from HCC. It is usually a well circumscribed, solitary mass, in the right lobe of the liver, which varies in size from 5 to 25 cm. The tumor often displays faint lobulation, cystic degeneration, necrosis, and hemorrhage. Microscopically, it consists of epithelial elements of various stages of maturation and a variable mesenchymal component. The epithelial component, which is always present and predominant, consists of two types of primitive cells: (1) "embryonal" type of cells, which may be arranged in ribbons and rosettes; these cells are small, fusiform, and darkly stained with uniform hyperchromatic nuclei and little cytoplasm; (2) "fetal" type of cells, which are generally organized in trabeculae or plates; these cells are larger with more cytoplasm, which may be granular or clear depending on the amount of glycogen or fat (Figure 23-7). Sinusoids and bile canaliculi may be formed. The mesenchymal component often consists of osteoid and rarely shows cartilaginous differentiation or muscular differentiation. α-Fetoprotein is consistently positive in the tumor cells.

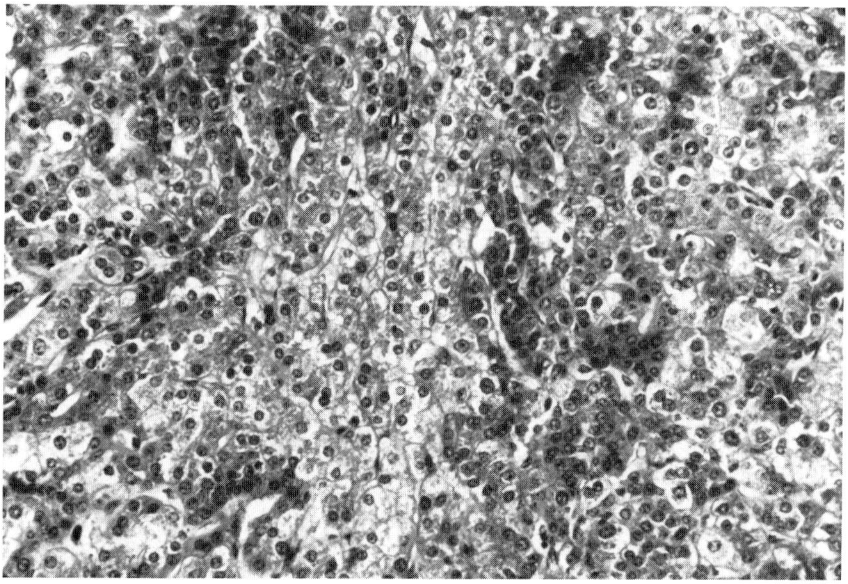

Figure 23-7
Hepatoblastoma containing both "embryonal" and "fetal" type of tumor cells.

Angiosarcoma

The malignant tumor angiosarcoma may be confined to the liver or may be part of a multicentric process involving other reticuloendothelial organs. Its relation to several carcinogens, i.e., Thorotrast, inorganic arsenicals, and vinyl chloride, is well established. In the liver, it is usually multicentric, appearing as ill-defined, hemorrhagic, spongy nodules. Microscopically, the tumor cells line sinusoids or cavernous spaces or produce solid masses. These cells have pleomorphic, hyperchromatic, and sometimes multiple nuclei and elongated scanty, ill-defined cytoplasm. The solid tumor nodules may have polyhedral cells indistinguishable from HCC or other types of sarcoma. The pattern of coarse reticulin fibers separating attenuated plates of liver cells is characteristic and helpful in the distinction of angiosarcoma from HCC. The tumor cells may be positive for factor VIII–related antigen.

Hepatocellular Adenoma

The benign tumor hepatocellular adenoma occurs almost exclusively in women on oral contraceptives. It is usually a single, large nodule up to 15 cm in diameter (Figure 23-8). Multiple small tumors may also be seen. The tumor is well-defined but not or only partially encapsulated. It is very vascular and has a soft, hemorrhagic, and yellow-tan cut surface. Histologically, it consists of tightly packed liver cell plates, often two to three cells thick, separated by slit-like

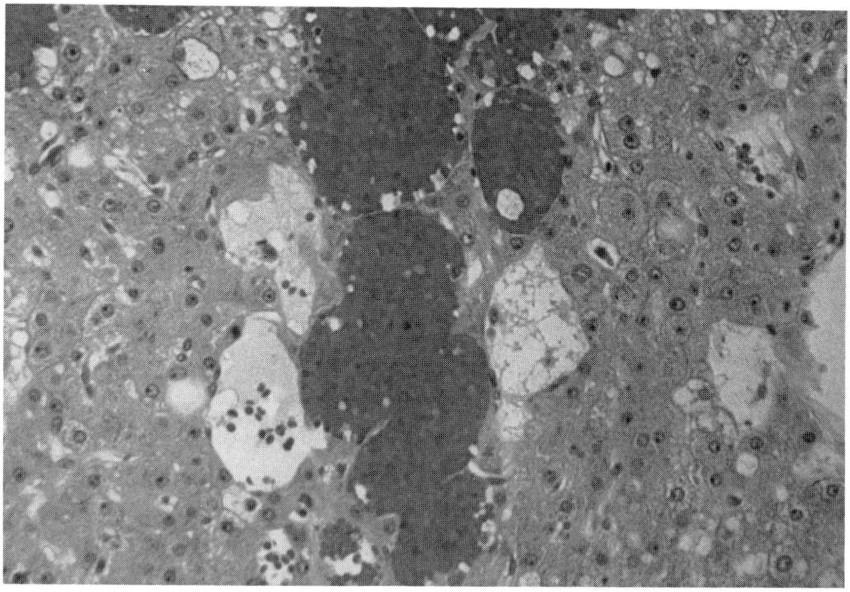

Figure 23-8
Hepatocellular adenoma with areas of peliosis (blood-filled cysts), which may result in hemorrhage.

sinusoids. The tumor cells are larger than normal hepatocytes. They have uniform nuclei and eosinophilic or clear cytoplasm because of excess glycogen or fat. Large thin-walled vessels are present. There are no portal tracts within the tumor. Irregular scars resulting from previous infarction may be seen. Hepatocelluar adenoma has to be differentiated from focal nodular hyperplasia and from well-differentiated HCC.

Focal Nodular Hyperplasia

The benign liver tumor focal nodular hyperplasia forms a rounded, solitary, well-circumscribed mass with a characteristic central scar (Figure 23-9). Fibrous septa radiate from the central scar and dissect the parenchymal component, which consists of relatively normal liver tissue. Cholestasis may be present. Portal tracts with well-formed bile ducts are lacking, though proliferated bile ductules are usually seen within the fibrous septa. An important diagnostic feature in distinguishing focal nodular hyperplasia from cirrhosis is the presence of disproportionately large, thick-walled, and structurally abnormal arteries. Focal nodular hyperplasia must also be differentiated from hepatocellular adenoma (see Figure 23-8) and diffuse nodular regenerative hyperplasia, which involves the entire liver. Although in some cases spontaneous rupture or an increased rate of growth may be attributable to oral contraceptives, there is no definite evidence of an etiologic association with steroids.

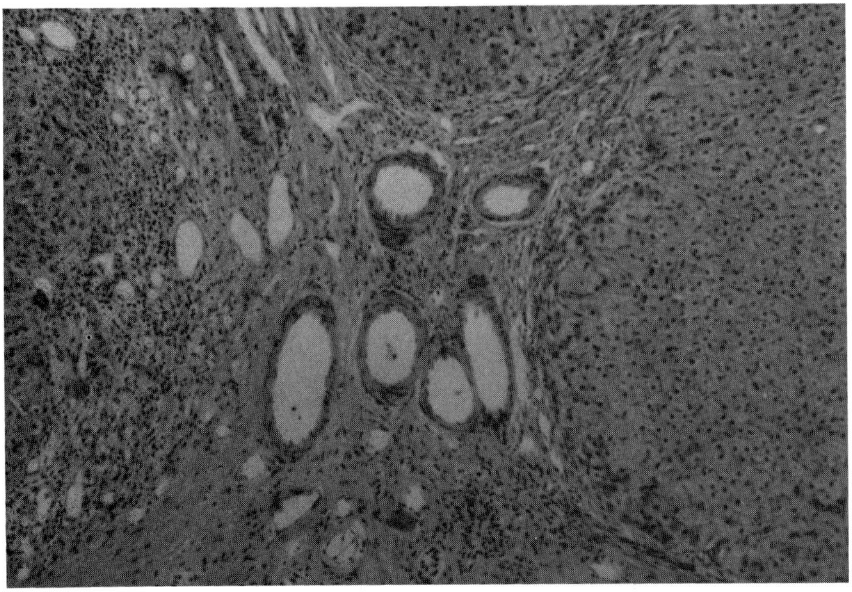

Figure 23-9
Focal nodular hyperplasia showing the characteristic central scar with large thick-walled arteries.

Diffuse Nodular Regenerative Hyperplasia

The benign condition diffuse nodular regenerative hyperplasia may be idiopathic or may be associated with long-term use of drugs or diseases such as rheumatoid arthritis and CRST (calcinosis, Raynaud's phenomenon, sclerodactyly, telangiectasis) syndrome. The hepatic parenchyma is almost entirely replaced by nodules varying from 0.1 to 4 cm in diameter. The nodules may be smaller or larger than one lobule in diameter and therefore may preserve or distort the lobular architecture. The nodules are not encapsulated, are yellow tan in color, and are visible on the capsular and cut surfaces. They consist of hyperplastic hepatocytes which are occasionally binucleated or multinucleated and are arranged in plates more than one cell thick. Atrophic hepatocytes are commonly found in a narrow rim around the expanding nodules. Sinusoidal dilatation, sometimes with congestion, accompanies the atrophic hepatocytes. These changes are best seen on a reticulin stain. Portal inflammation and fibrosis, when present, are mild. Although clinically it often mimics cirrhosis with portal hypertension, pathologically diffuse nodular regenerative hyperplasia is associated with little or no fibrosis or hepatocellular damage.

DIAGNOSIS

Serologic Markers

α-Fetoprotein (AFP) elevation in serum is seen in about two thirds of patients with HCC. A progressive rise in the level of AFP in the absence of hepatocellular necrosis, or an AFP level above 500 ng/ml is consistent with HCC. AFP is always elevated in hepatoblastoma. Elevation of carcinoembryonic antigen (CEA) is seen in 50% to 75% of patients with metastatic carcinoma or intrahepatic cholangiocarcinoma, but elevated values may also be found when the tumor is extrahepatic. Low levels of CEA elevation are observed in a variety of nonneoplastic conditions.

Imaging Techniques

Radionuclide scanning or scintigraphy using ^{99m}Tc-labeled sulfur colloid is noninvasive and is widely available. Most primary and metastatic neoplasms are visualized as areas of decreased uptake. Lesions must be at least 1.5 to 2 cm in diameter to be detected. The overall accuracy has been reported to be as high as 90%, though it is lower in most series. Both false-positive and false-negative results may occur.

Ultrasonography is noninvasive, and since it does not employ ionizing radiation, it is perhaps the safest of diagnostic procedures. Modern equipment has a resolution of 2 mm, but most detectable lesions are 2 cm or larger. Solid lesions are often echogenic and appear as areas of increased density. Necrosis or cystic degeneration within a tumor may be detected as an area of decreased echogenicity. The accuracy is as high as 90% depending on the skill and expertise of the ultrasonographer. False-negative and false-positive scans are found.

Computerized tomography (CT) is noninvasive and has gained a reputation for extreme accuracy and sensitivity. Lesions as small as 5 mm in diameter can be detected with up to 95% accuracy, though, as with other techniques, false-positive and false-negative findings occur. The procedure costs more than ultrasonography or scintigraphy. Therefore it is usually reserved for patients with suspected tumor in the liver in whom other techniques are negative or equivocal.

"Guided" fine-needle aspiration in conjunction with ultrasonography or any other imaging technique is often performed for tissue diagnosis. Despite claims to the contrary, this method is more suitable for the diagnosis of metastatic liver tumors and the recognition of HCC remains difficult. The distinction of a well-differentiated HCC, in which assessment of the growth pattern is necessary for the diagnosis, from normal hepatocytes, may pose a problem in fine-needle aspiration material. Immunohistochemical staining for CEA to delineate structures analogous to normal bile canaliculi formed between tumor cells in HCC is helpful in differentiating it from cholangiocarcinoma or metastatic adenocarcinoma.

Nuclear magnetic resonance imaging is a tool of chemical analysis that has been applied to medical imaging with extremely promising results. This technologic modality employs magnetism and radio waves to generate data that are processed by computer to form an image. It is comparable to computerized tomography in the detection of focal liver lesions.

Hepatic angiography is both invasive and expensive and is used in selected cases to provide useful information unobtainable by other means. It is particularly helpful in defining the vascular supply of a tumor nodule when one is considering surgical resection.

Biopsy

The definite diagnosis of malignancy in the liver requires biopsy and microscopic examination. Percutaneous "blind"-needle biopsy is most frequently used and can establish the diagnosis in up to 75% of patients with suspected malignancy. "Guided" biopsies, utilizing ultrasonography or other imaging modalities or biopsy performed during laparoscopy, are necessary for small tumors deep within the liver and can improve the yield.

PROGNOSIS

The overall survival of patients with HCC from the time of diagnosis ranges from several weeks to 6 months. Treatment such as tumor resection or chemotherapy may prolong survival, but early detection offers the greatest hope for a better outcome. Early diagnosis of HCC in patients with chronic liver disease, particularly in carriers of HBsAg, increases the chances of resectability and the time of survival. Patients at high risk for the development of HCC are screened regularly by serial measurement of serum AFP and by ultrasound examination of the liver.

Among the different types of HCC, fibrolamellar carcinoma progresses slowly and has a favorable prognosis. The average survival in these patients was 32 months. The cure rate after resection for fibrolamellar carcinoma is 48%, in contrast to HCC, which varies from 9% to 23%.

Hepatoblastoma in children is rapidly progressive and kills the patient by rupture, liver failure, or metastases. Early surgical resection combined with chemotherapy or radiation, or both, has improved the prognosis, and about 25% of the cases are alive and free of disease 9 years later.

SUMMARY

Although metastases are the most frequent tumors in the liver in the Western world, hepatocellular carcinoma represents the most common visceral cancer on a worldwide basis. The major risk factors predisposing to the development of HCC are geography, race, increasing age, male sex, chronic infection of the liver by hepatitis B virus and also hepatitis C virus, and many chronic liver diseases of almost any cause, particularly in association with cirrhosis. A variety of chemicals and some drugs also represent hepatocarcinogens. Oral contraceptives are associated with the development of benign hepatocellular adenomas. On liver biopsy specimens, hepatocellular carcinoma can usually be distinguished from cholangiocarcinoma and metastatic carcinoma, particularly with the help of immunohistochemical staining for α-fetoprotein and cytokeratins. Early detection of hepatocellular carcinoma offers the best hope for effective treatment. This may be accomplished by the screening of patients at risk, such as hepatitis B virus carriers and cirrhotics, with periodic measurement of serum α-fetoprotein levels and selected imaging studies.

ACKNOWLEDGMENT

We are grateful to Mrs. Leslie Wulfekühler for secretarial help.

SUGGESTED READING

Beasley RP et al: Hepatocellular carcinoma and hepatitis B virus, Semin Liver Dis 4:113, 1984.

This is a review of a Taiwan study of relative risk of HCC in relation to HBV.

Berman MA, Burnham JA, and Sheahan DG: Fibrolamellar carcinoma of the liver: an immunohistochemical study of nineteen cases and a review of the literature, Hum Pathol 19:784, 1988.

This report describes a large series of this uncommon but important liver tumor.

DiBisceglie AM: Hepatocellular carcinoma: molecular biology of its growth and relationship to hepatitis B virus infection, Med Clin North Am 25:985, 1989.

This report provides a discussion of HBV and other risk factors of HCC and mechanisms of hepatocarcinogenesis.

Gerber MA: Recent studies on the developing human hepatocellular carcinoma, Cancer Surveys 5:741, 1986.

This paper provides a demonstration of the precursor lesions of HCC.

Ishak KG: Hepatic lesions caused by anabolic and contraceptive steroids, Semin Liver Dis 1:16, 1981.

This is a concise summary of complications of steroid therapy.

Kew MC et al: Relationship between hepatocellular carcinoma and cirrhosis, Semin Liver Dis 4:136, 1984.

A discussion of the association between cirrhosis and HCC is given.

Lai Y-S et al: Expression of cytokeratins in normal and diseased livers and in primary liver carcinomas, Arch Pathol Lab Med 113:134, 1989.

A recent immunohistochemical study of different liver diseases, including HCC is reported.

Newberne PM: Chemical carcinogenesis: mycotoxins and other chemicals to which humans are exposed, Semin Liver Dis 4:122, 1984.

This report provides an in-depth description of aflatoxins and other chemical carcinogens.

Popper H, Gerber MA, and Thung SN: The relation of hepatocellular carcinoma to infection with hepatitis B and related viruses in man and animals, Hepatology (suppl) 2:1, 1982.

This is a review of the pathogenesis of HCC and a hypothesis of hepatocarcinogenesis.

Popper H et al: Development of hepatic angiosarcoma in man induced by vinyl chloride, Thorotrast, and arsenic, Am J Pathol 92:349, 1978.

This is a classic paper on the development of hemangiosarcoma of the liver.

Popper H et al: Hepatocarcinogenicity of the woodchuck hepatitis virus, Proc Natl Acad Sci USA 84:866, 1987.

This is a classic paper of the development of HCC in woodchucks.

Stromeyer FW and Ishak KG: Nodular transformation (nodular "regenerative" hyperplasia) of the liver; a clinicopathologic study of 30 cases, Hum Pathol 12:60, 1981.

This is an in-depth description of a large series of diffuse nodular hyperplasia of the liver.

24 Therapy of Hepatic Neoplasms

Charles E. Riggs, Jr.

Neoplasms of the liver encompass both benign and malignant primary hepatic tumors and metastatic cancers from other primary sites. Metastases from primary carcinomas of the colon, rectum, lung, breast, and upper digestive tract, lymphomas, melanomas, and sarcomas are the most commonly encountered liver cancers in the United States. In Asia, India, and Africa, however, hepatocellular carcinomas are the predominant liver cancers. Treatment strategies that have been developed for primary and metastatic cancers of the liver overlap considerably. Thus, despite its relative infrequency in North America, many of the therapeutic approaches to hepatoma apply nicely to palliative- and curative-intent treatments of hepatic metastases. In this chapter, hepatoma is the model employed to illustrate applications of surgery, irradiation, and medical therapies to the problem of liver cancers, with appropriate references to differences among hepatoma, metastases from other primary sites, and benign neoplasms.

THE APPROACH TO HEPATOCELLULAR CARCINOMA

Hepatoma may be suspected in persons who present with complaints of right upper quadrant pain, whose physical examinations disclose ascites, portal hypertension, or liver enlargement (frequently a hard, nodular edge), or who have elevations of hepatocellular enzymes or bilirubin (Table 24-1). The clinical history of preexisting cirrhosis, chronic active hepatitis, hemochromatosis, or chronic exposure to anabolic steroids should raise the index of suspicion. Measurement of the serum α-fetoprotein (AFP) is a sensitive means of screening high-risk populations, which may aid in the identification of persons harboring clinically occult hepatomas at a time when the tumor is small and potentially more curable. Values for AFP in excess of 300 ng/ml should prompt one to obtain hepatic imaging, preferably with computerized tomography or magnetic resonance imaging. A very high AFP and a suggestive imaging study are sufficient to make the diagnosis in some patients. However, very small hepatomas may be associated with only small increases in serum AFP, and so any imaging abnormalities should be aggressively pursued to exclude hepatoma.

Surveillance testing of patients at high risk for the development of hepatoma is recommended. Although there exists some controversy as to exactly whom to

Table 24-1 Diagnostic evaluation for hepatic neoplasms

Patient presents with abdominal pain, upper abdominal mass, weight loss, or ascites

↓

Perform screening: liver function tests; HBsAg, HBsAb; α-fetoprotein; prothrombin time, activated partial thromboplastin time: general biochemical screen, complete blood cell count; chest radiograph

↓

Perform imaging: liver ultrasonogram, abdominal computerized tomographic scan, liver magnetic resonance imaging

↓

If mass is found, assess resectability (may require hepatic arteriography)

← →

Isolated lesion or disease confined to one lobe

↓

1. Wedge resection
2. Partial hepatectomy

Multilobar disease or evidence of regional or distant spread

↓

1. Percutaneous or transvenous biopsy
2. Open biopsy
3. Consider liver transplant if no regional or distant spread

The patient presenting with persistent abdominal pain, upper abdominal or liver mass, ascites, or unexplained weight loss must be screened for hepatic neoplasm. Benign disease may present in identical fashion to malignancy, including the possibility for massive intraabdominal hemorrhage from ruptured peliosis hepatis or vascular hepatoma. If a hepatic mass is found, resectability is assessed by noninvasive imaging. Apparently benign neoplasms can still harbor a small focus of hepatoma, and open biopsy with resection can be recommended for any suspicious mass. If hepatoma is suspected preoperatively, based on very high α-fetoprotein (AFP) or abnormal hepatitis serologic results, consideration for aggressive resection or even transplant should begin. Needle biopsies of isolated masses of hepatoma are discouraged because spread of tumor in the peritoneum and along the needle tract has been documented. Open biopsy also allows for definitive control of hemorrhage, which can complicate needle biopsy. If the AFP is very high and the patient is a poor surgical candidate, presumption of the diagnosis of hepatoma is acceptable. Abbreviations: *HBsAg,* hepatitis B surface antigen; *HBsAb,* antibody to HBsAg.

screen, the precise tests to perform, and the intervals at which screening evaluations are most beneficial, the following is suggested as a reasonable approach. Patients with chronic hepatitis (types B and C) and hemochromatosis with cirrhosis are at particularly high risk. Performing biochemical liver function tests and serum AFP analyses at 6-month intervals and a hepatic ultrasound examination annually is a cost-effective means to identify early hepatocellular carcinomas and has the attraction of low morbidity and good patient acceptance.

In the majority of suspected cases, confirmation of the diagnosis by tissue exam-

Table 24-2 Staging of hepatocellular carcinoma

Stage	AJCC criteria	Revised criteria for African patients
I	Tumor <2-3 cm confined to one lobe without lymph nodal or distant metastases	No ascites, weight loss, or portal hypertension; serum bilirubin <2 mg/dl
II	Single tumor >2-3 cm or multiple tumors of any size confined to one major lobe without lymph nodal or distant metastases	Ascites with or without moderate weight loss (<25% normal body weight); no portal hypertension; serum bilirubin <2 mg/dl
III	Tumor, any size, involving both major lobes with or without regional lymph nodes, without metastases	Severe weight loss (>25% of normal body weight); portal hypertension; serum bilirubin >2 mg/dl
IV	Tumor invading adjacent organs or distant lymph nodal or other metastases	Not represented in this system

The American Joint Commission on Cancer (AJCC) stage designations are further modified by adding "A" after the roman numeral (e.g., IA, IIIA) to indicate absence of cirrhosis and "B" (e.g., IB, IIB) to indicate presence of cirrhosis. The revised criteria for African patients include only three stage groupings based on the features of disease as shown. The stage designations are further modified by "+" or "−" to indicate presence or absence, respectively, of cirrhosis. Neither system is currently accepted as standard for staging. (From Primack A, Vogel CL, Kyalwazi SK, et al: A staging system for hepatocellular carcinoma: prognostic factors in Ugandan patients, Cancer 35:1357, 1975).

ination is desirable. For those in whom imaging studies demonstrate accessible lesions in the liver, adjacent tissues, or metastatic sites (lung, skin), needle biopsy is often sufficient. The exception would be those tumors of relatively small size (10 cm or less) confined to one liver lobe, with no apparent metastases. These potentially curable tumors should be approached by liver resection. Attempts to establish the diagnosis by needle biopsy preoperatively in curative-intent cases may seed tumor cells along the needle tract or intraperitoneally, and these vascular tumors may bleed.

The initial treatment planning for the patient with biopsy-proved or clinically suspected hepatoma must be directed by the stage of disease at presentation (Table 24-2). Stage I patients, whose disease is confined to a single liver lobe and who maintain reasonably normal liver function, should undergo curative-intent liver resection. The surgical result is influenced by the extent of cirrhosis, both in the ability to achieve hemostasis and acceptable surgical margins and in the incidence of perioperative complications because of the impact of liver function and reserve. Recent technical advances that have enhanced the success rates of surgical resections include intraoperative ultrasonography, which allows precise delineation of the malignant lesion, ultrasonic aspiration dissectors, and water-jet dissectors.

Stage II and III hepatoma patients are frequently unable to withstand the rigors of hepatic resection, which may involve a lobectomy for larger tumors, and are more likely to have bilobar or metastatic disease, which eliminates the curative potential of hepatic resection. These persons may be candidates for radiation therapy, chemotherapy, or combined modality therapy. Selection of therapy depends on the functional status of the patient, the expectations and goals of treatment, the extent of the primary lesion, and the sites of metastases (lymph nodes, lung, bone, skin, peritoneum, vena cava, adrenal glands, brain).

In evaluating the results of a therapeutic intervention, one must consider improvements in survival and symptoms. The perioperative mortality for hepatic resections has reported to be as high as 25%, with an average of 10% to 15% being most commonly cited. For those undergoing successful resection, 5-year survivorships of 20% to 30% are reported, with the majority of deaths being attributable to local or distant recurrence of hepatoma. Survival for those with unresectable or metastatic hepatoma is much worse, with some studies indicating 2- to 3-month medians for survival after diagnosis. These dismal figures are not appreciably improved by chemotherapy, irradiation, or immunotherapy. It is worth noting that there are individuals who enjoy prolonged survival, in excess of 2 years for some, despite the presence of advanced disease at diagnosis. There tends to be longer survival for those who respond to a therapeutic intervention, but whether the prolongation of life reflects an effect of the treatment on the natural history of the tumor or is merely a consequence of lead-time bias in the survival calculation remains unknown.

Prognostic factors correlating with prolonged survival have been sought in an effort to identify the populations of advanced hepatoma patients who might benefit the most from systemic therapies. Three that seem reliable are the presence of disease confined to the liver in an ambulatory, nonjaundiced patient; the presence of the fibrolamellar carcinoma pathologic variant; and longer doubling time for the primary tumor. The patient with fibrolamellar carcinoma is typically a younger white patient who, despite a tumor that may metastasize early and frequently, seems to have a slower growing tumor and a longer survival than one found with age-matched persons without that pathologic condition. The impact of hepatoma doubling times has been noted mostly in those undergoing hepatic resection, and median survivals are briefest for those with shorter doubling times. However, there are correlations between early, aggressive hepatic resections and longer durations of survival noted in numerous surgical series.

CHEMOTHERAPY OF HEPATOMA

Hepatocellular carcinomas have generally been found to have only moderate sensitivity to single chemotherapeutic agents. The availability of murine and human hepatoma cell lines that can be studied in clonogenic (Hamburger-Salmon) chemosensitivity assays has permitted screening of candidate agents for activity. With this technology the most promising new agents can preferentially be brought to clinical trials, and combinations of theoretical interest can be tested for the possibility of synergistic anticancer activity.

Results of numerous phase II trials of single-agent therapy of hepatoma are summarized in Table 24-3. It can be seen that the overwhelming majority of responses are only partial. As such the impact of these therapies on the quality of

Table 24-3 Summary of phase II chemotherapy trials in patients with hepatocellular carcinoma

Drug	Number of trials reported	Total number of patients	Number of responders	Overall response rates
Doxorubicin (Adriamycin)	22	430	18 CR, 84 PR	24% (4% CR, 20% PR)
Zinostatin (Neocarzinostatin K)	6	70	12 PR	17%
Cisplatin (Platinol)	4	21	3 PR	14%
Dichloromethotrexate (investigational)	2	23	3 PR	13%
Etoposide (VePesid; VP16-213)	2	70	7 PR	10%
5-Fluorouracil	6	111	9 PR	8%
Mitoxantrone (Novantrone)	2	61	1 CR, 3 PR	7% (2%CR, 5% PR)
Amsacrine (*m*-AMSA)	7	120	5 PR	4.2%
Mitomycin C (Mutamycin)	1	30	11 PR	37%
Hexamethylmelamine	4	9	2 PR	22%
Prednimustine	1	1	1 PR	100%

From data accumulated by the Investigational Drug Branch of the National Cancer Institute, NIH, as part of the Phase II reporting system. For responses, *CR* is complete regression and *PR* is partial regression of measurable disease.

life and survival in hepatoma patients would be expected to be minimal. Doxorubicin (Adriamycin) stands out as the single drug with the greatest antitumor activity, and several dosages and schedules for its use are indicated. Individual studies with zinostatin (Neocarzinostatin K), etoposide, cisplatin, amsacrine, and dichloromethotrexate have reported response rates in excess of 10%, but the aggregate experiences with these agents fail to support any consistent anticancer action after systemic administration.

Hormonal therapy of hepatocellular carcinomas has been attempted, based on the observations that some of these tumors, like breast and other carcinomas, bear receptors for estrogens, progesterone, androgens, or corticosteroids. The levels of receptor activity are typically lower for hepatomas than for other hormone-dependent tumors. Responses of hepatomas to hormonally directed therapy are poor and infrequent. Progestogen therapy with megesterol acetate induced partial regressions of tumor in two of five (40%) hepatoma patients but for brief durations. Cyproterone acetate, an antiandrogen, may be of benefit in cirrhotic patients with hepatoma, but further trials are required. The close association of estrogen use, hepatic adenoma, and hepatoma prompted a recently reported phase II study of the antiestrogen tamoxifen in 33 hepatoma patients with good-performance status. The estrogen receptor status of these patients was unknown, and one third had failed prior to chemotherapy. No complete or partial regressions of hepatoma were observed. Thus it appears that although there are occasional patients whose hepatocellular carcinomas will shrink during a hormonal intervention, the overwhelming majority will not benefit from such therapy.

One final consideration for hormone therapy must always be kept in mind in the patient with advanced, symptomatic hepatoma. Corticosteroids, usually prednisone or dexamethasone, can afford considerable relief of nausea, anorexia, and the generally poor performance status of some of these patients. The beneficial effects are the same as those observed in patients with a variety of other solid tumors, and there is no certain explanation for the temporary but gratifying responses to this form of intervention. Low doses (10 to 25 mg of prednisone-equivalent per day) are usually sufficient to achieve the desired improvement and are less likely to be attended by the unwanted consequences of steroid therapy in a hepatically impaired population—fluid retention, electrolyte imbalances, hypoproteinemia, and infections.

Randomized trials of various anticancer drugs in patients with hepatocellular carcinoma provide additional perspectives on whether the physician or oncologist should recommend chemotherapy routinely in this population. In one trial with a small number of patients, induction therapy with either doxorubicin or etoposide (VP16-213) was assigned; in cases of progressive disease with the originally assigned drug, crossover to the alternative drug was permitted. Partial remissions were recorded in 3 of 14 etoposide patients and 5 of 35 doxorubicin recipients. In those crossing over after initial failure to therapy or relapse, 3 of 10 etoposide-to-doxorubicin and 1 of 8 doxorubicin-to-etoposide patients responded. Longer durations of response occurred with doxorubicin, the longest being only 7 months. Only 10 of the 35 participants lived longer than a year, and so the impact of therapy on survival is questionable.

Two other trials report the responses of doxorubicin alone compared to multidrug regimens. The larger study, from the Eastern Cooperative Oncology Group, found response rates of 9% to 22% to doxorubin and three 5-fluorouracil–containing programs. The highest response rate occurred in the group who received a three-drug, doxorubicin plus 5-fluorouracil–containing regimen, but no substantial differences in median survivals resulted. As has been noted in several types of cancer, the best correlation with survival in this study was the performance status of the patient at the time of therapy. The second study compared doxorubicin to a four-drug, 5-fluorouracil–containing combination. A 25% complete (3 patients) plus partial (8 patients) remission rate was achieved with doxorubicin monotherapy, whereas none of the 19 combination therapy patients responded. The median survival in this study was only 14 weeks, again raising the question of whether a chemotherapy response produced any meaningful advantage. A recent, randomized comparison of mitoxantrone and cisplatin demonstrated response rates of 8% and 17%, respectively, with a 14-week median survival.

Results of systemic therapy with single agents or combination regimens would be strong evidence against recommending routine use of standard chemotherapy in advanced hepatoma patients. Symptomatic patients, if they achieve response after one or at most two cycles of therapy, may experience improved quality of life, but durations of response would be expected to be short. Such persons may be considered to be reasonable candidates for local therapies—irradiation of painful liver or metastatic sites and surgical resection or intravascular embolization of a painful or bleeding lesion. Radiation therapy to a symptomatic area of disease has appeal for several reasons. First, the usual course of radiation to the maximally tolerable liver dose (2100 cGy) can be delivered in 7 days and to metastatic sites in 10 days, minimizing the time that the person has to be in the clinic setting. Second, there is ordinarily little systemic toxicity from localized irradiation. Third, the improvement in general status from this form of therapy can make it feasible to consider other forms of systemic or operative therapy. Embolization or surgical resection have been employed for lesions in the liver or other organs. Although embolization of the feeding blood supply to a metastatic site would seem to offer the advantage of avoiding a surgery, the technique can induce severe systemic toxicities—fever, hypotension, organ dysfunction, or increased pain in the embolized area.

REGIONAL CHEMOTHERAPY OF HEPATOMA

In cancer treatment, there is an intuitive appeal to introducing high concentrations of a therapeutic agent directly into the disease-bearing region. It may be hypothesized that more tumor cytotoxicity would be observed as the relatively resistant tumor cells are exposed to the higher drug concentrations, which would be present in the selectively perfused region. Less systemic toxicity to the patient would occur because of sequestration or inactivation of the drug in the perfused tissue with resulting lower systemic drug concentrations. Because of the dual blood supply afforded the normal liver tissue via the portal venous and hepatic arterial systems and the observations that most hepatomas are supplied exclusively by the hepatic arterial system, hepatic intraarterial chemotherapy has been the object of intensive and extensive study.

The theoretical advantage to regional perfusion chemotherapy is a function of the relative rate of clearance of the agent or agents of interest from the circulation and the rate of blood flow in the perfused region. In the case of liver, the extraction rate of an anticancer drug also influences the theoretical advantage. When most or all of a drug is removed from the blood the first time it circulates through the liver ("first-pass effect"), it will not reach the systemic circulation in sufficient quantities to be toxic. Unfortunately, the hepatic arterial flow is relatively high, and only a few candidate chemotherapeutic agents fulfill the requirement of rapid enough clearance to warrant their use in regional perfusion schemes—5-fluorouracil, floxuridine (FUdR), cisplatin, and mitomycin. Because of its single-agent activity against hepatoma after intravenous injection, doxorubicin has also been studied in the regional perfusion setting. The relative advantage of hepatic intraarterial infusion of doxorubicin compared to intravenous injection of it is small because of its slow clearance from the circulation.

Another factor contributing to the proliferation of hepatic arterial chemotherapy protocols has been the development of indwelling (subcutaneous, intraabdominal) and percutaneous drug delivery systems. Such devices include the Infusaid implantable pump, a variety of subcutaneous vascular-access ports through which portable, external pumps can deliver single or multiple drugs, and sophisticated pumps that can deliver single or multiple drugs in schedules directed by preprogramed microchips. These devices permit outpatient delivery of complex drug regimens, contributing to cost effectiveness and patient acceptance. As will be discussed later in this chapter, their use may be extended to therapy of metastatic lesions of the liver.

In the most common scenario, the catheter from an Infusaid pump or a subcutaneous port is inserted into that artery feeding the tumor-containing liver tissue at the time of laparotomy. The artery is ligated in the process, and there may be some contribution of this interruption of the tumor blood supply to the success of therapy. The accessible injection site of the implanted device is usually located in the subcutaneous tissues of the anterior abdominal wall. One may ascertain the correct positioning of the catheter in the operating room by injection of the device with a fluorescing material and visualizing the tumorous hepatic tissue for fluorescence under ultraviolet light, or by injecting the system postoperatively with radiolabeled material and confirming the distribution of the label in the region of interest scintigraphically.

Despite the sophistication, pharmacologic advantages, and benefits suggested for this mode of therapy by preclinical models, there are no convincing data that regional chemotherapy of hepatoma prolongs survival. Response rates that exceed 50% in some series are hopeful, but observer bias, in terms of patient selection and definition of response, have hampered the interpretion of these results. The best advice for the clinician is to seek out an investigational trial of regional hepatic therapy to which hepatoma patients can be referred before one resorts to routine use of this expensive, potentially dangerous mode of treatment.

COMBINED MODALITY THERAPY OF HEPATOMA

The ability to give various drugs in regional fashion has led to some interesting clinical experiments of combined modality therapy. Three that have been shown to be feasible are radiation therapy combined with hepatic arterial drug infusion, embolization of the microcirculation in the perfused region with tiny particles of latex or albumin simultaneously with the injection of the anticancer drug or drugs, and attachment or admixture of the anticancer drug or drugs to microspheric particles.

The appeal of combining irradiation of the liver with medications derives from the limited tolerance of normal hepatic tissue for irradiation, the high doses of irradiation required to kill most hepatoma cells in vitro, and the potential of a variety of chemicals to sensitize hepatoma cells to the cytotoxic effects of ionizing radiation. Both standard antineoplastic agents and chemical compounds with or without inherent antitumor actions have been demonstrated to be effective as radiosensitizers and are usually most effective when infused intraarterially into the tumor bed. Combinations of doxorubicin and 5-fluorouracil have received the most attention because of initial reports of the effectiveness of this form of multimodality therapy. Subsequent trials of these and other standard anticancer drugs used as radiosensitizers, in which control groups receiving irradiation alone were included, failed to duplicate the high response rates and to confirm any survival advantage over hepatic irradiation alone. The latest attempts at exploiting radiosensitization techniques have focused on halogenated nucleoside analogs that are incorporated into DNA. The sites of incorporation are more sensitive to ultraviolet or gamma irradiation, depending on which halide (fluorine, iodine, bromine) is attached to the nucleoside. Prolonged hepatic arterial infusions can increase the incorporation of halogenated nucleoside, and the systemic effects of these agents, which possess some cytotoxic potential of their own, are minimized by first-pass catabolism. However, the limitations of combining external beam irradiation with chemical sensitizers will remain (1) the intolerance of normal liver tissue to sterilizing radiation doses and (2) the local nature of radiation therapy, which will leave any extrahepatic metastases untreated by the combination.

As discussed in the section on regional chemotherapy, the high flow rates of blood in the hepatic arterial system decrease the theoretical advantage of giving anticancer drugs directly into the tumor's vascular bed. One scheme for altering blood flow has been to inject small, spheric, degradable particles into the region to be perfused. These particles will occlude the tiniest arterioles, venules, and capillaries, producing stagnation of blood flow in the region. This prolongs the presence of the perfused agents in the tumor vasculature, presumably increasing cellular uptake and increasing cytotoxicity. Materials that have been utilized as particulates include gelatin powder, microfibrillar collagen, and albumin microspheres. Earlier reports described experience with latex particles.

Typical results are illustrated by a recent paper that described the percutaneous hepatic arterial infusion of a mixture of Gelfoam (The Upjohn Co., Kalamazoo, Michigan), contrast medium (for assessment of hepatic blood flow), and a mixture of doxorubicin, cisplatin, and mitomycin in 50 patients with advanced, unresectable, untreated hepatoma. Twelve (24%) of the patients had greater than 50% shrinkage of tumor, and another 13 (26%) had 25% to 50% shrinkage of tumor. One fourth of the patients had progressive disease. Although the survival of a highly selected population of patients such as this cannot be readily compared to the general hepatoma population, there was survival for 3 years in at least one patient.

The toxicities of embolization therapy are substantial, and these alone should caution one to seek a clinical trial for any hepatoma patient who seems to be a reasonable candidate for consideration of this form of therapy. All patients manifest temporary elevations of hepatic biochemical tests, and virtually all suffer significant right upper quadrant or abdominal pain. Nausea, vomiting, and fever are nearly universal, but these may be as related to the antineoplastic drugs as to the embolization. Those with cirrhosis may have considerable worsening of their symptoms and signs of liver disease. Causes of death after embolization have included hepatorenal syndrome, venoocclusive disease of the liver, and hemorrhage, in addition to the more typical, tumor-related death.

The third method differs slightly from the embolization method in which an anticancer agent is admixed with the occluding medium or injected immediately after occlusion. With this third technique, the anticancer agent is directly attached to or is suspended in the carrier medium, which is then site-specifically directed to the vascular bed of interest. The oily contrast medium lipiodol has been shown to persist in tumor vessels longer than in those of surrounding normal liver, suggesting the possibility of selective delivery of agents to tumor cells, sparing the normal hepatocytes from toxicity. Drugs dissolved in lipiodol can be infused intraarterially, and the selectivity can be further enhanced by simultaneous embolization. In another approach, doxorubicin has been attached to magnetic albumin microspheres, which are injected intravenously or into the hepatic artery. A strong magnet placed over the site of the tumor in the liver causes the microspheres to collect in the magnetic field, and biodegradation of the albumin from which the spheres are made releases doxorubicin into the tumor. This approach has the advantage of avoiding percutaneous arterial cannulations, for which some hepatoma patients may not be suitable. Finally, radionuclides can be incorporated into albumin or glass microspheres, for site-directed delivery of high-intensity irradiation of tumors, which would not be feasible with current external beam techniques. Yttrium-labeled glass spheres have been studied in dogs, and radiation doses of 10,000 cGy, five times the normal liver tolerance, have been successfully delivered to tumors, without the devastating consequence of fatal hepatic necrosis.

Most of the foregoing discussion of combined modality techniques has concerned the approach to patients with unresectable hepatic neoplasms. It is clear that any technique that benefits these patients would be desirable for evaluation in the population of patients whose hepatomas are resectable. The best combined treatment for the resectable patient remains to be defined, and those hepatoma patients with the good fortune to have resectable disease should be offered entry onto clinical trials.

NEW APPROACHES TO THERAPY OF HEPATOMA

The exciting technologies that have been developed in response to the problem of hepatocellular carcinoma lend themselves to innovative combinations and to their inclusion as part of even newer technologies. The potential for delivering very high radiation doses with yttrium-90 microspheres has been mentioned, and similar approaches with other radionuclides and other, more selective, delivery systems can be expected. A few of the ongoing experimental approaches to hepatoma therapy are described in this section.

In vitro studies on human hepatoma cells indicate their sensitivity to high temperature and possible synergy of hyperthermia along with anticancer drugs. There now exist microwave-heating and hemoperfusion techniques for inducing temperatures of 42° C in the liver while maintaining body temperature at near-normal levels. Injection of candidate medications, which have included doxorubicin, mitomycin C, and 5-fluorouracil, at the time of peak liver temperature is being pursued to determine if this technique results in greater and more selective cytotoxicity to the hepatoma than to surrounding normal liver and other tissues. One potential advantage of this form of local-plus-systemic therapy is the opportunity to kill extrahepatic tumor cells, and the slight increases in whole-body temperatures accompanying certain forms of localized hyperthermia may offer additional benefit in the accomplishment of this goal.

The expression of high levels of immunoreactive ferritin by hepatoma cells led to a novel form of directed therapy. Polyclonal sera to ferritin were prepared, and the antibodies were labeled with one of several radionuclides, the most successful being radioiodine (I-131). These radioactive antibodies were shown to localize in the areas of tumor and thus had the potential to deliver high doses of radiation to the cells to which they bound. A protocol for treating unresectable hepatoma was initiated, with previously treated patients receiving the radioactive antiserum alone and untreated hepatoma patients receiving combined modality therapy. The latter consisted of external beam irradiation to the tolerance dose of the liver, simultaneously with doxorubicin and 5-fluorouracil. Subsequent cycles of intravenous doxorubicin and 5-fluorouracil were given for 2 to 4 months, and then radioactive antiserum was administered. Overall, one half of the 79 evaluable patients treated on the protocol (of the 105 entered altogether) achieved complete (7%) or partial (43%) remissions from this approach. Of interest was the group of previously treated persons, in whom radioactive antibodies alone appeared sufficient to induce responses. Several factors were examined for prognostic value, and the presence of measurable serum AFP was associated with an average survival of only one half of that found in patients lacking this serum marker. The durations of responses could be long, with documented 3- to 5-year remissions. However, the median survival of those participants achieving remission was only 11 months, and only 15% of the entered population survived for 2 years. Whether such statistics in a highly selected group of hepatoma patients differ from those of similar persons receiving external beam irradiation with chemotherapy is the objective of a current study by the Radiation Therapy Oncology Group.

The future of antibody-based therapies for hepatoma has much potential. Radioligands different from I-131 are being evaluated for their usefulness, both in terms of relative specificity for antibody binding and for the nature of their radioactive emissions. Alpha- and beta-particle emitters would have a theoretical advantage because of their limited tissue penetrations, compared to gamma-ray emitters, but have the disadvantage of poor visualization by external imaging techniques. Monoclonal antibodies would seem to offer the advantages of high specificity for unique hepatoma antigens, but the few available antibodies have proved to be less efficacious than the polyspecific sera to ferritin. A truly hepatoma-specific monoclonal antibody could be a great advance.

The oily fatty acid ester lipiodol, mentioned earlier, can also be labelled with iodine 131 or yttrium 90. Studies of these radioactive agents, which seem to traverse the tumor vasculature more slowly than that of the normal liver, are in progress in Korea, Japan, and the United States. Preliminary results indicate that focal, small-volume disease tends to respond, whereas multicentric or infiltrative disease, or bulky disease, is resistant to this form of radiation delivery.

Biological agents—interferons, interleukins, tumor necrosis factor—have been the subjects of intense study in hepatocellular carcinomas, stimulated in part by the presumed viral cause of many cases and the antiviral properties of many biological agents. Interleukin-2 (IL-2) has received the most attention. One hepatoma patient treated with IL-2 plus lymphokine-activated killer (LAK) cells failed to respond. In 28 patients receiving IL-2 via the splenic or the hepatic artery, two partial responses were observed. Therapy with LAK cells did not correlate with the two objective tumor regressions. In another trial, no objective responses occurred in patients with bulk disease, though several manifested declines in serum AFP. The patients undergoing successful hepatic resection followed by IL-2/LAK cell therapy did not experience recurrences during a very brief observation period. There are numerous leads to follow in combining IL-2 and other biologicals with some of the therapeutic modalities already discussed, and clinical trials of the more promising strategies are underway.

Certainly the most dramatic of the investigational approaches to curative-intent therapy of hepatoma is total hepatectomy and allogeneic liver transplantation. The rationale for this aggressive approach is based on observations that total surgical extirpation of the malignancy has been the only therapy inducing long-term, disease-free status, that early detection of small lesions may be possible in screening programs in high-risk persons, and that immunosuppressive therapies may be managed successfully to ensure prolonged survival of the allografted liver. Summary results in transplanted patients up to now indicate a 30% early (3-month) mortality, a 50% 1-year survival, and a 30% 3-year survival. Almost three fourths of the patients dying have recurrent disease, a reflection of the fact that most hepatomas produce micrometastases to other organs early in their development. The ultimate success of liver transplantation as a reasonable form of intervention will depend on continued improvements in the ability to detect disease early and on the identification of more effective systemic therapies, to sterilize extrahepatic metastases before the actual transplant procedure.

THERAPY OF OTHER LIVER TUMORS AND OF HEPATIC METASTASES

Cancers of the biliary system are approached in fashions similar to those for hepatocellular carcinoma. As with hepatoma, early surgical removal of all disease is the only sure means to produce long-term relief from disease. There is some argument that irradiation postoperatively may be of greater benefit than for hepatoma, but so few cases are localized enough to warrant aggressive local therapy that it is difficult to conclude that any adjuvant radiotherapy or chemotherapy would be of benefit.

Other primary liver tumors include lymphomas, sarcomas, mixed mesenchymal tumors, germ cell tumors, and the rare endodermal sinus tumor. These are approached initially as for hepatoma, to assess resectability and surgical curability. Those tumors that are recurrent or are unresectable can be treated with the therapeutic program appropriate for that tumor type. For instance, liver sarcomas may be treated with doxorubicin-dacarbazine–based regimens as for any soft-tissue sarcoma. The general experience is that despite the histological similarity to the same neoplasm in other primary sites hepatic primaries of these tumor types tend to respond less favorably.

Two tumors deserve special mention. Angiosarcoma of the liver is an aggressive mesenchymal, soft-tissue tumor, that is usually quite rare. Exposure of persons to the radioactive diagnostic imaging agent Thorotrast was associated with a striking incidence of hepatic angiosarcomas. This sarcoma has also been observed to be more frequent in those exposed to other thorium-containing materials, as well as to arsenic and vinyl chloride compounds. Eliciting a history of such exposures should prompt one to evaluate carefully for evidence of biochemical or structural liver abnormalities, with subsequent biopsy and surgery as dictated by the results of screening studies.

The other situation in which one should pay extra attention to screening for hepatoma is the patient with adenomatous hyperplasia. Although any process stimulating liver regeneration—liver injury, hepatitis, iron overload, cirrhosis, chronic inflammatory disease—should raise concerns about subsequent hepatoma, nodules of adenomatous hyperplasia may contain small nodules of hepatocellular carcinoma, presenting the special problem of finding a "lesion within a lesion." Extreme vigilance is required to pursue each abnormality in these select patient groups because the curability of the hepatoma that may ultimately be discovered depends directly on how early it is detected.

Metastases to the liver from other primary sites of carcinoma can be approached for treatment with the same rationale as for primary hepatocellular carcinoma. Long remissions from resected hepatic metastases occurring with carcinomas of breast, lung, colon, and other sites, melanomas, and occasional sarcomas are documented, but lesions resectable for cure comprise fewer than 5% of hepatic metastases. Recent suggestions of survival advantages for hepatic arterial chemotherapy of colon carcinoma metastases have renewed interest in long-term regional infusions for that disease process. It appears that the best results are achieved when as much or preferably all of the metastatic colon cancer can be resected before the hepatic arterial infusions. Current results indicate that 25% to 35% of those rendered disease-free by an aggressive, combined-modality program will remain alive without disease for 2 to 3 years, and some are undoubtedly cured by this approach. Recurrences are distant from the liver in two thirds of those who fail, usually in the lungs, and one third will suffer hepatic recurrence. As with the other neoplasms mentioned, a major impediment to successful outcomes is failure to diagnose extrahepatic metastasis before the aggressive local therapy, or low specificity in determining the earliest stages of recurrence of disease. Clinical trials of new monoclonal antibody-based imaging techniques for colon and breast carcinomas may allow for identification of those most likely to benefit from hepatic resection and postoperative adjuvant therapy.

THERAPY OF BENIGN HEPATIC NEOPLASMS

Focal nodular hyperplasia, adenomatous hyperplasia, and peliosis hepatis are the chief benign neoplasms encountered in the diagnostic evaluation for hepatocellular carcinomas. The relationship of these lesions to the evolution of hepatocellular carcinoma is suspected but not conclusively proved. One-third of women with hepatoma will give histories of prolonged estrogen use, usually administered as oral contraceptive or replacement therapy. There is a less striking association between androgen supplementation and hepatoma induction, and the case for anabolic steroids in the genesis of hepatoma is an area of current debate. As has been noted, some hepatomas bear receptors for sex steroids, supporting the notion of steroid action in the neoplastic process.

It is recommended that the offending steroid hormone be discontinued in those cases of peliosis hepatis and hepatic adenoma, usually resulting in resolution of the benign neoplasm. Because these benign lesions may hemorrhage spontaneously or after trauma, prompt recognition and intervention are important. Hypotensive crises or death may occur from bleeding surface adenomas or peliosis hepatis.

Although the associations between focal nodular hyperplasia and steroid use are less certain than those for adenomas, extreme caution and vigilance must be urged whenever a steroid-linked hepatic disorder is identified. The usual case will be a contraceptive-related benign neoplasm, and appropriate therapy is to discontinue the steroid agent. Persistence of the hepatic tumor can occur, and a single examination of the lesion pathologically may not be sufficient for long-term management of a persistent adenoma or hyperplastic nodule. There are sporadic reports of hepatomas occurring after steroid withdrawal and apparent resolution of a hepatic adenoma or area of focal nodular hyperplasia. Close monitoring of demonstrable lesions is advised, and surgical excision may be justified in cases in which there is not a significant reduction in the size of the nodule after steroid withdrawal.

SUMMARY

A variety of benign and malignant tumors can arise in or metastasize to the liver. Early identification of hepatic cancers is difficult, and many are not resectable or curable at the time of diagnosis. Hepatocellular carcinoma serves as model for surgical, radiotherapeutic, chemotherapeutic, and biological-agent treatment of malignant liver tumors in general. The best chances for long-term relief of liver cancers result from aggressive surgical resection, followed by chemotherapy and irradiation. Most patients will die from recurrence, however, and better modes of dealing with distant disease are desperately needed. Benign lesions of the liver are usually related to prolonged ingestion of sex steroid hormones, and most regress after withdrawal of the offending hormone. However, there may be an etiologic link between hormone use and subsequent cancer development, and high-risk persons should be subjected to frequent screening procedures. One should make attempts to treat isolated hepatic metastases from primary colon, breast, and lung cancers, employing techniques similar to those used for hepatomas. New modalities and therapies involving antibodies, biological agents, and allogeneic liver transplantation may improve the diagnostic sensitivity and the long-term outlook for victims of hepatic cancers.

SUGGESTED READINGS

Di Bisceglie AM, Rustgi VK, Hoofnagle JH, et al: Hepatocellular carcinoma, Ann Intern Med 108:390-401, 1988.

This NIH conference report reviews the relevant epidemiology, pathology, and treatment advances in hepatoma.

Ensminger W: Hepatic arterial chemotherapy for primary and metastatic liver cancers, Cancer Chemother Pharmacol 23:S68-S73, 1989.

Dr. Ensminger provides an excellent review of regional chemotherapy of hepatoma and includes considerations of combined modality therapies.

Kim BS, Yoo HS, Park YJ, and Loh JJK: Current status and future aspects on treatment of liver cancer, Cancer Chemother Pharmacol 23:S118-S120, 1989.

This report describes the combined modality therapy of 80 patients. In addition to regional chemotherapy, hyperthermia and radioactive fatty acids were shown to contribute positively to response rates and survival.

Luna G, Florence L, and Johansen K: Hepatocellular carcinoma: a 5 year institutional experience, Am J Surg 149:591-594, 1985.

The presenting features of hepatoma at a major university medical center are reviewed, and the results of therapy detailed. Of interest was the observation that 30% of hepatomas were found incidentally.

Order SE, Stillwagon GB, Klein JL, et al: Iodine 131 antiferritin, a new treatment modality in hepatoma: a Radiation Therapy Oncology Group study, J Clin Oncol 3:1573-1582, 1985.

In addition to a description of this new therapeutic approach, this report provides overviews of combined modality schemes for hepatoma therapy.

Patt YZ, Claghorn L, Charnsangavej C, et al: Hepatocellular carcinoma. A retrospective analysis of treatments to manage disease confined to the liver, Cancer 61:1884-1888, 1988.

This review of 73 hepatoma patients indicates that hepatic resection, either before or after chemotherapy, improved survival. Hepatic artery infusion of chemotherapy, with or without liver resection, was associated with longer survivals.

Venook AP, Stagg RJ, Lewis BJ, et al: Chemoembolization for hepatocellular carcinoma, J Clin Oncol 8:1108-1114, 1990.

This recent paper describes the typical format for chemoembolization protocols and is a review of the state of other investigations in this area.

25 Vascular Disorders

J. Michael Henderson

The liver is a highly vascular organ weighing approximately 2% to 2.5% of total body weight but receiving 20% to 25% of cardiac output. Its vasculature is complex but must be briefly reviewed to understand the pathophysiology of vascular disorders.

The hepatic artery usually arises from the celiac axis as the common hepatic artery and provides 20% to 30% of total liver blood flow. It divides into right and left branches before entering the liver. This arterial anatomy is abnormal in about 30% of the population, with the most common anomalies being replaced or accessory right or left hepatic arteries arising from the superior mesenteric or left gastric arteries respectively. Anomalies, many of which are more complex, are of importance to the surgeon when operating in the liver hilum on the bile duct, when resecting the liver, or when removing a donor liver for liver transplantation.

The portal vein is formed behind the neck of the pancreas by the union of the superior mesenteric and splenic veins and carries a liter or more of blood to the liver per minute. Anomalies of the vein are unusual, and it divides close to the hepatic parenchyma, with the left portal branch usually having a longer extrahepatic course.

The hepatic artery and portal vein provide blood flow into the liver at widely disparate pressures: the arterial inflow pressure approximates 100 mm Hg, whereas the portal venous inflow pressure is 7 to 10 mm Hg. Downregulation of the arterial pressure to a sinusoidal pressure of 4 to 7 mm Hg is achieved through complex mechanisms, as is the balance of hepatic arterial and portal venous flow.

The venous drainage of the liver is by the hepatic veins. These begin as the central veins of the lobule, which join to form sublobular veins, lobular hepatic veins, and finally right, left, and middle hepatic veins, which enter the inferior vena cava while it is still within the liver substance.

In a clinical context, the blood supply to the liver should be considered by its functional components as well as by this gross anatomic configuration. The segmental anatomy of the liver (Figure 25-1) subdivides the liver into eight segments based on their distinct hepatic veins. Each of these segments, however, also have their own hepatic arterial and portal venous inflows—a factor of significant importance in consideration of therapeutic interventions such as resection or embolization. Further, in consideration of vascular disorders of the liver, at a microscopic level the functional unit of the aci-

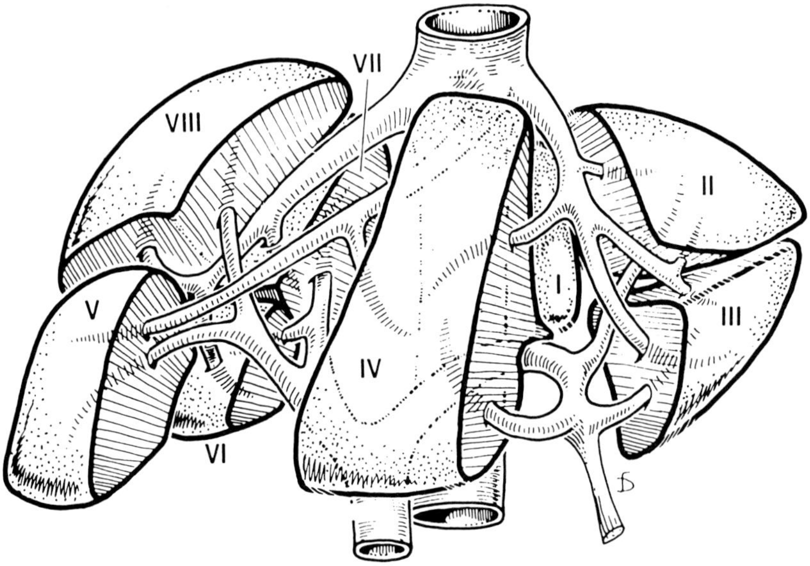

Figure 25-1
Segmental anatomy of the liver after Couinaud. The portal venous inflow and hepatic venous outflow to the eight liver segments can be seen. (From Bismuth H: Anatomical surgery of the liver. In Bluegart LH, ed: Surgery of the liver and biliary tract, Edinburgh, 1988, Churchill Livingstone.)

nus is key in the pathophysiology of these disorders. The anatomic configuration of the acinus has been described elsewhere, but in addressing injury and therapy it is important to differentiate if the portal tract or central vein is the primary site of insult.

In considering vascular disorders of the liver, this chapter broadly breaks these down into "inflow" and "outflow" disorders as outlined in the box at right.

VASCULAR DISORDERS OF THE LIVER

Inflow
- Hepatic artery
- Anteriovenous fistula
- Portal vein
- Ischemia
- Hepatic denervation

Outflow
- Budd-Chiari syndrome
- Veno-occlusive disease
- Congestive heart failure

INVESTIGATIVE METHODS

Pertinent points in the history, physical examination, and standard laboratory tests are emphasized with specific disorders. A liver biopsy may be required for definitive diagnosis. Radiologic imaging, using both noninvasive and invasive techniques, are required in the diagnosis of many of these disorders and is briefly reviewed.

Ultrasound imaging of the portal vein, hepatic artery, and hepatic veins combined with the Doppler flowmeter has evolved as useful technology in the evaluation of anatomic obstructive lesions. These methods continue to improve each year and will play an increasing role in patient evaluation. It has the merit of being totally noninvasive, with no irradiation, but is highly observer dependent. Figures 25-2 and 25-3 illustrate the imaging capability of this technique.

Computerized axial tomographic (CAT) scan is particularly useful in providing morphologic data or in defining localized intrahepatic lesions. The ability to Scan using different enhancement modalities, e.g., without contrast, with intravenous bolus enhancement, with specific hepatic arterial or portal venous enhancement, or finally with scanning delayed 4 to 6 hours after contrast administration has lead to greatly improved diagnostic capability by CAT scan.

Hepatic angiography is both invasive and complex but can provide essential diagnostic information. It can be broadly divided into inflow and outflow studies. Selective hepatic arteriography will define hepatic arterial anatomy, allow identification of anomalies, and be diagnostic of specific hepatic arterial pathologies. Selective superior mesenteric angiography followed through the venous phase is the standard method for angiographic imaging of the portal vein. Hepatic venography is of particular importance in evaluation of the outflow disorders under discussion in this chapter. Usually done by the transfemoral approach, the catheter is manipulated into the right hepatic vein under fluoroscopic control. If there is suspicion of a segmental pathologic condition, the middle and left hepatic veins should also be cannulated. Both pressure measurement and imaging should be done. Pressure is measured (1) with the

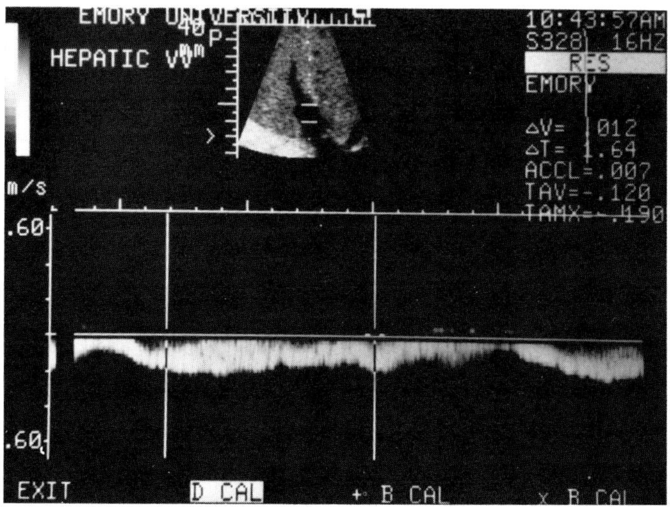

Figure 25-2
Ultrasound imaging of the middle hepatic vein, which can be seen entering the inferior vena cava.

A

B

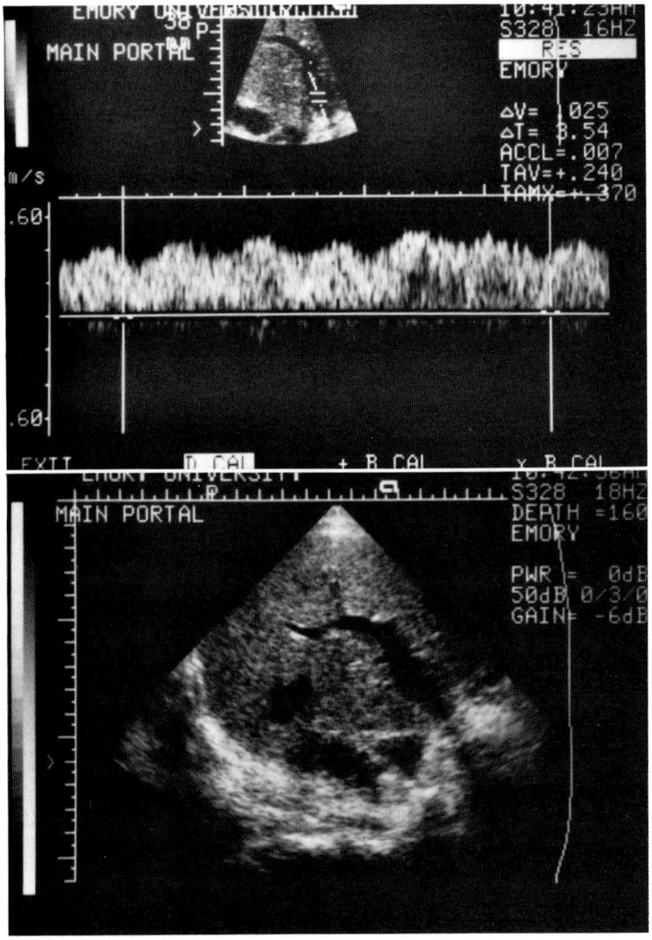

Figure 25-3
A, Doppler flowmetry. **B,** Ultrasound imaging of the main portal vein. The flow in this patient is prograde toward the transducer *(above the line)* and hence toward the liver.

catheter in the "wedged" position, or by balloon occlusion of a peripheral hepatic vein, (2) in the free hepatic vein, (3) in both the infrahepatic and intrahepatic parts of the inferior vena cava, and (4) in the right atrium. Contrast, 5 to 10 ml, should be injected in (1) the wedged position for evaluation of portal reflux and sinusoidal washout and (2) the free hepatic vein to exclude major vein obstruction.

INFLOW DISORDERS

The Hepatic Artery

Occlusion of the hepatic artery most commonly results from trauma but may rarely be seen with collagen vascular disease such as polyarteritis nodosa or with emboli. Iatrogenic traumatic occlusion of the artery may occur with an intimal flap at angiography, or at the time of biliary surgery. The most common injury, often unrecognized, is ligation of the right hepatic artery at the time of cholecystectomy. The basic rule is that, provided that the liver is normal and has good portal venous inflow, occlusion of a major branch of the hepatic artery will have minimal effect. Transient elevations of LDH and AST may be observed. However, when cirrhosis is present, increased hepatic arterial inflow is a compensatory mechanism that helps maintain hepatocyte perfusion, and occlusion of the hepatic artery may have a significant detrimental effect. Similarly hepatic arterial occlusion in the first 2 months after orthotopic liver transplantation usually results in patchy infarction of the liver, bile duct necrosis, and the need for retransplantation. A protective feature of hepatic arterial occlusion in the otherwise normal patient is the rapid development of adequate collaterals around the occlusion, thus reestablishing good arterial inflow. No therapy is required with the exceptions cited above.

Aneurysm of the hepatic artery is rare but is a diagnosis that must be considered for an unexplained mass either at the hilum of the liver or located in an intrahepatic position. Frequently a history of trauma, prior surgery, or liver biopsy may be elicited, but spontaneous hepatic artery aneurysm has been reported. Presentation ranges from vague pain in the right upper quadrant to profound hypovolemic shock secondary to free intraperitoneal rupture. In some cases of intrahepatic aneurysm rupture into the biliary tree may give profuse hemobilia and biliary colic.

The diagnosis may be indicated by ultrasonography, CT scanning, or magnetic resonance imaging (MRI), but the definitive study is angiography. The risk of enlargement and rupture mandate therapy when the diagnosis is made. Small aneurysms, particularly intrahepatic, can be occluded by angiographic embolization of spring coils and Gelfoam. Larger aneurysms may require surgical intervention, particularly when extrahepatic.

A patient with an intrahepatic artery aneurysm is illustrated in Figures 25-4 and 25-5. This aneurysm occurred after liver biopsy in a patient who had had a liver transplant. It ruptured into the biliary tree giving profuse hemobilia. Management was by angiographic occlusion of the feeding artery. This method controlled bleeding without further morbidity.

An *arteriovenous fistula* between a branch of the hepatic artery and the portal vein occurs in up to 5% of liver biopsy specimens. The majority are asymptomatic and probably close spontaneously. Occasionally they may persist, enlarge, and become symptomatic with "arterialization" of the portal tree. Portal hypertension can result, and if symptomatic, the fistula can be occluded by a transvascular approach. Figure 25-6 illustrates such a case, which occurred after liver biopsy in a patient with cirrhosis. Occlusion of the segmental feeding artery closed this fistula.

A less common cause of arteriovenous fistula in the liver is tumor. This is usually a hepatocellular carcinoma, but occasionally a large hemangioma or multiple telangiectasia may result in an arteriovenous fistula. If large, a bruit may be heard over the liver. Large fistula leading to

A

B

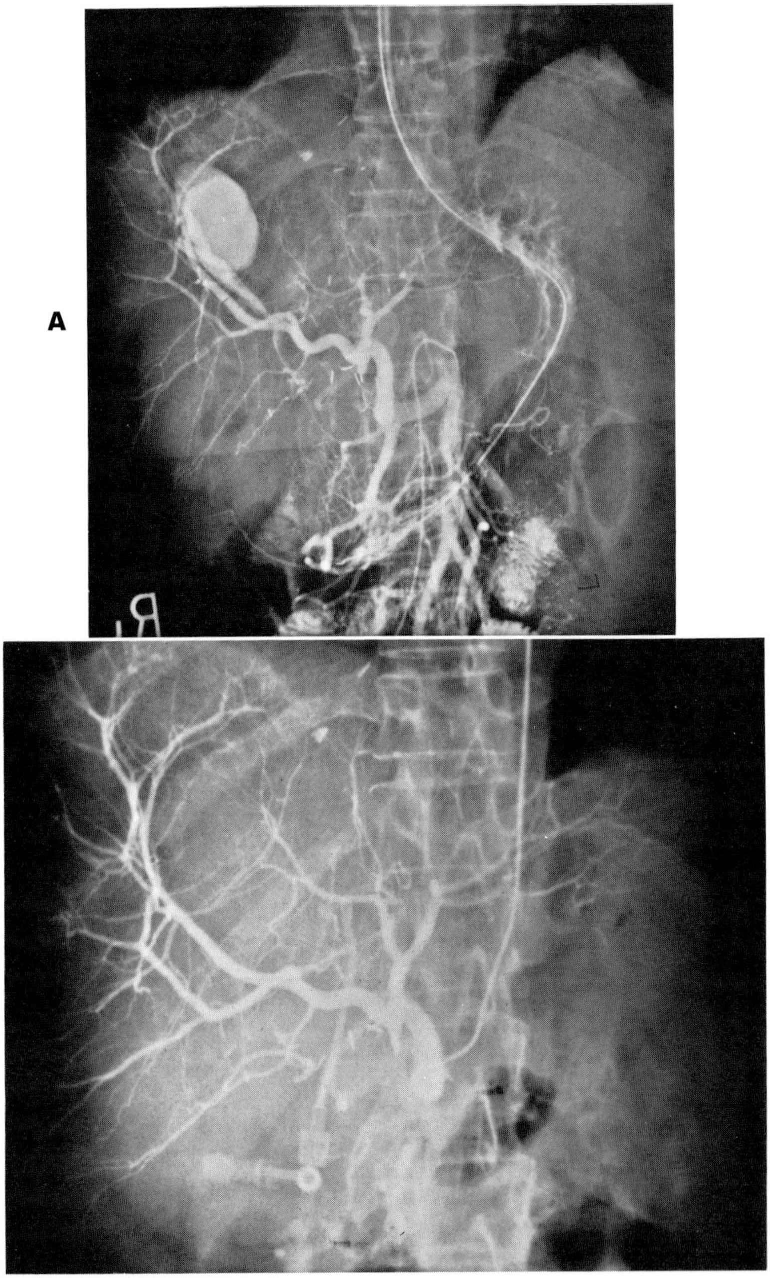

Figure 25-4

A, An intrahepatic hepatic artery aneurysm is shown on the hepatic arteriogram. This occurred after liver biopsy in a patient who had a liver transplantation. Clinically the patient had profuse hemobilia requiring transfusion. **B,** Arteriography after occlusion of the feeding vessel with a steel coil shows no further filling of the aneurysm.

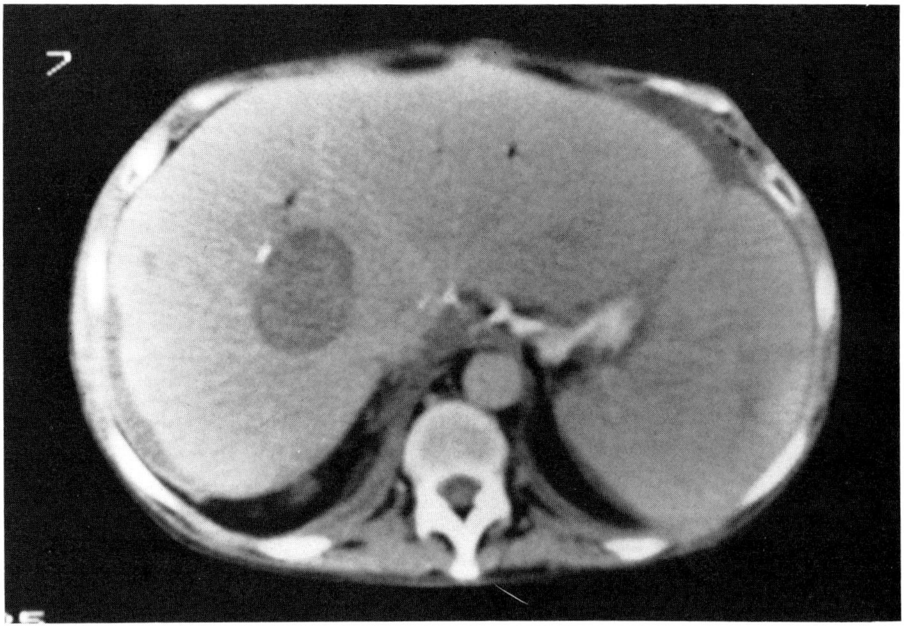

Figure 25-5
CAT scan of the same patient as in Figure 25-4 showing the intrahepatic aneurysm after thrombosis following occlusion of the feeding vessel.

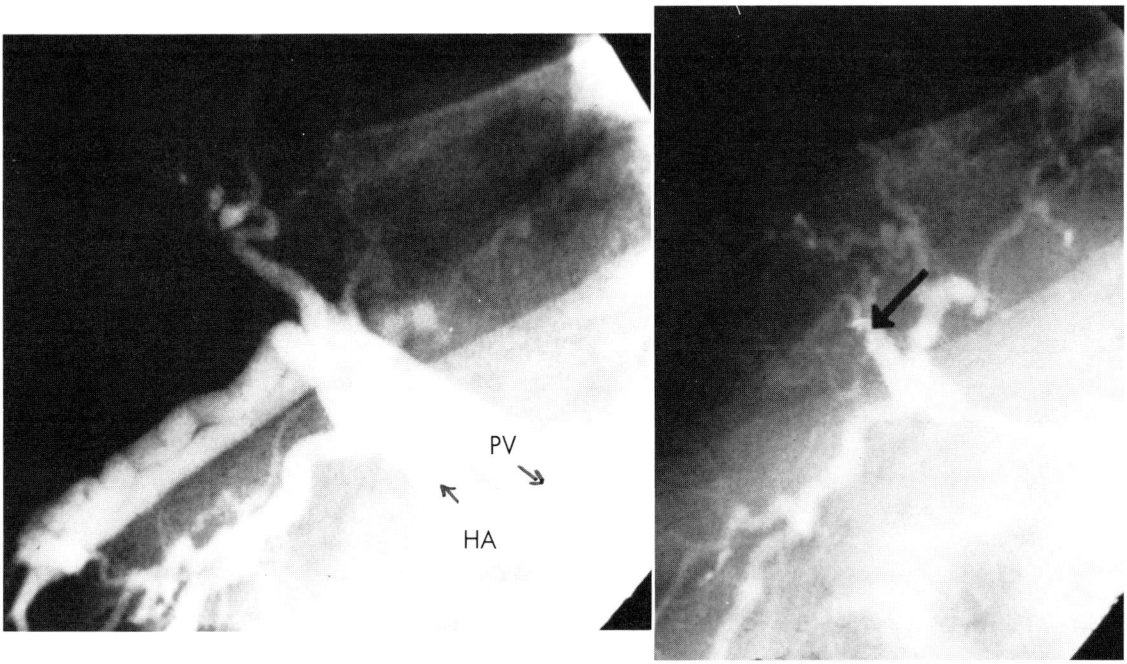

B

Figure 25-6
A, Hepatic arteriogram showing early direct filling and retrograde flow in the portal vein through an arteriovenous fistula. **B,** Occlusion of the feeding branch of the right hepatic artery shows occlusion of the fistula *(arrow)*. *HA,* hepatic artery; *PV,* portal vein.

congestive heart failure may require embolization of the tumor mass.

Portal Vein

Congenital anomalies. The portal vein develops from the vitelline and umbilical veins. Considering the complexity of this process, it is surprising that anomalies of the portal venous system are rare. Agenesis and atresia have been reported, as have persistence of major fetal tributaries such as umbilical and inferior mesenteric vessels. However, most clinical problems leading to portal vein thrombosis and portal hypertension have other definable causes.

Portal vein thrombosis. As a cause of variceal bleeding, portal vein thrombosis differs from most other pathoses leading to variceal bleeding in that the liver is normal. Prognosis is therefore much improved, and therapy must be focused on stopping bleeding.

The causes of portal vein thrombosis that can lead to portal hypertension and variceal bleeding are listed in the box below. In evaluating a patient for variceal bleeding in whom there is no known liver disease and in whom the picture "does not fit," the physician should always consider this diagnosis.

CAUSES OF EXTRAHEPATIC PORTAL VEIN THROMBOSIS

- Umbilical sepsis with or without catheterization
- Induced thrombosis
  - Trauma
  - Dehydration
- Hypercoagulable state
  - Protein C, protein S deficency
  - Antithrombin III deficency
  - Myeloproliferative disorder

Pathophysiology. Occlusion of the portal vein leads to increased venous pressure in the splanchnic bed (portal hypertension). The spleen enlarges, leading to a secondary hypersplenism. It is not unusual for the hematologist to see such patients first because of severe thrombocytopenia ($>50{,}000/mm^3$) and leukopenia in conjunction with massive splenomegaly. However, the platelets work normally, and injudicious splenectomy can deprive the patient of the best therapeutic option for their varices. Full evaluation is required.

The major difference in the pathophysiologic condition of these patients compared to that of most patients with portal hypertension is in the hemodynamics and function of their normal liver. Hemodynamically the normal (low) sinusoidal pressure encourages collateral formation from the high-pressure splanchnic bed back to the low-pressure sinusoids to the same degree as the high splanchnic pressure drives the development of varices. These collaterals are seen as "cavernous transformation" of the portal vein, which provides excellent continuing portal perfusion to the liver. However, gastroesophageal varices do develop and can bleed, leading to the need for therapy.

The liver is histologically and functionally normal. This feature should be documented as part of the evaluation. The liver is usually below normal size for body weight but in our experience shows normal functional capacity for its size.

Clinical features. The main clinical presentation is variceal bleeding, though some patients may present with splenomegaly or hematologic abnormalities. The young patient with variceal bleeding and no known liver disease has portal vein thrombosis (PVT) till proved other-

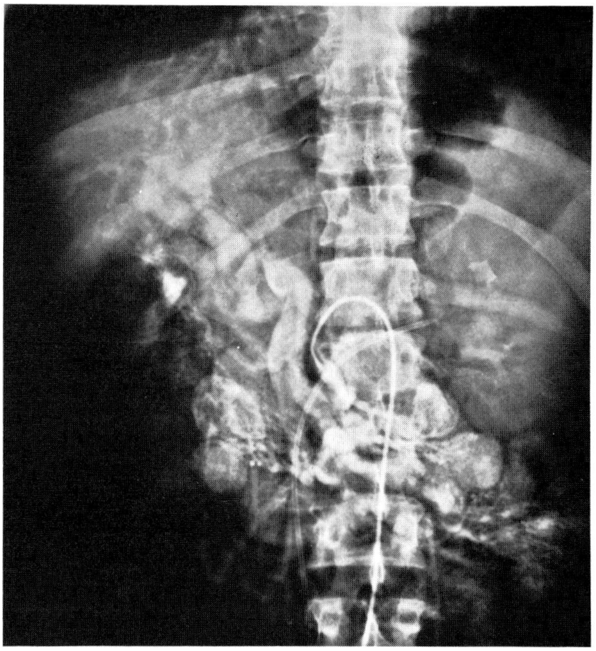

Figure 25-7
Superior mesenteric arteriogram showing in the venous phase the typical cavernous transformation of a patient with portal vein thrombosis.

wise. Bleeding rarely occurs before 4 years of age, and most commonly from 8 to 16 years in those with a neonatal origin for the PVT. However, I have seen patients up to 70 years of age present with variceal bleeding secondary to PVT.

The bleeding episode is usually well tolerated because the liver is normal. If the patient develops jaundice, ascites, or encephalopathy, a diagnosis other than PVT must be sought.

Diagnosis. Definitive diagnosis of portal vein thrombosis is made by arteriography. Figure 25-7 illustrates the typical cavernous transformation in such a patient who presented with variceal bleeding. Although presumptive or supportive evidence of this diagnosis can be reached with ultrasonography, CAT scanning or MRI angiography should be performed. Beyond allowing the diagnosis to be made, angiography also provides useful information on the patency of the portal vein tributaries, which may influence management decisions.

Liver biopsy should document normal liver histology findings before variceal bleeding can be ascribed solely to PVT. Occasionally intrahepatic pathosis such as cirrhosis, hepatic fibrosis, or portal sclerosis may accompany PVT and significantly affect prognosis.

Endoscopy will define the severity and bleeding risk of varices in both patients who have bled and in those who have not yet bled. It is important to perform endoscopy on this latter group because variceal bleeding may in the end prove to be their greatest life-threatening event. Varices will influence therapy choice.

Hematologic assessment should focus on hypercoagulable states, particularly in patients with no other definable risk factors. As in our Budd-Chiari patients (see p. 432) the incidence of such abnormalities has increased, since our department instituted the evaluation given in the box below.

Management. The three main factors that must be considered are (1) variceal bleeding (or the threat of such bleeding), (2) the splenomegaly and hypersplenism, and (3) the underlying etiologic disease if any.

Variceal bleeding in these patients is best treated by decompression of their varices. In our experience, more than 75% of such patients have patent splenic veins, which are suitable for selective variceal decompression by distal splenorenal shunt. The advantages of this operation in these patients are as follows: (1) Variceal bleeding is controlled in over 90% of patients. Careful follow-up observation is required, particularly in the first year, because there is a risk of shunt stenosis requiring dilatation in this group. (2) Portal perfusion of the liver is maintained through the cavernous collaterals, obviating the risk of late hepatic dysfunction secondary to loss of portal flow. (3) The spleen is reduced to approximately half its preoperative volume with a concomitant rise in platelet and white blood cell count.

Alternative methods of managing variceal bleeding have been used in this population. Total portal systemic shunts, such as mesocaval shunts, deprive the liver of portal blood, which, even in the normal liver, can lead to hepatic insufficiency over time. Endoscopic variceal sclerosis is a temporizing measure that does not address the pathophysiologic problem. It is useful in the emergent setting and in patients in whom a selective shunt is not an option.

Splenomegaly and hypersplenism can be satisfactorily treated by distal splenorenal shunt. Splenectomy is not a good option unless the splenic vein is totally thrombosed (about 20% to 25% of patients). The incidence of recurrent variceal bleeding or initial hemorrhage in those in whom splenectomy has been performed for splenomegaly is high. Splenectomy deprives such patients of their optimal therapeutic choice. Do not just treat the thrombocytopenia!

The final consideration in managing these patients must be therapy for any underlying pathosis. A clear history of neo-

HEMATOLOGIC EVALUATION IN BUDD-CHIARI SYNDROME

- Hemoglobin and hematocrit
- White blood count
- Platelet count and aggregometry
- Blood smear
- Bone marrow
  - Routine microscopy
  - Reticulin stain
  - Cytogenetic analysis
- Leukocyte alkaline phosphatase
- Red blood cell mass with chromium-51 labeling
- Sucrose hemolysis for paroxysmal nocturnal hemoglobinuria
- Vitamin B_{12} binding capacity
- Protein C, protein S, antithrombin III

natal sepsis or umbilical catheterization defines a cause and eliminates the need for further therapy. The risk of further venous thrombosis and particularly shunt thrombosis must be evaluated in patients with no other risk factors. If a hypercoagulable state is defined, anticoagulation, or treatment of an underlying myeloproliferative disorder should parallel other therapy.

Ischemia

The liver is remarkably resistant to shock, with recognized ischemic hypotensive injury being rare. The key factors that contribute to the occurrence of a significant hepatic ischemic injury are presence of concomitant liver disease and the duration of hypotension. The liver's remarkable reserve capacity may well mask lesser degrees of a significant ischemic injury. The ability to detect liver dysfunction with standard tests such as serum bilirubin, AST, and lactate dehydrogenase is notoriously insensitive. Methods of quantitatively measuring impaired function in the patient with shock are beginning to be applied in clinical practice and may well give new insight into the effect of ischemia on the liver.

The classic teaching, that prolonged hypotension with a systolic blood pressure below 80 mm Hg for 10 hours or greater is required for significant liver ischemia, must be called into question. This degree of ischemia will result in a measurable rise in standard liver tests and is histologically associated with a central zonal necrosis. Recovery is dependent on resolution of the underlying cause.

In patients with cirrhosis in whom the liver is more dependent on an increased hepatic arterial perfusion for adequate function, the ischemic effect may be more pronounced. This may often be aggravated in clinical practice by therapeutic interventions, which further reduce liver perfusion. An example is the use of pitressin in the management of variceal bleeding. A patient who is already hypotensive from a gastrointestinal blood loss is given a potent splanchnic vasoconstrictor drug to lower portal pressure, but in so doing the liver receives less blood and further ischemia can result. The relative contributions of bleeding, hypotension, the underlying liver pathosis, and the pitressin in causing hepatic ischemia in such patients are hard to determine but should be considered in patient management.

The ischemic injury of cardiac failure is discussed in more detail on p. 442-443.

The amazing resistance of the liver to ischemic injury is further seen in liver transplantation. In this ultimate ischemia, when the liver is maintained unperfused at 4° C for up to 24 hours, a remarkable return of function can be seen within an hour of reperfusion. The visual evidence for this is the production of bile in the operative field and the return of blood clotting in a patient with a good functioning graft. Objective data showing return of function are the increase in coagulation factors and the rapid clearance of elevated bilirubin in the subsequent 24 to 48 hours. The major determinant of the "harvest injury" of the transplanted liver appears to relate more to events in the donor before or during harvest than to the actual ischemia of the explanted liver.

Hepatic Denervation

A new area of interest and investigation in considering "inflow" vascular disorders of the liver is the denervated liver. This has become a pertinent question in light of the increasing clinical application of liver transplantation.

Increased blood flow in the transplanted liver has been suggested to occur by a combination of loss of normal sympathetic vasomotor regulation and persistence of the systemic hyperdynamic cardiovascular state, which is a feature of the patient with cirrhosis. Studies by our group have shown an increase in low-dose galactose clearances (a liver blood flow–dependent clearance measurement) in the first 6 months after transplantation. The relative roles of hepatic arterial and portal venous inflows and of systemic hemodynamic abnormalities to this finding have still to be defined but pose intriguing questions on the regulation of liver blood flow.

The clinical importance of this lies in the metabolic and pharmacologic implications. For highly extracted substances the "first pass" through the liver is the metabolic rate–limiting step, leading to an increased metabolism of such substances. Nutritional and pharmacologic therapy in patients after transplantation should be kept in mind.

OUTFLOW DISORDERS

Budd-Chiari Syndrome (BCS)

The Budd-Chiari syndrome group of disorders brings together many causes of hepatic vein obstruction that may occur at the smallest vein of the lobule, in the main hepatic veins, or in the vena cava or right atrium. The common feature is venous outflow block: although blood can get into the liver through the hepatic artery and portal vein, it cannot get out, and congestion results. Budd described the pathologic features in 1857 but did not recognize the clinical picture. Chiari reported on the clinical picture in 1899.

Definition. The clinical syndrome comprises hepatomegaly, ascites, and abdominal pain. The histologic features are centrilobular sinusoidal dilatation, pooling, and congestion, which may lead to hepatocyte necrosis and ultimately fibrosis.

Pathophysiology. The main causes are listed in the box below. They should be considered by their sites of obstruction, though these may overlap. Until recently it was believed that the majority of patients presenting with Budd-Chiari syndrome had no recognizable cause. However, increasing recognition of the role of myeloproliferative disorders and their associated hypercoagulable state has led to recognition of this as a cause in 9 of our last 14 patients with Budd-Chiari syndrome. The role of oral contraceptives should probably be viewed against other

CAUSES OF BUDD-CHIARI SYNDROME

Site of occlusion	Etiologic factors
Lobule	Venoocclusive disease Sclerosing hyaline necrosis
Hepatic vein	Hypercoagulable state (myeloproliferative) Oral contraceptives Paroxysmal nocturnal hemoglobinuria Infection Webs Trauma Tumor

etiologic factors. Paroxysmal nocturnal hemoglobinuria is a cause that should be considered and investigated.

The other listed etiologic factors in the box on p. 432 usually cause a secondary Budd-Chiari syndrome because of mechanical obstruction either of a single hepatic vein, all the hepatic veins, or the final outflow of the intrahepatic vena cava or right atrium. The highest incidence of web obstruction is reported in the Orient.

Clinical features. The range of clinical presentations of Budd-Chiari syndrome may be from an acute fulminant course to an insidious chronic form evolving over several years. The rapidity of presentation is primarily a function of how complete and sudden the onset of the outflow obstruction is.

An acute presentation may occur with sudden complete thrombosis of all hepatic veins. This thrombosis can be secondary to trauma, tumor, or an underlying coagulable state. Right upper quadrant pain secondary to liver swelling, massive ascites, hepatomegaly, and rapid deterioration into hepatocellular failure can occur over several days to weeks. This presentation, though less common than the chronic form, requires rapid evaluation, accurate diagnosis, and urgent therapy.

The more common and less acute form of Budd-Chiari syndrome has an insidious onset over weeks or months. This is associated with occlusion of one or two hepatic veins initially, sparing some hepatic parenchyma but then usually running a progressive course with involvement of other outflow paths. Symptoms and signs are more subtle than in the acute form. Abdominal swelling secondary to ascites is usually present, but because it is not sudden and massive, the patient may have simply ascribed it to "weight gain." General malaise may be a feature. Hepatomegaly can usually be detected on physical examinations, and on occasion lower-limb edema is found because of inferior vena caval obstruction. The patient rarely shows jaundice or other stigmas of chronic liver disease till very late in the course. The diagnosis can easily be overlooked, and frequently there is a delay of several months before the correct diagnosis is made. A high index of suspicion must be present to detect the subtle clinical signs and symptoms in the patient with a subacute course. Early diagnosis can lead to earlier therapy, which may save both liver and life.

A small percentage of patients present with a late chronic form of Budd-Chiari syndrome, with a picture of advanced liver disease. These patients have progressed through the sequence just outlined and have evolved to a full-blown cirrhosis. They may present with variceal bleeding or hepatic failure.

Laboratory data. There are no classic diagnostic laboratory tests for Budd-Chiari syndrome (BCS). Standard biochemical tests are usually normal until there is severe hepatocellular necrosis. In acute BCS the serum aminotransferases may rise, as may the bilirubin. However, normal or mild elevations of these do not rule out a diagnosis of BCS. In subacute or chronic BCS the standard liver tests are usually normal or show mild elevation. In my experience with 21 patients requiring a decompressive shunt for ongoing hepatocyte necrosis the mean bilirubin was 2 mg/dl, albumin 3.5 gm/dl, AST 60 μg/L, and alkaline phosphatase 250 μg/L. Quantitative measurement of hepatocyte function in this group of patients showed large liver volume (2000 cc) and mild reduction in galactose elimination capacity (350 mg/min, with normal being 500 mg/min).

Chronic BCS may lead to changes in biochemical data as the continuing liver damage leads to progressive fibrosis and cirrhosis. This is most noticeably documented by reduction in quantitative hepatic function.

Hematologic laboratory data similarly are normal or show minor changes. Coagulation (measured by prothrombin time prolongation, partial thromboplastin time, and platelet count) is usually normal. As discussed below, this normalcy may however be deceptive because many of these patients do have an underlying myeloproliferative disorder as the cause of their BCS. The combination of hepatic dysfunction and splenomegaly may mask subtle changes, and it is only with more sophisticated studies that the underlying disorder may be defined. This evaluation is presented below.

Pathology. In acute Budd-Chiari syndrome the liver is enlarged, purple, and smooth, often being two to three times normal size. The surface of the liver shows "pitting edema" and has a distinct sponge-like texture. The surface lymphatics may be prominent. A liver needle biopsy core from such a liver looks like blood because of the severe parenchymal congestion.

The hepatic veins may contain thrombus through their full extent or in a segmental fashion depending on the cause and site of involvement. The age of the thrombus dictates its appearance, varying from fresh in the acute case to organized or even recanalized in the chronic case. In cases caused by malignancy the thrombus may contain malignant cells. The vein wall may become thickened in chronic cases with increasing distortion. In the course of the disease there is an inexorable attempt by the liver to drain the congested sinusoids through the development of capsular collaterals to the diaphragm. The caudate lobe drains directly into the vena cava through several small direct veins, which are usually spared the thrombotic process. For this reason, the caudate lobe is usually spared in BCS, and in an attempt to compensate for damage to the rest of the liver it hypertrophies.

Histologically, BCS shows characteristic changes depending on the stage of the disease. Biopsy is a mandatory step in evaluation (see p. 436), and a core should be taken from both the right and left lobes because there may be differential involvement. The principal features on biopsy revolve around centrilobular (zone 3) changes. The progression of severity is initial sinusoidal dilatation and congestion, which may lead to hepatocyte necrosis and ultimately to fibrosis and lobular collapse. Thrombus may be identified in the central veins. The late findings of chronic BCS are of central fibrosis, which if associated with lobular collapse will proceed to a frank cirrhosis. However, in acute BCS the periportal hepatocytes may be remarkably spared the otherwise severe injury. Figures 25-8 and 25-9 illustrate these histologic changes.

Diagnosis. The two essential steps in establishing a diagnosis of BCS are liver biopsy and hepatic venography. Other adjunctive investigations such as ultrasound imaging (with or without Doppler flowmetry), CT scanning, or MRI scanning may provide helpful information but do not provide definitive diagnostic data or guide therapy.

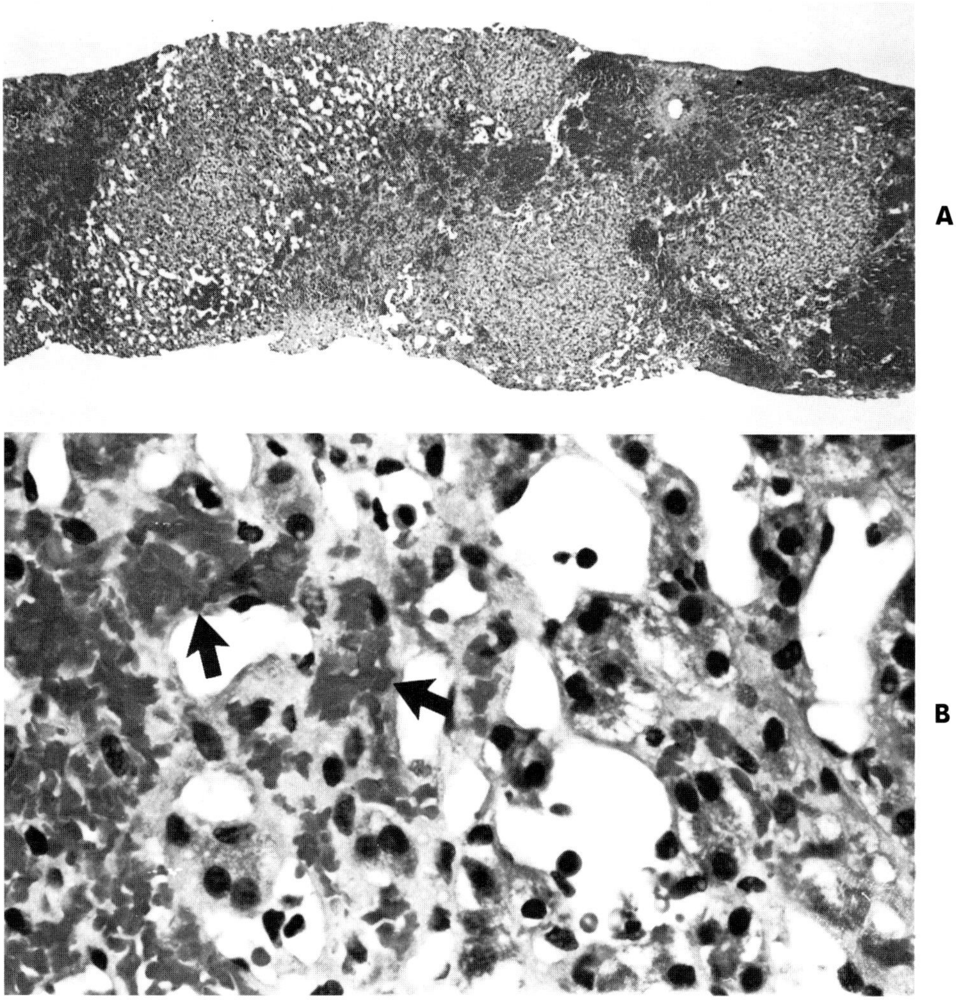

Figure 25-8
Acute Budd-Chiari syndrome. **A,** Confluent dark areas of severe zone 3 congestion and confluent hepatocytic dropout surround pale-staining islands of intact zone 1 parenchyma. **B,** Sinusoidal dilatation extends into zone 2 and is associated with entrapment of erythrocytes in the space of Disse and hepatocytic loss, *arrows*. Remaining hepatocytes are atrophic. (Courtesy Dr. Gary Hertzler, Department of Pathology, Emory University Hospital, Atlanta, Ga., 1990.)

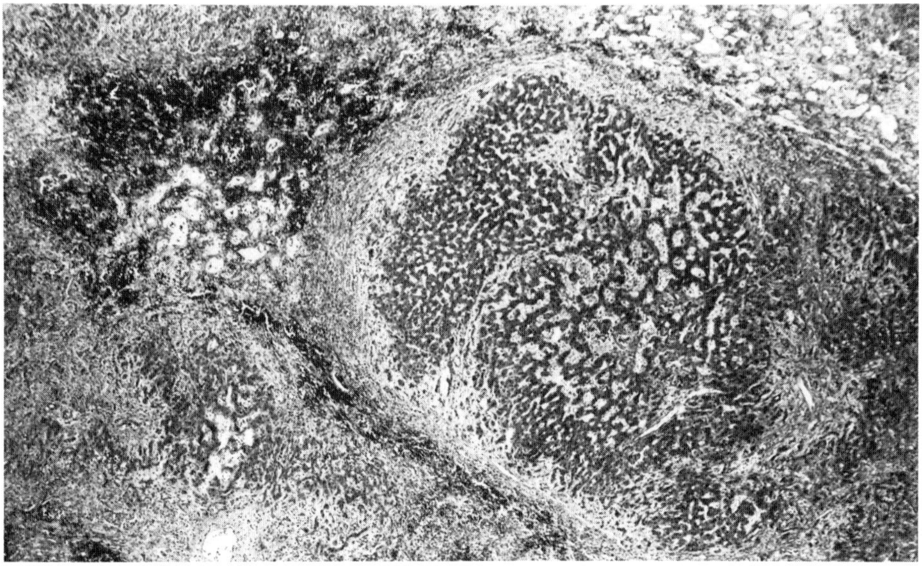

Figure 25-9
Chronic Budd-Chiari syndrome. Dark hemorrhage and dilated sinusoids lie in confluent areas of collapse and fibrosis. A regenerative hepatocytic nodule surrounded by a pale fibrotic band denotes transformation into frank cirrhosis. (Courtesy Dr. Gary Hertzler, Department of Pathology, Emory University Hospital, Atlanta, Ga., 1990.)

Hepatic venography is done by the transfemoral route. Failure to cannulate any of the three main hepatic veins provides diagnostic information. More typically, a short segment of abnormal vein can be cannulated, and injection of contrast medium shows the classic spider-web pattern that illustrates the liver's attempt to provide venous drainage through collaterals (Figure 25-10). It is important that the radiologist does define involvement or normality of the three major hepatic veins. Venography can provide other diagnostic information such as inferior vena cava occlusion by either intraluminal obstruction or extraluminal compression. From a subsequent management point of view, measurement of pressure in the infrahepatic and intrahepatic sections of the vena cava and in the right atrium may dictate subsequent surgical therapy (Figure 25-11).

Liver biopsy of both right and left lobes should be done under either CT or ultrasound guidance. The rationale that "the patient is too sick for liver biopsy" is untenable because the sicker the patient the more urgent the biopsy. Massive ascites may require paracentesis, and clotting deficits may require correction. It is determination of the degree of ongoing injury that dictates therapy, and there is no other way of determining the degree of hepatocyte necrosis. The features of liver biopsy that help define appropriate management

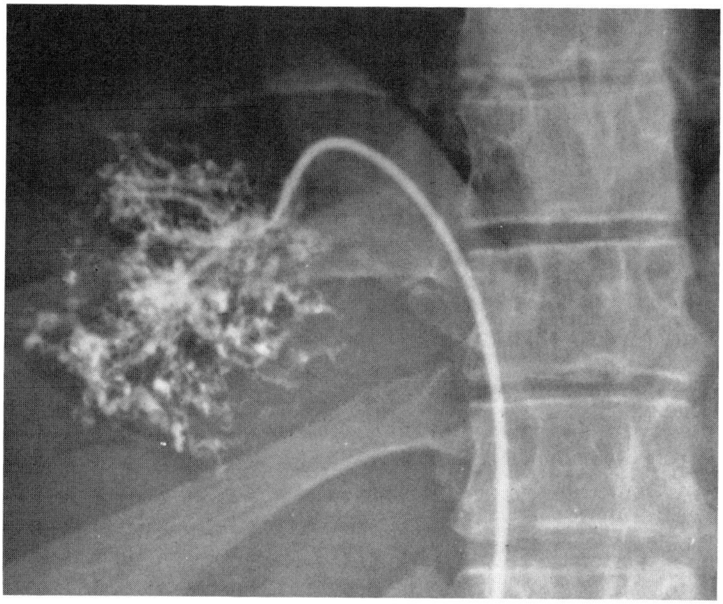

Figure 25-10
Hepatic venogram in a patient with acute Budd-Chiari syndrome showing the spider-web pattern. Multiple small intercommunicating veins indicate the attempt to provide drainage. No major hepatic veins could be found.

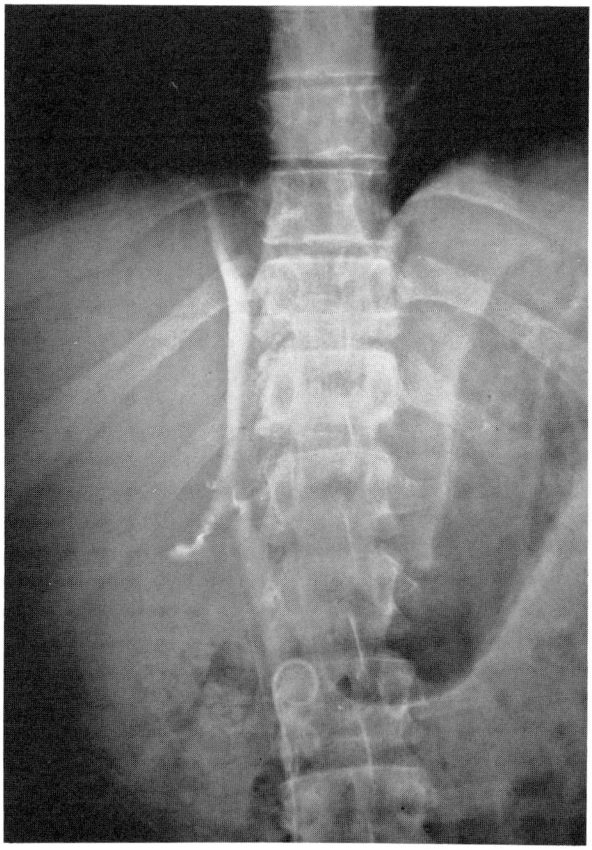

Figure 25-11
Inferior vena cavagram in a patient with Budd-Chiari syndrome. The enormously swollen and congested liver has obliterated the intrahepatic vena cava. A pressure gradient of 22 mm Hg from the right atrium to the infrahepatic vena cava led to a mesoatrial shunt.

are the degree of ongoing necrosis and the amount of fibrosis.

Etiology should be investigated early in the course of evaluation. Imaging of the major hepatic veins, inferior vena cava, and right atrium as described in the prior section should define intraluminal lesions leading to outflow block, or may be suggestive of a local intrahepatic lesion if a single vein is compressed. One should perform CT scanning of the liver and abdomen to look for intrahepatic or intraabdominal malignancy.

Hematologic abnormalities should be assiduously sought as causative in BCS. The box on p. 430 summarizes the hematologic work-up. Early identification and treatment of hypercoagulable states will minimize the chance of further thrombosis when therapy is instituted. The classic definition of polycythemia rubra vera based on the criteria of the Polycythemia Rubra Vera Study Group may not be fulfilled, in that the presence of liver disease or bleeding may result in a normal hematocrit. The splenomegaly associated with portal hypertension may also mask thrombocytosis. Additional criteria that our group has found useful have been increased reticular fibrosis on bone marrow biopsy and the occurrence of an abnormal marrow karyotype. Since instituting this evaluation in 1985, 9 of the last 13 patients we have evaluated with BCS have had an underlying myeloproliferative disorder.

Management

The aims of therapy with BCS are first to halt or prevent ongoing hepatocyte damage and second to treat the underlying problem. An algorithm for management is given in Figure 25-12.

Early diagnosis is the key to optimal management. It is therefore important to institute the above evaluation steps on suspicion of the diagnosis. Therapy for the liver is based on the liver biopsy findings. Ongoing hepatocyte necrosis requires decompression by establishment of a venous outflow.

Mild disease is defined as centrilobular dilatation and congestion on liver biopsy without hepatocyte necrosis or fibrosis. It is difficult to tell at a single time point if this is likely to be progressive or will resolve. A period of observation, with appropriate dietary and diuretic management of ascites, with follow-up liver biopsy in 2 to 6 months is indicated. Clinical deterioration should lead to earlier reevaluation. Etiologic factors should be sought and if identified be treated.

Acute disease is defined as severe centrilobular congestion with ongoing hepatocyte necrosis but usually without significant fibrosis on liver biopsy. This congestion requires urgent decompression to halt the hepatocyte destruction. Such decompression is achieved by use of the portal vein as an outflow track from the obstructed sinusoids. The operative choices are an infrahepatic side-to-side portal systemic shunt such as a portacaval or mesocaval shunt (Figures 25-13 and 25-14), or a suprahepatic shunt, which is usually a mesoatrial shunt (Figures 25-15 and 25-16). The surgical decision as to whether an infrahepatic shunt will suffice or a suprahepatic shunt is required is based on pressure-gradient measurements from the right atrium to the infrahepatic cava. If the enlarged liver has compressed the intrahepatic cava sufficiently to obstruct the infrahepatic flow back to the heart, a portacaval or mesocaval shunt will not be decompressive. Under these conditions a mesoatrial shunt is required. Again, it is important to emphasize the need to fully evaluate the patient for an

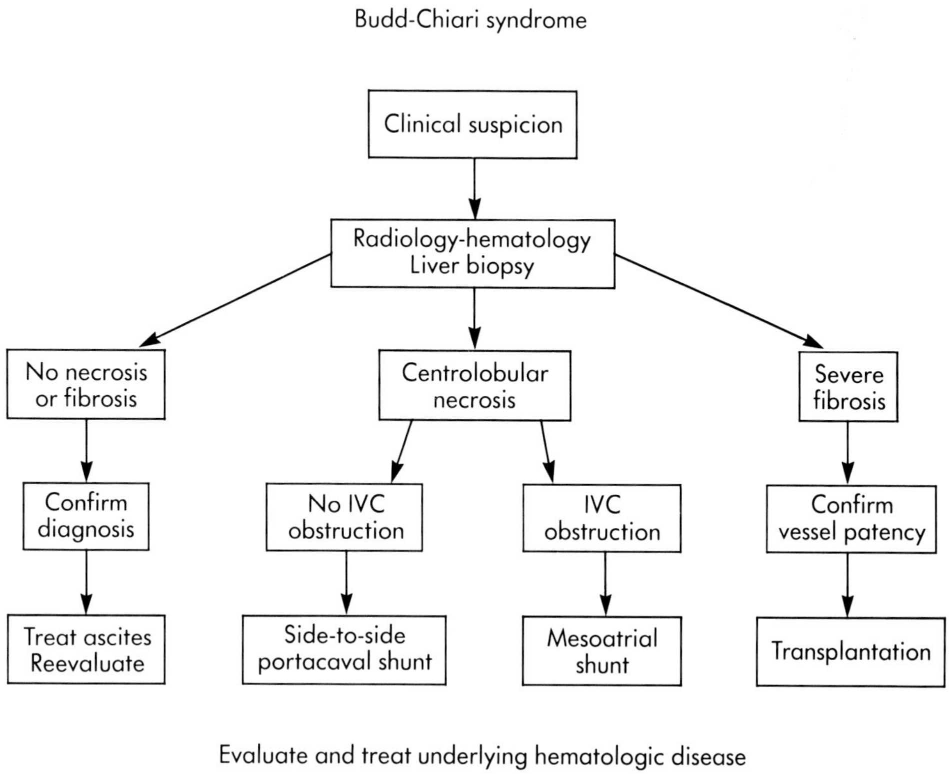

Figure 25-12
Algorithm for management of Budd-Chiari syndrome. (From Henderson JM, Warren WD, Millikan WJ Jr, et al: Surgical options, hematologic evaluation, and pathologic changes in Budd-Chiari syndrome, Am J Surg 159:41, 1990.)

underlying hypercoagulable state. Failure to identify and treat a myeloproliferative disorder will increase the risk of thrombosis in the shunt.

Severe disease is defined on the liver biopsy when there is significant fibrosis, often with lobular collapse, bridging, and cirrhosis. This may or may not be accompanied by ongoing hepatocyte necrosis. In these patients the best treatment option is liver transplantation. By the time there is established, irreversible damage, as indicated by fibrosis on the liver biopsy, it is unlikely that a decompressive shunt will be adequate therapy. Additional information as to the adequacy of hepatocyte reserve can be obtained by quantitative liver function testing. In our experience, a galactose elimination capacity (GEC) in excess of 300 mg/min in such patients, even in the presence of some fibrosis, may be useful in indicating use of a shunt rather than a transplant. On the other hand, we have found that when the GEC is less than 250 mg/min in BCS and there is severe fibrosis on the liver biopsy, liver transplantation appears to be indicated.

Is liver transplantation contraindicated in patients with an underlying myeloproliferative disorder? This question should

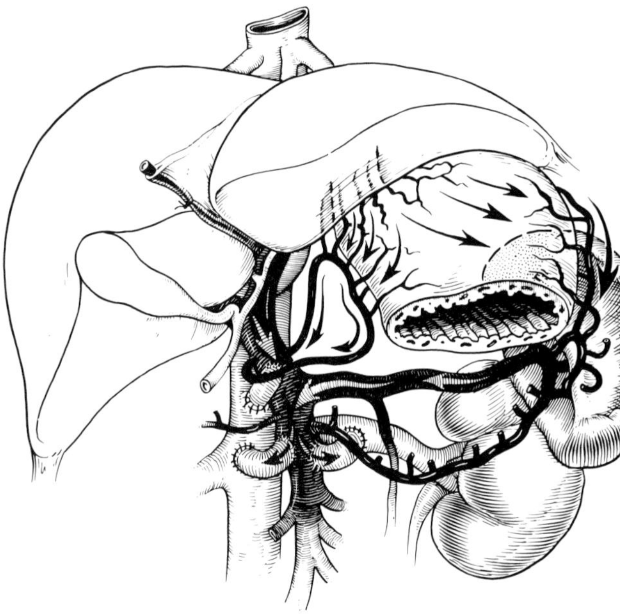

Figure 25-13
Infrahepatic total side-to-side portal systemic shunts that may be used to decompress the liver retrograde via the portal vein in patients with Budd-Chiari syndrome and no intrahepatic vena cava obstruction. Interposition portacaval H-graft and mesocaval and mesorenal shunts are shown. (From Henderson JM and Warren WD: Portal hypertension, Curr Probl Surg 25(3):149, 1988.)

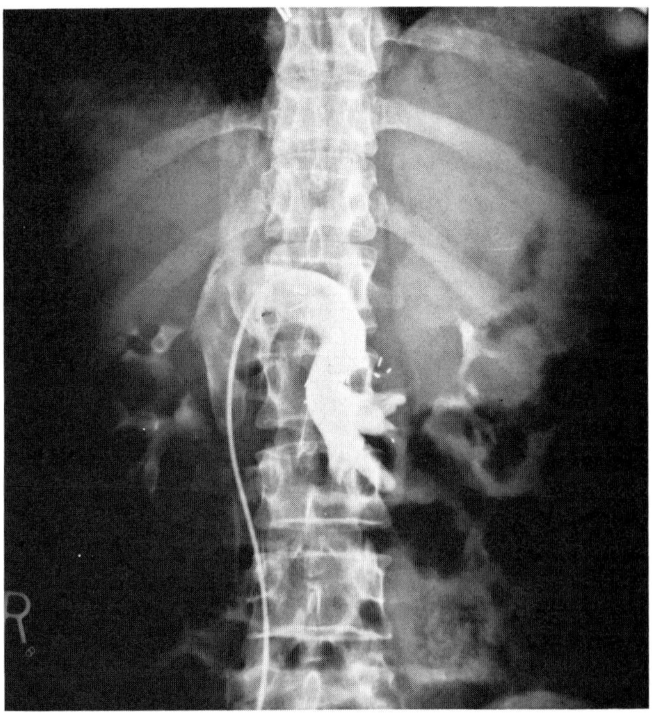

Figure 25-14
Direct catherization of a portacaval H-graft (16 mm) showing total diversion of superior mesenteric, splenic, and portal venous flow to the vena cava. The portal vein serves as an outflow track from the liver.

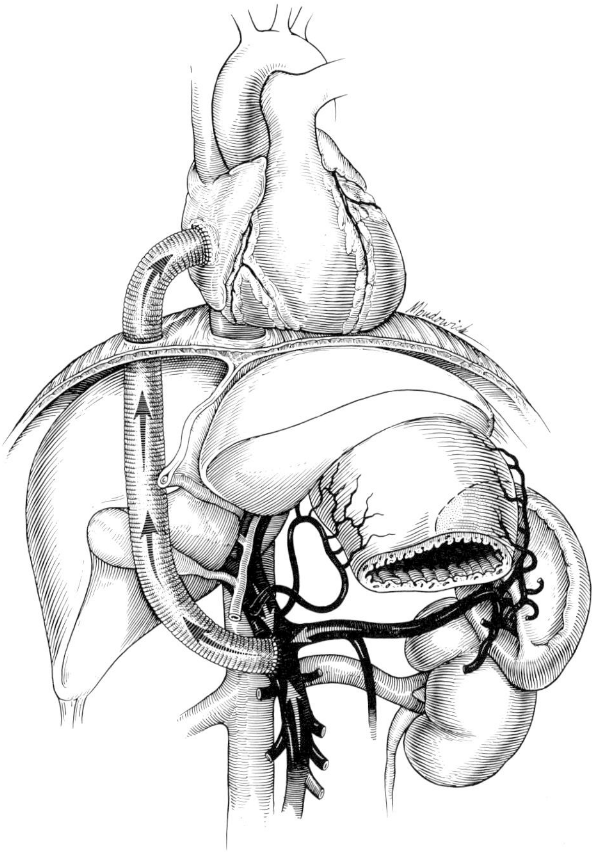

Figure 25-15
Diagrammatic illustration of a mesoatrial shunt. The principle is to use the portal vein for outflow from the congested liver and then bypass the obstructed intrahepatic vena cava with the long mesoatrial shunt. (From Henderson JM and Warren WD: Portal hypertension, Curr Probl Surg 25(3):149, 1988.)

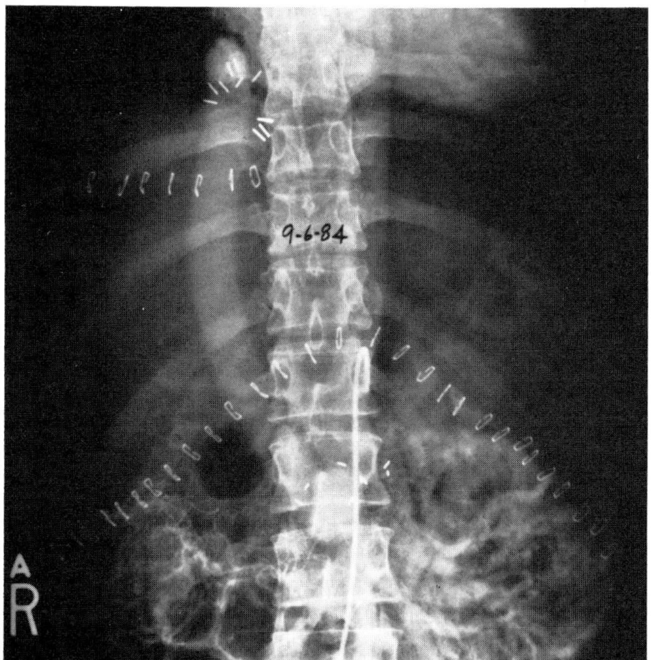

Figure 25-16
Superior mesenteric angiogram in the venous phase showing a patent mesoatrial shunt.

be carefully evaluated and discussed with a hematologist experienced in managing such patients. If it is believed that the myeloproliferative disorder can be readily treated and the only available therapy for the liver disease is transplantation, it is reasonable to proceed. On the other hand, if the myeloproliferative disorder is aggressive, with other thrombotic manifestations and unlikely to respond to therapy, liver transplantation is probably not indicated.

Follow-up study. Longitudinal follow-up observation of patients with BCS should allow one to monitor both the course of the liver disease and the patient's hematologic status. Progression of the liver disease may lead to the eventual need for transplantation. However, in our experience, adequate decompression of the liver in acute BCS has been associated with remarkable stability of quantitative liver function up to 5 years after shunt.

Development of clinical or laboratory evidence of a myeloproliferative disorder has been defined at various time points in the postdecompressive stage. Again, early detection and appropriate therapy will minimize the risk of further thrombotic problems.

Veno-occlusive Disease

Veno-occlusive disease is characterized by occlusion of the small hepatic veins, leading to hepatic injury by centrizonal congestion and necrosis. The medium and large-sized hepatic veins are usually spared. There are several described etiologic factors.

Pathophysiology. The pyrrolizidine alkaloids were originally implicated in the 1950s in medicinal bush decoctions in Jamaica. The toxic injury at that time was recognized histologically as being veno-occlusive and was ascribed to *Senecio* poisoning. Further outbreaks in the Middle East and Arizona have been recognized since. Lumped into the same disease group are histologically similar injuries secondary to liver irradiation, azathioprine, chemotherapy for acute leukemia, and a graft vs. host reaction seen after some allogeneic bone marrow transplants.

Clinical features. The clinical features may present either acutely, subacutely, or in a chronic stage. The acute presentation is of right upper quadrant pain with acute hepatomegaly and ascites. This may resolve, prove rapidly fatal, or pass into a subacute phase. Persistent hepatomegaly and persistent or intermittent ascites characterize the subacute phase, which if persistent over several months will pass into the chronic stage. Fibrosis and scarring like any other chronic liver disease are the features of untreated and unresolved veno-occlusive disease.

Diagnosis and management. Investigation and management of veno-occlusive disease should parallel the studies laid out for Budd-Chiari syndrome. Progressive damage to the liver is determined by the presence of ongoing hepatocyte necrosis, which can be determined only by liver biopsy. Minimizing the injury, if there is ongoing necrosis, can be achieved only if one provides an outflow route for the obstructive liver. If indicated, this can be achieved by a side-to-side total portal systemic shunt. Ultimate prognosis is determined by (1) the severity of the veno-occlusive disease and (2) the underlying pathosis.

Cardiac Failure and the Liver

Pathophysiology. The congestion of the liver in cardiac failure is reminiscent of the changes in Budd-Chiari syndrome,

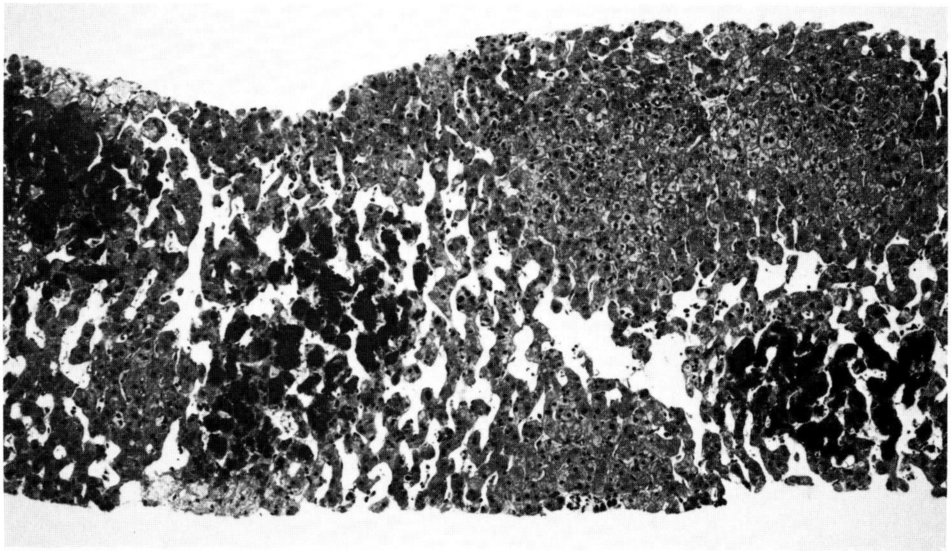

Figure 25-17
Acute passive congestion. Zone 3 sinusoids are dilated and blood-filled in a patient with right ventricular failure. Intervening hepatocytic cords are compressed and partially necrotic. (Courtesy Dr. Gary Hertzler, Department of Pathology, Emory University Hospital, Atlanta, Ga., 1990.)

but the mechanisms are somewhat different. The two main factors leading to liver damage are (1) hepatic congestion secondary to high right-sided heart pressures and (2) reduced blood flow into the liver because of low cardiac output.

Pathology. Grossly, the liver is enlarged and usually purple. It has a similar appearance to that in the Budd-Chiari syndrome. In the patient with chronic cardiac failure, the liver may progress to a frank cirrhosis. Microscopically, the hepatic lobules show dilated central veins with a centrilobular congestion (Figure 25-17). As with BCS, the degree of injury may vary from mild to destructive. Severe congestion may progress to hepatocyte necrosis, which in end-stage cardiac failure is compounded by poor prograde perfusion. In the long-standing chronic setting, the development of cirrhosis can lead to the classic "nutmeg" liver of chronic congestive cardiac failure.

Clinical features. Right upper quadrant pain secondary to hepatomegaly and distention of the liver capsule is the most consistent feature. Acute distention is more painful than the slow enlargement of chronic congestive failure. Ascites may well be present and may be a feature of an anasarca state. The patient may have jaundice, varying from mild to moderate. Jaundice is attributable to a combination of hepatocellular damage and an increased bilirubin load from hemolysis in other poorly perfused tissue. The poorly perfused liver cannot handle the extra bilirubin load. Hepatojugular reflux can be shown with right upper quadrant pressure over the congested liver giving a visible pulse wave in the neck veins. Such reflux cannot be elicited in BCS where there is a outflow-path block.

Acute hepatic failure can occasionally develop with severe cardiac failure but is usually a manifestation of end-stage multiorgan failure.

In the patient with chronic cardiac failure, the persistent injury combined with the liver's attempts at repair may lead to "cardiac" cirrhosis. This in turn may be manifested with the clinical problems of portal hypertension.

Diagnosis. The diagnosis is based on clinical findings and physical examination. The features of this are given on p. 434. There are no specific diagnostic tests. The serum bilirubin may be elevated, the degree of it being proportional to the severity of the process and having prognostic value. The serum transaminase value may rise, a finding more associated with an acute injury. Reduction of serum albumin is an indication of more chronic disease.

Management. Therapy must aim to treat the cardiac failure. Failure to improve cardiac function will not help the liver. Prognosis is entirely dependent on the success of treating the cardiac problem. Provided that this can be successfully achieved before there is fibrosis in the liver, the hepatic changes are reversible. The worst prognostic sign from the liver standpoint in such patients is a rising bilirubin value.

Constrictive Pericarditis

Pathophysiology. Constrictive pericarditis affects the liver by acting as an outflow block. It is the failure of blood to pass normally through the right side of the heart, which leads to passive congestion in the liver and a picture similar to that described in detail for Budd-Chiari syndrome.

Clinical features. Hepatomegaly is found, with the liver often being tender. A prominent hepatojugular reflex can be demonstrated. Ascites may often be significant, but in contrast to the patient with cardiac failure there may not be significant peripheral edema. Jaundice is not usually present.

Diagnosis. Evaluation should again be focused on the underlying cardiac cause. Clinical, electrocardiographic, and cardiac catheterization studies will define constrictive pericarditis.

Management. Management requires correction of the underlying problem, which with established constricture pericarditis requires complete operative resection of the pericardium. Resolution of the liver symptoms will be complete provided that there has been no irreversible damage.

SUMMARY

Vascular disorders of the liver have been viewed as either inflow or outflow disorders in this chapter. Hepatic arterial occlusion, aneurysm, and fistula require anteriographic study, possible radiologic interventive therapy, and in some instances surgery. Hepatic ischemia is an unusual clinical problem except when there are other risk factors. Portal vein thrombosis usually presents with variceal bleeding and presents a different investigation and management challenge compared to other causes of variceal bleeding. The denervated, transplanted liver poses a new challenge.

Outflow disorders fall into the broad category of outflow block with varying degrees of hepatic congestion. Liver biopsy is the key in both diagnosis and management decisions. The aim should be to preserve the liver by halting active necrosis, but if end-stage liver damage results, a liver transplant may be required.

SUGGESTED READINGS

Henderson JM, Warren WD, Millikan WJ, et al: Surgical options, hematologic evaluation, and pathologic changes in Budd-Chiari syndrome, Am J Surg 159:41, 1990.

This paper presents data on a consecutive series of 33 patients with Budd-Chiari syndrome. It details an investigation and management strategy that has evolved from this experience.

Klein AS and Cameron JL: Diagnosis and management of the Budd-Chiari syndrome, Am J Surg 160(1):128, 1990.

This review of Budd-Chiari Syndrome gives an opinion on the investigation and management of this disorder from a group with extensive experience.

Languas AN, Stratta RJ, Shaw BW, and Wood RP: Vascular complications following orthotopic liver transplantation, Am J of Surg 161:76, 1991.

This paper critically reviews the vascular complications in 391 liver transplants. Etiologic factors and management method for the 36 complications are reviewed.

Okuda K: Frequency of intrahepatic arteriovenous fistula as a sequel to percutaneous needle puncture of the liver. Gastroenterology 74:1204, 1978.

This paper reviews the frequency, cause, and sequelae of arteriovenous fistula after percutaneous needle biopsy of the liver.

Stuart KL and Bras G: Veno-occlusive disease of the liver, Q J Med 26:291, 1957.

This original classic description of veno-occlusive disease secondary to medicinal bush decoctions remains a classic paper. The clinical and pathologic features are clearly recognized and described.

Warren WD, Henderson JM, Millikan WJ, et al: Management of variceal bleeding in patients with noncirrhotic portal vein thrombosis, Ann Surg 207:623, 1988.

This paper reviews an 18-year experience with 70 patients managed for variceal bleeding secondary to portal vein thrombosis. It provides an investigation and management strategy based on this experience.

Weaver DH, Fleming RJ, and Barnes WA: Aneurysm of the hepatic artery: the value of arteriography in surgical management, Surgery 64:891, 1968.

This paper reviews a collected series of 175 patients with hepatic artery aneurysm. It defines location and management methods, indicating improvement in outcome with newer techniques.

26 Cirrhosis of the Liver

Rowen K. Zetterman

Cirrhosis is a diffuse lesion characterized by architectural distortion of the liver because of collagen deposition and development of nodules of regenerating hepatocytes. It is an irreversible change that results from diseases characterized by chronic liver injury. Cirrhosis alters the pattern of blood flow through the liver and results in impaired perfusion of hepatic lobules with intrahepatic and extrahepatic shunting of blood. This deprives hepatocytes of uniform perfusion by arterial and portal venous blood resulting in both portal hypertension and other consequences of cirrhosis including impaired protein synthesis and altered drug metabolism. The histologic diagnosis of cirrhosis requires the presence of regenerative nodules or pseudolobules completely encircled by fibrosis. The presence of fibrosis alone is not sufficient because diseases with extensive fibrosis such as congenital hepatic fibrosis can result in portal hypertension in the absence of cirrhosis.

The events leading to the development of cirrhosis are generally those of chronic injury with hepatocyte destruction. Acute severe liver injury as in fulminant viral hepatitis does not result in cirrhosis and the liver generally returns to normal after recovery. Cirrhosis can be classified by macroscopic appearance, by cause, and by histologic appearance and location of liver damage. Micronodular cirrhosis is composed of uniform nodules less than 3 mm in diameter, whereas macronodular cirrhosis has varying size nodules greater than 3 mm diameter. Mixed nodular cirrhosis has nodules of both sizes. Some liver diseases such as alcoholic liver disease may present as micronodular cirrhosis and develop larger nodules with subsequent regeneration of hepatocytes. For this reason, many prefer etiologic classification (e.g., alcoholic cirrhosis). The designation of cirrhosis as postnecrotic, biliary and portal are still commonly used and imply predominant histologic location of fibrosis.

Etiology

The mechanism for collagen deposition in response to liver damage is unknown. Accumulation of fibroblasts with collagen formation may occur as a nonspecific response to hepatocyte damage, to drugs and toxins or to release of cytokines from infiltrating mononuclear cells. Cirrhosis can be a consequence of many liver diseases including: chronic viral hepatitis B, C and D (in association with B); autoimmune chronic active hepatitis; ethanol; metabolic disorders such as hemochromatosis, Wilson's disease, alpha-1-antitrypsin deficiency, tyrosinemia, galactosemia, diabetes mellitus and Indian childhood cirrhosis; diseases with prolonged cholestasis such as biliary obstruction of any cause, cystic fibrosis and destructive bile duct disorders including primary biliary cirrhosis, sclerosing cholangitis and biliary atresia; vascular or congestive liver injury including Budd-Chiari syndrome, veno-occlusive disease and cardiac cirrhosis from congestive heart failure and constrictive pericarditis; and other liver disorders including jejunoileal bypass-induced liver disease, toxin-related liver injury and cryptogenic cirrhosis (see box at right). Malnutrition may coexist with liver disease but does not cause cirrhosis. The cirrhosis of alcohol, hemochromatosis, Wilson's disease, biliary cirrhosis, and jejunoileal bypass-induced liver disease are typically micronodular, whereas chronic viral hepatitis, autoimmune chronic active hepatitis and α_1-antitrypsin deficiency are usually macronodular.

CAUSES OF CIRRHOSIS

- Chronic hepatitis
  - Chronic viral hepatitis B, C, D
  - Autoimmune chronic active hepatitis
  - Chronic drug-induced hepatitis, e.g., oxyphenisatin
- Ethanol
- Metabolic causes
  - Hemochromatosis
  - Wilson's disease
  - α_1-Antitrypsin deficiency
  - Tyrosinemia
  - Galactosemia
  - Diabetes mellitus
  - Glycogen storage disease
- Diseases of prolonged cholestasis
  - Primary biliary cirrhosis
  - Primary sclerosing cholangitis
  - Biliary atresia
  - Chronic bile duct obstruction
  - Cystic fibrosis
  - Hyperalimentation-induced cholestasis
- Toxic exposure
  - Carbon tetrachloride
  - Hypervitaminosis A
  - Methotrexate
- Vascular/congestive
  - Budd-Chiari syndrome
  - Veno-occlusive disease
    - Idiopathic
    - Drug-induced
    - Toxin-induced
    - Ethanol?
  - Cardiac cirrhosis
- Miscellaneous
  - Jejunoileal bypass–induced liver disease
  - Indian childhood cirrhosis
  - Cryptogenic

EXAMINATION MODES

Clinical Observations

The patient's history may provide clues to the cause or causes including a history of alcohol consumption, chronic medication use, intravenous drug abuse, prior blood transfusions or hepatitis exposure, or a family history of liver disease. The clinical features of cirrhosis are generally a result of either portal hypertension or the diversion of portal blood flow past functioning hepatocytes. Patients may complain of profound weakness, fatigue, and malaise often of such proportions as to interfere with normal daily living and serve as an indication for intervention with liver transplantation. Anorexia, weight loss, and proximal muscle wasting are often present in advanced liver disease. Malnutrition may be present in the alcoholic. Fever occurs in diseases with active hepatocyte necrosis such as alcoholic hepatitis, though it can also indicate infectious complications including pneumonia or spontaneous bacterial peritonitis. Hypothermia may be present in deep hepatic coma and in some patients with infection. Jaundice, dark urine, and light-colored stools develop with cholestasis and hyperbilirubinemia. Bleeding from gums and venipuncture sites and peripheral edema may result from hypoprothrombinemia and hypoalbuminemia caused by impaired protein synthesis. There is an increased risk of peptic ulcer disease and its symptoms. Although the prevalence of pigmented gallstones is increased with cirrhosis, they are usually asymptomatic and rarely require intervention. Abdominal swelling from ascites is typical of end-stage liver disease and is often associated with peripheral edema. Secretory diarrhea can occur from portal hypertension with passive congestion of the bowel. Decreased libido is frequent in those with alcoholic cirrhosis or hemochromatosis. However, the patient with cirrhosis may also be asymptomatic.

A careful physical examination can provide clues to the presence of cirrhosis, its complications, or its cause. Fetor hepaticus is a sweet odor of the breath associated with end-stage liver disease. Examination of the head should include observation for parotid enlargement especially in the alcoholic, for icteric sclera, and for the red tongue of vitamin deficiencies. Dermovascular signs of chronic liver disease include hyperpigmentation in primary biliary cirrhosis (PBC) and hemochromatosis, periorbital xanthelasma and eruptive xanthomas over extensor surfaces in PBC, Dupuytren's contracture of the palmar fascia in the alcoholic, and signs of bruising and loss of body hair with development of a female escutcheon. Palmar erythema may be prominent over the thenar and hypothenar eminences and can be observed on the soles of the feet. Palmar erythema may also occur in rheumatoid arthritis, the elderly, during pregnancy and as a familial trait. Spider angiomas develop over the distribution of the superior vena cava and are most frequent in cirrhosis because of chronic active hepatitis and alcoholism. Spiders also develop in pregnancy, with birth control pills and hyperthyroidism. Numerous cutaneous telangiectasias may develop over sun exposed areas in the cirrhotic person. Nail changes include Muehrcke's lines, white nails from hypoalbuminemia, loss of lunulae, and clubbing. The examination of the chest may demonstrate gynecomastia (especially common in hemochromatosis and alcoholic liver disease), and high diaphragms with basilar atelectasis from ascites. The cardiovascular examination may indicate a hyperdynamic circulation with tachycardia, prominent pulses, and peripheral vasodilatation. Pulmonary hypertension can cause an increased P_2 heart sound. Rarely, peripheral cyanosis develops from right to left intravascular shunts within the lung, especially in those with autoimmune chronic active hepatitis who have undergone portosystemic shunts. Hepatomegaly is virtually always present in cirrhosis and may be the only clue to its presence. The liver edge is firm, and regenerative nodules may be palpable. Those with cryptogenic cirrhosis can present with their liver disease so late that the liver is small. Liver size is best estimated by light percussion of the upper border and palpation of the lower edge in the right midclavicular line. Although splenomegaly is frequent, very large spleens are unusual except in chronic active hepatitis. Ascites may cause bulging flanks, a fluid wave, right-flank dullness to percussion, or shifting dullness. The puddle sign is the most sensitive physical finding of ascites. Umbilical and inguinal hernias can develop with ascites. Hypogonadism and feminization are especially common in alcoholic cirrhosis and hemochromatosis. Hepatic encephalopathy can cause asterixis and altered consciousness. Asterixis is a flapping tremor of the hands when held in extension with outstretched arms. It can also be demonstrated as a pulsating "milk maid's" grip as the patient's hand grasps the examiner's fingers and attempts to sustain a steady clasp. Asterixis is not specific for hepatic encephalopathy occurring in renal, pulmonary, and cardiac failure. Deep tendon reflexes are enhanced in early hepatic encephalopathy and hyporeflexic with deep coma. Clonus may also be present. Wernicke's encephalopathy should be considered if malnutrition is present. Peripheral neuropathy develops from coexisting vitamin deficiencies such as thiamine deficiency, diabetes mellitus, or xanthomatous involvement of peripheral nerves. Transverse myelitis rarely develops in conjunction with chronic encephalopathy.

Laboratory Evaluation

The initial laboratory evaluation should include an etiologic profile. Viral studies for hepatitis B, C, and D and disease-specific markers including serum iron and iron binding capacity, ferritin, ceruloplasmin, and protease inhibitor (Pi) typing may assist in diagnosis. Autoantibodies such as antinuclear (ANA), smooth muscle (SMA), and antimitochondrial (AMA) antibodies are frequently present in chronic active hepatitis (ANA and SMA) and primary biliary cirrhosis (AMA). Elevated levels of IgG and IgM immunoglobulins are typical of chronic active hepatitis and primary biliary cirrhosis respectively, and IgA and IgG may be increased in alcoholic cirrhosis. Serum cholesterol levels are increased in diseases with prolonged cholestasis and then fall with advanced cirrhosis because of synthetic dysfunction. Hypoalbuminemia and hypoprothrombinemia may occur. Thrombocytopenia and leukopenia result from hypersplenism, and hemolysis can be associated with alcoholic hepatitis and chronic active hepatitis. Macrocytic red blood cell indices may develop with cirrhosis or from folic acid deficiency. Spur cells occur with alcoholic cirrhosis. Primary biliary cirrhosis is associated with both pancreatic insufficiency and celiac disease, and steatorrhea may be a result.

A liver biopsy should be performed to establish the presence of cirrhosis and provide clues to the cause. The diagnosis of cirrhosis requires demonstration of regenerative nodules or pseudolobules completely encircled by fibrosis. Other findings may include ground glass cells (hepatitis B), coarse granular cytoplasm of hepatocytes (hepatitis C), periportal hepatocyte and bile duct cell iron accumulation (hemochromatosis), periportal copper (Wilson's disease), periportal α_1-antitrypsin globules with α_1-antitrypsin deficiency (which can also occur as a nonspecific finding in cirrhosis), bile duct loss (PBC), lamellar fibrosis circumscribing bile ducts (sclerosing cholangitis), terminal hepatic venule occlusion (veno-occlusive disease), reversed lobulation with portal areas at the center of cirrhotic nodules (cardiac cirrhosis), fatty metamorphosis of hepatocytes with Mallory bodies and pericellular polymorphonuclear leukocyte accumulation (ethanol), and changes of storage disorders. It is important to obtain an adequate liver biopsy specimen to make the diagnosis of cirrhosis. Laparoscopy can also assist in defining the presence of cirrhosis through visual observation of regenerative nodules.

Radiography

Plain chest radiographs of the patient with cirrhosis may demonstrate elevated diaphragms and basilar atelectasis and a ground glass appearance of the abdomen when ascites is present. As pigmented gallstone prevalence is increased in cirrhosis, right upper quadrant calcification may be observed. Bony demineralization can develop in any patient with advanced liver disease, especially primary biliary cirrhosis. Esophagrams may indicate esophageal varices. However, sensitivity of barium studies for varices is only 65% to 80%. Esophagoscopy is considered the best examination to document the presence of esophageal and gastric varices. Technetium radionuclides are taken up by Kupffer cells and may demonstrate a shift in uptake to the spleen and bone marrow because of portal hypertension and intrahepatic and extrahepatic shunting of hepatic blood flow. Liver scans can document size, contour, and the patchy hepatic uptake of nuclide characteristic of cirrhosis. HIDA (dimethyl iminodiacetic acid) or biliary scans are of little use in the routine evaluation of cirrhosis. Ultrasonography can assist in the diagnosis of cirrhosis and its complications such as portal hypertension by allowing one to observe portal vein collaterals, splenomegaly, and ascites. Size and shape of the liver can be estimated, and change of ultrasound attenuation may indicate fibrosis. Doppler studies of liver vasculature can determine portal vein flow and direction, hepatic artery flow, and the presence of hepatic or portal vein occlusion. These studies are useful in pretransplant evaluation to ensure that vessels are adequate for anastomosis. Hepatocellular carcinoma may also be identified as intrahepatic nodules. Computerized tomography (CT) provides similar hepatic information as ultrasound. However, early changes of cirrhosis and some vascular abnormalities may not be well seen. Regenerative nodules have similar density to normal liver. Hepatocellular carcinoma may appear as hypodense nodules. Enlarged perihepatic nodes may indicate metastasis or granulomas. Hemochromatosis is associated with an increase in Hounsfield units at CT. Vascular collaterals may be seen as serpiginous retroperitoneal densities with contrast enhancement. Vascular changes may also be observed by magnetic resonance imaging (MRI). Both cirrhosis and iron accumulation will change MRI density. Visualization of the portal circulation can be accomplished by the venous phase of abdominal arteriography or by direct injection into the portal venous circulation through splenoportography or transhepatic portal venography. Measurement of portal vein pressure is easiest by wedged hepatic vein pressures. In presinusoidal portal hypertension, however, portal venous pressures cannot be determined by this method. Techniques to directly document pressures include percutaneous transhepatic cannulation of portal vein radicles and cannulation of the umbilical vein.

Course and Prognosis

The clinical course depends on the cause of cirrhosis and precipitating events leading to presentation. Cirrhosis is an irreversible disease, and attempts should be made to stabilize the patient and to control the cause. Factors that indicate a poor outcome include an elevated prothrombin time that does not correct itself with parenteral vitamin K, upper gastrointestinal bleeding caused by varices, ascites refractory to therapy, increased age of the patient, severe malnutrition, spontaneous bacterial peritonitis, a pronounced increase of serum bilirubin in the absence of hemolysis, and hepatocellular carcinoma. In general, all causes of upper GI bleeding are associated with an increased mortality in patients with cirrhosis. For those with alcoholic cirrhosis who lack portal hypertension, survival is similar to an age-matched cohort if alcohol intake is stopped. If ethanol consumption continues, mortality is higher.

Treatment

Treatment should be directed at the cause and at the complications of cirrhosis. Corticosteroids may improve survival in women with cryptogenic cirrhosis. In one study of patients with cirrhosis (mostly alcoholic), there was a reduction in deaths and a suggestion of decreased severity of cirrhosis in patients who took daily colchicine for up to 9 years. No other medications are of proved benefit except those directed at the underlying cause or complications. Suspect toxins and medications should be stopped. Those with hemochromatosis require weekly phlebotomy until the excess iron is removed. Although controversial, it appears that adequate phlebotomy and prevention of cirrhosis will also reduce the occurrence of hepatocellular carcinoma in patients with hemochromatosis. Wilson's disease should be treated with D-penicillamine. Zinc therapy alone may not be effective. It is unclear if patients with cirrhosis caused by hepatitis B or C should be treated with α-interferon. Additional studies of this group are required. Corticosteroids may cure or slow progression of autoimmune chronic active hepatitis. Complications of cirrhosis must be treated as they occur. Liver transplantation should be considered for patients with end-stage liver disease and life-threatening complications. Patients should be referred early before they are severely ill because postoperative mortality is less with earlier intervention.

ALCOHOLIC LIVER DISEASE

Chronic ethanol intake can cause fatty liver, alcoholic hepatitis. and cirrhosis. At clinical presentation of alcoholic hepatitis, 50% of patients already have cirrhosis, and 50% of the remainder will develop cirrhosis during recovery and abstinence. This indicates that alcoholic hepatitis may be a precirrhotic lesion of alcoholic liver disease. Many potential mechanisms for development of alcoholic hepatitis have been suggested including malnutrition, a direct toxic effect of ethanol, ethanol-induced centrilobular hypoxia, and autoimmunity. Signs of malnutrition may occur simultaneously with alcoholism. However, no conclusive evidence links malnutrition to the pathogenesis of alcoholic liver disease. The epidemiology of alcoholism indicates that the intake of the equivalent of more than 160 gm of absolute ethanol daily (about 12 ounces of 80 proof whiskey) for men and 80 gm daily for women for more than 10 years may be associated with an increased prevalence of cirrhosis. Beverage type does not appear to influence hepatotoxicity. Ethanol is metabolized by alcohol dehydrogenase to acetaldehyde, a highly reactive intermediate that can bind to lysine residues on proteins to form acetaldehyde-protein adducts. These adducts may interfere with cell function and cause membrane alteration and result in cell wall injury. Redox changes occurring during ethanol metabolism may also interfere with hepatocyte function. Ethanol metabolism increases oxygen consumption by the liver and may decrease oxygen tension in the centrilobular region of the lobule to add to hepatic injury. The role of genetics in alcoholic liver disease is unclear. There may be a genetic predisposition for alcoholism. Male offspring of alcoholics are more likely to develop alcoholism, and the A1 allele of the dopamine D2 receptor gene occurs in 77% of alcoholics as compared to 28% of nonalcoholics. Women seem to be at greater risk than men to develop liver disease. This may be attributable to a relative lack of alcohol dehydrogenase in the stomach mucosa, which decreases ethanol metabolism by the stomach and increases ethanol delivery to the liver. With less metabolism by the stomach, a greater concentration of acetaldehyde is available within the hepatocyte to form adducts. Autoimmune mechanisms of liver injury may have a role in chronic alcoholic liver disease. Acetaldehyde-protein adducts and alcoholic hyalin have been proposed as antigens with sensitization of T-cells causing hepatic injury and its sequelae.

Clinical Features

Not all patients with chronic alcohol intake develop liver disease. Some have hepatomegaly with normal histologic features by light microscopy. When evaluated by electron microscopy, hepatocyte enlargement with smooth endoplasmic reticulum hypertrophy is observed. Serum γ-glutamyl transpeptidase (GGTP) levels may be increased in the alcoholic because of enzyme induction. Ethanol can cause bone marrow suppression with thrombocytopenia and leukopenia that resolves with 7 to 10 days of abstinence.

Fatty metamorphosis of the liver is the most common histologic abnormality and affects up to 50% of chronic alcoholics. Patients may be asymptomatic or present with mild nausea, vomiting, and right upper quadrant (RUQ) pain from hepatomegaly. The liver may be tender to palpation. Hepatic enzymes may be normal or increased. The ratio of aspartate aminotransferase (AST) to alanine aminotransferase (ALT) is typically greater than 2 and usually reverses during recovery. Hypertriglyceridemia with pancreatitis or hemolysis may occur. Fatty liver will resolve with 4 to 6 weeks of abstinence. Although rare, pronounced fatty liver from ethanol can present as encephalopathy and jaundice associated with severe cholestasis. Liver biopsy typically shows foamy degeneration of hepatocytes from microvesicular fatty change and little inflammation. Death occurs from complications of encephalopathy, hypoglycemia, or fatty pulmonary emboli.

Patients with alcoholic hepatitis may be asymptomatic or have severe fatigue, malaise, anorexia, weight loss, fever, and RUQ pain. Age at onset is variable but is usually between 35 and 45 years. Clinical presentation often follows a recent increase in daily ethanol intake. Fever, hepatosplenomegaly, and RUQ tenderness are typical. The fever is typically low grade, but spiking and remitting fevers can develop. A bruit over the liver occurs in 25%. Hepatic decompensation with ascites, encephalopathy, and GI bleeding can dominate presentation. The AST/ALT ratio remains greater than 2 even during recovery. Cholestasis is typical with elevations of alkaline phosphatase, GGTP, and bilirubin. Leukocytosis is present in 50%. Leukemoid reactions may occur. Hypersplenism from portal hypertension can develop. Elevations of IgG and IgA occur as a polyclonal hypergammaglobulinemia. The clinical course of alcoholic hepatitis is variable. Hepatic decompensation can develop. Because these patients frequently present with fever, RUQ pain, and jaundice associated with leukocytosis, a mistaken impression of acute cholecystitis can be made. Correct diagnosis is essential because any operation in the patient with alcoholic hepatitis carries a high mortality.

The patient with alcoholic cirrhosis may be asymptomatic— present during acute alcoholic hepatitis or because of the complications of portal hypertension. The physical abnormalities that are frequently associated include parotid enlargement, proximal muscle wasting, Dupuytren's contracture of the palmar fascia, spider angiomas, and hepatomegaly with predominant left lobe enlargement of the liver. Changes of feminization including gynecomastia, testicular atrophy, female escutcheon, and loss of body hair are common in alcoholic cirrhosis. The patient with alcoholic cirrhosis has at least a 30% risk of developing hepatocellular carcinoma. Half of the cirrhotics who develop carcinoma will do so within 4.5 years of diagnosis.

Laboratory Findings

The alcoholic may have increases of mean red cell volume (MCV), γ-glutamyl transpeptidase (GGTP) and uric acid as nonspecific markers of excess ethanol intake. MCV is also increased in patients with cirrhosis. Serum GGTP is a marker of enzyme induction from ethanol but can also be increased by cholestasis. Aminotransferase levels are elevated with alcoholic liver disease. The aspartate aminotransferase (AST) value is generally at least two times the alanine aminotransferase (ALT). The reason that the AST level exceeds the ALT is unknown. It may be a consequence of pyridoxine deficiency or the greater release of AST from subcellular hepatocyte organelles than of ALT from the cytosol with ethanol injury. This ratio usually reverses during recovery of patients with fatty liver but not those with alcoholic hepatitis or active cirrhosis. Alcoholic hepatitis is a cholestatic disorder. Cholestasis may also predominate in severe alcoholic fatty liver of foamy degeneration. Signs of parenchymal cell dysfunction associated with alcoholic hepatitis or cirrhosis include hypoalbuminemia, hypoprothrombinemia, and hyperbilirubinemia. Polyclonal hypergammaglobulinemia with increased IgG and IgA is frequent in patients with alcoholic cirrhosis. Delayed hypersensitivity skin reactions may be impaired.

The liver biopsy of the patient with fatty liver demonstrates perivenular accu-

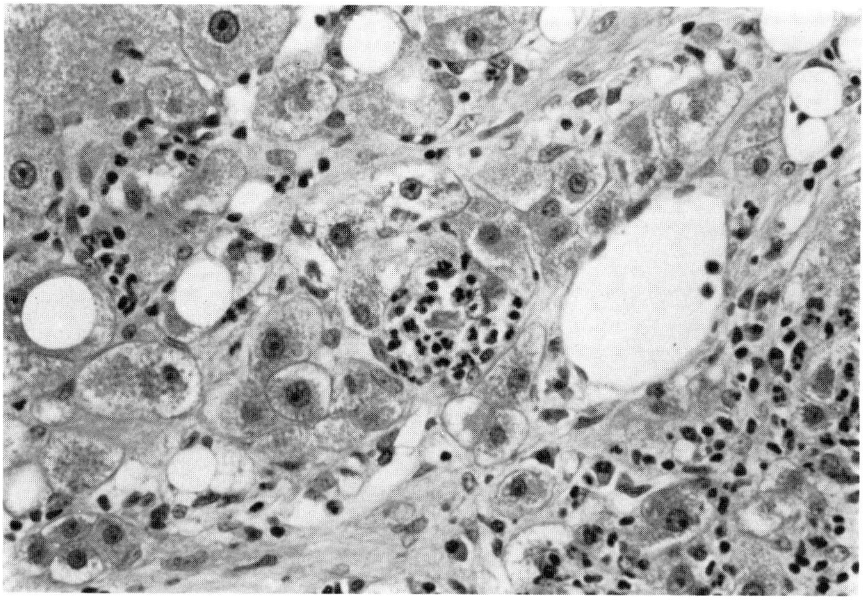

Figure 26-1
Alcoholic hepatitis. Collections of neutrophils surround degenerating hepatocytes and ballooned hepatocytes that contain alcoholic hyalin. (Hematoxylin and eosin, ×100.) (From Markin RS and Zetterman R: The pathology of alcoholic liver disease. In Gitnick G, editor: Current hepatology, vol 10, Chicago, 1990, Year Book Medical Publishers.)

mulation of intracellular fat, which displaces the hepatocyte nucleus. Little inflammation is observed. In alcoholic hepatitis, perivenular hepatocellular necrosis and polymorphonuclear leukocyte infiltration of the sinusoids predominate (Figure 26-1). Intracellular accumulation of alcoholic hyalin (Mallory bodies) may be present. Polymorphonuclear leukocytes may encircle hepatocytes containing alcoholic hyalin. Patients with alcoholic hepatitis who have intracellular hyalin are typically more ill and have a greater mortality. Hyalin is not specific for alcoholic hepatitis, however, and is also noted in Wilson's disease, diseases with severe cholestasis such as sclerosing cholangitis and primary biliary cirrhosis, chronic active hepatitis, hepatocellular carcinoma, and hepatocellular adenoma (see box on p. 456). Fatty metamorphosis of the hepatocytes may also be present. Portal inflammation is common, and an increase of T-cells is noted. Megamitochondria may occur in the liver cells of patients with alcoholic hepatitis and tend to indicate a better clinical prognosis. Perivenular fibrosis and collagenization of the space of Disse are common. Veno-occlusive disease can also develop from the perivenular injury. This has been called "sclerosing hyalin necrosis" and can result

> **DISEASES THAT CONTAIN MALLORY BODIES (ALCOHOLIC HYALIN)**
>
> Alcoholic hepatitis
> Wilson's disease
> Diseases with cholestasis
>   Sclerosing cholangitis
>   Primary biliary cirrhosis
>   Extrahepatic bile duct obstruction
> Nonalcoholic steatonecrosis
> Jejunoileal bypass
> Indian childhood cirrhosis
> Abetalipoproteinemia
> α_1-Antitrypsin deficiency
> Chronic active hepatitis
> Short bowel syndrome
> Weber-Christian disease
> Hepatocellular carcinoma
> Hepatic adenoma
> Medications
>   Perhexilene maleate
>   Betamethasone
>   Coralgil (hexestrol bis[β-diethylaminoethyl ether] dihydrochloride)
>   Amiodarone
>   Griseofulvin
> Alveolar cells in asbestosis

in central vein occlusion and portal hypertension. The lesion of alcoholic hepatitis may resolve with return of the liver to normal. Chronic active hepatitis may also occur from ethanol. The potential role of hepatitis C in these cases is unclear. Cirrhosis from alcohol is typically micronodular but can become macronodular with abstinence and regenerative activity (Figure 26-2). This transition is also associated with development of hepatocellular carcinoma.

Course and Prognosis

Fatty metamorphosis of the liver generally has a good prognosis. With abstinence from ethanol and adequate nutrition, fatty liver will resolve within 4 to 6 weeks. However, severe fatty metamorphosis and foamy degeneration of hepatocytes can lead to cholestasis and encephalopathy with an increased risk of death. In autopsy series of adult males with sudden death, an increased prevalence of fatty liver is also described.

The prognosis of alcoholic hepatitis is variable and does not directly correlate with histologic findings. Alcoholic hyalin may indicate a worse prognosis. Only the presence of intracellular megamitochondria correlates with a better clinical outcome. Poor prognostic clinical factors include azotemia, bilirubin elevations above 10 mg/dl, hypoprothrombinemia unresponsive to parenteral vitamin K, ascites, spontaneous encephalopathy, and gastrointestinal bleeding. For those with bilirubins under 2.0 mg/dl, a normal prothrombin time, and no ascites, the mortality is still 1% to 2%. With an increase of bilirubin to greater than 5.0 mg/dl, mortality approaches 20% and if the prothrombin time also exceeds 17 seconds and ascites is present, the mortality approaches 50%. The operative mortality is also increased in patients with alcoholic hepatitis and may be as high as 65%.

For the patient with alcoholic cirrhosis and no portal hypertension, there is no difference in mortality when compared to an age-matched cohort. Factors that influence mortality include gender (women may have a higher mortality), alcohol consumption (5-year survival for those

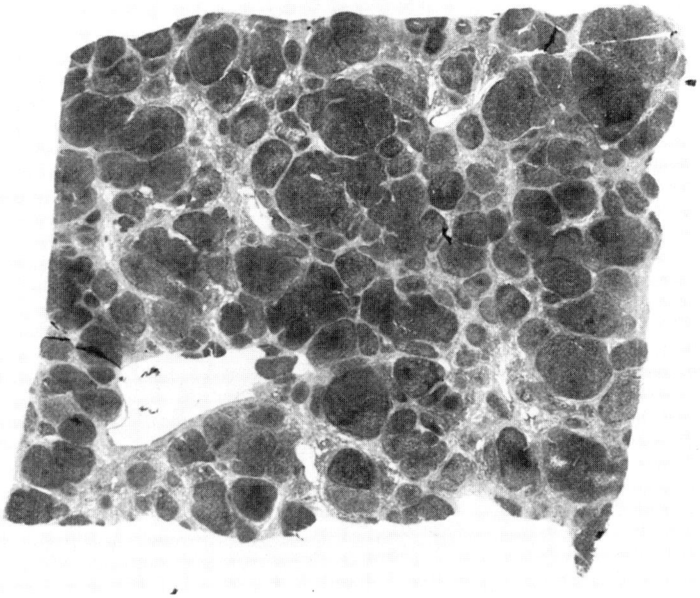

Figure 26-2
Alcoholic cirrhosis. Whole mount of liver showing a mixed micronodular-macronodular pattern of cirrhosis. (Masson's trichrome.) (From Markin RS and Zetterman R: The pathology of alcoholic liver disease. In Gitnick G, editor: Current hepatology, vol 10, Chicago, 1990, Year Book Medical Publishers.)

that stop is 60% but only 40% if ethanol intake continues), the presence of extensive perivenular fibrosis, the complications of gastrointestinal bleeding, encephalopathy, and ascites, and abnormalities of synthetic function including hypoprothrombinemia and hypoalbuminemia.

Treatment

The treatment of the patient with alcoholic liver disease should include attempts to improve nutritional deficiencies, encourage abstinence, and correct complications. Administration of anabolic steroids to the patient with fatty liver will clear hepatocyte fat more quickly but is not recommended because fat will dissipate with abstinence alone. Augmentation of nutrition through use of amino acid supplements may improve survival of the patient with alcoholic hepatitis. The use of medications in the treatment of alcoholic hepatitis is controversial. Although large studies of corticosteroid administration have not demonstrated an effect, smaller studies of select populations, including those who are female, have hypoprothrombinemia and spontaneous encephalopathy. An improvement of survival has been described. Although the data are limited, anabolic steroids may also affect long-term survival. In the VA Cooperative Trial, there was a better long-term survival in those receiving anabolic steroids than in those receiving placebo or corticosteroids. However, the 30-day mortality was unaffected. Because of the hypermetabolic state of the perivenular hepatocytes, which may occur with alcoholic liver disease, propylthiouracil (PTU) has been evaluated to see if it will improve outcome. Although no effect is observed in death rates of acute severe alcoholic hepatitis, long-term outcome may be better in those alcoholics receiving PTU, especially if they continue to drink.

In a study of patients with cirrhosis, most of whom were alcoholic, colchicine appears to improve long-term survival. PTU has also been suggested to improve survival of alcoholic cirrhotics. However, for many, the treatment is largely controlling the complications of cirrhosis including ascites, variceal bleeding, encephalopathy, and spontaneous bacterial peritonitis. Liver transplantation for severe complications should be considered. However, there may be an increased perioperative mortality in those with alcoholic hepatitis.

PRIMARY BILIARY CIRRHOSIS

Primary biliary cirrhosis (PBC) is a chronic destructive injury of the interlobular bile ducts within the liver characterized by mononuclear inflammation and their eventual disappearance. The pathogenesis of primary biliary cirrhosis is unknown. Several theories have been suggested including immune complex disease, cell-mediated immunity, copper retention, and genetic predisposition. Circulating immune complexes injected into animals can result in granuloma formation. However, immune complexes appear to be nonspecific and not to play a role in PBC. The cellular immune system seems a better candidate for its pathogenesis. PBC is characterized by portal inflammation with duct injury and mononuclear cell infiltration and frequently with granulomas containing cytotoxic T-cells. Cytotoxic T-cells may cause ductular destruction because of increased MHC class II expression on bile duct cells. In vitro, a reduction of suppressor T-cell activity and depressed mitogen responsiveness is also observed. Furthermore, the morphology of bile duct damage is similar to graft vs. host disease and transplant rejection with bile duct destruction. These observations have led to the postulation that PBC may result from a similar mechanism as graft vs. host disease. Copper retention occurs in the periportal region of the hepatic lobule because of an interruption of the enterohepatic circulation of copper by cholestasis. This pattern of deposition is similar to Wilson's disease and indicates that copper may be toxic in PBC as well. However, the lack of response to D-penicillamine and the predominance of bile duct damage in PBC indicate that copper retention may not be pathogenic. Antimitochondrial antibodies are also more frequent in relatives of patients with PBC, and familial clustering is described. However, PBC affects all ethnic groups, and HL-A similarity between patients has not been observed, a finding suggestive of genetic factors playing little role in the pathogenesis of primary biliary cirrhosis.

Clinical Features

Primary biliary cirrhosis typically presents in middle-aged women between 25 and 80 years of age. Diagnosis after 60 years of age is uncommon. Only 10% of cases occur in men. Most patients come to diagnosis because of cholestasis with pruritus. Jaundice may be initially present in some patients but typically follows pruritus. PBC may come to diagnosis during pregnancy or with use of birth control pills. The differential diagnosis of pruritus includes reactions of medications, skin allergies, hyperthyroidism, intrahepatic cholestasis of pregnancy, benign recurrent intrahepatic cholestasis, and occasionally extrahepatic biliary obstruction. Because of the increased use of routine laboratory screening, more patients come to diagnosis because of asymptomatic elevations of alkaline phosphatase. These patients may remain asymptomatic for years before onset of symptoms and typically do not develop complications of their disease for 10 years or more. Other symptoms may include malaise and fatigue. In later stages, fatigue can be so severe as to interfere with daily living. Patients may also notice dark urine and light- or clay-colored stools caused by cholestasis. Sicca complex is present in the majority of patients with PBC producing symptoms of dry eyes and mouth. Some patients do not present until they have advanced liver disease, presenting with complications such as upper gastrointestinal bleeding or ascites. Physical findings include hyperpigmentation of the skin and consequences of itching, including scratch marks. These may occur in a butterfly pattern over the back marking the places where the patient can reach. Xanthelasmas are common in the periorbital regions, and xanthomas frequently develop over elbows and knees and along palmar creases. Peripheral neuropathy from xanthomatous nerve infiltration may occur. Several associated disorders may be present including the CRST syndrome, scleroderma, rheumatoid arthritis, mixed connective tissue disease, systemic lupus erythematosus, dermatomyositis, Hashimoto's thyroiditis, renal tubular acidosis, glomerulonephritis, celiac disease, pancreatic insufficiency, pernicious anemia, and clubbing. There are similarities between PBC and sarcoid with interstitial pulmonary granulomas and bronchoalveolar lavage findings of increased mononuclear cells. Both sarcoid and PBC have been described in the same patient. There is also a syndrome of bile duct loss from granulomatous destruction in patients with sarcoidosis who are usually male and are usually antimitochondrial antibody (AMA) negative. Most patients with PBC eventually develop significant hepatic osteodystrophy similar to osteoporosis with vertebral collapse and spontaneous fractures.

The differential diagnosis of primary biliary cirrhosis includes sarcoidosis, chronic active hepatitis, sclerosing cholangitis, secondary biliary cirrhosis, and drug-induced cholestasis. If PBC becomes symptomatic during pregnancy, intrahepatic cholestasis of pregnancy must also be considered. In its early stages, the histology and biochemical picture of PBC may be similar to chronic active hepatitis, since both can have predominant portal and periportal injury with piecemeal necrosis of hepatocytes. The biochemical changes of sclerosing cholangitis are similar to PBC. Both can occur in association with ulcerative colitis, though the prevalence of sclerosing cholangitis is much greater. Secondary biliary cirrhosis should be suspected in patients who present early with jaundice, lack significant pruritus, and have intermittent RUQ pain. Cholangiography may be helpful in differential diagnosis. Long-term use of chlorpromazine can induce a chronic liver injury similar to primary biliary cirrhosis. These patients are typically AMA negative. Medications such as chlorpromazine can also bring subclinical cases of primary biliary cirrhosis to diagnosis through aggravation of cholestasis. This generally occurs within 30 days of initial administration of the drug.

Laboratory Findings

The use of chemistry screens has led to earlier diagnosis of the asymptomatic patient. PBC is characterized by cholestasis with elevations of alkaline phosphatase and GGTP. Serum bilirubin levels are initially normal or minimally elevated at clinical presentation. A progressive rise in bilirubin is a poor prognostic sign. Some patients initially present with hyperbilirubinemia and usually have more advanced disease. Other features include hypercholesterolemia and pronounced elevations of IgM and sedimentation rate. Circulating immune complexes may occur. Albumin levels are normal early and indicate development of advanced disease as they fall. Steatorrhea from pancreatic insufficiency or celiac disease may occur. Serum bile acid levels are increased.

The antimitochondrial antibody (AMA) test is positive in more than 90% of females but only 25% of males with primary biliary cirrhosis. The AMA represents a heterogeneous group of antibodies that react with mitochondrial membranes. The M2 antimitochondrial antibody is the most specific and reacts with the inner membrane of the mitochondrion. The M2 antibody is virtually 100% positive in patients with PBC. Other AMA subtypes also occur. The mechanism of their occurrence is unknown. It has been suggested they are a response to bacterial mitochondria. They can also be observed in drug-induced liver injury, autoimmune chronic active hepatitis, and collagen vascular diseases but not bile duct obstruction.

To establish the diagnosis of primary biliary cirrhosis, a liver biopsy is required. There must be a sufficient number of portal areas to permit an estimation of the quantity of bile ducts present. Biliary radiography is no longer routinely required to exclude secondary causes of bile duct injury or primary sclerosing cholangitis but should be considered in patients with atypical presentations. It might also be considered in some males, because sclerosing cholangitis is much more common. The histologic duct abnormalities of PBC include swollen bile duct cells, duct cell necrosis, and mononuclear infiltration of bile ducts. These are the earliest changes of PBC and are referred to as the "florid duct lesion of PBC" (Figure 26-3). Ductular proliferation develops in the portal area followed by eventual loss of the interlobular bile duct. Accumulation of mononuclear cells and histiocytes within portal areas is typical. Periportal hepatocyte necrosis may occur and with early presentation of PBC can mimic chronic active hepatitis. Portal granulomas may be observed in early stages of PBC and seem to indicate a better overall prognosis. Periportal copper accumulation can be documented by copper stains. These stains can be a useful adjunct for the diagnosis of PBC. Mallory's hyalin is also observed in 20% to 25% of patients in periportal hepatocytes. Portal and periportal fibrosis develop, and fibrous septa extend from the portal areas into the lobules with eventual development of cirrhosis. Primary biliary cirrhosis may be histologically staged into stage I, the florid duct lesion; stage II, the stage of ductular

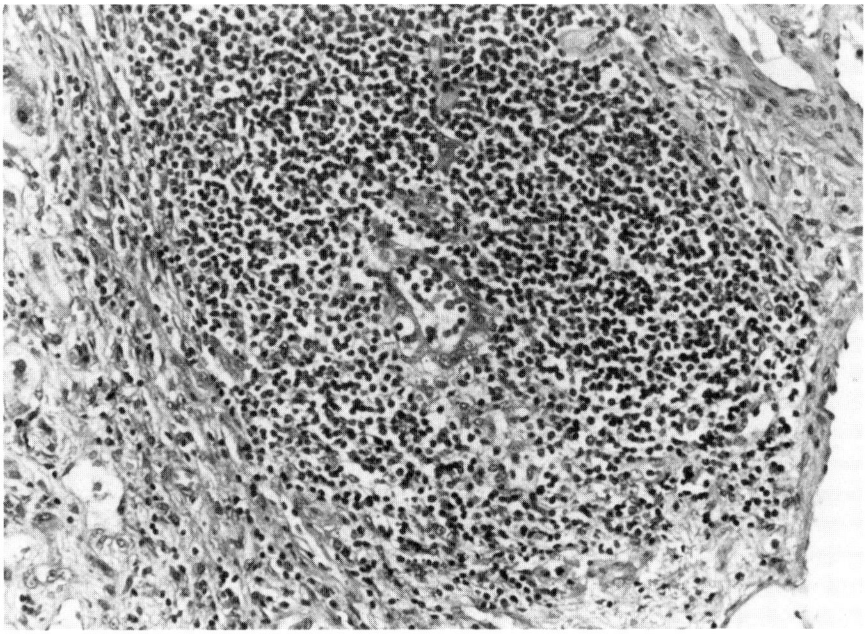

Figure 26-3
Primary biliary cirrhosis. Increased mononuclear inflammation of the portal areas with destruction of the interlobular bile duct.

proliferation; stage III, periportal fibrosis; and stage IV, cirrhosis (see box at right). Cirrhosis is characterized by uniform nodules with a micronodular pattern. Features of each of these stages may coexist within the same biopsy.

Radiology

With an adequate liver biopsy, bile duct radiography is rarely needed to exclude sclerosing cholangitis or secondary biliary cirrhosis. In atypical cases, however, endoscopic retrograde cholangiography should be performed.

Radiographs may document hepatic osteodystrophy and pulmonary changes of interstitial fibrosis and pulmonary hypertension. Pigmented gallstones occur. The evaluation of the liver by ultrasound or computerized tomography may reveal typical changes of advanced liver disease. CT scans for bony mineralization are helpful to assess osteodystrophy.

Course and Prognosis

The course of primary biliary cirrhosis is variable. Those asymptomatic at diagno-

HISTOLOGIC STAGES OF PRIMARY BILIARY CIRRHOSIS

Stage I	Florid duct lesion
Stage II	Bile ductular proliferation
Stage III	Periportal and bridging fibrosis
Stage IV	Cirrhosis

sis will typically be followed for greater than 12 years before the rate of death exceeds an age-matched cohort, whereas those who are symptomatic will survive 5 to 7 years. Signs of poor prognosis at diagnosis include hyperbilirubinemia, ascites, hypoalbuminemia, and hypoprothrombinemia. Other complications of cirrhosis including variceal bleeding, spontaneous bacterial peritonitis, and azotemia also indicate a poor prognosis. Patients with advanced age at diagnosis and those with hepatic granulomas seem to have a better prognosis. Variceal bleeding is also a poor prognostic sign but does not always indicate the presence of cirrhosis because portal hypertension can be presinusoidal because of portal tract inflammation and fibrosis. The development of progressive weight loss, hyperbilirubinemia, ascites, and frequent variceal bleeding are predictive of a poor outcome. The loss of pruritus and xanthomas and reductions in albumin and cholesterol are also signs of poor prognosis (see box at right).

INDICATORS OF POOR PROGNOSIS IN PATIENTS WITH PRIMARY BILIARY CIRRHOSIS

Progressive hyperbilirubinemia
Ascites
Spontaneous bacterial peritonitis
Hypoalbuminemia
Hypoprothrombinemia
Variceal bleeding
Progressive weight loss

Treatment

At present there are no specific treatments that conclusively improve or slow progression of the liver disease in patients with primary biliary cirrhosis. Pruritus can usually be controlled with 4 gm of cholestyramine given up to 4 times per day. Rifampicin and phenobarbital have also been used to assist in control of pruritus. Antihistamines may also be helpful. Fat-soluble vitamins, folic acid, and supplemental calcium should be prescribed. Utilization of 1,25-dihydroxyvitamin D does not prevent the development of hepatic osteodystrophy. Steatorrhea occurs in some patients with primary biliary cirrhosis and is usually attributable to pancreatic insufficiency. Pancreatic enzyme supplements should be administered. Celiac disease is uncommon in PBC but should also be considered in patients with diarrhea or steatorrhea, or both, and treated with a gluten-free diet.

Azathioprine and D-penicillamine do not appear to prevent progression of primary biliary cirrhosis. Corticosteroids are not recommended because of their potential to aggravate the bone disease of PBC. Colchicine has been shown to improve liver biochemical tests of patients with PBC but does not seem to alter progression of the histologic lesion. It has been suggested that one use a small trial of chlorambucil so that it can improve the prognosis, but the potential for significant toxicity has prevented its further evaluation. At present, trials of ursodeoxycholic acid, methotrexate, and cyclosporin A are being completed. Although preliminary results have appeared promising, they are too preliminary to recommend routine use and should be administered only within controlled trials.

Complications of advanced primary biliary cirrhosis must be aggressively treated. In those bleeding from varices with presinusoidal portal hypertension attributable to portal fibrosis, portosystemic shunts should be considered. However, with advanced disease, and especially if other complications of portal hypertension such as ascites or portosystemic encephalopathy are present, liver transplantation may be a better approach. Profound fatigue that interferes with a normal life style can also be an indication for liver transplantation. There is no evidence that primary biliary cirrhosis will recur in the allograft.

SECONDARY BILIARY CIRRHOSIS

Secondary biliary cirrhosis develops from the fibrotic reaction to obstruction of the biliary system. This can be a consequence of bile duct obstruction from cystic fibrosis, bile duct strictures, biliary calculi, and some tumors with bile duct obstruction. Biliary cirrhosis also occurs with primary biliary cirrhosis, sclerosing cholangitis, arteriohepatic dysplasia, and biliary atresia. In general, complete obstruction of the bile duct is more likely to result in biliary cirrhosis and generally takes 6 or more months to develop.

Clinical Features

The clinical features of secondary biliary cirrhosis are related to the underlying cause and may include jaundice, RUQ pain and tenderness and fever for the patient with common bile duct stones, and recurring cholangitis and jaundice in those with bile duct strictures. In complete bile duct obstruction, cholangitis is less likely to occur. Signs of cholestasis including clay-colored stools, dark-colored urine, and pruritus may develop.

Laboratory Findings

The laboratory values in biliary cirrhosis may reflect bile duct obstruction with elevated levels of alkaline phosphatase, γ-glutamyl transpeptidase, and bilirubin. Leukocytosis usually occurs with cholangitis.

Liver biopsies are helpful in the differential diagnosis of causes of secondary biliary cirrhosis. It is typically a micronodular cirrhosis with uniform portal to portal linkage from fibrosis. With time and hepatic regeneration, larger nodules develop, and a mixed nodular cirrhosis is evident. Bile duct changes may include intraluminal bile and polymorphonuclear leukocytes with biliary strictures or calculous disease and cholangitis, inspissation of eosinophilic material within bile ducts in cystic fibrosis, periductular lamellar fibrosis and portal mononuclear inflammation with sclerosing cholangitis, bile duct mononuclear inflammation and loss with primary biliary cirrhosis, and ductular proliferation with portal inflammation and bile duct plugs in neonates with biliary atresia.

Radiologic Findings

Biliary obstruction may be documented by radionuclide scans using radioactive technetium-labeled iminodiacetic acid (IDA) conjugates. These substances are taken up by the liver, excreted into the bile ducts, and transported with bile into the gallbladder and intestinal tract. These scans are nonspecific but can demonstrate bile duct obstruction by failure of passage of isotope into the intestine and may indicate the presence of cirrhosis by patchy distribution of isotope within the liver. Acute cholecystitis may also be suggested by the inability of isotope to enter the gallbladder. Direct instillation of radiopaque contrast into the bile ducts is the best technique to document bile duct disease. Biliary obstruction, strictures, and retained common bile duct stones can be identified by endoscopic retrograde or percutaneous transhepatic cholangiography. In those with suspected pancreatic disease, endoscopic retrograde cholangiopancreatography (ERCP) is preferred because a pancreatogram can also be obtained. At cholangiography, intrahepatic biliary radicles will appear "pruned" in patients with cirrhosis because of a reduction of size and number of intrahepatic branches.

Course and Treatment

The course of biliary cirrhosis is related to the development of complications. Early correction of disorders that can lead to biliary cirrhosis should be undertaken including evacuation of retained bile duct stones and correction of biliary strictures. Operative correction of bile duct strictures will prevent progressive hepatic injury. Balloon dilatation and prolonged stenting of strictures through nonoperative techniques may also be effective, though long-term follow-up studies are needed to document their effectiveness. In advanced cases, hepatic transplantation may be the only appropriate therapy.

POSTNECROTIC CIRRHOSIS

Postnecrotic cirrhosis is a designation for a mixed nodular cirrhosis characterized by broad bands of fibrosis and nodules of varying size. It can evolve from any liver injury as the liver attempts to replace lost hepatic mass with regenerative nodules of hepatocytes. It can result from chronic viral hepatitis, from autoimmune chronic active hepatitis, and in the late stage of Wilson's disease. Even the alcoholic can develop a pattern of postnecrotic cirrhosis with abstinence and hepatic regeneration. "Posthepatic cirrhosis" is a term used for the cirrhosis developing from chronic viral hepatitis. Cryptogenic cirrhosis is typically a postnecrotic cirrhosis of unclear cause, some cases of which are probably attributable to autoimmune chronic active hepatitis, α_1-antitrypsin deficiency, ethanol, or chronic viral hepatitis.

Clinical Features

There are no specific features to set postnecrotic cirrhosis apart from other forms of cirrhosis. The history may assist one in defining the cause. Palpable nodules on the liver surface may be noticed. There also is an increased prevalence of hepatocellular carcinoma with postnecrotic cirrhosis, which should be suspected in the patient with a palpable mass and corresponding hepatic bruit or sudden clinical deterioration. The liver biopsy specimen often demonstrates wide bands of fibrosis containing multiple portal areas from broad areas of hepatocyte loss and collapse. The course of postnecrotic cirrhosis will depend on the underlying cause and the presence of coexisting complications of portal hypertension or impaired synthetic function. Treatment of patients with postnecrotic cirrhosis is directed at the underlying cause and at control of complications.

SUGGESTED READINGS

Anthony PP, Ishak KG, Nayak NC, et al: The morphology of cirrhosis: definition, nomenclature, and classification. Bull WHO 55(4):521-540, 1977.

This article discusses the etiologic and morphologic classification of cirrhosis, chronic hepatitis and hepatic fibrosis. A table of morphologic markers of various etiologies is included.

Beswick DR, Klatskin G, and Boyer JL: Asymptomatic primary biliary cirrhosis: a progress report on long-term follow-up and natural history, Gastroenterology 89:267-271, 1985.

Thirty-six asymptomatic patients with primary biliary cirrhosis are discussed with a median follow-up observation of 11.4 years. Portal granulomas indicated a better long-term prognosis. Associations that had a poorer prognosis included thyroiditis, sicca syndrome, CRST syndrome, and Raynaud's syndrome. At this point in follow-up, almost one half have developed signs or symptoms of progressive disease.

Chedid A, Mendenhall CL, Tosch T, et al: Significance of megamitochondria in alcoholic liver disease, Gastroenterology 90:1858-1864, 1986.

Megamitochondria were observed in 20% of liver biopsy specimens of patients with alcoholic hepatitis. The majority of these patients had less severe disease with a decreased risk of death and fewer complications than those lacking megamitochondria.

Christensen E, Crowe J, Doniach D, et al: Clinical pattern and course of disease in primary biliary cirrhosis based on an analysis of 235 patients, Gastroenterology 78:236-246, 1980.

In a study of 235 symptomatic patients with primary biliary cirrhosis who were followed for 5 years, the frequency of cirrhosis increased from 30% to 82%. The feature that correlated best with progressive disease was the rapid development of cholestasis. Age, histologic stage, and serum bilirubin were additional prognostic factors.

Gines P, Quintero E, Arroyo V, et al: Compensated cirrhosis: natural history and prognostic factors, Hepatology 7(1):122-128, 1987.

This is a review of 293 patients with cirrhosis caused by ethanol, hepatitis B, or cryptogenic cirrhosis who never had ascites, variceal bleeding, jaundice, or encephalopathy before inclusion in the study. Median follow-up observation was 63 months. The probability of dying within 10 years was 53%, and 58% developed clinical signs of decompensation (ascites was the most common event). Factors that predicted poor outcome included elevated bilirubin, gamma globulin, and prothrombin time; advanced age; male gender; and elevated alkaline phosphatase.

Goodman ZD and Ishak KG: Occlusive venous lesions in alcoholic liver disease, Gastroenterology 83:786-796, 1982.

A review of occlusive central vein or terminal hepatic venule vascular lesions in liver specimens of patients dying with alcoholic liver disease indicates there are three types: (1) a lymphocytic phlebitis of the terminal hepatic venule in 17% of patients with alcoholic hepatitis; (2) a perivenular scarring with obliteration of the central vein frequent in all patients examined with alcoholic hepatitis; and (3) veno-occlusive lesions of the central veins in 52% of alcoholic hepatitis patients and 74% of cirrhotics.

Lischner MW, Alexander JF, and Galambos JT: Natural history of alcoholic hepatitis, Am J Dig Dis 16(6):481-494, 1971.

A study of the natural history of 169 patients with alcoholic hepatitis. The overall mortality of this group, all of whom could be biopsied for inclusion, was 4%.

MacSween RNM and Burt AD: Histologic spectrum of alcoholic liver disease, Semin Liver Dis 6(3):221-232, 1986.

This is a summary of the varying histologic features of alcoholic liver disease.

Orrego H, Blake JE, Blendis LM, et al: Prognosis of alcoholic cirrhosis in the presence and absence of alcoholic hepatitis, Gastroenterology 92:208-14, 1987.

In a follow-up study of alcoholic cirrhotic patients with and without alcoholic hepatitis, those with coexisting alcoholic hepatitis had an increased mortality, greater clinical severity, and bigger livers than those with cirrhosis alone.

Schenker S: Alcoholic liver disease: evaluation of natural history and prognostic factors, Hepatology 4(1):36S-43S, 1984.

A review of the natural history and prognostic factors in patients with alcoholic liver disease.

Sherlock S and Scheuer PJ. Medical intelligence: current concepts: the presentation and diagnosis of 100 patients with primary biliary cirrhosis, N Engl J Med 289(13):674-678, 1973.

This is a discussion of the presenting characteristics of 100 patients with primary biliary cirrhosis.

Uchida T, Kao H, Quispe-Sjögren M, et al: Alcoholic foamy degeneration: a pattern of acute alcoholic injury of the liver, Gastroenterology 84:683-692, 1983.

This study defines the clinical and morphologic features of 21 patients with alcoholic foamy degeneration.

27 Complications of Cirrhosis

Rowen K. Zetterman

Cirrhosis can be present without clinically significant complications and be identified only at autopsy or during evaluation of abnormal liver tests. However, for many patients the disease is slowly progressive resulting in one or more complications. The clinical manifestations of cirrhosis are a result of altered hepatic blood flow through the liver with intrahepatic shunting causing impaired perfusion of hepatocytes or portal hypertension with shunting of blood around the liver through portosystemic communications. The major complications of portal hypertension include esophageal or gastric varices, ascites, portosystemic encephalopathy, and hepatorenal syndrome. With impairment of hepatocyte perfusion or reduction of hepatocyte number, altered synthetic function can result in hypoalbuminemia, hypoprothrombinemia, and changes in drug metabolism.

PORTAL HYPERTENSION AND VARICEAL BLEEDING

The portal vein arises from the confluence of the splenic, inferior mesenteric, and superior mesenteric veins. It enters the hilum of the liver dividing into the right and left branches and subsequently into smaller venules to perfuse the sinusoids of the hepatic lobules. In normal persons, there is little resistance to sinusoidal outflow into the hepatic venous system. Portal venous flow is approximately 1L/minute. The hepatic artery supplies an additional 500 ml/minute to the liver.

Increasing pressure within the portal vein, portal hypertension, is a consequence of the resistance to blood flow within the portal system. Portal resistance can be attributable to changes of either the portal vein or its branches within the liver (presinusoidal portal hypertension), to collagenization or compression of the sinusoidal lumen (sinusoidal portal hypertension), or to obstruction of venous blood flow at or beyond the terminal hepatic venule (postsinusoidal portal hypertension). (see box on p. 468). Some disorders interfere with portal blood flow at more than one level. For example, cirrhosis can cause compression of both the sinusoids and terminal hepatic venules by large regenerative nodules. Portal pressure can also be elevated as a result of an increased volume of blood inflow into the portal circulation from some splenic disorders.

Presinusoidal portal hypertension results from resistance to flow in the portal

MECHANISMS OF PORTAL HYPERTENSION

Presinusoidal portal hypertension

Portal vein occlusion
- Hypercoagulable state (e.g., lupus)
- Infection
- Pregnancy
- Tumors
- Cirrhosis

Primary biliary cirrhosis
Congenital hepatic fibrosis
Schistosomiasis
Nodular regenerative hyperplasia
Granulomatous liver disease
- Sarcoid

Idiopathic portal hypertension
Arsenic-induced liver disease
Arterial-portal vein fistula

Sinusoidal portal hypertension

Cirrhosis of any type
Idiopathic portal hypertension

Postsinusoidal portal hypertension

Cirrhosis
Budd-Chiari syndrome
Veno-occlusive disease
Sclerosing hyalin necrosis (alcoholic hepatitis)
Constrictive pericarditis
Congestive heart failure

vein or its branches within the liver. Many of its causes are noncirrhotic and may not have significant liver disease as a component. Portal vein thrombosis initially causes total occlusion of portal flow. The thrombus usually recanalizes into multiple small channels and is identified as cavernous transformation at ultrasound or portal venography. Continuing resistance to flow is usual. Splenic vein thrombosis proximal to the portal vein from pancreatitis or tumor can cause gastric or esophageal varices as splenic vein flow drains through the short gastric veins. Hepatic artery–portal vein fistulas can develop within the liver parenchyma from tumors or after trauma or liver biopsy. The arterial inflow into the portal vein results in an increase of pressure that can result in varices and bleeding. Other diseases including Gaucher's disease, lymphoma, or myeloproliferative disorders can also raise portal pressure by increased blood inflow because of increased arterial flow to an enlarged spleen. Compression of portal vessels at the hilum from nodular regenerative hyperplasia or tumor will also cause portal hypertension. Intrahepatic diseases can compress or obliterate interlobular portal vein radicles. Such changes may be attributable to granulomatous inflammation (e.g., schistosomiasis or sarcoid) and diseases with pronounced portal inflammation (e.g., primary biliary cirrhosis). Presinusoidal portal hypertension may not result in other manifestations of portal hypertension such as ascites or hepatic encephalopathy until late in their course.

Sinusoidal portal hypertension occurs from compression of the sinusoids by regenerative nodules in cirrhosis or from obliteration of the sinusoids by collagenization of the space of Disse as in primary portal hypertension, alcoholic cirrhosis, and some drug-induced liver diseases (e.g., arsenicals and polyvinyl chloride). Sinusoidal compression from ethanol-induced enlargement of hepatocytes in alcoholic cirrhosis may add to portal resistance and portal hypertension.

Postsinusoidal portal hypertension occurs from resistance to outflow from the sinusoids and can follow compression or occlusion of the terminal hepatic veins from cirrhosis, sclerosing hyalin necrosis (alcoholic hepatitis), veno-occlusive disease, and thrombosis of the hepatic veins (Budd-Chiari syndrome), or from inferior vena cava webs or constrictive pericarditis. These disorders increase sinusoidal pressure and result in ascites and other manifestations of portal hypertension. Hepatocellular carcinoma can also develop in patients with inferior vena cava webs.

Clinical Features

When patients develop esophageal or gastric varices, cirrhosis is the most likely cause. Varices can also occur with some pre- and postsinusoidal disorders in the absence of cirrhosis. Midesophageal varices may be identified in congestive heart failure or during pregnancy because of intravascular volume expansion and increased pressure within the azygous venous system. They rarely result in bleeding. Superior vena cava occlusion can cause the formation of "downhill" varices, which flow from above the thrombosis into the submucosal plexus of the esophagus and stomach to anastomose with the inferior vena cava drainage below.

Portal hypertension opens many potential shunts between the portal and inferior vena caval systems. Intrahepatic shunts develop in the fibrous bands surrounding regenerative nodules. Collateralization may also occur at any potential communication between the portal and peripheral circulation including the anterior abdominal wall via the umbilical vein and phrenicocolic ligament, through any intra-abdominal adhesion to the abdominal wall, from the hilum of the spleen through the short gastric veins to the azygous vein via the submucosal plexus of the stomach and esophagus (varices), through the hemorrhoidal veins (perianal hemorrhoids), and in the retroperitoneum to the renal veins. Patients with ulcerative colitis and coexisting sclerosing cholangitis who have had a colectomy with ileostomy may develop bleeding from ileal varices at the stoma.

There may be several clues to the presence of cirrhosis with bleeding because of varices. Variceal bleeding is often large in volume and lacks associated abdominal discomfort other than nausea and vomiting. Signs of chronic liver disease and of portal hypertension may also be present including splenomegaly, ascites, prominent abdominal wall venous collaterals (caput medusae), and a venous hum above the umbilicus (Cruveilhier-Baumgarten syndrome).

The diagnosis of portal hypertension can be established by the presence of esophageal or gastric varices with documentation of increased portal pressures. Esophagoscopy is the single best examination to document varices because esophagrams are only 65% to 80% sensitive. Esophagoscopy permits assessment of varix size and can also identify changes suggestive of potential bleeding including red wales and lines, adherent clots, thinning of the varix wall, and erosive mucosal changes. Large varices are more likely to bleed than small varices. Portal pressures can be estimated by measurement of wedged hepatic venous pressure. An end-hole catheter is passed via the inferior vena cava into the hepatic vein and wedged into the hepatic parenchyma. The wedged pressure is measured and compared to the free pressure in the midhepatic vein or inferior vena cava. The wedged pressure should not exceed the hepatic vein or IVC pressure by more than 5 mm Hg. If the difference is greater than 5 mm, portal hypertension may be present. Wedged hepatic vein pressures are invariably more than 12 mm Hg above hepatic vein pressure in those who bleed from varices. This technique measures changes in portal pressure as a consequence of sinusoidal or postsinusoidal causes. In presinusoidal portal hypertension, the wedged hepatic venous pressure will not reflect true portal vein pressure because the blockage to flow is between the sinusoid and the portal vein. It can also underestimate portal pressures in cryptogenic and posthepatic cirrhosis and tends to work the best for alcoholic liver disease. Direct measurement of portal pressures can be accomplished by transhepatic entry into branches of the portal vein, by surgical placement of a catheter through the umbilical vein into the portal circulation, and by cannulation of a branch of the superior mesenteric vein at operation. By insertion of a needle into the spleen, splenic pulp pressure (and consequently portal pressure) can be determined. These techniques are useful in determining the pressures of all causes of portal hypertension, and simultaneous injection of contrast permits excellent visualization of the portal system. Recent studies have indicated that catheterization with thermal dilution determination of azygous vein flow directly correlates to portal pressure. A reduction of azygous flow in response to somatostatin, vasopressin, and propranolol was observed.

Laboratory and Radiology Findings

The laboratory findings of portal hypertension are few. Thrombocytopenia and leukopenia are frequently present with hypersplenism. Changes of cirrhosis may also be observed.

Ultrasound of the liver with Doppler flow studies of the portal venous circulation can document changes of cirrhosis, portal vein size, and direction and volume of portal venous flow. The portal vein is often enlarged with portal hypertension, and an enlarged umbilical vein may be seen. Portal vein thrombus can be present with stagnant portal flow. Cavernous transformation of the portal vein may follow thrombosis. In addition, other signs including ascites and splenomegaly can indicate portal hypertension. In those with prior portosystemic shunts, shunt patency can be assessed. Computerized tomography (CT) will determine liver and spleen size and the presence of ascites. With contrast enhancement, retroperitoneal collaterals may also be observed. However, CT cannot readily document portal vein patency or flow. Arteriography may assist in determination of portal vein patency and presence of collaterals through use of venous phase radiography. Direct portal venography can be accomplished by transhepatic entry into the portal vein, by umbilical vein catheterization, or by splenoportography with injection of contrast into the splenic hilum. With good opacification of the portal circulation, portosystemic shunts and other collaterals can be documented. A "pruned tree" appearance of intrahepatic portal vein radicles is typical of cirrhosis. Radiographs of the hepatic veins obtained by injection of contrast during hepatic vein catheterization may establish the diagnosis of Budd-Chiari syndrome. Magnetic resonance imaging (MRI) can also assist in determining portal vein, hepatic vein, and portosystemic shunt patency.

Clinical Course and Prognosis

The site of esophageal variceal bleeding is invariably within 2 cm of the esophagogastric mucosal junction. Portal pressures are usually in excess of 12 mm Hg, though there is no absolute correlation of the likelihood of variceal bleeding to the degree of portal pressure above this level. Increased intravascular volume (e.g., overtransfusion) and ascites can increase portal pressure and the risk of subsequent variceal hemorrhage. Nonsteroidal antiinflammatory drugs also increase the risk of bleeding. At endoscopy, some patients with variceal hemorrhage will have associated esophagitis. Lower esophageal sphincter pressures are reduced with cirrhosis. However, it is unclear if esophagitis is a major factor in the initiation of bleeding from varices. Reflux studies utilizing 24-hour pH monitoring do not identify a greater frequency of reflux in patients with cirrhosis, the control of acid reflux with H_2 receptor antagonists does not prevent rebleeding, and at autopsy, severe esophageal ulceration in association with variceal hemorrhage is unusual.

Once variceal hemorrhage has occurred, there is a 75% likelihood of rebleeding. This risk is greatest within the first 24 hours, occurring in 60%. At endoscopy, signs of a greater likelihood to rebleed include red wales or stripes along varices, adherent clots, and varices with thin appearing walls. Large varices greater than 5 mm in diameter are also more likely to rebleed.

The prognosis of the patient with variceal hemorrhage is partially dependent on the underlying cause. Patients with alcoholic cirrhosis fare less well than other groups, possibly because of associated alcoholic hepatitis. Patients who have presinusoidal portal hypertension (e.g., primary biliary cirrhosis) tend to do better because the underlying liver disease may be less severe. However, in end-stage primary biliary cirrhosis, variceal hemorrhage is a poor prognostic sign. When the risk of dying from variceal hemorrhage is compared to the severity of the underlying liver disease, there is greater mortality with increasing severity. Using the Child-Pugh classification (Table 27-1), Child's A patients have a 75% 1-year survival after variceal hemorrhage, but Child's C patient has only a 30% survival. With end-stage liver disease of any cause, up to 25% of patients will die with each episode of variceal bleeding. In addition, any cause of upper gastrointestinal bleeding will carry a higher mortality in the patient with cirrhosis, especially if the cause is alcohol.

Table 27-1 Child-Turcotte-Pugh classification

	A	B	C
Serum bilirubin (mg/dl)	<2	2-3	>3
Serum albumin (gm/dl	>3.5	3-3.5	<3
Prothrombin time (seconds prolonged)	Normal	>3 seconds	>3 seconds
Ascites	None	Easily controlled	Poorly controlled
Encephalopathy	None	Minimal	Coma

Treatment

When the patient with cirrhosis presents with upper gastrointestinal bleeding, he or she must be quickly evaluated and resuscitated. Not all will be bleeding from varices. In the patient with alcoholic cirrhosis who was continuing to consume ethanol before admission for bleeding, one of the acute mucosal diseases such as esophagitis, gastritis, and peptic ulcer is a more likely cause than variceal hemorrhage. Emergent esophagogastroduodenoscopy (EGD) is generally indicated and can allow assessment of varices for signs of hemorrhage, looking for other sources of bleeding, and providing emergent therapy. The presence of portal hypertensive gastropathy manifesting as a reticular pattern of submucosal gastric vessels can also be determined. It is increasingly recognized as a frequent cause of upper gastrointestinal bleeding in the cirrhotic.

Variceal hemorrhage can result in massive blood loss. With significant hypotension, splanchnic and hepatic perfusion are reduced, and necrosis of regenerative nodules can further compromise hepatic function. Hypovolemia must be quickly corrected. Other medical complications should also be controlled. The presence of ascites will increase portal pressure and may be associated with a greater risk of rebleeding. Patients should receive medications such as H_2 blockers, sucralfate or antacids to control coexisting acute mucosal inflammation.

Intravenous infusion of vasopressin can induce splanchnic vasoconstriction and assist in decreasing variceal perfusion and bleeding. It can be given as a bolus or as a continuous infusion. The efficacy of both is controversial, though bolus infusion has been suggested to control bleeding in up to 50% of patients. Myocardial infarction, cerebrovascular accidents, and small bowel necrosis in association with vasopressin have been described. The simultaneous administration of nitroglycerin may decrease portal venous resistance and further reduce portal pressure. It will also produce systemic vasodilatation and reduce cardiac side effects of vasopressin. Systolic blood pressure should be maintained at about 90 mm Hg during their simultaneous use. Other agents that have been utilized include the longer-acting 1-triglycyl-8-lysine vasopressin and the somatostatin analogue octreotide. The mechanism of action of somatostatin is also believed to be as a vasoconstrictor.

If these measures do not result in rapid cessation of hemorrhage, emergent sclerotherapy should be considered. Although it will acutely control 90% of variceal bleeding, sclerotherapy does not affect long-term outcome. Possible complications of sclerotherapy include chest pain, fever, pleural effusions, esophageal perforation, and stricture. Endoscopic banding of varices similar to the treatment of hemorrhoids has also been utilized. If bleeding persists, introduction of a Sengstaken-Blakemore tube may control hemorrhage. It should be placed through the mouth and must include a catheter above the esophageal balloon to continuously suction the upper esophagus and prevent pulmonary aspiration of secretions. After placement, its satisfactory location should be confirmed by a plain radiograph. Potential complications of the Sengstaken-Blakemore tube include aspiration pneumonia, esophageal rupture from intraesophageal insufflation of the gastric balloon, esophageal or gastric erosions, and perioral ulcerations. Percutaneous transhepatic variceal embolization can also be utilized to control hemorrhage by placement of a catheter through the liver into the portal circulation. An increased risk of portal vein thrombosis has been described.

Long-term management of variceal hemorrhage includes chronic sclerotherapy, administration of beta-adrenergic receptor blockers, and surgically created portosystemic shunts. With repetitive sclerotherapy, obliteration of varices can be achieved. Patients should be periodically reendoscoped as varices reform. In controlled trials, there are fewer bleeding episodes in those treated with repetitive sclerotherapy than among controls. Prophylactic sclerotherapy of varices that have never bled is not recommended. Beta blockers have also been utilized for long-term control of bleeding varices in portal hypertension. At a dose sufficient to decrease base-line heart rate by 25%, splanchnic and portal blood flow are reduced. Their efficacy for the prevention of variceal bleeding remains controversial. A recent study suggests they may be useful in controlling varices after initial elimination by repetitive sclerotherapy. Surgically created portosystemic shunts can prevent rebleeding from varices. They should not be used as prophylaxis to prevent initial bleeding and may not affect hypersplenism. The choice of operation is partially dependent on the surgeon's training and skill. Portacaval shunts can be created as end-to-side or side-to-side anastomoses of the portal vein to the inferior vena cava (IVC) or as a graft between the superior mesenteric vein and the IVC (the mesocaval shunt). With splenectomy, the proximal end of the splenic vein can be anastomosed to the left renal vein as a splenorenal shunt. The thrombosis rate of proximal splenorenal shunts is 40%. The spleen can also be left intact with the distal end of the splenic vein transected from the portal vein and anastomosed to the left renal vein as a distal splenorenal shunt. This shunt selectively drains the gastric and esophageal varices via the short gastric veins into the splenic hilum and subsequently the IVC. It causes less disruption of portal venous blood flow than portosystemic shunts because the superior mesenteric inflow remains. The operative mortality of surgical shunts correlates with underlying clinical severity of the liver disease. Although variceal bleeding is controlled by shunts, chronic hepatic encephalopathy may complicate some patients. Many patients who bleed from varices are at a time of accelerated decompensation of their liver disease and should be considered for liver transplantation instead of portosystemic shunts. Sclerotherapy can be used to control hemorrhage until a suitable donor is identified.

ASCITES

The development of ascites in patients with cirrhosis represents a balance of sodium retention, increased intrasinusoidal pressure as a consequence of portal hypertension, the reduction of oncotic pressure from hypoalbuminemia, and the capacity of the lymphatics to handle excess lymph formation. The elevation of pressure at the end of the sinusoid produces an increase in hydrostatic pressure resulting in transudation of fluid into the space of Disse. The transudate drains to the lymphatics. When the quantity exceeds the capacity of the lymphatics, ascites will weep from the hepatic surface into the abdominal cavity. At laparoscopy, small blebs of fluid can be observed on the hepatic surface of those forming ascites. Abdominal absorption of ascites occurs principally through the lymphatics along the diaphragmatic surface. Renal changes that occur in association with ascites formation include decreased perfusion of the renal cortex, diminished glomerular filtration, intense proximal tubular reabsorption of sodium, and impaired free water clearance.

Two mechanisms have been proposed to account for the retention of sodium and subsequent ascites formation. The hypovolemia theory indicates that there may be a renal response to decreased "effective" intravascular volume that results in sodium and water retention. This increases intravascular volume and consequently portal pressure to cause transudation of fluid into the space of Disse. When patients with ascites are immersed to the neck in water, there is an increase of core intravascular volume equivalent to the infusion of 2 liters of fluid, and spontaneous diuresis will follow. The other possibility is the overflow theory, which proposes that cirrhosis causes an intense retention of sodium by the proximal renal tubule with reduced delivery of sodium to the distal renal tubule. The retention of sodium results in an increased intravascular volume with a corresponding rise of sinusoidal pressure and transudation of fluid into the space of Disse. A reduction in sodium at the distal tubule may contribute to impaired free water clearance.

Other factors that play a role in sodium and water retention include increased circulating aldosterone and antidiuretic hormone activity. Aldosterone levels may be normal in well-compensated cirrhotics and increased in the decompensated patient with ascites, adding to the potassium depletion and sodium retention of cirrhosis. Increased levels of antidiuretic hormone decrease free water clearance and result in water retention. Reduction of serum albumin decreases oncotic pressure but contributes little to the development of ascites until levels are very low. Increased sympathetic activity in the kidney may also contribute to sodium retention. Renal prostaglandin E activity may also determine sodium retention and distribution of intrarenal blood flow. Administration of nonsteroidal antiinflammatory drugs reduces glomerular filtration and sodium excretion. With head-out immersion of the patient with cirrhosis in water, there is an increase of urinary excretion of prostaglandin E that correlates with enhanced natriuresis. There does not appear to be a role for atrial natriuretic factor in the pathogenesis of ascites.

The differential diagnosis of ascites includes portal hypertension, peritoneal disease, pancreatic disorders, some causes of presinusoidal and postsinusoidal portal hypertension, and hypothyroidism (see box on p. 475). Cirrhosis is the most frequent cause. All patients with new onset or changing ascites must be evaluated with paracentesis to look for infection or to establish the reason for occurrence.

Clinical Features

The onset of ascites may be insidious or rapid with exaggerated sodium input during dietary indiscretion or resuscitation of the bleeding patient with blood, plasma, and intravenous sodium-containing crystalloid solutions. Physical findings include a protuberant abdomen with bulging flanks, a fluid wave, shifting dullness as the patient is rolled from side to side, and right-flank dullness. The most reliable physical sign of ascites is the puddle test, in which a patient is placed on his hands and knees and the hyperresonance above

CAUSES OF ASCITES

Portal hypertension

Presinusoidal portal hypertension
- Portal vein occlusion
- Granulomatous liver disease
- Some diseases of hepatic fibrosis

Cirrhosis

Acute severe liver disease
- Viral hepatitis

Hepatocellular carcinoma

Metastatic liver disease

Postsinusoidal portal hypertension
- Budd-Chiari syndrome
- Veno-occlusive disease
- Constrictive pericarditis
- Congestive heart failure

Peritoneal disease

Tumor
- Mesothelioma
- Metastatic disease

Infection
- Tuberculosis

Pancreatic disease

Pancreatitis

Pancreatic pseudocyst

Tumor

Renal disease

Renal failure

Nephrotic syndrome

After dialysis
- Hemodialysis
- Peritoneal dialysis

Hypothyroidism

Lymphatic obstruction (chylous ascites)

the ascites is percussed while one listens with a stethoscope on the other side of the abdomen. Lower extremity peripheral edema is frequently present, and scrotal swelling may occur with advanced ascites. Umbilical hernias are common and can ulcerate, leading to rupture of ascites. The mortality of umbilical perforation is high, in part because of the development of peritonitis. Staphylococcal infection of umbilical ulcerations is frequent. The increase of intraabdominal pressure from ascites may also result in elevation of the diaphragm with lower lobe atelectasis. Communications between the abdominal cavity and the pleural space may lead to pleural effusion. Other causes of effusion should also be considered. Congestive heart failure could produce both ascites and pleural effusion, or both heart failure and liver disease can have the same cause (e.g., ethanol).

Spontaneous bacterial peritonitis (SBP) is a frequent complication of ascites, occurring in 10% or more of patients with alcoholic cirrhosis and ascites. There may be few clinical signs of peritonitis. It should be suspected in any patient with worsening ascites or encephalopathy, fever, abdominal tenderness, nausea, diarrhea, anorexia, ileus, or azotemia. Fever is present in less than 50% of cases. Up to 30% may be asymptomatic. The mortality of SBP is high and partly dependent on the severity of underlying liver disease. Patients with hyperbilirubinemia and azotemia will have up to 50% mortality despite treatment. Most patients (90%) have a single organism to account for infection. In patients with multiple organisms, enteric perforation should be considered. The mechanism of infection is unclear but may result from passage of the bacteria across the intestinal wall or from bacteremia attributable to urinary tract infection and respiratory sources. Upper and lower endoscopy are also associated with SBP. Some patients present after paracentesis, raising questions of inadvertent contamination. Decreased opsonization of ascites fluid, impaired Kupffer cell function, and decreased leukocyte chemotaxis may permit infection to progress. The bacteria are generally gram negative enteric organisms or gram positive cocci. Anaerobes are infrequent, probably because the pO_2 content of ascites fluid is similar to that of venous blood. Patients with either new onset ascites or a change in the status of their ascites should have a diagnostic paracentesis. At the bedside, blood culture bottles should be inoculated with ascitic fluid. This will increase the yield of positive ascitic cultures by at least 10% over the plating of fluid in the bacteriology laboratory. Blood culture results may also be positive in 50% of patients with SBP. If infection is suspected, broad spectrum antibiotic therapy that will treat potential organisms should be administered. A third-generation cephalosporin such as cefotaxime will cover most bacterial infections with less nephrotoxicity than combinations with aminoglycosides. When cultures are available, antibiotic coverage can be modified.

Laboratory Findings

The laboratory abnormalities of the patient with ascites will reflect the presence of cirrhosis. Urinary sodium levels are typically less than 10 mEq/L. Paracentesis should be performed in all patients with any change in their ascites or with any symptoms suggestive of SBP. A site away from abdominal vessels or spontaneous portosystemic anastomoses should be chosen. This is best accomplished in the midline midway between the umbilicus and pubis at a point of dullness from fluid. It may be helpful to have the patient sitting during paracentesis to float the bowel away from the entry site. Ascites fluid should be evaluated for cell count and differential, pH, protein, amylase, gram stain, bacterial cultures, and cytologic features. If tuberculosis is suspected, 1 liter of fluid can be removed and concentrated for culture. The yield from this technique is as good as a Cope needle biopsy of the peritoneum looking for granulomas. Laparoscopy is the preferred diagnostic study for peritoneal tuberculosis. The white blood cell count of uncomplicated ascites is typically less than 300 cells/ml, with the majority of cells being lymphocytes. With diuresis, the percentage of mononuclear cells will rise in ascitic fluid. In patients with spontaneous peritonitis, the white blood cell count is usually increased with a polymorphonuclear leukocyte increase of greater than 25%. Approximately 10% of patients with SBP will have a WBC cell count of less than 300 cells/ml. A large increase of ascites fluid neutrophil count will also occur in pancreatic ascites. Red blood cells may result from trauma during the tap but can also indicate underlying carcinoma or tuberculosis. The ascitic fluid pH should be greater than 7.3 and may signal infection if reduced. Elevated lactate levels can also be used as an indicator of SBP. Ascitic fluid protein is generally less than 2.0 gm/dl in patients with cirrhosis, though levels of greater than 3 are observed in 10%. Up to 40% of patients with tuberculosis or carcinoma also have transudative ascites. Gram stains may be positive in 25% of cases of SBP. Acid-fast stains are rarely positive in tuberculous peritonitis. The presence of ascitic fluid amylase in excess of serum levels can be an indicator of a pancreatic origin of ascites. Chylous ascites can form from disruption of abdominal lymphatics, producing a milky-appearing ascitic fluid. Measurement of triglyceride content will confirm the presence of fat. Elevated ascitic triglyceride content is frequent in intraabdominal malignancy. Cytologic studies should be completed when malignancy is suspected.

Radiology

Plain abdominal films of patients with ascites show haziness of the abdomen with separation of bowel loops. Elevated diaphragms with basilar atelectasis of the lungs and pleural effusions may be observed in chest radiographs. Use of ultrasound is important in establishing the differential diagnosis of ascites and its presence. It will demonstrate the hepatic changes of cirrhosis, enlarged lymph nodes of metastatic disease, intrahepatic tumors, or the occlusion of portal or hepatic veins. Computerized tomography can also document ascites, intrahepatic or pancreatic tumors, and changes of cirrhosis.

Course, Prognosis, and Treatment

The development of ascites in conjunction with cirrhosis is a poor prognostic sign, and up to 50% will die within 2 years of ascites onset. The development of spontaneous bacterial peritonitis is also a grave sign, with only a 21% to 38% 1-year survival. Prompt treatment of ascites is important because other complications related to ascites such as bleeding varices and spontaneous peritonitis may be aggravated.

The patient with ascites should have an initial diagnostic paracentesis, urine and serum electrolytes, serum BUN and creatinine, and daily weights. A low-sodium diet of 250 to 500 mg/day should be provided during hospitalization with dietary instruction for 500 to 1000 mg/day at home. Protein restriction is added only if portosystemic encephalopathy is present, and fluid restriction should not be used unless the serum sodium is less than 125 mEq/L. The goal of weight loss is 0.5 kg/day. With peripheral edema, greater loss is possible because of simultaneous reabsorption of edema fluid. In the absence of peripheral edema, only 400 ml of ascites can be mobilized daily. Approximately 25% of patients with their initial bout of ascites will spontaneously diurese with sodium restriction alone. If not, the aldosterone antagonist spironolactone can be started at 50 mg bid. Spironolactone has a half-life of approximately 12 hours. Amiloride can also be used. Approximately 50% of patients will diurese with this regimen. If a sustained weight loss of 0.5 kg/day does not occur after 3 days, the dose of spironolactone can be increased to 100 mg twice daily. In 3 more days, furosemide or hydrochlorothiazide can be added if necessary. Additional diuretic dosage is dependent on response. Serum sodium and potassium should be periodically monitored. Complications of diuretic management can include prerenal azotemia, hyponatremia, hyperkalemia, metabolic alkalosis, hepatic encephalopathy, and possibly hepatorenal syndrome. Gynecomastia can develop from spironolactone. Hyponatremia should be treated with water restriction if necessary. Demeclocycline can induce renal failure in cirrhosis and should not be used to control hyponatremia. Nonsteroidal antiinflammatory drugs should also be avoided because they can reduce renal blood flow and glomerular filtration.

Therapeutic paracentesis has been used in place of diuretics. Up to 3 liters of ascites is removed each day for several consecutive days. It will permit faster control of ascites than diuretics can. Patients should be carefully selected for therapeutic paracentesis. Those who are Child's class C or have alcoholic hepatitis or azotemia are better treated conservatively. Although it may be unnecessary for many patients, administration of intravenous albumin equal in amount to that removed at paracentesis may assist in decreasing the potential of renal failure. The risks of large volume paracentesis include intravascular volume loss, renal failure, infection, and protein loss.

Refractory ascites may develop with end-stage liver disease or in the presence of excess sodium intake. When ascites becomes refractory, the patient's diet must be reviewed and spontaneous bacterial peritonitis excluded. Albumin infusions may help some patients. The LeVeen shunt has also been used for refractory ascites. Although the LeVeen shunt is initially effective in ascites control in most patients, it does not improve survival over conventional diuretic therapy and is not effective in the treatment of hepatorenal syndrome. Potential complications of LeVeen shunts include disseminated intravascular coagulation, congestive heart failure, bleeding varices, superior vena cava thrombosis, infection, and difficulty maintaining shunt patency. Side-to-side portacaval shunts decrease intrahepatic sinusoidal pressure and control ascites but have a risk of hepatic coma from impaired sinusoidal perfusion.

PORTOSYSTEMIC ENCEPHALOPATHY

Hepatic encephalopathy is a reversible alteration of consciousness that may develop in association with either cirrhosis or acute severe liver injury such as fulminant hepatitis. In most patients, a precipitating factor will be present. These include large dietary protein loads, azotemia, gastrointestinal bleeding, infections, or metabolic changes such as hypokalemia, hyponatremia, hypomagnesemia, hypocalcemia, or alkalosis. Administration of sedatives may also induce hepatic coma.

The pathogenesis of hepatic coma is unclear and has been attributed to production of excess ammonia or the accumulation of false neurotransmitters, γ-aminobutyric acid (GABA), or endogenous benzodiazepine-like substances. Serum levels of ammonia tend to correlate with the degree of encephalopathy once the patient is at stage II or greater. Ammonia can be formed in the intestine from protein and urea, portal vein levels are increased in patients with encephalopathy, and ammonia avoids extraction by the liver in cirrhosis by passing through portosystemic shunts to reach the brain. In the cerebrospinal fluid, it combines with glutamic acid to form glutamine. A synergistic effect of short chain fatty acids and ammonia has been suggested. Ammonia may also induce coma in noncirrhotic diseases such as the disorders of urea synthesis and after ureterosigmoidoscopy.

In patients with advanced liver disease, there is an increase of serum aromatic amino acids such as methionine and phenylalanine and a decrease of branched chain amino acids such as leucine, isoleucine, and valine. It has been suggested that the aromatic amino acids can cross the blood-brain barrier and cause encephalopathy.

It has also been proposed that a true neuroinhibitory neurotransmitter, GABA may be formed in the intestine and bypass the liver of patients with cirrhosis to reach the brain and cause coma. The GABA receptor in the brain shares a chloride channel with the benzodiazepine receptor. However, serum levels of GABA do not correlate with the degree of encephalopathy, and other substances that can bind to the GABA receptor may be formed in cirrhosis and cause coma. The manifestations of hepatic coma can be reversed by the benzodiazepine antagonist flumazenil. This reversal indicates that an endogenous benzodiazepine may be formed and cause coma in the patient with advanced liver disease. Although these theories explain features of hepatic coma, at present, there is no unifying hypothesis.

Clinical Features

The early symptoms of hepatic encephalopathy may be difficult to distinguish in the patient with cirrhosis and include lethargy, personality changes, a reversal of the day-night sleeping pattern, apathy, and slow mentation. Cognitive function may also be impaired. In acute hepatic encephalopathy from fulminant hepatic failure, agitation, and delirium are common. Delirium is rarely observed in the hepatic coma of cirrhosis. With increasing encephalopathy, patients become progressively more sleepy until they cannot be aroused. Sedative drugs that require hepatic metabolism will have a longer half-life and can induce or worsen encephalopathy.

Asterixis is usually present in the patient with hepatic coma. It is demonstrated by having the patient attempt to maintain dorsiflexion of the hands while holding the arms outstretched. When present, it produces a flapping action of the hands and represents an inability to hold this posture because of incoordination. It can also be demonstrated as a "milk maid's" grip when the patient is asked to steadily grasp the fingers of the examiner, producing a rhythmic grasp-relaxation sequence. Asterixis is not specific for hepatic coma and can be observed with kidney, heart, or lung disease and with drug overdose. Other signs of hepatic coma include impaired cognitive function such as subtracting serial 7's and the loss of spatial orientation, including constructional apraxia, impaired handwriting, and difficulty in completing the Reitan trail test. In deep coma, respirations are deep and even (Kussmaul's respirations) and may result in respiratory alkalosis. Reflexes are initially hyperreactive in stages I and II and may include clonus. With deeper coma, the reflexes become hypoactive, and in stage IV, the patient is flaccid. Babinski's sign may also develop in advanced encephalopathy. The breath of the patient with hepatic coma may have a fruity odor, termed "fetor hepaticus," because of respiratory excretion of mercaptans. Electroencephalographic changes of hepatic encephalopathy include diffuse slowing and triphasic waves. They are invariably present by stage II coma and may be observed in stage I. Triphasic waves are absent in deep coma. Visual evoked potentials can also be used to monitor hepatic coma. Diffuse slow wave changes are typi-

Table 27-2 Stages of hepatic coma

	Consciousness	Asterixis	Reflexes	EEG
Stage O:	Normal	None	Normal	Normal
Stage I:	Day-night reversal Agitation Personality changes	None	Increased	Normal to slow waves
Stage II:	Lethargic Arousable	Present	Increased	Slow waves Triphasic waves
Stage III:	Poorly arousable	±	Decreased	Slow waves Triphasic waves
Stage IV:	Unarousable	Absent	Flaccid	Slow waves

cal of any metabolic encephalopathy and are also seen in uremia, CO_2 retention, drug-induced coma, and hypoglycemia. Hepatic coma can be graded as to severity (Table 27-2). Grading is useful for documentation and for interobserver assessment of patients.

Laboratory Findings

If desired, ammonia levels can be measured in patients with hepatic encephalopathy. Arterial and not venous ammonia levels should be utilized because of ammonia formation by muscle. Ammonia levels may lag behind the clinical events of encephalopathy, remaining normal in early encephalopathy and then staying elevated longer than the patient is clinically encephalopathic after recovery. Cerebrospinal fluid glutamine and α-ketoglutarate levels also correlate with the presence of hepatic coma. Measurement of serum amino acid profiles is not helpful in the diagnosis of hepatic encephalopathy. Precipitating events of hepatic coma include hypokalemia, profound hyponatremia, hypomagnesemia, hypocalcemia, and alkalosis and should be assessed in any patient who develops coma.

With chronic recurring encephalopathy, the brain may develop Alzheimer's type II astrocytosis, a thinning of the cerebral cortex and demyelinization of pyramidal tracts. Cerebral edema is not believed to occur in chronic hepatic encephalopathy. Demyelination of long tracts can result in motor deficits such as paraplegia or hemiplegia. Cerebellar and basal ganglion changes may also occur, creating a clinical picture similar to Wilson's disease with choreoathetoid movements and an unstable gait. The basal ganglia will show patchy neuronal necrosis and spongy degeneration.

Course, Prognosis and Treatment

The development of encephalopathy in the patient with cirrhosis generally includes a precipitating event such as prerenal azotemia or electrolyte abnormalities from diuresis, diarrhea, vomiting, paracentesis, or gastrointestinal bleeding. It may also be a consequence of infection, operation, excess dietary protein, or severe constipation. Other causes of coma in addition to hepatic encephalopathy should also be considered. The prognosis depends on the precipitating event and the ease of control. If no obvious event is quickly identified, the patient should have cultures of blood, ascites, urine, and sputum, and a nasogastric tube should be inserted into the stomach to look for blood. Laboratory studies of potassium, sodium, magnesium, calcium, venous pH, and a drug screen should be completed. Dehydration and electrolyte abnormalities should be corrected and the gastrointestinal tract purged with magnesium citrate to rid the intestine of any possible blood. Antibiotics should be considered even if no obvious infection is identified. They can be stopped or modified when the results of the cultures are known. If the patient develops stage III or greater coma, he or she should be intubated with assisted ventilation to prevent respiratory arrest. Administration of lactulose or nonabsorbable antibiotics such as neomycin can assist in controlling encephalopathy. As patients recover, they can be started on a 20 gm protein, sodium-restricted diet, with the protein increased by 10 to 20 gm every 3 days as tolerated. Vegetable protein is better tolerated in hepatic encephalopathy than meat protein. It is imperative to avoid all sedative drugs in agitated patients with early hepatic encephalopathy. The half-life of drugs requiring hepatic metabolism will be increased in patients with cirrhosis. The deepening of coma that results from sedatives may increase the risk of fatal complications.

With chronic relapsing hepatic encephalopathy, continuous administration of lactulose in a dose sufficient to produce 2 or 3 stools daily may be helpful. Neomycin should not be used over a long term because of potential nephrotoxicity. Lactulose is a nondigestible carbohydrate that is degraded by the bacteria of the colon, making the colonic contents more acidic and changing the quantity of urea-splitting bacteria. Serum ammonia levels will decrease with lactulose treatment. Dietary protein should be increased to the quantity the patient can tolerate. There does not appear to be a specific benefit of hepatic encephalopathy from the administration of high-branched-chain amino acid supplements. In patients with end-stage liver disease and recurring hepatic encephalopathy, liver transplantation should be considered.

HEPATORENAL SYNDROME

Hepatorenal syndrome is a progressively oliguric, azotemic renal failure that develops in the presence of end-stage liver disease or acute hepatic failure. It is a functional renal failure characterized by normal renal tubular function and histologic features and is more common in advanced alcoholic liver disease. It may develop after hospitalization. The pathogenesis of hepatorenal syndrome is unknown. It is associated with decreased renal perfusion with shunting of blood away from the renal cortex in the presence of a normal cardiac output. The renin-angiotensin system may be activated by the decline in "effective" intravascular volume, and angiotensin could contribute to intrarenal vasoconstriction. Bradykinin levels are reduced in cirrhosis and could permit intrarenal vasoconstriction. It might also occur as a response to altered prostaglandin E (PGE) or thromboxane levels. Urinary prostaglandins are reduced in hepatorenal syndrome. PGE_2 can affect renal blood flow and decrease tubular reabsorption of sodium, resulting in enhanced natriuresis. Use of nonsteroidal antiinflammatory drugs can decrease renal blood flow and glomerular filtration. Increased thromboxane synthesis could contribute to intrarenal vasoconstriction. Other candidates as intrarenal vasoconstricting substances include substance P and vasoactive intestinal polypeptide (VIP).

Clinical Features

There are no specific symptoms for hepatorenal syndrome. Patients experience weakness, fatigue, and anorexia. With increasing azotemia, nausea, vomiting, and worsening hepatic encephalopathy will follow. Progressive oliguria is characteristic, and ascites is invariably present. The differential of hepatorenal syndrome includes volume depletion and prerenal azotemia, acute tubular necrosis, nephrotoxic drugs, and diseases that affect both the liver and kidney such as glomerulonephritis from ethanol, vasculitis, leptospirosis, and *Amanita* poisoning.

Laboratory and Radiology Findings

Hepatorenal syndrome is characterized by progressive azotemia and an increased urine osmolality, with a sodium of less than 10 mEq/L. A urinary sodium alone is not sufficient to establish the diagnosis of hepatorenal syndrome, because sodium retention in cirrhosis is intense and frequently produces urine sodium levels in this same range. Serum sodium levels may also be low from impaired free water clearance. Pronounced azotemia rarely develops as the patients succumb to the complications of coexisting hepatic coma.

There are no specific radiologic features that are helpful in the diagnosis of hepatorenal syndrome. Ultrasound can exclude ureteral obstruction and thrombosis of renal veins. If arteriography of the kidney is completed, impaired perfusion of the renal cortex from intrahepatic shunting is observed. In general, the use of radiographic contrast in the patient with cirrhosis should be avoided because it may result in renal failure.

Course, Prognosis and Treatment

Hepatorenal syndrome is a progressive disorder that usually does not reverse itself unless the hepatic injury improves. The patients rarely die of uremia. Rather, hepatorenal syndrome is associated with progressive encephalopathy, and the complications of hepatic coma lead to a fatal outcome. With liver transplantation and a return of hepatic function to normal, hepatorenal syndrome will recover. Furthermore, since the kidney is histologically normal in hepatorenal syndrome, it can be successfully transplanted into patients with chronic renal failure and resume normal function.

When progressive oliguria or azotemia develops in the patient with cirrhosis, prompt correction of intravascular volume deficiencies may lead to an improvement of renal function. A Swan-Ganz catheter should be placed and pulmonary capillary wedge pressures determined. If hypovolemia is present, correction with red blood cell transfusions (if needed) and infusion of 25% albumin may stabilize or improve renal function. Nonsteroidal antiinflammatory drugs should be avoided. In selected patients, paracentesis may decrease intraabdominal pressure and result in an increase of cardiac output and renal perfusion. With large volume paracentesis, however, cardiac output begins to fall as the ascites reforms and renal perfusion will decline. If paracentesis is utilized to increase cardiac output, albumin infusions should follow paracentesis in an attempt to maintain intravascular volume. Total body immersion in water up to the neck will also increase core intravascular volume, cause increased secretin of PGE, and may improve renal perfusion and function. Administration of low-dose dopamine does not improve renal function. There is no evidence that placement of a LeVeen shunt will reverse hepatorenal syndrome. Hemodialysis is not effective in management of patients with hepatorenal syndrome. They rarely develop complications of uremia.

MISCELLANEOUS COMPLICATIONS

Infections

The alcoholic is especially prone to infections with encapsulated organisms such as pneumococci or *Klebsiella*. This is partly a consequence of impaired polymorphonuclear leukocyte chemotaxis, diminished opsonizing capacity, reduced intracellular killing of bacteria, and abnormal clearance of bacteria by Kupffer cells. *Enterobacter* infections are frequent in cystic disorders of the liver. Pulmonary tuberculosis is also more common in the alcoholic patient, because cell-mediated immunity is decreased in patients with advanced alcoholic liver disease. Tuberculous peritonitis may cause ascites with few systemic signs such as fever or abdominal pain. The ascites of TB peritonitis is characterized by lymphocytosis, red blood cells, a low glucose level, and an elevated protein level.

Endocarditis is more common in the patient with cirrhosis, and both gram-negative organisms and *Staphylococcus aureus* are likely. Spontaneous bacterial peritonitis (see earlier) can develop in any patient with ascites. With any deterioration in hepatic function or increase of ascites, paracentesis should be performed.

Neurologic Complications

Wilson's disease may present with neurologic complications including choreoathetoid movements, dysarthria, tremor, drooling and personality changes. Neurologic presentation predominates after 25 years of age.

Nonwilsonian hepatolenticular degeneration can occur with cirrhosis and repeated episodes of hepatic encephalopathy. It is manifest by choreoathetoid movements, dysarthria, confusion, disorientation, apathy, ataxia, and a spongy degeneration of the basal ganglia from focal neuronal necrosis. There is no therapy.

Transverse myelitis and demyelinization of pyramidal tracts can also occur with chronic hepatic encephalopathy and may result in hemiplegia or paraplegia. Most of these patients will have had prior portosystemic shunts.

Pulmonary Complications

Patients with sarcoid and primary biliary cirrhosis may have impaired diffusing capacity. Right-to-left shunts can occur in patients with advanced cirrhosis. These arteriovenous communications are typically present in the bases of the lungs with desaturation aggravated by upright posture. Portal circulation–pulmonary artery shunts and pleural nevi may also develop but contribute little to desaturation. Patients with chronic active hepatitis and cirrhosis who have undergone a portacaval shunt can develop cyanosis from right-to-left shunts. Clubbing may also be present. Administration of oxygen to some patients with intrapulmonary shunts results in total correction of hypoxemia. There is a recent report that desaturation from right-to-left shunts may also improve with administration of the somatostatin analog octreotide.

Pulmonary hypertension can develop in any form of cirrhosis with a prevalence of approximately 1 case per 140 cirrhotics. It occurs in the absence of cardiac or parenchymal pulmonary disease. Physical findings include an increased P_2 and eventual development of cardiac failure. The mechanism of pulmonary hypertension is unknown and may be a consequence of multiple pulmonary emboli, vasoactive hormones, increased intravascular volume, or inflammatory effects on pulmonary vasculature.

Pleural effusions may develop in patients with ascites as a result of diaphragmatic defects. The negative intrathoracic pressure will pull ascites into the chest, even when little intraabdominal ascites is present. Effusions can be large and interfere with lung mechanics.

Cardiovascular Effects

The patient with cirrhosis typically has a hyperdynamic circulation with increased cardiac output, bounding pulses, and reduced systemic vascular resistance. Congestive heart failure is rare. The pathogenesis is unknown and may be attributable to increased intravascular volume and circulating vasodilatory factors. With pronounced ascites, inferior vena caval blood return to the right heart may be decreased. After paracentesis and a corresponding decrease in intraabdominal pressure, an increase in venous return and cardiac output may occur.

Gastrointestinal Effects

Secretory diarrhea can complicate the patient with portal hypertension because of increased superior mesenteric venous pressure causing transudation of fluid across the bowel. Diarrhea can also develop in the malnourished alcoholic with niacin deficiency. Ethanol may affect jejunal mucosal cells. Peptic ulcer disease occurs in 15% of patients with cirrhosis. Gastroesophageal reflux is aggravated by increased intraabdominal pressure from ascites and a reduction of lower esophageal sphincter pressure in cirrhosis. Medical therapy of esophagitis should be administered as needed. Portal hypertensive gastropathy may develop in the patient with portal hypertension and be a significant cause of upper gastrointestinal bleeding.

Hematologic Complications

Patients with cirrhosis may present with anemia as a consequence of hemolysis, blood loss, anemia of chronic disease, or vitamin deficiency. Hemolysis develops in Wilson's disease from release of copper into the circulation after hepatocyte necrosis. Zieve's syndrome occurs in alcoholic fatty liver in association with hypertriglyceridemia, with a peripheral blood smear that demonstrates spur cells. The pathogenesis of hemolysis from ethanol is unclear and may be attributable to a stiffening of the red blood cell membrane from crosslinking of membrane proteins by acetaldehyde or from alteration of the cholesterol-phospholipid ratio. Hemolysis may also complicate chronic active hepatitis. The development of polycythemia should alert the clinician to the possible presence of a complicating hepatocellular carcinoma.

Coagulopathy from impaired hepatic production of vitamin K–dependent coagulation factors occurs in advanced cirrhosis. Disseminated intravascular coagulation (DIC) may rarely develop. Measurement of factor VIII levels will help to separate the patient with impaired coagulation factor production attributable to liver disease from DIC. Factor VIII is made by endothelial cells and remains normal in cirrhosis. DIC may also complicate the placement of a LeVeen shunt. If bleeding develops, the shunt requires ligation. The resolution of laboratory signs of DIC after a LeVeen shunt is placed usually means the shunt is occluded. Thrombocytopenia can occur from the hypersplenism of portal hypertension. Antithrombin III and protein C levels are often reduced in cirrhosis, though clinically significant thrombosis is rare. Reduced protein C levels may predispose children to an increased frequency of hepatic artery thrombosis immediately after liver transplantation.

Hepatocellular Carcinoma

Hepatocellular carcinoma can develop in the patient with cirrhosis. It is common in those with alcoholic cirrhosis, chronic hepatitis B or C, hemochromatosis, and heterozygous or homozygous α_1-antitrypsin deficiency and rare in those with Wilson's disease and primary biliary cirrhosis. It should be suspected in any stable cirrhotic who suddenly deteriorates with worsening ascites or encephalopathy or develops a fever, abdominal mass, or polycythemia. α-Fetoprotein levels are increased in approximately two thirds of cirrhotic patients with hepatocellular carcinoma.

Liver Transplantation

Patients with end-stage liver disease who develop complications of their disease should be considered for liver transplantation. They should be referred early before becoming moribund because the mortality of liver transplantation is less in the patient with good nutrition, little weight loss, better coagulation factors, and no infection. Indications for transplantation include poorly controlled ascites, variceal hemorrhage, especially if it is recurrent, spontaneous peritonitis, hepatorenal syndrome, and recurring cholangitis in those with sclerosing cholangitis and some patients with fatigue and malaise that interfere with their life-style. Alcoholic liver disease is not considered a contraindication to transplantation. Those with coexisting acute alcoholic hepatitis may have increased operative mortality. Patients should ideally have 6 months of abstinence from ethanol. Advanced age is not a contraindication to transplantation, though the elderly patient may do poorly if postoperative complications occur.

SUGGESTED READINGS

Burroughs AK, Jenkins WJ, Sherlock S, et al: Controlled trial of propranolol for the prevention of recurrent variceal hemorrhage in patients with cirrhosis, N Engl J Med 309(25):1539-1542, 1983.

This is a randomized trial of propranolol for prevention of recurrent variceal hemorrhage. There was no difference in the rate of rebleeding between the groups.

Cello JP, Grendell JH, Crass RA, et al: Endoscopic sclerotherapy versus portacaval shunt in patients with severe cirrhosis and variceal hemorrhage, N Engl J Med 311(25):1589-1594, 1984.

In this trial of Child's C cirrhotics, patients were randomized to either sclerotherapy or portosystemic shunts. There was no difference in survival rates. Initially, there was a decrease in total health care costs for the sclerotherapy patient, though subsequent studies have shown that the recurrent bleeding rate and consequent hospitalizations will eventually equalize medical care expenditures.

Conn HO, Leevy CM, Vlahcevic ZR, et al: Comparison of lactulose and neomycin in the treatment of chronic portal-systemic encephalopathy, Gastroenterology 72:537-583, 1977.

This double blind trial of lactulose vs. neomycin plus sorbitol for treatment of chronic or recurrent hepatic encephalopathy demonstrated equal clinical efficacy of both treatments.

Edell ES, Cortese A, Krowka MJ, et al Severe hypoxemia and liver disease, Am Rev Resp Dis 140(6):1631-1635, 1989.

Six patients with chronic liver disease (3 of 6 biopsied and cirrhosis confirmed) with hypoxemia, upright desaturation, and no overt lung disease were studied. Right-to-left shunts ranged from 4% to 28% and were believed attributable to capillary dilatation within the pulmonary parenchyma. They could not exclude a potential component of impaired diffusing capacity.

Gabuzda GJ: Cirrhosis, ascites and edema: clinical course related to management, Gastroenterology 58(4):546-553, 1970.

This is a classic review of the management of ascites.

Guadalupe G-T, Conn HO, and Lerner E: The diagnosis of bacterial peritonitis: comparison of pH, lactate concentration, and leukocyte count, Hepatology 5(1):91-96, 1985.

This study of initial parameters to assist the diagnosis of spontaneous bacterial peritonitis (SBP) indicates that a polymorphonuclear leukocyte count of greater than 500 cells/ml coupled with an arterial-ascitic fluid pH gradient of more than 0.10 is often observed in SBP. An ascitic fluid pH of less than 7.35 was also frequent.

Henderson JM, Kutner MH, Millikan WJ, et al: Endoscopic variceal sclerosis compared with distal splenorenal shunt to prevent recurrent variceal bleeding in cirrhosis: a prospective, randomized trial, Ann Intern Med 112:262-269, 1990.

When sclerotherapy was compared to the distal splenorenal shunt for the management of variceal hemorrhage, initial sclerotherapy with utilization of the shunt as a rescue for continued variceal bleeding was the most effective therapy.

Hoefs JC, Canawati HN, Sapico FL, et al: Spontaneous bacterial peritonitis, Hepatology 2(4):399-407, 1982.

In 43 patients with spontaneous bacterial peritonitis, single organisms were isolated from 38 and multiple organisms from 5. Of those with single organisms, Escherichia coli was isolated in 21. Early death was more frequent in those with azotemia, hyperbilirubinemia, and leukocytosis >25,000/ml.

Hoefs JC: Diagnostic paracentesis, Gastroenterology 98:230-236, 1990.

This is a review of the usefulness of diagnostic paracentesis in the assessment of causes of ascites.

Iwatsuki S, Popovtzer MM, Corman JL, et al: Recovery from hepatorenal syndrome after orthotopic liver transplantation, N Engl J Med 289(22):1155-1159, 1973.

Three patients with hepatorenal syndrome recovered renal function after liver transplantation.

Jensen LS and Krarup N: Propranolol may prevent recurrence of oesophageal varices after obliteration by endoscopic sclerotherapy, Scand J Gastroenterol 25:352-356, 1990.

When propranolol was administered after obliteration of varices by sclerotherapy, there was a significant reduction in rebleeding as compared to no additional therapy.

Koppel MH, Coburn JW, Mims MM, et al: Transplantation of cadaveric kidneys from patients with hepatorenal syndrome, N Engl J Med 280(25):1368-1370, 1969.

Kidneys from 6 patients dying of hepatorenal syndrome were transplanted into 7 patients with end-stage renal disease with improvement in renal function in 6 of 7. Later articles have noted the risk of development of severe hypertensive crises when hepatorenal kidneys are utilized, and they are no longer transplanted.

Lebrec D, Poynard T, Hillon P, et al: Propranolol for prevention of recurrent gastrointestinal bleeding in patients with cirrhosis: a controlled study, N Engl J Med 305(23):1371-1374, 1981.

In this study of 74 patients with cirrhosis and at least one episode of upper gastrointestinal bleeding caused by varices or acute gastric erosions, propranolol significantly reduced the frequency of rebleeding. The majority of patients were alcoholic.

MacDougall BRD, Westaby D, Theodossi A, et al: Increased long-term survival in variceal haemorrhage using injection sclerotherapy: results of a controlled trial, Lancet 1(8264):124-127, Jan 16, 1982.

Sclerotherapy was compared to expectant care in the follow-up observation of patients who bled from varices. In those patients with variceal obliteration by sclerotherapy, a reduction of episodes of bleeding varices was observed.

Pérez-Ayuso RM, Arroyo V, Planas R, et al: Randomized comparative study of efficacy of furosemide versus spironolactone in nonazotemic cirrhosis with ascites: relationship between the diuretic response and the activity of the renin-aldosterone system, Gastroenterology 84:961-968, 1983.

In comparing spironolactone to furosemide for the treatment of nonazotemic patients with ascites, spironolactone was significantly more effective in inducing natriuresis than furosemide was, especially in those with high circulating renin levels.

Rikkers LF, Rudman D, Galambos JT, et al: A randomized, controlled trial of the distal splenorenal shunt, Ann Surg 188(3):271-282, 1978.

When distal splenorenal shunts were compared to portosystemic shunts as therapy for bleeding varices, there was no difference in survival, shunt occlusion, or episodes of rebleeding. However, there were more episodes of postoperative encephalopathy in those receiving portosystemic shunts.

Runyon BA and Hoefs JC: Culture-negative neutrocytic ascites: a variant of spontaneous bacterial peritonitis, Hepatology 4(8):1209-1211, 1984.

Seventeen patients with ascites characteristics typical of spontaneous bacterial peritonitis but who were culture negative indicated that this group has similar signs, symptoms, and mortality to those who are culture positive. This indicates that culture negative patients with parameters indicative of infection should receive a full course of antibiotics.

Stassen WN, McCullough AJ, Bacon BR, et al: Immediate diagnostic criteria for bacterial infection of ascitic fluid, Gastroenterology 90:1247-1254, 1986.

In patients with cirrhosis and ascites, the occurrence of an ascites fluid pH of less than 7.34 was highly indicative of infection. When ascitic fluids from patients with malignancy were included with those with cirrhosis, the best tests of infection were a polymorphonuclear leukocyte count of more than 500 cells/ml and blood–ascitic fluid gradient of more than 0.10.

van Leeuwen DJ, Howe SC, Scheuer PJ, et al: Portal hypertension in chronic hepatitis: relationship to morphological changes, Gut 31(3):339-343, 1990.

Anatomic factors that can interfere with sinusoidal resistence were compared to wedged hepatic venous pressures in patients with chronic active hepatitis or alcoholic liver disease. Multiple factors to account for portal hypertension were frequently present in each patient including collagenization of the space of Disse, hepatocyte enlargement, and histologic evidence of cirrhosis. Portal hypertension was often present before there was evidence of cirrhosis.

Zeppa R, Hensley G, Levi JU, et al: The comparative survivals of alcoholics versus nonalcoholics after distal splenorenal shunt, Ann Surg 187(5):510-514, 1978.

In patients treated for bleeding varices by distal splenorenal shunts, there was a greater mortality in alcoholics than in nonalcoholics.

28 Metabolic and Systemic Diseases

Charles F. Gholson and Bruce R. Bacon

Liver diseases attributable to metabolic or systemic abnormalities are common problems that constitute an important part of the practice of medicine. Although the spectrum of liver abnormalities related to metabolic and systemic conditions is broad, the major categories encompassing most disorders are non alcoholic fatty liver, liver disease associated with total parenteral nutrition, vitamin-related liver disease, thyroid-liver interactions, the porphyrias, metal-storage diseases, and liver disease associated with collagen vascular diseases. An understanding of these conditions is essential because specific therapy is available for many of these disorders. This discussion is a review of diseases that fall into these broad categories with an emphasis on pertinent aspects of hepatic metabolism and pathophysiology.

NONALCOHOLIC FATTY LIVER (NAFL)

Traditionally the term "fatty liver" (or hepatic steatosis) is associated with alcoholic liver disease. Although excessive intake of ethanol accounts for many of the patients who have fatty liver, a wide variety of conditions other than alcohol are associated with fatty infiltration of the hepatic parenchyma. Because this lesion is so common and so often asymptomatic, it is tempting to attribute it to occult ethanol abuse or to dismiss its significance. However, one must keep in mind that both acute, severe hepatocellular dysfunction as well as chronic, progressive, irreversible hepatic dysfunction can be associated with nonalcoholic fatty liver.

The central role of the liver in lipid and lipoprotein metabolism is well recognized. Normal hepatic lipogenesis is a complex process regulated by dietary (starvation, obesity), hormonal (prandial status, insulin, thyroid hormone, sex, pregnancy), and environmental (drug therapy, ethanol consumption) factors. In the normal situation, hepatic triglycerides are combined with apoproteins and secreted as very low-density lipoproteins (VLDL), a complex process under similar dietary, hormonal and environmental controls. Whenever an imbalance of triglyceride synthesis and VLDL secretion develops, hepatic accumulation of fat (usually triglycerides in cytoplasmic vesicles) occurs, which eventually finds morphologic expression as fatty liver. The fact that so many intrahepatic and extrahepatic disorders can result in hepatic steatosis is

Table 28-1 Nonalcoholic fatty liver: clinical characteristics

	Macrovesicular steatosis	Microvesicular steatosis
Usual patient age	>30	<30
Usual severity	Minimal	Pronounced
Fulminant course	Rare	Common
Fatalities	Rare	Common
Histochemical demonstration	Hematoxylin and Eosin	Oil Red O
Associated histologic features		
Mallory bodies	Common	Rare
Necrosis	Occasional	Rare
Cirrhosis	Occasional	Never

CAUSES OF NONALCOHOLIC FATTY LIVER (NAFL)

Macrovesicular steatosis
- Obesity
- Diabetes mellitus
- Protein-calorie malnutrition
- Hyperlipidemia
- Drug therapy (e.g., corticosteroids, methotrexate)
- Jejunoileal bypass surgery
- Parenteral hyperalimentation

Microvesicular steatosis
- Acute fatty liver of pregnancy
- Jamaican vomiting sickness
- Reye's syndrome
- Drug therapy (e.g., valproate, tetracycline)

probably attributable to the diffuse, multifactorial regulation of hepatic lipogenesis and VLDL export with resultant sensitivity to a wide variety of disease processes.

The causes of nonalcoholic fatty liver (NAFL) can be divided into macrovesicular and microvesicular categories (see box above and Table 28-1), based on the pattern of hepatocellular fat accumulation. The pathophysiologic reason for these two morphologic forms of steatosis is unclear. One hypothesis suggests that macrovesicular fat is the result of hepatocellular injury, whereas microvesicular fat is a cause of cell injury. Unlike the lipid droplets in macrovesicular steatosis, which are composed of noncytotoxic neutral triglycerides, biochemical analysis of microvesicular fat from one patient with acute fatty liver of pregnancy disclosed free fatty acids, which are potentially hepatotoxic.

Macrovesicular steatosis is characterized histologically by accumulation of neutral triglycerides within the hepatocellular cytoplasm. These eventually form fat droplets, which, as they grow, displace the nucleus and other cytoplasmic structures to the cell periphery. In histologic sections, this results in a clear, empty "hole" in the hepatocyte because lipid is digested away in formalin-fixed, paraffin-embedded specimens (Figure 28-1). Large fat droplets may coalesce to form fatty cysts, which can subsequently rupture, leading to phagocytosis and for-

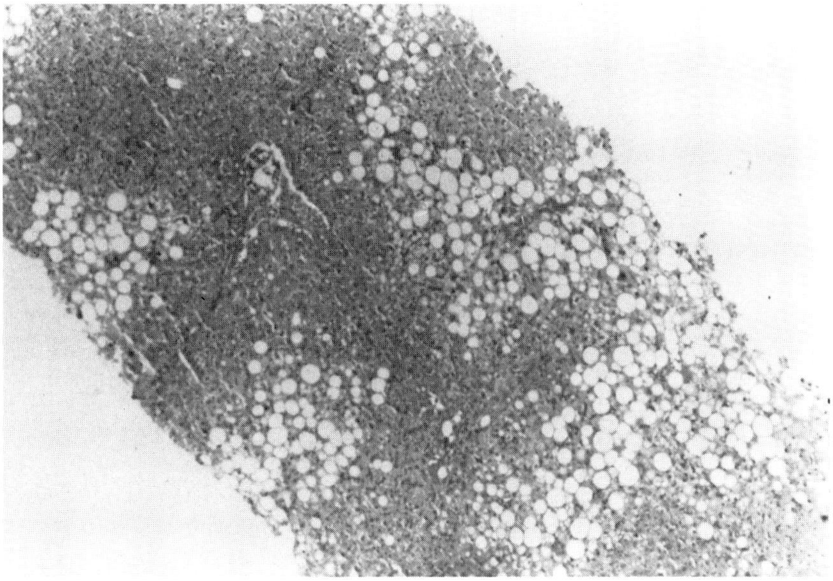

Figure 28-1
Macrovesicular steatosis in liver. This liver biopsy specimen was obtained from an asymptomatic 52-year-old male who was referred for evaluation of elevated serum transaminases. He was 30 pounds overweight with mild glucose intolerance. Hepatic steatosis is seen in a pericentral (zone 3) distribution. There are no inflammatory infiltrates, Mallory bodies, or hepatocellular necrosis. (Hematoxylin and eosin stain, ×50.)

mation of lipid granulomas. Varying degrees of hepatocellular necrosis may be present. Mallory bodies are also occasionally seen and are by no means pathognomonic for alcoholic liver disease.

Nonalcoholic macrovesicular steatosis is traditionally considered a benign process, unlike its alcoholic counterpart. However, several recent studies have indicated that cirrhosis may develop in 15% to 30% of asymptomatic obese, nonalcoholics biopsied because of abnormal liver enzymes. Perivenular fibrosis and micronodular cirrhosis, indistinguishable from the histologic picture seen in alcoholic liver disease, are well documented, underscoring the importance of a thorough understanding of these disorders.

The histologic features of microvesicular steatosis are quite distinct when compared with macrovesicular steatosis. In early lesions, hepatocytes often have a ballooned appearance, reminiscent of viral hepatitis, and accumulated lipid is inapparent on routine hematoxylin and eosin stains. Accordingly, when a disorder causing microvesicular steatosis is suspected, prebiopsy coordination with an experienced pathologist to obtain an Oil Red O stain is essential for diagnosis of these conditions at an early stage. Late lesions exhibit the characteristic fine-droplet steatosis on routine hematoxylin and eosin sections. Associated hepatocellular necrosis, Mallory bodies, and inflammation are distinctly absent, and progression to cirrhosis has not been described.

SELECTED DISORDERS ASSOCIATED WITH NAFL

Obesity

The majority of patients with NAFL are obese. Most studies indicate that over 60% of obese subjects have macrovesicular steatosis, whereas the actual incidence in the general population is unknown. Likewise it is unclear whether the amount of excess body weight correlates in a predictable way with the amount of fat in the liver. The relevance of most published studies to the average patient with NAFL is equally unclear because most data were derived from series of morbidly obese subjects, which comprise a minority of patients who are overweight. Patients with NAFL are usually asymptomatic, and fatty liver may persist for up to 30 years without progression to more serious liver disease. There is no evidence that accumulated intracellular triglyceride is inherently hepatotoxic or stimulates fibrogenesis. Accordingly, the central issue regarding macrovesicular steatosis in obese patients is its natural history and prognostic significance.

Several clinical syndromes have been described in patients with NAFL attributed to obesity (see box at right). Most patients are asymptomatic, and steatosis is usually discovered in the course of an evaluation of abnormal serum liver enzymes. Physical examination usually reveals only mild hepatomegaly, or may be entirely normal, aside from obesity. Two

CLINICAL SYNDROMES ASSOCIATED WITH OBESITY-INDUCED NONALCOHOLIC FATTY LIVER

- Asymptomatic incidental finding
- Hypodense hepatic parenchymal lesion on CT scan (diffuse or focal)
- Asymptomatic transaminase elevation
- Nonalcoholic steatonecrosis
- Micronodular cirrhosis

recent studies have demonstrated NAFL as one of the most common causes (21% to 63% of cases) of asymptomatic transaminase elevation, particularly when abnormal physical findings are absent. Hepatic steatosis can also cause hypodense areas on computerized tomographic scans, which may be diffuse or localized (Figure 28-2). The latter situation may lead to confusion with neoplastic lesions, resulting in biopsy with demonstration of only fatty liver.

Although NAFL attributable to obesity is usually benign, it leads to progressive necroinflammatory infiltrates or cirrhosis in up to a third of patients when other identifiable causes of liver disease are absent. These patients are usually middle-aged women who may have other chronic medical conditions such as hypertension or arthritis. When a liver biopsy is performed to evaluate abnormal serum liver enzymes, histologic lesions identical to alcoholic hepatitis or micronodular cirrhosis can be seen (Figure 28-3). Mallory bodies may be present in zone 3 hepatocytes, though they are less abundant than in patients with true alcohol-induced liver disease. Fortunately, despite their histo-

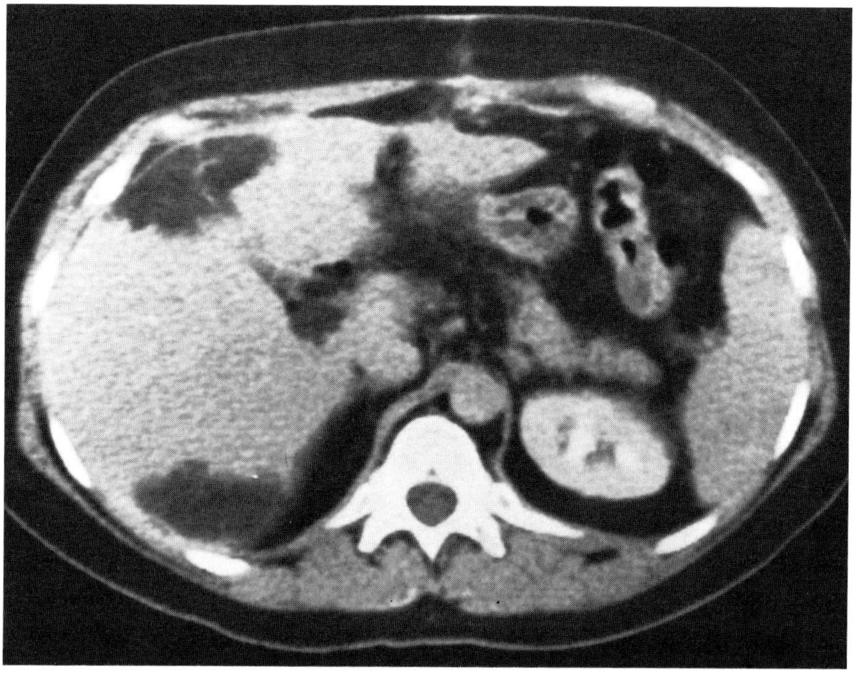

Figure 28-2
Computerized tomography in focal fatty liver. This CT scan is from a 34-year-old female who was referred for evaluation of hepatomegaly. Several hypodense areas are seen in the liver. Laparoscopic biopsy revealed fatty infiltration.

logic similarities, clinical and biochemical features can be used to separate alcoholic from nonalcoholic steatohepatitis. Patients with alcoholic steatohepatitis tend to have more pronounced symptoms and biochemical abnormalities, whereas obese patients with "pseudo-alcoholic lesions" or "nonalcoholic steatohepatitis" are typically asymptomatic, jaundice is rare, and the AST/ALT ratio is less than 3. Alkaline phosphatase and γ-glutamyl transpeptidase levels may be elevated in both entities, though pronounced elevation of the latter is more consistent with an alcoholic cause.

Weight reduction is obviously desirable in obese patients for a variety of reasons unrelated to the liver. Unfortunately, its efficacy in preventing, reversing, or retarding the progression of obesity-induced NAFL or nonalcoholic steatohepatitis is unproved. Indeed, starvation can cause steatosis, as described below. These issues are further complicated by the typically subtle clinical manifestations and lack of striking biochemical abnormalities; thus serial liver biopsy specimens would be required for adequate assessment of improvement with weight reduction.

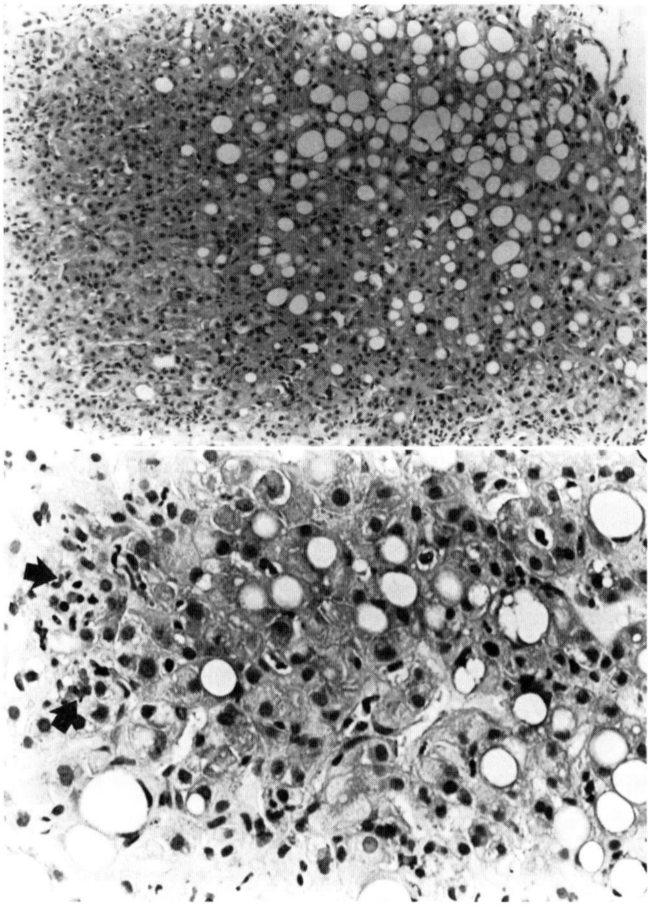

A

B

Figure 28-3
Nonalcoholic steatohepatitis in liver. This liver biopsy specimen was from a 54-year-old female who was referred for evaluation of elevated serum liver enzymes. She was obese and had hypertension and osteoarthritis. **A,** Macrovesicular and occasional microvesicular steatosis is seen with preservation of the hepatic architecture. **B,** at higher power, inflammatory cells, arrows, can be seen in addition to the steatosis. (**A** and **B,** Hematoxylin and eosin stain; **A,** ×125; **B,** ×320.)

Considering these issues, the decision to perform a liver biopsy at all in a greatly obese patient becomes difficult. A recent study has clarified some of these issues. Histologic findings on wedge biopsy specimens obtained before bariatric surgery were correlated with preoperative clinical and biochemical features in 98 morbidly obese subjects. Patients with lesions other than uncomplicated steatosis (e.g., steatonecrosis, fibrosis, or cirrhosis) were correctly predicted in 78% of patients by clinical features that included age over 40 years, more than 120% overweight, female, elevated serum ALT levels, and triglyceride levels exceeding 120 mg/dl. From these observations, it can be reasoned that obese patients with these characteristics should undergo liver biopsy. In one recent study, a direct correlation between the amount of excess body weight and the severity of hepatic histologic abnormalities was demonstrated. Thus weight reduction may arrest the progression of steatonecrosis and fibrosis. Prospective studies will be necessary to confirm this hypothesis.

Protein Calorie Malnutrition

Paradoxically, famine as well as feast causes NAFL. Liver disease has been associated with various forms of starvation but is most predictably associated with protein-calorie malnutrition (kwashiorkor). Although this condition is prevalent in underdeveloped countries, it can complicate numerous disease entities associated with severe anorexia, making an understanding of the pathophysiologic mechanisms essential to all physicians.

The majority of patients with kwashiorkor exhibit macrovesicular steatosis. The pathogenesis has been studied extensively and appears to be attributable to defective secretion of lipid by the hepatocyte. In several animal models of kwashiorkor, impaired hepatic protein synthesis with reduced apolipoprotein production has been demonstrated. This results in impaired formation and secretion of VLDL in the midst of massive peripheral lipolysis. These factors, together with reductions in lipoprotein lipase, all promote hepatocellular accumulation of neutral triglycerides.

Clinically an enlarged liver is the most common hepatic manifestation of protein-calorie malnutrition. Biopsy reveals macrovesicular steatosis, most prominent in periportal hepatocytes. Necroinflammatory infiltrates and Mallory bodies are relatively uncommon. Serum liver enzymes are usually normal or only minimally elevated. Although progression to hepatic failure is reported, this is distinctly unusual and probably relates to the underlying condition. There is no good evidence that chronic liver disease results from protein-calorie malnutrition, and successful nutritional repletion totally reverses hepatic abnormalities. The initial clearance of steatosis is from centrilobular hepatocytes, followed by periportal hepatocytes.

Diabetes Mellitus

The association of diabetes mellitus and NAFL is not surprising when one considers the high frequency of obesity among type 2 diabetics. Several factors are involved in the development of hepatic steatosis in diabetics. Virtually all type 2 diabetics are hyperinsulinemic with peripheral insulin resistance, enhancing peripheral lipolysis and delivery of free fatty acids to the liver. Insulin-induced hepatic triglyceride synthesis ensues with accumulation of triglycerides, resulting in macrovesicular steatosis. In addition, insulin itself may promote steatonecrosis. Continuous ambulatory peritoneal dialysis patients with type 1 diabetes receiving intraperitoneal insulin have subcapsular hepatic steatonecrosis in a third of the cases, suggestive of a role for insulin in hepatocellular necrosis as well as steatosis.

Thorough evaluation of hepatic dysfunction in diabetics is important to exclude progressive liver disease associated with diabetes as well as disorders such as hereditary hemochromatosis, which can present with hepatomegaly, liver enzyme abnormalities, and glucose intolerance. Asymptomatic hepatomegaly attributable to fatty liver and mild abnormalities of serum liver enzymes are seen in 30% to 75% of diabetics. Liver biopsy may reveal a wide variety of histologic findings, particularly among type 2 diabetics (see box at right). Macrovesicular steatosis is the most common histologic finding, though precirrhotic lesions have also been described. Pericentral fibrosis, occasionally accompanied by Mallory bodies, has been well documented, particularly in obese, diabetic females. Although this lesion would appear precirrhotic, cirrhosis strictly attributable to diabetes has only rarely been reported. Other findings include steatonecrosis and increased hepatic glycogen stores with glycogenated nuclei.

Although correction of obesity and maintenance of euglycemia are desirable for any diabetic, their effect on hepatic abnormalities associated with diabetes is unclear. Reversal of steatosis, but not fibrosis, has been described with a closely supervised, supplemented diet. In contrast, fatal progressive steatosis and cirrhosis have been reported after repeated attempts at dramatic weight reduction. Thus careful supervision is recommended in the management of these delicate patients.

HISTOLOGIC FINDINGS IN THE LIVER IN DIABETES

Glycogenated nuclei
Macrovesicular steatosis
Mallory bodies
Steatonecrosis
Pericentral fibrosis
Cirrhosis

The incidence and natural history of biliary disease in diabetics has been recently clarified. Diabetics are at increased risk for the formation of gallstones. Insulin therapy can create lithogenic bile by increasing biliary cholesterol secretion and by reducing bile acid secretion. Furthermore, diabetics may have biliary stasis and impaired gallbladder emptying because of autonomic dysfunction. These considerations and the predisposition to infection and postoperative cardiac complications in diabetics led physicians in the past to recommend "prophylactic" cholecystectomy for diabetics with cholelithiasis. This position has been challenged by studies demonstrating no significant difference in postoperative complications or mortalities for patients with diabetes and those without. Accordingly, it appears that cholelithiasis can be managed the same in diabetics as in nondiabetics.

Liver Disease After Jejunoileal Bypass

Macrovesicular steatosis is a common complication of jejunoileal bypass surgery for morbid obesity. Reports of more severe liver lesions complicating jejunoileal bypass have led to the virtual abandonment of this procedure. The spectrum of related histopathologic lesions closely resembles alcoholic liver disease. Bacterial production of toxins such as lithocholic acid in the defunctionalized limb and rapid weight loss are believed to be important pathogenetic factors. This hypothesis stems from the observations that early liver lesions are reversed by administration of metronidazole or restoration of intestinal continuity and that liver disease is often most evident during the period of rapid postoperative weight loss.

A spectrum of postoperative hepatic abnormalities may result. Nonspecific elevation of serum transaminases and alkaline phosphatase are common and usually indicate the presence of NAFL. A more serious liver pathologic condition is present when they fail to improve within 3 months. Coagulopathy and jaundice are more ominous and predict hepatic failure which occurs in 5% of patients, usually within the first postoperative year because of hepatic histologic anomalies mimicking alcoholic hepatitis. Accordingly, restoration of intestinal continuity is advisable when prothrombin time prolongation or icterus is detected. Another 5% to 10% of patients insidiously develop portal fibrosis and cirrhosis over 5 to 10 years. Because clinical and biochemical abnormalities in this group may be minimal or absent, liver biopsy is advisable at 6- to 12-month intervals postoperatively. Restoration of intestinal continuity should be strongly considered when hepatic fibrosis or a histologic condition similar to alcoholic hepatitis is observed.

Miscellaneous Causes of NAFL

There are several other miscellaneous causes of hepatic steatosis that are discussed elsewhere in this text. These include drug-induced fatty liver, which can present as both macrovesicular and microvesicular steatosis. Patients with Reye's syndrome usually have microvesicular steatosis.

HEPATIC COMPLICATIONS OF TOTAL PARENTERAL NUTRITION

Total parenteral nutrition (TPN) is a commonly employed means of providing nutrition in a wide variety of clinical settings. With its increasing use, complications of TPN have become more precisely characterized and their effective management, more important. As a result, it has become clear that liver disease is a major complication of TPN. In general, TPN-related hepatotoxicity is very similar to NAFL related to obesity and (as in obesity) may be associated with more advanced lesions such as steatonecrosis, portal fibrosis, and cirrhosis. In addition, a unique, severe cholestatic syndrome may complicate the use of TPN.

The pathophysiologic mechanisms of TPN-related hepatotoxicity have been recently clarified. Hepatic steatosis results from a combination of factors related to both the infused nutrients and the baseline catabolic state; these factors accelerate lipogenesis and reduce hepatic export of triglycerides. Hyperinsulinism, resulting from infusions rich in glucose, along with varying degrees of protein-calorie malnutrition contribute to this phenomenon. In essence, the patient receiving TPN resembles diabetics as well as patients with protein-calorie malnutrition, both of whom are metabolically prone to hepatic steatosis.

The pathogenesis of severe cholestasis related to TPN is more complex, involving numerous etiologic factors including hepatotoxins in or derived from stagnant enteric bacteria, deficiency states (choline, taurine, essential fatty acids, etc.), lack of first-pass detoxification of potentially hepatotoxic infusates, excessive TPN carbohydrate content, and lack of enteral stimulation by enteric hormones. Among the putative hepatotoxins, lithocholate

(LCA), and endotoxin derived from stagnant gut bacteria are probably the most important. A striking histologic similarity exists between the cholestatic lesions seen in animals fed LCA and in patients with TPN-related cholestasis. Furthermore, serial examinations of biliary bile acid composition before and during a course of TPN revealed that biliary LCA levels rose from less than 1% to a range of 7% to 15% of total biliary bile acids within 11 to 22 days in patients who developed cholestasis. These observations have led to the hypothesis that TPN-associated cholestasis results from hepatotoxic effects of excessive LCA produced by anaerobic organisms that flourish in the stagnant intestinal contents resulting from prolonged fasting.

Clinically, asymptomatic transaminase elevations (three- to fivefold increase) occur in 32% to 90% of patients during the early weeks of TPN, especially when high-concentration dextrose is administered without lipid infusions. These findings are often transient or resolve after lipid infusions are begun. Macrovesicular steatosis occurs shortly after TPN is initiated in up to 90% of patients, though its relation to serum liver enzyme abnormalities is uncertain. Furthermore, the significance of hepatic steatosis seen in association with TPN is also uncertain because metabolic alterations caused by TPN (hyperglycemia, carnitine deficiency, essential fatty acid deficiency), as well as disease processes for which TPN is administered (Crohn's disease, secondary cachexia, associated septicemia) are themselves associated with hepatic steatosis.

After 3 to 4 weeks of TPN, 30% to 50% of patients develop intrahepatic cholestasis. Bilirubin and alkaline phosphatase elevations can be striking (more than tenfold), with periportal lymphocytic infiltrates, cholestasis, and duct proliferation seen on biopsy. Advanced forms of liver disease may evolve with continued TPN. Progressive liver disease (steatonecrosis and cirrhosis) may develop in 5% to 15% of these patients after 3 to 4 months of TPN. In addition, patients receiving TPN for prolonged periods of time have lithogenic bile and gallbladder stasis, primarily as a result of prolonged fasting. Thus they are prone to biliary lithiasis and its attendant cholestatic complications.

Patients receiving TPN who develop hepatic dysfunction tend to be extremely complex with multiple comorbid factors, making a thorough, objective evaluation essential. One should keep in mind that only a relatively small fraction of patients on TPN develop progressive liver disease, making exclusion of other causes important. If cholestasis develops, it is particularly important to exclude biliary obstruction with ultrasonography or, if necessary, ERCP. Acalculous cholecystitis should always be considered in the presence of vague abdominal pain or unexplained fever. Because these patients are frequently on multiple medications and may have had blood transfusions, drug hepatotoxicity and hepatitis C infection become important considerations as well.

Patients who develop serum liver enzyme elevations early in the course of TPN are best managed by alteration of the infusate (Table 28-2). Reevaluation of the patient's caloric requirements and provision of approximately one third of nonprotein calories as lipid emulsion can reverse the hepatotoxicity. Also, reduction in the amount of glucose infused should be considered. Some authorities advocate "cyclic" TPN, where the glucose infusion

Table 28-2 Useful therapeutic measures for TPN-associated hepatic dysfunction

Early asymptomatic transaminase elevation
Reduce glucose infused
Provide a third of nonprotein calories as lipid
Cyclic infusions
Progressive cholestasis (more than 4 weeks into therapy)
Rule out extrahepatic obstruction
Intermittent small volume feedings
Cyclic infusions
Consider alternative nutritional means
Trial of metronidazole

is discontinued for 8 to 12 hours daily. This approach allows the patient to develop a metabolic state similar to the postabsorptive state, which continuous TPN eliminates.

Patients developing cholestasis present later and require exclusion of extrahepatic obstruction. The hypothesis that cholestasis results from hepatotoxic substances derived from stagnant gut bacteria has led to trials of antibiotics to reduce the enteric anaerobic population. In one small series of Crohn's disease patients receiving TPN, metronidazole effectively prevented or reversed biochemical cholestasis. The efficacy of metronidazole for prophylaxis and for reversal of more advanced hepatic lesions will need to be established with more complete studies. However, until more effective therapy is developed, a therapeutic trial of metronidazole, 500 mg intravenously 3 or 4 times daily, is worthwhile for patients with TPN-associated cholestasis. Intermittent small volume feeding is also useful to reduce gallbladder stasis.

Management of patients with evidence of progressive hepatocellular necrosis on long-term TPN is more difficult, and recommendations must be individualized. In this situation, it is essential to exclude extrahepatic obstruction and focal parenchymal lesions with ultrasonography or ERCP, or both. If the biliary tree is patent, a liver biopsy is advisable to document the severity of the hepatic lesion. Cyclic manipulation of TPN and metronidazole may be tried, but in the final analysis, the demonstration of steatonecrosis and fibrosis in a patient who has no possible cause other than TPN should lead to careful reexamination of the indications for TPN. If possible, an alternative means of nutrition should be used.

VITAMIN-RELATED LIVER DISEASE

The use of vitamin A in the treatment of alcohol-related hypogonadism and dermatologic conditions and its common inclusion in food faddisms has increased its importance as a hepatotoxin. Although it was once believed that massive doses (over 100,000 IU/day) ingested for periods of weeks were required to induce toxicity, ingestion of "common" doses (20,000 to 50,000 IU/day) over longer periods of time may be hepatotoxic. Hepatotoxicity probably stems from storage of excess vitamin A in hepatic lipocytes (Ito cells). Accumulated vitamin A has several potential cytotoxic effects including disruption of membranes, mitochondrial swelling, and reduced membrane fluidity. With excessive ingestion, lipocytes proliferate and enlarge, thus obliterating the space of Disse. After formation of numerous lipid vacuoles, the lipocyte transforms into a fibroblastic cell and increased collagen is deposited in the hepatic sinusoids. Progressive hepatic fibrosis and eventual nodular regeneration can rarely result.

Clinically, hypervitaminosis A occurs after ingestion of large doses of vitamin A for weeks to months, or after more chronic ingestion of smaller amounts. Extrahepatic manifestations include increased intracranial pressure with papilledema and headache, neuropsychiatric changes, nausea, vomiting, and dermatologic changes (alopecia, scaling skin). Hepatic manifestations vary with dose and chronicity. Chronic ingestion of less than 50,000 IU/day can result initially in mild hepatitis with modest transaminase elevation and occasional prothrombin prolongation in the absence of hepatomegaly or jaundice. Acute, larger ingestions cause hepatomegaly, jaundice, and hypoprothrombinemia, though fulminant hepatic failure has not been described. Portal hypertension attributable to fibrosis and cirrhosis may occur rarely. Serum levels of vitamin A and related retinols are not useful in diagnosis. Comorbid factors believed to potentiate the hepatotoxicity of vitamin A include concomitant liver disease, renal failure, hypertriglyceridemia, regular excessive consumption of animal liver, and, most importantly, excessive ethanol consumption.

Histologically, in very early vitamin A hepatotoxicity, clear, lipid-laden lipocytes enlarge in the sinusoids with surrounding chronic inflammation. Continued ingestion results in accumulation of perisinusoidal lipocytes and progressive fibrosis, sinusoidal congestion, and dilatation with eventual central vein sclerosis. Progression to cirrhosis is very rare but has been described.

The diagnosis of vitamin A hepatotoxicity is based on exclusion of other causes, a history of excessive ingestion, and a typical hepatic histologic lesion. Dietary restriction of vitamin A is the only known therapy. Unfortunately, depletion is slow, and there is no known pharmacologic means of accelerating the process. Prevention by avoidance of food fads and excessive vitamin A consumption in patients with potentiating comorbid features (renal failure, ethanol consumption, hyperlipidemia) are essential.

There are no other known hypervitaminosis syndromes that cause liver disease.

THYROID-LIVER INTERACTIONS

Liver Disease and Thyroid Function

The liver and thyroid gland are critically interdependent from a metabolic standpoint because the liver plays a key role in the peripheral metabolism of thyroid hormone. Conversion of tetraiodothyronine (T_4) to its more potent physiologically active derivative triiodothyronine (T_3) occurs mainly in the liver and kidney. When this conversion is defective, the physiologically inert isomer of T_3, that is, rT_3, accumulates. In addition, the liver synthesizes proteins that bind circulating thyroid hormone and help regulate the free, physiologically active fraction. Accordingly, diseases of the liver and thyroid are inherently intertwined (Table 28-3).

Hepatic-thyroid relationships may alter circulating thyroid hormone levels in the absence of thyroid hyperfunction or hypofunction. Transient elevations of T_4 in clinically euthyroid patients with acute viral hepatitis are common and probably re-

Table 28-3 Thyroid-liver interactions

Liver disease and thyroid function
Altered peripheral conversion of T_4 to T_3
Altered levels of transport protein (TBG)
High rT_3 and rT_3/T_3 ratios indicate brief short-term survival in chronic liver disease
Hashimoto's thyroiditis associated with primary biliary cirrhosis (PBC)
Thyroid disease and liver function
Transaminase elevation
Jaundice and thyroid storm
Ascites and myxedema

sult from thyroxine binding globulin (TBG) release by necrotic hepatocytes. Curiously, depressed T_4 levels are the rule in alcoholic hepatitis. Additionally, severe liver disease alters rT_3 levels in a prognostically important way. For example, the short-term prognosis for prospective liver transplant patients can be predicted by serum thyroid hormone levels. Patients with the worst prognosis exhibit considerably defective peripheral conversion of T_4 to T_3, have high rT_3 levels and rT_3/T_3 ratios, and are likely to die awaiting transplantation. For reasons that are unclear, the T_3/T_4 ratio does not correlate directly with survival, as one might expect.

Specific hepatic diseases that are associated with pathologic alteration or dysfunction of the thyroid include primary biliary cirrhosis (PBC) and autoimmune chronic active hepatitis. Antithyroglobulin and antimicrosomal antibodies are common in both of these autoimmune liver diseases. Indeed, up to one fifth of patients with PBC have coexistent Hashimoto's thyroiditis. Accordingly, when one is evaluating patients with liver disease, measurement of free T_4, TSH, and the response of TSH to TRH infusion are often essential in determining the functional significance of abnormal circulating hormone levels.

Thyroid Disease and Liver Dysfunction

Liver dysfunction may have several causes in patients with thyroid disease, which may be reflected by direct effects of aberrant thyroid hormone levels on the liver, or, alternatively, the liver may be altered in an indirect way, such as thyroid-induced dysfunction of another organ like the heart. Fortunately, most hepatic abnormalities resolve when a euthyroid state is restored. Abnormalities of serum liver enzymes are seen in over two thirds of patients with hyperthyroidism. Minor elevations of transaminases and alkaline phosphatase are commonly observed, though the latter can be attributable to increased osteoclastic activity. Jaundice associated with thyroid storm may have several causes. For example, associated heart failure and possibly the hepatotoxic effect of thyroid hormone itself may lead to jaundice. Alternatively, thyrotoxicosis can unmask Gilbert's disease and lead to hyperbilirubinemia. In these situations, bilirubin returns to normal when a euthyroid state is restored. In the absence of cardiac failure, hepatic dysfunction is unusual in hypothyroidism, though abnormal enzymes resulting from muscle necrosis can be confused with hepatic abnormalities. In patients with advanced cardiac failure caused by myxedema, hepatomegaly with ascites with a high protein concentration may occur. The association of the latter with nonpitting peripheral edema is a useful clinical clue to the presence of hypothyroidism.

THE PORPHYRIAS

The porphyrias are a group of metabolic disorders characterized by various inherited or acquired enzyme deficiencies that result in abnormalities in heme biosynthesis. Specific enzyme deficiencies have been identified for each of the several types of porphyria (Table 28-4). Synthesis of heme is required of all cells (Figure 28-4), but the bone marrow and the liver are the only organs that are quantitatively important in the overproduction of the porphyrins and porphyrin precursors in these various conditions. The major clinical manifestations of the porphyrias are dermatologic, neurologic, and hepatic disorders. Dermatologic conditions result from the photosensitizing effects of accumulated porphyrins, which are deposited in the skin or are found in the dermal circulation. The dermatologic response to porphyrin-induced photosensitivity is increased fragility of light-exposed skin, as seen in porphyria cutanea tarda, or acute erythema and burning of light-exposed skin, as occurs in protoporphyria. Neurologic disturbances occur in those types of porphyria that are complicated by acute attacks of abdominal pain, which are believed to be caused by an autonomic neuropathy that affects the gastrointestinal tract.

There are few if any histologic abnormalities in the liver in acute intermittent porphyria, and liver enzymes are typically normal. In patients with hereditary coproporphyria, increased concentrations of coproporphyrin can be found in the liver using fluorescent techniques, but there are no structural hepatic abnormalities. Similarly, variegate porphyria and porphyria attributable to ALA dehydrase deficiency do not have hepatic structural involvement. Excess hepatic iron deposition can be found in patients with congenital erythropoietic porphyria, and macronodular cirrhosis has been described. In hepatoerythropoietic porphyria there is a severe deficiency in uroporphyrinogen decarboxylase activity. Increases in serum transaminases are seen, and histologically the liver shows nonspecific lobular or portal inflammation. A small number of patients with protoporphyria have developed severe liver disease with death caused by hepatic failure. Once jaundice develops, progressive hepatic deterioration ensues. At autopsy the liver is cirrhotic with excessive amounts of dark brown pigment caused by protoporphyrin deposition.

Porphyria cutanea tarda (PCT) is the most common cause of hepatic porphyria and is distinct from several of the other forms mentioned, in that acute abdominal pain is not seen and hepatic dysfunction with structural damage can occur. PCT occurs in both an acquired form, which is more common, and a rarer, inherited form. The biochemical defect in PCT is a deficiency in the activity of the enzyme uroporphyrinogen decarboxylase, which results in an increase in tissue and urinary uroporphyrins and heptacarboxyl porphyrins.

Patients with PCT have a variety of cutaneous manifestations including blisters, vesicles, and sores that develop at sites of mild trauma and in sun-exposed areas like the hands, forehead, ears, and neck. In addition to accumulation of porphyrin in the liver, PCT is associated with excessive hepatic iron deposition in about 75% of patients. The cause of iron

Table 28-4 Classification and diagnosis of the porphyrias

Disease	Enzyme defect	Structural hepatic involvement	Acute abdominal pain	Diagnostic findings: Urinary ALA	Urinary PBG	Urinary Uro	Urinary Copro	Fecal Uro	Fecal Copro	Fecal Proto
ALA dehydrase deficiency	ALA dehydrase	−	+	↑↑	↑	↑	↑↑	nl	nl	nl
Acute intermittent porphyria (AIP)	Porphobilinogen deaminase	−	+	↑	↑	nl-↑	nl-↑	nl-↑	nl-↑	nl-↑
Congenital erythropoietic porphyria (CEP)	Uroporphyrinogen III synthase	+	−	nl	nl	↑↑	↑	↑↑	↑↑	nl
Porphyria cutanea tarda (PCT)	Uroporphyrinogen decarboxylase	+	−	nl	nl	↑↑	↑	↑	↑	nl
Hepatoerythropoietic porphyria (HEP)	Uroporphyrinogen decarboxylase (severe)	+	−	nl	nl	↑↑	↑	↑	↑	↑
Hereditary coproporphyria (HCP)	Coproporphyrinogen oxidase	−	+	nl-↑↑	nl-↑↑	nl-↑	↑↑	nl	↑	↑
Variegate porphyria (VP)	Protoporphyrinogen oxidase	−	+	nl-↑↑	nl-↑↑	nl-↑	↑↑	nl	↑	↑↑
Protoporphyria (PP)	Ferrochelatase	+	−	nl	nl	nl-↑	nl-↑	nl	nl-↑	↑↑
Normal (nl) values:				<3*	<2.5*	10-60†	50-250†	0-5‡	Tr-50‡	Tr-120‡

*mg/gm of creatinine.
†μg/gm of creatinine.
‡μg/gm of dry-weight stool.
Tr = Trace.

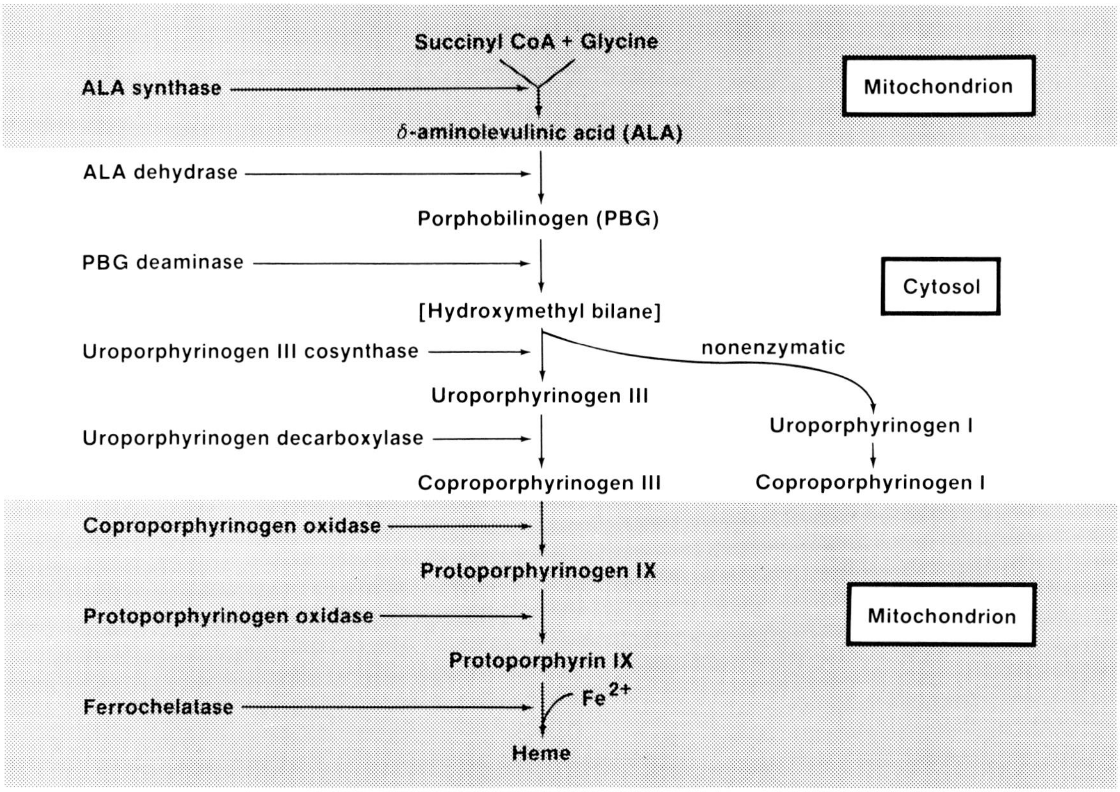

Figure 28-4
Biosynthesis of heme.

overload is unknown, but one study has suggested that some patients with PCT are heterozygous for hereditary hemochromatosis (HHC), whereas another has disproved this contention. In addition to excess iron, focal lobular hepatocellular necrosis and steatosis, hepatocyte hyperplasia and periductal lymphocytic aggregates have been described. The role of the increased iron in the pathogenesis of symptomatic PCT is well established because diminution of iron stores by phlebotomy therapy ameliorates the biochemical and symptomatic manifestations of the disease and replenishment of iron stores after successful phlebotomy therapy causes biochemical relapse. The mechanisms by which a synergistic interaction of the increased hepatic iron and porphyrin accumulation produce the symptomatic and biochemical manifestations of the disease are unknown.

Excessive ethanol ingestion and the intake of estrogens have also been implicated in the clinical expression of the disease. Thus the mainstays of therapy have been to discontinue alcohol or estrogen ingestion and to remove excess iron by phlebotomy. Excess iron stores are usually on the order of 4 to 6 gm, and so phlebotomy requirements are not as extensive as in hemochromatosis. Chloroquine has also been advocated in low doses (125 mg two to three times a week) for those patients not responding to phlebotomy. Chloroquine enhances the removal of porphyrins from tissues with subsequent urinary excretion. Patients with long-standing untreated PCT may develop cirrhosis and hepatocellular carcinoma.

A diagnosis of porphyria is made by the demonstration of increased amounts of porphyrins or their precursors (ALA, PBG) in the urine, stool, or blood (Table 28-4). If a screening Watson-Schwartz test is positive for porphobilinogen, quantitative determinations of PBG should be obtained. A variety of drugs including barbiturates, estrogens, ethanol, griseofulvin, sulfonamides, oral contraceptives, meprobamate, and hydantoin have been reported to exacerbate the acute hepatic porphyrias, and thus these medications should be avoided in patients in whom porphyria has been diagnosed.

METAL STORAGE DISEASES

Iron Metabolism

The liver plays a central role in iron metabolism. It is one of the body's major storage organs for iron, and the plasma iron transport protein transferrin is synthesized by the liver. The average daily Western diet contains 10 to 20 mg of iron, of which approximately 10% is absorbed in normal persons. In the absence of blood loss, iron excretion is very limited and usually amounts to 1 to 2 mg/day, which is lost mainly in desquamated gut mucosal cells, sweat, and bile. Because the excretory capacity for iron is limited, body homeostasis for iron is regulated by absorption, which occurs primarily in the duodenum and proximal jejunum and which appears to be regulated by the enterocyte. Iron is absorbed in both ionic forms and as heme, which is derived principally from red meat. Factors in the lumen of the intestine affect the bioavailability of nonheme iron but do not play a physiologic role in the regulation of iron absorption.

To enter the body, iron passes through the enterocyte and into the submucosal capillary network in three basic steps: uptake into the enterocyte, storage or intracellular transport of iron to the basolateral surface and subsequent transfer of the iron to the circulation. Separate pathways exist for the uptake of heme and nonheme iron. Heme iron constitutes only 5% to 10% of dietary iron, but it accounts for nearly one third of the iron absorbed each day because heme is more readiiy absorbed than nonheme sources of iron. Heme taken up by the enterocyte is degraded by heme oxygenase with release of inorganic iron, which then enters a common iron pool. Iron is transported to the portal blood by a carrier-mediated, energy-dependent process, in which the final transport of iron across the serosal surface to the portal blood appears to be the rate-limiting step. Newly absorbed iron is transported in the blood bound to transferrin. Approximately 80% of absorbed iron is utilized in the bone marrow for incorporation into developing erythrocytes. Most of the remainder is transported to muscle and to the liver for storage.

In the circulation, iron is transported primarily bound to transferrin but can also be found as heme bound to hemopexin, hemoglobin bound to haptoglobin, and circulating ferritin. Hepatocellular uptake of iron proceeds by receptor mediated endocytosis with specific receptors for iron-transferrin, hemehemopexin, hemoglobin-haptoglobin, and ferritin. Within the liver, iron is found in hemoproteins (e.g., cytochromes, catalase), in storage forms (ferritin, hemosiderin), and in a poorly characterized intracellular transit pool that serves to move iron from the plasma membrane to sites of utilization or storage (Figure 28-5).

Iron Storage Disorders

The various types of hemochromatosis can be divided into four major categories based on the cause of the increased iron stores (Table 28-5). These are as follows: (1) hereditary hemochromatosis (HHC), which has also been referred to as genetic,

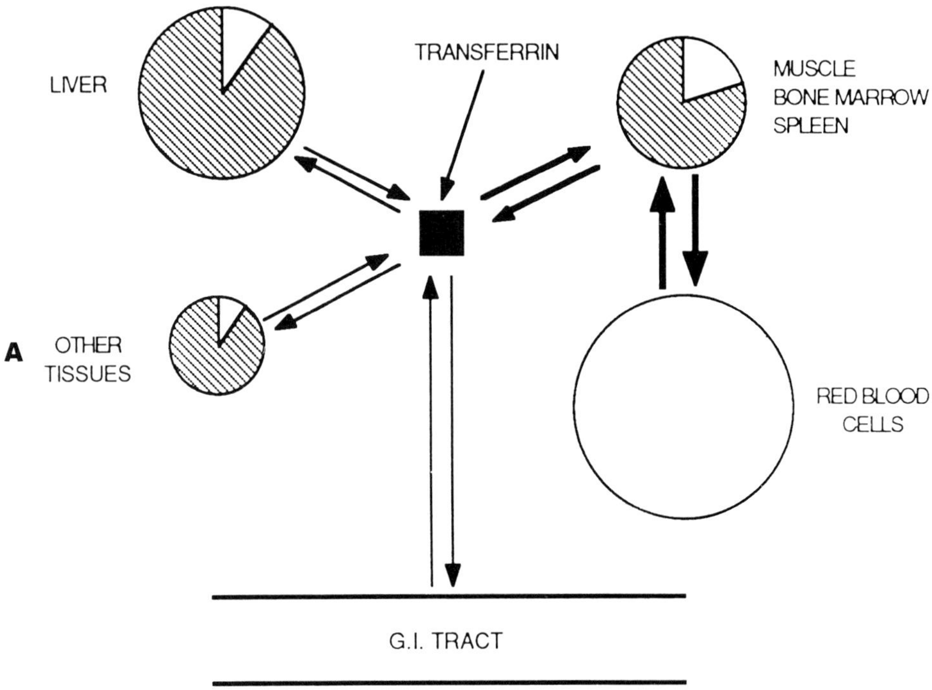

Figure 28-5
Whole body iron distribution and exchange in normals, **A,** and in patients with hemochromatosis, **B** and **C.** In hemochromatosis, there is an increase in absorption of iron from the gastrointestinal tract with progressive deposition of storage iron mainly in parenchymal cells of the liver and to a lesser degree in other tissues. Total body iron is increased as a result of increases in the storage compartments, *hatched,* without any changes in iron found in hemoproteins (e.g., hemoglobin, myoglobin, and cytochromes), *open.* All iron exchange is channeled through plasma transferrin, which becomes highly saturated in patients with hemochromatosis.

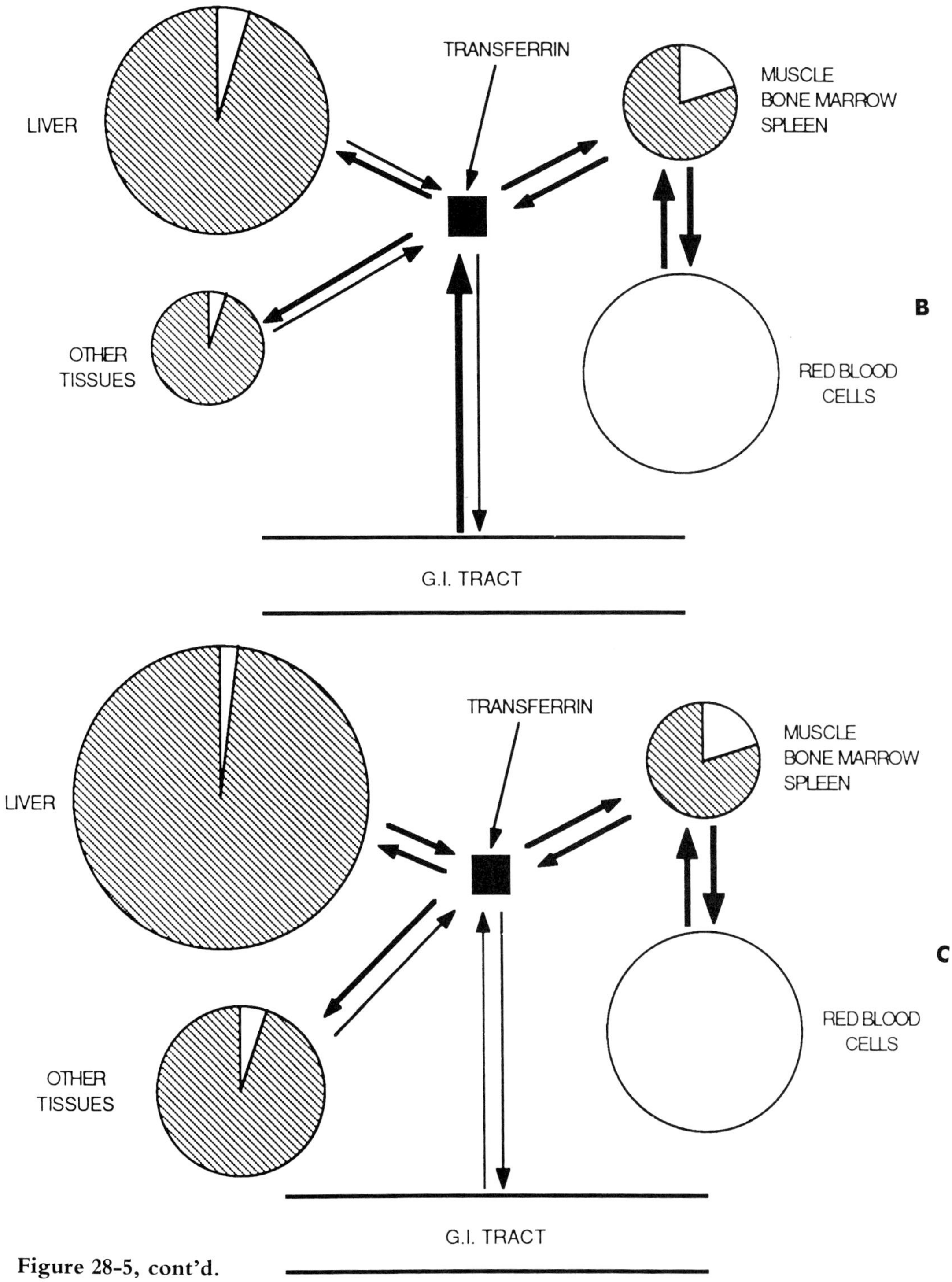

Figure 28-5, cont'd.

Table 28-5 Classification of iron overload disorders

Hereditary hemochromatosis (idiopathic, genetic, primary)
Secondary iron overload
Anemia attributable to ineffective erythropoiesis
β-Thalassemia
Sideroblastic anemia
Pyruvate kinase deficiency
Liver disease
Alcoholic cirrhosis
After portacaval anastomosis
Porphyria cutanea tarda
Increased oral intake of iron
Dietary iron overload in the Bantu
Prolonged excessive medicinal iron ingestion
Congenital atransferrinemia
Parenteral iron administration
Blood transfusions
Iron dextran injections
Chronic hemodialysis
Neonatal iron overload
Neonatal hemochromatosis
Hereditary tyrosinemia
Zellweger's cerebrohepatorenal syndrome

primary, or idiopathic hemochromatosis, in which there is an inherited defect resulting in increased absorption of dietary iron. (2) Secondary iron overload, in which an underlying disorder or an enormous dietary intake of bioavailable iron can result in an increase in intestinal iron absorption. Disorders of ineffective erythopoiesis, such as sideroblastic anemia or β-thalassemia, are common underlying conditions, and iron overload may occur without prior transfusion. Secondary iron overload may also be seen in patients with porphyria cutanea tarda, in those after having a portacaval shunt, and in many patients with various causes of cirrhosis. (3) Parenteral iron overload, in which the excessive body iron is obtained from blood transfusions or from iron injections. In this setting, iron is initially deposited in the reticuloendothelial system, but with enough iron loading, iron is redistributed into parenchymal cells, where it is potentially more toxic. (4) There are also several forms of neonatal iron overload.

Hereditary Hemochromatosis

Hereditary hemochromatosis (HHC) is an autosomal recessive disorder of iron metabolism characterized by excessive intestinal iron absorption leading to parenchymal iron overload with subsequent tissue damage. The hemochromatosis gene is located on the short arm of chromosome 6 and is strongly associated with HLA haplotypes A_3 and B_{14}. HLA haplotyping and pedigree analysis have shown the homozygote frequency among whites to be about 1 in 250, with a heterozygote frequency of approximately 1 in 10; thus HHC is one of the most common inherited disorders. The disease is more pronounced and presents at an earlier age in males than females, partly because physiologic iron loss (menstruation, pregnancy) delays iron accumulation in women. The liver, heart, pancreas, joints, and pituitary are the main organs affected. Excessive alcohol consumption is believed to accentuate the liver disease in homozygotes, though this contention has not been rigorously proved. Heterozygotes may have minor increases in hepatic iron stores but do not develop tissue damage.

The pathophysiologic mechanism or mechanisms underlying the increased intestinal absorption of iron in HHC are unclear, partly because the regulation of normal iron absorption is so poorly understood. Nevertheless, increased iron absorption leads to excess iron accumulation in the liver, where iron concentrations up to 30 to 50 times normal can be seen. In early HHC virtually all excess iron is found within periportal hepatocytes, with very little in Kupffer cells (Figure 28-6). Later, in more established HHC, excess iron can be found in Kupffer cells, endothelial cells, and bile ductular cells, as well as in hepatocytes. The majority of stored iron is found as hemosiderin within secondary lysosomes, called "siderosomes," with increased amounts of soluble ferritin found in the cytosol of the hepatocyte. Recent clinical and experimental studies indicate that hepatic injury and fibrosis occur after a "toxic threshold" of iron is exceeded. In most patients, fibrosis or cirrhosis, or both, occur when hepatic tissue levels of iron exceed 22,000 μg/gm, dry weight, (normal <1,500 μg/gm, dry weight). The major mechanistic theories of hepatocellular injury and fibrogenesis in chronic iron overload revolve around knowledge that iron is a potent pro-oxidant that can catalyze peroxidative damage to polyunsaturated fatty acids of organelle membrane phospholipids leading to organelle and cellular dysfunction and damage. In addition, breakdown products of peroxidized phospholipids have been shown to stimulate collagen synthesis in experimental systems.

The clinical presentation of patients with hemochromatosis is variable, and patients often have subtle, vague complaints resulting in delayed diagnosis (up to 5 years). Most patients present with clinically evident disease after 40 years of age, at which point total body iron stores often exceed 20 gm (normal is 1 gm). Frequent presenting symptoms are weakness and malaise (75%), abdominal pain (60%), arthralgias (50%), and impotence and loss of libido (40%). Approximately 75% of patients have hepatomegaly, and when patients present with symptomatic HHC, 69% have cirrhosis, 21% have fibrosis without cirrhosis, and only 10% have no fibrosis or cirrhosis. Serum transaminases (ALT, AST) are mildly elevated (twice normal) in about 50% of patients.

Patients with HHC usually have extrahepatic manifestations. Arthritis is commonly an initial symptom, occurring in up to 50% of patients and typically involving the second and third metacarpophalangeal joints, the proximal interphalangeal joints, and the knees, back, and neck. Radiographic findings show joint space narrowing, osteosclerosis, subchondral cysts, and chondrocalcinosis. Pancreatic endocrine deficiency is manifested as glucose intolerance, which can be seen in up to two thirds of patients and is more prevalent in patients with cirrhosis (71%) than in those without cirrhosis (20%). Many patients require insulin, but some can be managed with oral hypoglycemic agents. Patients with HHC do not have pancreatic exocrine deficiency. About 50% of patients show evidence of anterior pituitary dysfunction, with deficiencies of gonadotropin and prolactin secretion. Additionally, there may be primary gonadal failure caused by iron deposition in the testes. The increased awareness of hemochromatosis in recent years has made presentation with cardiac failure much less common than 40 or 50 years ago. Congestive heart failure, when

A

B

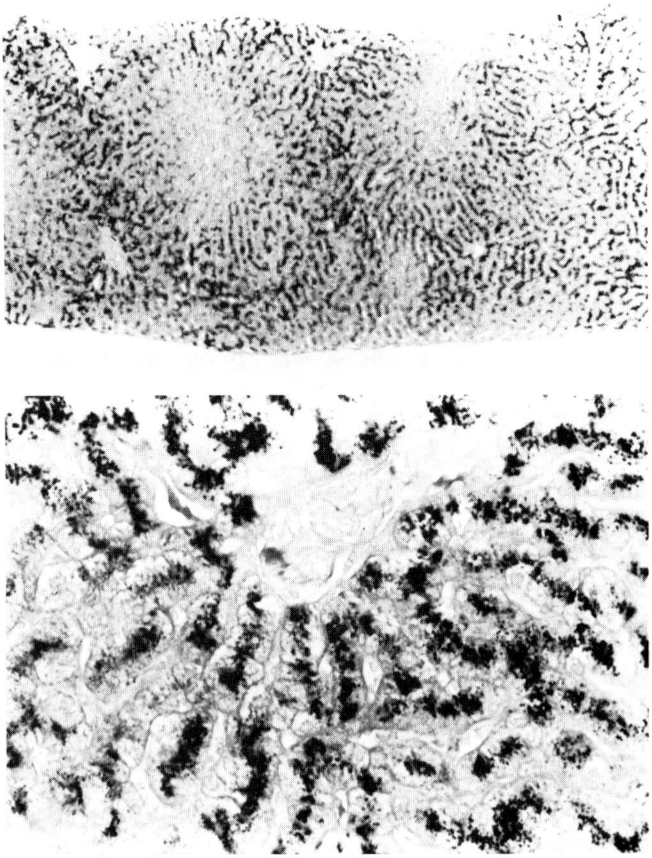

Figure 28-6
Hemochromatosis in liver. This liver biopsy specimen was obtained from an asymptomatic 34-year-old male who was referred for evaluation of an elevated serum iron level found on routine screening. The hepatic iron concentration was 17,300 μg/gm, dry weight. **A,** Iron deposition is seen in a periportal distribution with normal hepatic architecture. (Perls' Prussian blue stain, ×50.) **B,** At higher power, iron deposition is found predominantly in hepatocytes with very little found in reticuloendothelial cells. (Perls' Prussian blue stain, ×320.)

present, is usually attributable to a dilated cardiomyopathy, but restrictive cardiomyopathy has also been described. Cardiac arrhythmias (atrial tachycardia, ventricular premature beats and ventricular tachycardia) can be life threatening. Cardiac involvement should be regarded as an emergency because, without treatment, cardiac disease may progress rapidly to death within 1 year. Abnormal skin pigmentation, which is often mild but distinct, occurs in up to 80% of patients. A grayish skin color is attributable to iron deposits in the basal cells of the epidermis and sweat glands, whereas a bronze pigmentation is attributable to increased melanin production.

Many patients with HHC are never diagnosed. This potentially fatal disease often escapes detection for three reasons. First, there is relatively little awareness of the disorder by the public or the medical profession. Physicians have been exceptionally aware of the symptoms and physical findings of iron deficiency for many decades; however, only in recent years have physicians become aware of iron overload and its manifestations. Second, patients frequently do not develop symptoms until late adulthood, and when symptoms develop, they mimic other common disorders in this age group, such as diabetes, arthritis, and congestive heart failure. Third, there is variability in the expression of the disease, and it is unclear whether all homozygotes or only a fraction of them eventually develop symptoms. Environmental factors such as the quantity of dietary iron and the ingestion of agents that enhance iron absorption (e.g., ethanol and ascorbate) affect the phenotypic expression of the disease. Pronounced variations in iron stores occur among homozygotes of approximately the same age, and the degree of iron loading is not always constant within a pedigree. Unfortunately, it is unclear which patients with the genetic disease will develop clinical symptoms.

Fifty years ago, HHC was recognized only by the classic triad of bronzing of the skin, diabetes, and hepatomegaly with liver disease. Today, iron overload is easily detected before symptoms or physical findings develop. Because neither the gene causing iron-loading nor its protein product have been identified, phenotypic tests for iron overload are used for diagnosis. Once hemochromatosis is suspected, the diagnosis is reasonably straightforward. Blood studies that should be obtained include the serum iron concentration, total iron binding capacity (TIBC), and ferritin concentration. These should be drawn in the fasting state. From the serum iron and the TIBC, the percent transferrin saturation (iron ÷ TIBC × 100%) can be calculated. Representative measurements can be found in Table 28-6. A combination of a transferrin saturation over 50% and an elevated serum ferritin concentration is 94% sensitive and 86% specific for the detection of hemochromatosis in young (less than 30 years) homozygotes (confirmed by HLA typing). From these observations in young homozygotes with HHC, it is reasonable to extend these guidlines to the evaluation of all patients suspected of having hemochromatosis.

If serum iron studies are abnormal, the diagnosis should be strongly considered and a liver biopsy performed for histologic interpretation (with iron stains) and biochemical determination of hepatic iron concentration. Quantitative hepatic iron levels permit a definitive initial diagnosis of HHC and serve as a reference point for

Table 28-6 Representative iron measurements in hereditary hemochromatosis (HHC)

Parameter	Normal	HHC
Serum iron (μg/dl)	50-150	180-300
Total iron binding capacity (μg/dl)	250-370	200-300
Transferrin saturation (%)	20-50	80-100
Serum ferritin (ng/ml)		
Males	20-300	600-6000
Females	15-250	
Liver iron concentration		
(μg/gm, dry weight)	300-1500	10,000-30,000
(μmoles/gm, dry weight)	5-30	180-535
Hepatic iron index		
(μmoles/gm, dry wt ÷ age in years)	<2	>2

future biopsy assessment of therapeutic efficacy. Patients with symptomatic HHC have hepatic iron concentrations exceeding 10,000 μg/gm dry weight and in some circumstances as high as 40,000 μg/gm dry weight (normal is <1500 μg/gm dry weight). In asymptomatic, younger patients with early precirrhotic HHC, quantitative hepatic iron levels will be increased, but to a lesser degree, with a mean of approximately 10,000 μg/gm. A recent study has shown that hepatic iron concentrations in excess of 22,000 μg/gm dry weight are associated with the development of fibrosis and cirrhosis. Histochemical stains for excess storage iron in HHC show deposition predominantly in parenchymal cells in a periportal distribution as illustrated in Figure 28-6. Grade IV staining, in which virtually all parenchymal cells show a positive Prussian blue reaction, is unequivocal evidence of iron overload. Lesser grades of staining on light microscopy do not adequately correlate with the quantitative iron determination.

Liver disease is manifested by variable degrees of fibrosis, ranging from minimal periportal or perilobular fibrosis, to fully developed micronodular cirrhosis. The degree of fibrosis probably depends on several factors, including the hepatic iron concentration, the length of time that the liver has been exposed to high iron concentrations, and parenchymal versus reticuloendothelial deposition. Intermediate iron levels may be difficult to interpret, especially in patients with alcoholic liver disease. In this situation, the hepatic iron index (HII), defined as the hepatic iron level (in μmoles/gm dry weight) divided by the age (in years) is useful. HII values greater than 2.0 are seen in patients homozygous for HHC, whereas heterozygotes and alcoholics with secondary iron overload have HII values less than 2.0.

Hepatocellular carcinoma (HCC) develops in up to 14% of patients with HHC. Virtually all hemochromatotic patients who have developed HCC have preexisting cirrhosis, though there have been a few recent case reports of patients developing hepatocellular carcinoma in the absence of cirrhosis. Overall, HCC and complications of chronic liver disease are the most common causes of death in patients with hemochromatosis.

Phlebotomy is the treatment of choice for HHC and should be carried out weekly or biweekly until iron stores are depleted. Serum iron studies are monitored during phlebotomy therapy and the ferritin level will gradually decrease with reduction of excess tissue iron stores. The percent transferrin saturation will not decrease until late in therapy. Each unit of blood represents 200 to 250 mg of iron; therefore, to adequately treat someone with 40 gm of excess storage iron, 160 units of blood will have to be removed. Thus initial depletion of iron stores in most symptomatic patients with HHC usually requires removal of more than 100 units of blood (greater than 25 gm of excess iron). Development of anemia earlier (i.e., after 10 to 15 units are removed) should be suggestive of some other form of liver disease (e.g., alcoholic cirrhosis) with secondary iron overload rather than homozygous hemochromatosis.

Once a patient has been effectively "de-ironed," phlebotomy of one unit of blood every 3 to 4 months is adequate to remain in normal iron balance. Recent studies demonstrate that noncirrhotic patients with hemochromatosis successfully depleted of excess iron by rigorous phlebotomy have a life expectancy similar to age- and sex-matched individuals in the general population. This finding, coupled with the evidence of a "toxic threshold" for iron in the liver, makes an excellent case for early phlebotomy in the management of patients with HHC in order to prevent cirrhosis as well as dysfunction to other organs and possibly hepatocellular carcinoma (HCC). In addition, these considerations underscore the importance of screening family members of probands with HHC in order to detect affected individuals in the precirrhotic state.

Screening asymptomatic first degree family members of probands is an important part of the management of patients with HHC. If serum iron and ferritin levels are normal and the percent transferrin saturation is less than 50%, HHC is unlikely (<3% chance). If any iron study is abnormal, a liver biopsy should be performed for histologic evaluation and quantitative iron determination. HLA typing is useful for comparison of family members with probands but is not used as a general screening tool.

Because hereditary hemochromatosis is a common treatable metabolic disorder, the index of suspicion should be high among physicians caring for patients with liver disorders. Early diagnosis is extremely important because phlebotomy treatment will prevent complications and allow a normal life span.

Copper Metabolism

As in iron metabolism, the liver plays a central role in body copper homeostasis. Hepatic copper concentrations are the highest of any organ and the main route of copper excretion is through the biliary tract. The average daily Western diet contains approximately 3 mg of copper, 50% of which is absorbed in the proximal small intestine. Copper is absorbed mainly in soluble complexes with histidine rich oligopeptides or amino acids. The mechanism of regulation of intestinal copper absorption is undefined, but intestinal metallothionein may play an important role in this process. Certain high molecular weight binding complexes in bile actually inhibit copper absorption. Once copper is absorbed it is bound primarily to albumin and transported to the liver, where it is rapidly cleared. Over two thirds of absorbed copper is subsequently excreted in the bile and almost all the remainder returns to the blood bound to ceruloplasmin. Although 94% of plasma copper is bound to ceruloplasmin, it appears that this protein does not play a major role in transporting copper to sites of utilization. It is the other 6% of the plasma copper bound to albumin and amino acids that is in a dynamic state. Copper excretion is mainly by bile, and both extrahepatic and intrahepatic cholestatic syndromes are associated with considerable accumulation of hepatic copper. The major clinical disorder of copper overload is Wilson's disease, which is discussed in detail below.

Wilson's Disease

Wilson's disease (hepatolenticular degeneration) is an uncommon autosomal recessive condition found in all races that usually presents with hepatic or neurologic abnormalities. Different studies place the prevalance from 1 in 30,000 to 1 in 200,000; the abnormal gene has been located on the short arm of chromosome 13. Although the exact pathophysiologic defects in the hepatocellular metabolism of copper in Wilson's disease are unknown, there is a defect in the transfer of hepatocellular lysosomal copper into bile, and this may involve an abnormal tissue metallothionein compound. Gradual accumulation of tissue copper results in subsequent toxicity to target organs, which include the liver, brain, eyes, kidneys, and red blood cells. Excess hepatic copper deposition has many potential hepatotoxic effects, which include the promotion of oxidative damage to plasma membranes, mitochondria, and microtubules. Damage to these subcellular organelles has been confirmed ultrastructurally and biochemically in experimental models of copper overload. Interestingly, despite the knowledge of the hepatotoxic effects of excess copper, liver disease attributable to copper overload is proved only in Wilson's disease and not in the other conditions associated with hepatic copper overload, such as primary biliary cirrhosis.

Clinically, hepatocellular dysfunction attributable to Wilson's disease is not seen before 6 years of age, whereas neurologic manifestations present in adolescence or in early adult life. By 15 years of age, almost half the patients with Wilson's disease have symptoms referable to the disease. Of these symptomatic patients, about 42% present initally with hepatic manifestations, 34% with neurologic manifestations, and 10% with psychiatric manifestations. About 12% present with hematologic or endocrine features and the remaining 1% with renal complications. In about 25% of patients, presenting signs and symptoms originate from two or more organ systems. It is important to emphasize that all patients presenting with neurologic disease have evidence of preexisting chronic liver disease.

Hepatic involvement in Wilson's disease may manifest itself in several ways: (1) steatosis, (2) chronic active hepatitis, (3) cirrhosis, and (4) fulminant hepatic failure. One of the earliest hepatocellular lesions is hepatic steatosis with increased glycogen deposits in enlarged nuclei. In the majority of patients, this lesion progresses gradually and silently to fibrosis and ultimately cirrhosis. Alternatively, in some patients, a picture of chronic active hepatitis may be present with histologic findings of inflammatory cell infiltration, piecemeal necrosis, erosion of the limiting plates of the lobules, and parenchymal collapse. It has been estimated that up to 5% of patients under 35 years of age with presumed idiopathic chronic active hepatitis have Wilson's disease. Therefore one should perform careful studies of copper metabolism on all young patients with chronic active hepatitis or other forms of chronic liver disease so as not to overlook this treatable disorder. A small number of patients may present with fulminant hepatic failure (FHF). The ability to differentiate FHF attributable to Wilson's disease from idiopathic or viral FHF has recently been demonstrated. Patients with FHF from Wilson's disease are usually younger than patients with other forms of FHF, most patients with FHF attributable to Wilson's disease have Kayser-Fleischer rings, and patients with Wilson's disease have higher serum urine and hepatic copper levels, less pronounced elevations of transaminases, higher levels of total bilirubin, and lower hemoglobin values. Serum copper is the most useful biochemical test in the diagnosis of FHF attributable to Wilson's disease before death.

As described above, numerous extrahepatic manifestations of Wilson's disease may be present. The neurologic manifestations typically occur during the early teens but may be seen in patients up to 40 years of age. Serum liver tests may be normal; however cirrhosis is usually present, as are Kayser-Fleischer rings. Initial symptoms may be limited to psychologic deficits, such as a worsening performance in school, behavioral problems, or trouble with authorities. Later, specific neurologic symptoms and signs such as tremor, slowness of movement, dysarthria, dysphagia, hoarseness, and choreic movements may be seen. As the disease progresses, patients develop more profound dysphagia, with drooling, rigidity, and slowness of movement of the limbs, fixed facial muscles, dysarthria, and a parkinsonian-like tremor, signifying copper-induced damage to the cerebellum and extrapyramidal nervous system.

The Kayser-Fleischer corneal ring is the golden-brown or greenish granular discoloration caused by copper deposition in the deepest layer of the cornea (Descement's membrane) (Figure 28-7). Kayser-Fleischer rings are invariably seen in patients with neurologic disease but may not be present in children or asymptomatic adults with liver disease. In addition to Wilson's disease, Kayser-Fleischer rings have been seen in patients with long-standing cholestatic liver diseases, such as primary biliary cirrhosis, intrahepatic cholestasis of childhood, and non-

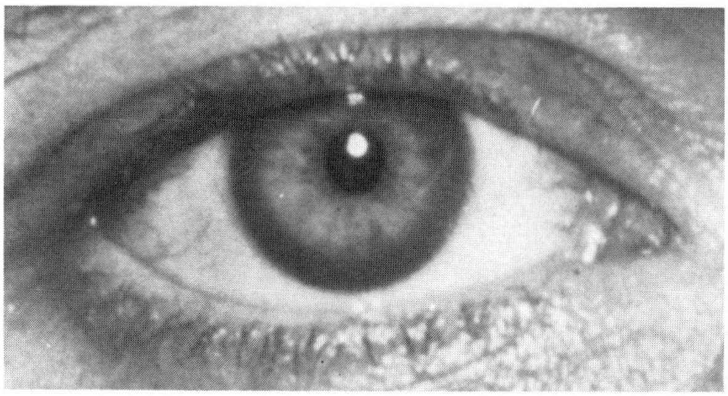

Figure 28-7
Kayser-Fleischer rings. Excess pigmentation caused by copper deposition is seen in the periphery of the cornea in this 16-year-old male with Wilson's disease.

wilsonian chronic active hepatitis and cryptogenic cirrhosis. In the presence of neurologic manifestations, however, Kayser-Fleischer rings are pathognomonic for Wilson's disease. "Sunflower" cataracts are a more pronounced later ophthalmologic finding in which vision is not affected.

A small number of patients may present with a Coombs'-negative hemolytic anemia. This is usually an acute and transient event. It has been postulated that a rapid hepatic release of copper into the bloodstream causes a sudden increase in plasma copper, which provides sufficient oxidant stress to red blood cell membranes to cause them to rupture. When hemolysis accompanies hepatic failure, the prognosis is poor. Abnormalities in renal function include proximal tubular dysfunction resulting in aminoaciduria, glucosuria, uricosuria, hyperphosphaturia, and hypercalciuria. Additionally, patients may develop a distal renal tubular acidosis, and many patients (16%) develop nephrolithiasis. Bony abnormalities seen in patients with Wilson's disease include osteomalacia, osteoporosis, premature osteoarthritis, spontaneous fractures, and osteochondritis dissecans with associated chondrocalcinosis. Hypoparathyroidism has been described, as has pancreatic exocrine insufficiency, amenorrhea in women, and gynecomastia in males.

The diagnosis of Wilson's disease should be considered in any patient under 40 years of age with noncholestatic liver disease, particularly in the presence of neuropsychiatric syptoms not attributable to portosystemic encephalopathy. Initial evaluation (Table 28-7) should include measurement of serum and urine copper and of serum ceruloplasmin and slitlamp examination for Kayser-Fleischer rings. Approximately 95% of all patients with Wilson's disease will have a decreased level of ceruloplasmin in the plasma. Because it is an acute-phase reactant, ceruloplasmin may be elevated to within the lower limits of normal in patients with active liver disease; thus a smaller percentage (85%) of patients with hepatic manifestations will show decreased levels. Decreased ceruloplasmin levels can also be seen in patients with malabsorption, malnutrition, nephrotic syndrome, or protein-losing enteropathy, or in a small percentage of persons who are heterozygous

Table 28-7 Laboratory evaluation in Wilson's disease

	Normal	Nonfulminant	Fulminant
Serum copper (μg/dl)	80-140	<80	>200
Urine copper (μg/24 hr)	<40	>100	>100
Serum ceruloplasmin (mg/dl)	20-40	<20	<20
Hepatic copper concentration (μg/gm, dry weight)	15-50	>250	>250
Hemolysis	Absent	Absent	Present
Alkaline phosphatase	—	Low normal	Absent-low

carriers of the disease. Therefore, in asymptomatic patients or in those with only hepatic manifestations, the ceruloplasmin level can be in the normal range in up to 15% of patients. In addition, even though a decreased ceruloplasmin level is highly suggestive of the disease, it alone is not sufficient for a definitive diagnosis. The serum non–ceruloplasmin bound copper level is usually elevated in patients with Wilson's disease, but it may be increased in patients with other types of liver disease as well, making it an unhelpful test except in patients with fulminant hepatic failure, in whom the increase in nonceruloplasmin copper may outweigh the fall in ceruloplasmin. Increased urinary excretion of copper can be a useful confirmatory test, and patients with Wilson's disease may excrete from 100 to 1000 μg per 24 hrs (normal <40 μg per 24 hours). If blood or urine studies are suggestive, liver biopsy for histologic staging and quantitative copper determinations should be performed. Because the histopathologic changes in a liver biopsy specimen can be quite diverse, histochemical staining for copper may be a helpful adjunct in support of the clinical diagnosis of Wilson's disease. Predominantly pericanalicular localization of copper-associated proteins may be visualized by the use of stains such as rubeanic acid, rhodanine, or orcein, but these methods lack sensitivity when compared with biochemical assessment of tissue copper concentration. Hepatic copper concentrations are typically greater than 250 μg/gm dry weight and may be as high as 3000 μg/gm (normal is 15 to 50 μg/gm). The hepatic distribution of copper may be patchy and thus a concentration of less than 250 μg/gm may be obtained on occasion. Elevated hepatic copper concentrations can be found in other types of chronic liver disease, such as primary biliary cirrhosis, intrahepatic cholestasis of childhood, Indian childhood cirrhosis, and extrahepatic biliary obstruction. However, the histologic, biochemical, and clinical features of these diseases can be readily differentiated from Wilson's disease.

A practical approach to the diagnosis of Wilson's disease is (1) to include it in the differential diagnosis when one is evaluating young patients with liver disease and (2) to look carefully (by including slit-lamp examination) for Kayser-Fleischer rings in young patients who present with compatible neurologic manifestations. If Kayser-Fleischer rings are identified in a patient with neurologic findings, a ceruloplasmin level should provide satisfactory confirmation and a liver biopsy is not necessary. In patients with hepatic manifestations without Kayser-Fleischer rings, the serum ceruloplasmin and copper concentration, 24-hour urinary copper excretion, and liver biopsy for histology and biochemical determination of copper should be obtained. When a proband is identified, family members (especially siblings) should be carefully evaluated. Serologic tests differ in fulminant and nonfulminant forms of Wilson's disease and are outlined in Table 28-7.

Therapy for Wilson's disease should be initiated as soon as the diagnosis is confirmed, no matter how advanced the disease. D-Penicillamine is the drug of first choice and should be given initially in a dose of 500 mg 3 times a day. Patients quickly develop a negative copper balance, and symptomatic patients generally respond within a few weeks to a few months of treatment. Some patients deteriorate before eventual improvement, and this possibility should be recognized and should not impede continued therapy. Therapy with D-penicillamine is usually effective and should be continued lifelong; however, some patients develop hypersensitivity or intolerance to D-penicillamine and can be treated with alternative copper chelating agents such as Trientine (triethylenetetramine), which has been used effectively in patients who cannot tolerate D-penicillamine. In addition, dietary supplementation with zinc has resulted in decreased copper absorption and negative copper balance in patients with Wilson's disease.

Fulminant hepatic failure attributable to Wilson's disease does not respond to medical therapy and is an indication for urgent orthotopic liver transplantation. Other indications for transplantation in Wilson's disease include patients who cannot be adequately decoppered on standard medications and those with decompensated cirrhosis at the time of diagnosis. Discontinuation of maintenance D-penicillamine may precipitate fulminant hepatic failure. Patients with neurologic disease may improve dramatically but are often left with residual effects of the disease, such as dystonia and spasticity. Likewise, fibrotic changes in the liver do not improve with removal of excess copper.

As in hemochromatosis, the key to successful treatment and a normal life is the early diagnosis of asymptomatic relatives and patients who have not yet developed irreversible complications. Increased awareness of these uncommon yet treatable diseases is one of the most important steps to successful preventive treatment.

COLLAGEN VASCULAR DISEASES AND THE LIVER (Table 28-8)

Considering the numerous extra-arthritic manifestations that characterize the collagen vascular diseases, it is surprising that associated severe liver disease is relatively uncommon. Serum liver enzyme abnormalities are seen frequently, however, and determination of their pathologic significance often poses a diagnostic challenge. Furthermore, these patients commonly require multiple potentially hepatotoxic drugs, which further complicate the differential diagnosis.

Table 28-8 Hepatic diseases associated with collagen vascular diseases

Rheumatoid arthritis	Biochemical cholestasis
Felty's syndrome	Noncirrhotic portal hypertension Nodular regenerative hyperplasia Nonspecific hepatitis
Still's disease	Nonspecific hepatitis Acute hepatitis Fulminant hepatitis
Lupus erythematosus	Chronic active hepatitis Granulomatous hepatitis Cirrhosis Canalicular cast lesion
Polyarteritis nodosa	Hepatitis B Hepatic infarction Hepatic artery aneurysm Spontaneous intrahepatic bleeding Cirrhosis Nodular regenerative hyperplasia

Rheumatoid Arthritis and its Variants

Clinically apparent liver disease is rare in rheumatoid arthritis (RA), but biochemical cholestasis is common. Elevations of alkaline phosphatase and γ-glutamyl transpeptidase are observed in 25% to 50% of patients. In this situation, liver biopsy reveals nonspecific abnormalities including Kupffer cell hyperplasia, fatty infiltration, and portal mononuclear infiltrates. Elevation of transaminases are unusual and should be suggestive of an alternative diagnosis.

Felty's syndrome is associated with a more impressive array of hepatic abnormalities. Serum liver enzymes are abnormal in over 25% of patients, and hepatomegaly is present in over two thirds. However, the correlation of these two findings appears to be poor. Histologically, diffuse lymphocytic infiltrates and Kupffer cell hyperplasia are seen. Portal hypertension and variceal hemorrhage accompanied by mild portal fibrosis without cirrhosis is a well-known complication of Felty's syndrome. Nodular regenerative hyperplasia is another well-known complication, which may explain the atypical cases of noncirrhotic portal hypertension.

Hepatic abnormalities are more common with Still's disease than with any other form of rheumatoid arthritis, afflicting up to 90% of pediatric cases and approximately one third of adult-onset Still's disease patients. Hepatomegaly and serum transaminase elevations are the usual hepatic manifestations. Histologically, only periportal lymphocytic infiltration and Kupffer cell hyperplasia are found, despite pronounced hepatomegaly. Two syndromes of acute hepatocellular disease have been described with Still's disease. In children, several cases of acute hepatitis followed by dramatic improvement in the arthropathy have been reported. It is unknown whether these represent manifestations of Still's disease itself or superimposed viral hepatitis. In adults, more alarming cases of acute, fulminant hepatic failure with life-threatening and fatal outcomes have been described. The possible role of aspirin and other nonsteroidal antiinflammatory agents is impossible to exclude.

Systemic Lupus Erythematosus

The true incidence of liver disease in systemic lupus erythematosus (SLE) is unknown because prospective studies have not been performed. However, one retrospective evaluation suggests that as many as 18% of patients with SLE have biopsy-documented abnormalities believed to be associated with SLE. Most patients present with anorexia, nausea, vomiting, hepatosplenomegaly, and elevated serum transaminases. Although the most common histologic lesion seen on biopsy is steatosis, more progressive lesions have been seen as well, including chronic active hepatitis, granulomatous hepatitis, and cirrhosis. Patients with cirrhosis often exhibit a seemingly unique "canalicular cast" lesion, where the canaliculi are filled with bile and appear as if they were injected with latex. Although some patients die of hepatic failure, most improve with corticosteroid therapy.

The patient with SLE and chronic active hepatitis presents a special problem in that one cannot be sure whether the entire disease process represents SLE or the patient has autoimmune chronic active hepatitis with systemic manifestations, or in combination with SLE. This problem is accentuated by the frequent presence of antinuclear antibodies and positive LE cell preparations in both entities. Although this problem is not resolved, the therapeutic solution should be a practical one. If diagnostic criteria for SLE as well as biopsy-proved chronic active hepatitis are both present, one should proceed with corticosteroid therapy based on traditional disease manifestations of autoimmune chronic active hepatitis, which is usually sufficient to treat most extrahepatic manifestations of SLE.

Polyarteritis Nodosa

Autopsy studies indicate that the hepatic arterial tree is involved in 60% of patients with polyarteritis nodosa (PAN). Of patients with PAN, 30% to 70% have a positive HBsAg and chronic persistent hepatitis, but the spectrum of histologic abnormalities is large and includes acute hepatitis B, chronic active hepatitis B, and postnecrotic cirrhosis. In general, however, the vasculitis, rather than the liver disease, dominates the clinical picture.

Severe, acute liver disease may complicate PAN because of the vasculitis and the multifocal hepatic artery aneurysms that are present in 60% of patients with PAN. This accounts for the fact that over 50% of cases of spontaneous hepatic infarction occur in PAN patients. In addition, intrahepatic hemorrhage occasionally progressing to hepatic rupture with intraperitoneal bleeding may occur. These patients present with acute epigastric or right upper quadrant pain with elevation of serum transaminases. Computerized tomography reveals intrahepatic hematomas. Angiography is advisable to define anatomic segments involved in the hemorrhage and to embolize lesions that are actively bleeding. Surgery should be considered in cases of overt hepatic rupture, intraperitoneal hemorrhage, active bleeding with hemodynamic instability, and severe abdominal pain. Smaller hematomas and infarctions can be managed conservatively.

Other hepatic lesions seen in PAN include cirrhosis and nodular regenerative hyperplasia. Because of the presence of multifocal hepatic artery aneurysms, liver biopsy entails a high risk of bleeding and is best avoided in patients with PAN.

Hepatotoxicity of Drugs used to Treat Rheumatic Disorders

Because a detailed discussion of drug hepatotoxicity is provided elsewhere in this volume, only general remarks are made here. Although all the commonly employed antirheumatic drugs have been implicated in hepatotoxicity, these complications are fortunately infrequent. The most commonly implicated drug is aspirin in patients with Still's disease. Although usually asymptomatic, over 50% of patients have transaminase elevations without hepatomegaly. Liver biopsy reveals a spectrum of lesions, which include hepatocellular necrosis, nonspecific hepatitis, and Kupffer cell hyperplasia. These resolve when the drug is discontinued. A wide variety of hepatotoxic reactions have been reported with other nonsteroidal anti-inflammatory agents; they are all rare but potentially severe. Case reports of severe cholestasis mimicking biliary obstruction have been described as being attributable to gold salts.

SUMMARY

There are a variety of liver diseases that are caused by systemic or metabolic problems and are important to all clinicians. Some are a result of primary hepatic defects (e.g., Wilson's disease), others are a response to systemic nutritional and metabolic abnormalities (e.g., diabetes, obesity, parenteral nutrition), and still others are caused by individual inherited defects that result in hepatic and other manifestations (e.g., hemochromatosis, the porphyrias). Many of these disorders can lead to life-threatening complications if not diagnosed promptly and managed properly. Fortunately, specific therapy is available for most of these disorders.

SUGGESTED READING

Bacon BR and Tavill AS: Role of the liver in normal iron metabolism, Semin Liver Dis 4:181, 1984.

This article provides an overview of normal hepatic iron metabolism and includes detailed sections of hepatic uptake and release of iron as well as sections on several aspects of intracellular iron metabolism.

Bassett ML, Halliday JW, and Powell LW: Value of hepatic iron measurements in early hemochromatosis and determination of the critical iron level associated with fibrosis, Hepatology 6:24, 1986.

This article emphasizes the positive correlation between hepatic iron concentration and the occurrence of liver disease, and the value of hepatic iron measurements in differentiating alcoholic liver disease with iron overload from HHC.

Bloomer JR and Bonkovsky HL: The porphyrias, Disease-a-Month 35:1, 1989.

This is a comprehensive review written by two authorities on the subject.

Bomford A and Williams R: Long-term results of venesection therapy in idiopathic hemochromatosis, Q J Med 45:611, 1976.

The beneficial value of long-term phlebotomy therapy is described in this paper.

Capron J-P et al: Metronidazole in prevention of cholestasis associated with total parenteral nutrition, Lancet 1:446, 1983.

Therapeutic options to consider in patients with hepatic complications of TPN are described in this paper.

Diehl AM, Goodman Z and Ishak KG: Alcohol-like liver disease in nonalcoholics: a clinical and histologic comparison with alcohol-induced liver injury, Gastroenterology 95:1056, 1988.

This study describes the clinical, biochemical, and histologic features of nonalcoholic steatohepatitis and makes useful comparisons with other types of liver disease, notably alcoholic liver disease.

Hay JE et al: The nature of unexplained chronic aminotransferase elevations of a mild to moderate degree in asymptomatic patients, Hepatology 9:193, 1989.

Hultcrantz R et al: Liver investigation of 149 asymptomatic patients with moderately elevated activities of serum amino transferases, Scand J Gastroenterol 21:109, 1986.

These two studies show that fatty liver is a very common finding in asymptomatic patients with elevated serum liver enzymes.

Klein S and Nealon WH: Hepatobiliary abnormalities associated with total parenteral nutrition, Semin Liver Dis 8:237, 1988.

Both the hepatocellular and the biliary complications of total parenteral nutrition are reviewed in this paper.

Matuchansky C et al: Cyclic (nocturnal) total parenteral nutrition in hospitalized adult patients with severe digestive diseases: report of a prospective study, Gastroenterology 81:433, 1981.

Cyclic administration of TPN is promoted in this paper.

McCullough AJ et al: Diagnosis of Wilson's disease presenting as fulminant hepatic failure, Gastroenterology 84:161, 1983.

This paper describes the laboratory differentiation of fulminant and nonfulminant Wilson's disease.

Mills PR and Sturrock RD: Clinical associations between arthritis and liver disease, Ann Rheum Dis 41:295, 1982.

This article provides well-referenced reviews of the association between liver disease and collagen vascular disease.

Minuk GY, Kelly JK, and Hwang WS: Vitamin A hepatotoxicity in multiple family members, Hepatology 8:272, 1988.

This recent paper describes the clinical, biochemical, and histologic findings in the liver in hypervitaminosis A.

Nichols GM and Bacon BR: Hereditary hemochromatosis: pathogenesis and clinical features of a common disease, Am J Gastroenterol 84:851, 1989.

This review article provides an authoritative summary of the clinical manifestations of patients with HHC.

Niederau C et al: Survival and causes of death in cirrhotic and in noncirrhotic patients with primary hemochromatosis, N Engl J Med 313:1256, 1985.

This article offers the strongest evidence that phlebotomy therapy initiated in the precirrhotic stage can lead to normal life expectancy.

Runyon BA, LaBrecque DR, and Anuras S: The spectrum of liver disease in SLE. Am J Med 69:187, 1980.

This study indicates that the prevalence of liver disease in SLE may be higher than previously suspected.

Salata R, Klein I, and Levey GS: Thyroid hormone homeostasis and the liver, Semin Liver Dis 5:29,1985.

The principal physiologic and pathophysiologic thyroid-liver interactions are described in this paper.

Schaffner F and Thaler H: Non-alcoholic fatty liver disease, Prog Liver Dis 8:283, 1986.

This comprehensive paper thoroughly reviews all aspects of nonalcoholic fatty liver.

Scheinberg IH and Sternlieb I: Major problems in internal medicine. Vol 23, Wilson's disease, Philadelphia, 1984, WB Saunders Co.

This review article highlights all the clinical and pathologic features exhibited by patients with Wilson's disease.

Sternlieb I: Copper and the liver, Gastroenterology 78:1615, 1980.

The author presents a classic review of hepatic copper metabolism.

Sternlieb I and Scheinberg IH: Chronic hepatitis as a first manifestation of Wilson's disease, Ann Intern Med 76:59, 1972.

Chronic hepatitis as a manifestation of Wilson's disease is described in this paper.

Stone BG and Van Thiel DH: Diabetes mellitus and the liver, Semin Liver Dis 5:8, 1985.

The hepatic biochemical and clinical manifestations of diabetes mellitus are completely reviewed in this paper.

Van Thiel DH et al: Prognostic value of thyroid hormone levels in patients evaluated for liver transplantation, Hepatology 5:862, 1985.

This paper describes the prognostic importance of thyroid hormone levels in patients with chronic liver disease.

Weinblatt ME, Tesser JRP, and Gilliam JH: The liver in rheumatic diseases, Semin Arthritis Rheum 11:399, 1982.

This is a well-referenced review of hepatic complications in patients with rheumatic disease.

Winge DR: Normal physiology of copper metabolism, Semin Liver Dis 4:239, 1984.

This review emphasizes the role of the liver in normal copper metabolism.

29 Jaundice

Cameron Ghent

CLASSIFICATION

Biochemists often classify hyperbilirubinemia on the basis of which molecular form of bilirubin is elevated in the blood. This is also a highly appropriate classification scheme in certain clinical situations (e.g., neonatal jaundice). However, it is inimical to the modus operandi of experienced clinicians who mentally classify the possible causes of a patient's jaundice after completing a history and physical examination and before resorting to the laboratory determination of the molecular form of the excess bilirubin. Accordingly, in this classification I pay scant attention to the details of bilirubin chemistry (See Chapter 2) but delve into the following distinctions of greatest importance to the clinician in deciding on appropriate further investigation and treatment of the patient with jaundice.

- Overproduction of bilirubin
- Congenital defects in bilirubin metabolism
- Hepatocellular diseases
- Cholestatic diseases
- Combined and complex causes of jaundice

DIAGNOSTIC APPROACH

The first distinction that must be made in a discussion of the causes of the jaundice is between overt icterus, noted by the patient, family, examining physician, or nurse, as a yellow color of the eyes or skin and biochemically determined but clinically inapparent hyperbilirubinemia. The differential diagnosis of mild hyperbilirubinemia, which is not clinically detectable, includes almost all the disease processes producing deep jaundice but the converse is not true; i.e., deep jaundice carries a shorter list of possible diagnoses than mild jaundice or hyperbilirubinemia without jaundice does. Thus, for example, Gilbert's syndrome must be included in the differential diagnosis of the latter but not of deep chronic jaundice, except as an antecedent factor contributing to and complicating the clinical picture (Table 29-1).

It is clinically useful to remember that yellow discoloration of sclerae and skin is usually detectable when the stable level of serum bilirubin exceeds 2.4 to 3.0 mg/dl. However, when the serum bilirubin is rapidly rising (as in acute bile duct obstruction) clinical jaundice may be absent with much higher levels of bilirubin. In contrast, jaundice may be detected at lower levels of bilirubin when serum is being rapidly cleared (as after surgical relief of biliary obstruction).

It is intellectually challenging and a good learning experience to commit one-

Table 29-1 Features of jaundice

	Usual significance
Abrupt onset	Viral hepatitis or biliary obstruction
Intermittent, mild	Hemolysis, Gilbert's or hepatocellular disease
Very pronounced	Cholestasis
Insidious onset	Chronic hepatocellular disease or medical cholestatic disease

Table 29-2 Associated symptoms

	Usual Significance
Pruritus	Cholestasis
Dark urine	Bilirubinuria
Pale stools	Cholestasis, carcinoma of pancreas
Abdominal pain	Choledocholithiasis (intermittent, severe)
Fever	Viral hepatitis, cholangitis (episodic)
Anorexia, nausea, vomiting	Cholangitis, viral hepatitis
Considerable weight loss	Carcinoma of pancreas, ampulla, bile ducts

self to a specific tentative diagnosis in each case of jaundice without the benefit of laboratory tests. This approach will direct further evaluation and frequently greatly reduces the number of tests necessary to resolve the clinical problem. Broad categories that are traditionally used to direct further diagnostic investigations are prehepatic, hepatocellular, and cholestatic causes of jaundice. Although there is considerable overlap in the last, these broad categories are useful in characterizing jaundice during the patient interview and physical examination. In doing so, clinical interviewing and physical examination must be skilled and directed. This frequently involves "detective work," not often encouraged in medical training. The features of the jaundice itself (Table 29-1 and 29-2), associated symptoms and signs, history of past illnesses, drug history, social history, and a search for past investigations may all be very rewarding.

The History

The history of the jaundice itself is crucial. The duration and fluctuations of jaundice may be difficult to establish. In reviewing historical features in a patient with jaundice, a cautious skepticism about the reliability of the patient's account is helpful. Patient's relatives may be more reliable in determining the time of onset and waxing and waning of jaundice. The date of onset of jaundice should be carefully corroborated with them. Although some patients are simply unobservant, patients who very obviously have jaundice but are oblivious to their own color should be strongly suspected of suffering from disease related to substance abuse—it is difficult to see yourself clearly in the mirror if you are constantly too intoxicated to stand up. Intermittent mild jaundice over months or years , particularly with fasting or intercurrent illness, which has no associated symptoms or signs, strongly suggests a benign defect in bilirubin metabolism of some type,

Table 29-3 Investigation of isolated mild jaundice

	Anticipated results	
	Gilbert's disease	**Hemolysis**
Unconjugated bilirubin	Elevated	Elevated
Conjugated	Normal	Elevated
Hb Hct	Normal	Normal or low
Reticulocyte count	Normal	Elevated
Blood Smear	Normal	Abnormal
Urine for bilirubin	Negative	Negative
Transaminases, alkaline phosphatase	Normal	Normal

most commonly Gilbert's Disease, with or without a concomitant compensated hemolytic process. In such individuals, diagnostic investigations can be safely limited to a few noninvasive tests. (Table 29-3) However, any associated symptoms such as dark urine, pruritus or abdominal pain, which are chronologically related to episodes of jaundice, strongly suggest that unconjugated (prehepatic) jaundice is not the etiology and further investigation is mandatory. Uncovering a history of drug or alcohol abuse, sharing of needles, or promiscuous (particularly male homosexual) sexual practices demands the suspicious mind of a sleuth and the diplomacy of a Kissinger but can provide important clues to an alternative diagnosis of viral or alcoholic hepatitis, which may not be accompanied by other symptoms or signs.

Associated symptoms or physical signs frequently allow characterization of jaundice as hepatocellular or cholestatic, or point to an even more specific diagnosis (see Table 29-2). Pruritus is often severe, progressive, and disabling in cholestatic disorders and may precede jaundice by months or years, particularly in primary biliary cirrhosis. The onset is usually insidious and accompanied by fatigue. An abrupt onset coincident with dark urine and abdominal pain is more suggestive of choledocholithiasis. Most patients do not associate itch with liver disease, and this symptom must therefore be carefully elicited by direct questioning. So pervasive is the advertising influence of Madison Avenue that most patients (and many physicians) attribute pruritus to "dry skin" and fail to mention it or relate this symptom when being assessed for jaundice. Dark urine noticed by the patient signifies bilirubinuria and may be seen in either cholestatic or hepatocellular causes of jaundice. Pale stool does not mean the absence of bilirubin breakdown products, but rather the absence of food-derived chromogens from the gut. These apparently undergo an enterohepatic circulation and require both bile and pancreatic secretions to be converted into brown pigment. Theoretically, pale stool can therefore result from pancreatic duct obstruction in the absence of cholestasis. Consequently, clinically pale stools that precede the development of jaundice, itch, and dark urine by weeks or months are strongly suggestive of carcinoma of the head of the pancreas.

Abdominal pain accompanies many diseases associated with jaundice, but characteristics of the pain allow some diagnostic discrimination. Severe intermittent upper abdominal pain coinciding with fever and chills, deepening jaundice, nausea, and vomiting is strongly suggestive of choledocholithiasis. A mild, dull, right upper quadrant ache is more characteristic of diseases such as viral hepatitis, or chronic active hepatitis, especially when accompanied by tender hepatomegaly on physical examination. Fever may also frequently accompany alcoholic hepatitis. Severe progressive weight loss is most characteristic of neoplastic causes of jaundice, particularly carcinoma of the head of the pancreas.

The detective work of finding a record of past laboratory tests, often done as part of a routine screen and then completely ignored, can be more useful diagnostically than any amount of current testing. A patient with mild jaundice without bilirubinuria was believed to have a pure hemolytic jaundice caused by a *Mycoplasma pneumoniae* infection. However, one telephone call established that mild unconjugated hyperbilirubinemia without jaundice had been present before the infection, at the time of a hysterectomy 4 years earlier, and thereby confirmed a diagnosis of Gilbert's disease, which had remained clinically silent until exacerbated by the intercurrent pneumonia. A similar aggressive search for results of past testing of liver enzymes can be equally rewarding. A 25-year-old woman who had abused intravenously administered drugs in 1983 and shared needles at that time began to abuse alcohol in 1986. She was found on such searching to have had elevated serum bilirubin and ALT levels in 1985, thus providing the clue that her recent presentation with jaundice might be attributable to alcoholic liver disease complicated by chronic hepatitis C, or vice versa. A test for hepatitis C antibody was positive, and a liver biopsy specimen showed severe alcoholic hepatitis, which made determination of concomitant viral injury difficult.

Review questions when one is taking the history to detect clues about risk factors for exposure to viral or toxic hepatic injury or liver injury–associated multisystem disease may range from the obvious to the ridiculously obscure. Although eating raw shellfish is frequently listed as a risk for developing type A viral hepatitis, exposure to undiapered infants in day-care centers is a more common source of this infection. Travel to areas of the world where viral hepatitis is endemic may be relevant in providing a clue to the presence of hepatitis B or E, but casual sexual indiscretions with a member of a high risk group are much more difficult to uncover and equally important. The occupational exposures of health-care workers may also be highly relevant. Among the more obscure causes of jaundice, poisoning by *Amanita phalloides* (a poisonous mushroom) and tularemia from exposure to wild rodents may be overlooked unless the appropriate history is elicited.

Physical Examination

Even though a tentative diagnosis of jaundice as prehepatic, hepatocellular, or cholestatic, or an even more precise etiologic diagnosis may be made by history alone, a thorough physical examination is vital and at times can provide either definitive supporting evidence (Virchow's node or hepatic friction rub in metastatic carcinoma) or a single physical indication to rethink the diagnosis. Two cases will illustrate.

> A 56-year-old white mechanic was referred for further investigation of jaundice that had been extensively scrutinized elsewhere. Serum bilirubin had been 60 to 90 μmol/L (3.5 to 5.2 mg/dl) for 5 months, and he denied itch, ab-

dominal pain, or fever. There was a small amount of ascites detectable; liver enzymes were nonspecifically mildly abnormal, and serum albumin levels were depressed at 2.8 gm/dl. A previous percutaneous liver biopsy specimen had been reported to show extensive pericentral fibrosis, consistent with remote alcoholic liver disease. The history indicated that jaundice had begun 8 months after the patient had ceased his significant alcohol abuse and had been progressively worsening. Jugular venous distention noted previously had been attributed to ischemic cardiomyopathy with a vague history of nonexertional chest pain and an abnormal cardiac wall motion study. An astute intern noticed that the jugular venous pressure rose with inspiration (Kussmaul's sign). Further investigation confirmed very severe constrictive pericarditis. Pericardectomy led to complete resolution of jaundice over a further 6 months.

A 62-year-old male alcohol abuser admitted with deep jaundice and abdominal pain was believed to have severe alcoholic hepatitis. However, persistent pruritus coincident with the onset of jaundice was believed to be unusual for this, and careful physical examination revealed dullness to percussion in the left lung base and a 12 cm tender immobile mass in the epigastrium. A chest radiograph, a serum amylase determination, and endoscopic retrograde cholangiopancreatography (ERCP) confirmed that this man's jaundice was attributable to common bile duct compression from a large pancreatic pseudocyst associated with chronic pancreatitis, rather than to alcoholic liver disease. Percutaneous drainage of the pseudocyst led to complete resolution of jaundice and itch, though the serum bilirubin remained mildly elevated.

The need to search for physical signs of chronic liver disease is obvious, but the interpretation of such signs is not always unambiguous. The most reliable indicators of antecedent long-standing liver disease in the patient with jaundice are probably the presence of multiple spider nevi, dilated abdominal venous collaterals, ascites indicated by shifting dullness and a fluid thrill, and the firm consistency of an enlarged and nodular liver edge, though the latter judgment is very subjective. Palpable splenomegaly may be an indicator of chronic hematologic disease leading to or associated with hemolysis rather than caused by portal hypertension.

Further Routine Investigations

There is much debate about the appropriate routine investigation of jaundice with serum and urine tests, imaging studies, and invasive diagnostic tests. The precise extent of investigation, appropriate sequence, and the timing of these tests will depend not only on the characteristics of the problem as identified by patient interview and physical examination, but also by the experience and expertise of the clinician and the ancillary services available to him or her. Nevertheless there exists a core of tests that can be recommended to be performed at least once for all cases. These are listed in the box on p. 530.

Most clinical laboratories use some modification of the diazo reaction to measure total bilirubin spectrophotometrically with reasonable precision and consistency, provided that interfering substances in serum are adequately extracted. However, measurement of conjugates by this method produces considerabe overestimation of their concentration in the presence of excess unconjugated bilirubin.

ROUTINE TESTS IN PATIENTS WITH JAUNDICE

Serum total bilirubin
Urinalysis
Complete blood count, blood film
ALT, AST, alkaline phosphatase
γ-Glutamyl transferase

More accurate film chromatographic systems are becoming widely available. The need for fractionation of serum bilirubin at all diminishes if one remembers that the presence of detectable bilirubin in urine implies an elevated serum conjugated bilirubin and absence of bilirubinuria in the presence of a stable total serum bilirubin above 68 μmol/L (4 mg/dl) implies that the latter is largely or entirely unconjugated. The usefulness of bilirubin fractionation is greatest when serum levels are one to five times normal because few conditions producing unconjugated hyperbilirubinemia result in higher serum levels than this. The exception is in the investigation of neonatal jaundice where the finding of a high serum conjugated bilirubin may lead one away from the diagnosis of "physiologic" jaundice or hemolysis to early detection of neonatal hepatitis or "obstructive cholangiopathy." In neonates, the measurement of unconjugated serum bilirubin likewise has great therapeutic implications for commencement of phototherapy to prevent kernicterus. For this purpose, the newer more accurate methods of bilirubin fractionation by chromatography, such as the Kodak Ectachem system, are recommended.

The predictive value of a ratio of conjugated-to-unconjugated bilirubin measurement, even by accurate laboratory methods, to distinguish hepatocellular from cholestatic causes of jaundice is very limited. In studying 50 patients with proven primary biliary cirrhosis, I have found several with a completely normal serum conjugated bilirubin by the Ectachem method.

The measurement of hemoglobin, hematocrit, and mean corpuscular volume and the review of a blood film on a routine basis can be justified to detect anemia associated with hemolysis, macrocytosis associated with occult alcohol abuse, chronic liver disease, or vitamin B_{12} or folic acid deficiency, or anemia of chronic disease. The reticulocyte count serves only to confirm hemolysis with appropriate marrow responses and is indicated only if the clinical diagnosis is jaundice caused by unconjugated hyperbilirubinemia.

Serum transaminases and alkaline phosphatase should be measured once in any patient presenting with jaundice for the first time. In Gilbert's disease, hemolysis, and ineffective erythropoesis, their normality is simply reassuring evidence of the absence of underlying liver disease. In hepatocellular disease or cholestasis, the expectation is that they will be abnormal, and the pattern of abnormalities may provide further direction to investigation, more appropriate than simply investigating jaundice. Thus very high levels of transaminases (greater than 10 times normal) are suggestive of hepatocellular injury such as viral hepatitis, whereas disproportionate elevation of alkaline phosphatase may be suggestive of cholestasis. However, there are pitfalls in such pattern interpretations. Early in the course of acute biliary obstruction, such as choledocholithiasis, serum transaminases may rise to more than 1000 IU and then progressively fall. Furthermore, congestion of the liver, infiltrative disorders, systemic sepsis, and metastatic neoplasms are all associated with an "obstructive" enzyme pattern. At times a patient with mild jaundice may have completely normal "liver enzymes" with an inactive cirrhosis—it is when the clinical diagnosis is hepatocellular disease but the enzymes are normal that fractionation of serum bilirubin to confirm the elevation of conjugated bilirubin may be most useful. One other unusual pattern of enzyme elevation is very suggestive of a precise diagnosis. This is the elevation of serum alkaline phosphatase unaccompanied by an elevation of γ-glutamyl transpeptidase. Such a clustering in a pruritic female using oral contraceptives or who is pregnant is strong supporting evidence for the diagnosis of familial cholestasis of pregnancy.

Further diagnostic testing is discussed in the following sections dealing with major categories of jaundice, as outlined in the introduction.

BILIRUBIN OVERPRODUCTION

- Extravascular red blood cell destruction
  - Trauma, hematoma resorption
  - Burns
  - Pulmonary infarction
- Intravascular hemolysis
  - Stored or mismatched blood transfusion
  - Defective heart valves
  - Drugs, e.g., α-methyldopa
  - Bacterial infections, e.g., *Mycoplasma pneumoniae*
  - Wilson's disease
  - Red blood cell defects, e.g., sickle cell disease

OVERPRODUCTION OF BILIRUBIN

Normal adult humans produce 250 to 350 mg of bilirubin daily. Most of this is from breakdown of senescent red blood cells in the reticuloendothelial system. A small proportion derives from ineffective erythropoeisis, which may be increased in patients deficient in vitamin B_{12} or folic acid. A somewhat larger proportion (25%) derives from the breakdown of hepatic hemoproteins, a fraction that may be greatly increased by the very rare inherited disorder called "shunt hyperbilirubinemia" and in erythropoetic protoporphyria.

Most causes of overproduction of bilirubin are readily apparent from the clinical setting (see box above). Trauma or surgery with hematoma resorption invariably produces a bilirubin load. Absorption of a 1 liter of hematoma leads to production of 5000 mg of bilirubin (if one assumes a normal hematocrit), and combined with transfusion of blood with a more rapid destruction than normal, the overproduction of bilirubin can easily exceed the normal liver's capacity for uptake and conjugation. Intravascular red blood cell destruction, especially with defective or leaky native, artificial, or bioprosthetic heart valves, can also lead to overproduction of bilirubin.

The list of congenital defects in red blood cell membranes leading to rapid cell turnover and bilirubin overproduction is extremely long and belongs in a hematology rather than a hepatology text. Although such diseases as thalassemia major or sickle cell disease seldom are diagnosed first with jaundice as the presenting feature, less florid red blood cell defects may produce subtle changes in hematologic parameters and present as jaundice attributable to bilirubin overproduction. The clue to all of these is the presence of abnormal red blood cell morphology, with or without anemia, and usually accompanied by reticulocytosis. The clinical setting will seldom provide clues to the exact cause of hemolysis, which can be investigated further if necessary depending on the results of examination of a blood film, e.g., hemoglobin electrophoresis if abnormal red blood cell forms are detected, or serum B_{12} and folate levels if macrocytosis with hypersegmented neutrophils are observed.

Even in individuals with apparently straightforward Gilbert's syndrome, a family history, review of medications, and social history with respect to risk factors for chronic liver disease may produce valuable ancillary information. If several members of a family are affected, a familial hemolytic process is more likely than an isolated defect in bilirubin conjugation. α-Methyldopa may convert anicteric Gilbert's syndrome into overt jaundice by increasing bilirubin production. Similar increased bilirubin production frequently contributes to jaundice in sepsis, falciparum malaria, and burns and after blood transfusions. Hemolysis is also a frequent, but seldom an isolated, feature of Wilson's disease.

The jaundice is typically mild, intermittent, and painless and is associated with no other symptoms or signs. The urine tests negative for bilirubin, and the liver enzymes are normal, unless the liver is secondarily damaged by ischemia (sickling crisis) or by viral hepatitis, transmitted by transfusions to treat the hematologic disorder. Serum lactate dehydrogenase may be elevated, serum haptoglobin decreased, and bone marrow examination will show erythropoetic hyperplasia, but these tests are seldom necessary to explain the jaundice.

A list of common causes of bilirubin overproduction is given in the box on p. 531.

CONGENITAL DEFECTS IN BILIRUBIN METABOLISM

Gilbert's Disease

Gilbert's disease is by far the most common congenital defect in bilirubin metabolism, occurring in 3% to 7% of the population. The exact cause of the defect, and indeed the existence of a distinct defect common to all persons labeled as having Gilbert's disease, is disputed. There appear to be individuals with a decreased affinity of unconjugated bilirubin on hepatic Y protein (ligandin), which is believed to be necessary for holding unconjugated bilirubin within hepatocytes and presenting it to the conjugating enzyme bilirubin UDP glucuronyl transferase. This conjugation step is also slower than normal in at least some individuals with Gilbert's disease.

Clinically Gilbert's disease is frequently diagnosed because of an incidental finding of mild hyperbilirubinemia during the course of an intercurrent illness or during investigations of mild intermittent jaundice. The patients may have a family history of a similar disorder, but the inheritance pattern is not definitively known.

Patients are often misdiagnosed as having viral hepatitis despite the absence of characteristic symptoms, signs, or laboratory tests. Bilirubin is absent from the urine and transaminase levels are normal. Fasting and intercurrent illnesses raise serum bilirubin levels to the point where jaundice may be appreciated, possibly by inhibition of hepatic bilirubin uptake by serum fatty acids and by increased bilirubin production with fasting. Tests for the defect by fasting have little clinical utility and are not specific. There is often a mild hemolytic defect as well, but this may be fortuitous—people with bilirubin overproduction and decreased bilirubin clearance are more likely to develop overt jaundice than those with only one defect.

Provided that the clinical examination is consistent with Gilbert's disease and the tests outlined in Table 29-3 are confirmatory, adult patients can be confidently diagnosed as having Gilbert's disease, reassured, and dismissed without further tests. Similar patients in the pediatric age group, however, especially if serum bilirubin exceeds 6 mg/dl, should be investigated further for possible Crigler-Najjar disease, type II.

Crigler-Najjar Disease

Crigler-Najjar disease is an extremely rare but severe and often fatal disorder. Arias divided the original description of the disease into two, type I and a milder type II, based on clinical features and responsiveness to treatment. Although the basic defect is undoubtedly complex, almost complete failure of bilirubin conjugation is a cardinal feature of both types. As a result, unconjugated bilirubin accumulates and bilirubin encephalopathy is severe. In type I disease, unconjugated bilirubin levels of 20 to 40 mg/dl develop in the neonatal period and fail to fall with phenobarbital therapy. In contrast, patients with type II disease have milder jaundice, survive into adulthood, and show a pronounced decline in serum bilirubin levels with phenobarbital. Type I disease has been successfully treated by phototherapy and plasma exchange, followed by early liver transplantation. Type II disease need not be treated at all except for cosmetic purposes.

Dubin-Johnson and Rotor's Syndromes

The extremely rare and similar disorders Dubin-Johnson and Rotor's syndromes are characterized by defective hepatic excretion of conjugated bilirubin. Clinically, both present as mild fluctuating jaundice with bilirubinuria and serum bilirubin levels of up to 20 mg/dl. These defects may be uncovered by intercurrent illnesses or drugs, usually present in adulthood, and are autosomal recessive traits. There are characteristic patterns of bromosulfophthalein kinetics and urinary coproporphyrin excretion in Dubin-Johnson syndrome but not present in Rotor's syndrome. The other difference is the presence of a dark granular pigment in hepatocytes in Dubin-Johnson syndrome. In both conditions the liver architecture is preserved.

These conditions are benign, require no treatment, and are the most common in Iranian Jews (Table 29-4).

HEPATOCELLULAR DISEASES

Hepatocellular causes of jaundice are common, multitudinous, and often difficult to diagnose with precision. The direction of investigation, if any investigation is needed at all, will usually depend more on the associated clinical and labora-

Table 29-4 Congenital disorders of bilirubin metabolism

	Gilbert	Crigler-Najjar Type I	Crigler-Najjar Type II	Dubin-Johnson	Rotor
Serum bilirubin					
Conjugated	Normal	Normal	Normal	2-16	2-16
Unconjugated	1-16	20+	2-8	Normal	Normal
Age of presentation	Teens-adult	Neonate	Child-teen	Adult	Adult
Liver histology	Normal	Bile plugs	Bile Plugs	Pigment	Normal
Liver enzymes	Normal	Normal	Normal	Normal	Normal
Defect	Uptake	Conjugation	Conjugation	Excretion	Excretion
Incidence	Common	Very rare	Rare	Rare	Rare

tory abnormalities than on the level of bilirubin or the jaundice itself. Thus a patient with a history of recently sharing needles for intravenous heroin abuse, a moderate degree of recent-onset jaundice, systemic symptoms of fever, nausea, anorexia, and vomiting, transaminases of greater than 10 times normal, a normal alkaline phosphatase, and bilirubinuria need not raise suspicions of extrahepatic biliary obstruction, and imaging of the liver and biliary tree is neither necessary nor appropriate. Likewise, it would be highly inappropriate to *not* test for known hepatotrophic viruses in such a patient. The major clinical difficulty comes when there are no such clear-cut clinical clues to the cause of the jaundice, when the jaundice persists for many weeks, or when *too* many clues are present, producing conflicting evidence. A case illustration will outline some principles.

> A 28-year-old married male school teacher with no antecedent history of liver disease or risk factors underwent an emergency proctocolectomy for toxic megacolon complicating ulcerative colitis of 9 months' duration. He received four units of blood intraoperatively and developed jaundice 3 days later. This was attributed to hemolysis (bilirubin overproduction) and sepsis and subsided in a further week. Bilirubin was not fractionated, and urinalysis was not done, but it was noted that his liver enzymes were "mildly abnormal."
>
> Three months postoperatively he developed jaundice, dark urine, anorexia, nausea, and malaise. Transaminases were found to be greater than 10 times normal, and his liver was tender to percussion. A clinical diagnosis of posttransfusional hepatitis C was considered. However, deep jaundice persisted, and 2 months later he was tested for hepatitis B and was found to be positive for HBsAg, HbeAg, and anti-HBc. Retrospectively a donor of one unit of blood was found to be positive for anti-HBc, and a diagnosis of acute hepatitis B was entertained.
>
> He failed to improve and continued to have deep jaundice 6 months after surgery with a serum total bilirubin greater than 20 mg/dl but transaminases of less than 3 times normal.
>
> 1. What is the most likely diagnosis?
> 2. Will fractionation of serum bilirubin help?
> 3. Will ultrasound of his liver and bile ducts help?
> 4. What detective work is likely to be most rewarding?

In fact, the detective work included locating serum from preoperative tests and determining that it was negative for all markers for hepatitis B but showed a serum bilirubin of 2.1 mg/dl, an ALT of 120, an AST of 64, and an alkaline phosphatase of 1140 IU. Further inquiry disclosed that he had been pruritic for 1 year before his surgery but had not told his physician, attributing it to "dry skin."

With this additional information, his attending physician thought that the most likely diagnosis was primary sclerosing cholangitis associated with ulcerative colitis. Bilirubin fractionation was not done, and so the answer to this question remains moot. An ultrasound examination was done and was reported to be completely normal. Because of this, a liver biopsy was done, and the specimens showed "extensive patchy portal fibrosis with piecemeal necrosis and lobular hepatitis, consistent with chronic hepatitis B." Eventually, after another 2 months, ERCP was performed and showed a very irregular ductal system without dilatation (hence the normal ultrasound results) with a dominant stricture in the common hepatic duct. Endoscopic dilatation of the stricture led to complete resolution of his jaundice.

CHOLESTATIC DISEASE

The preceding case history illustrates the difficulty in differentiating hepatocellular and cholestatic causes of jaundice. However, clinical features commonly allow one to clearly categorize jaundice as cholestatic, (see Tables 29-1 and 29-2) or arrive at a more precise diagnosis. In such cases, it is usually necessary or desirable to do some further investigation to confirm the diagnosis or to treat the cause (Table 29-5). The exceptions are those situations in which cholestasis is chronologically so closely linked to administration of a drug known to cause cholestasis that withdrawal of the drug and waiting is all that is necessary. A second situation where imaging of the liver and biliary tree may not be necessary is in the patient with a very typical history, physical examination, and laboratory profile of primary biliary cirrhosis. In a middle-aged woman with the insidious onset of itch, fatigue, painless jaundice, and laboratory evidence of cholestasis, elevated IgM, and positive antimitochondrial antibody tests, liver biopsy is more appropriate than an image of the liver.

Table 29-5 Investigation of cholestasis

Feature	Action
1. History of drug use	Stop drug; reassess
2. History is suggestive of PBC	Test AMA, IgM If positive, do liver biopsy
3. History is suggestive of mechanical obstruction (stone, stricture, tumor)	Do ultrasonography, endoscopic retrograde cholangiopancreatography (ERCP)

With the proliferation of imaging modalities, the clinician is faced with too many choices in determining the cause of what he or she believes is "obstructive jaundice" in a patient. Ultrasonography? ERCP?, CT scan? MRI scan? HIDA scan?" endoscopic ultrasonography?, transhepatic cholangiogram?. There is a tendency to do them all, though that is likely to lead to confusion. The general consensus at present is that ultrasound is the initial best imaging modality and that direct cholangiography either by endoscopic retrograde cannulation or by transhepatic puncture of ducts in the liver produces the most precise anatomic detail. ERCP is preferred in most centers because of the potential to treat the cause of the obstruction at the same time by endoscopic sphincterotomy, stone extraction, stricture dilatation or placement of a stent.

An occasional patient with deep jaundice and cholestatic features will present a formidable diagnostic challenge. When all tests have been done and have yielded normal or equivocal results, it is time to return to basics. A fresh complete history and physical examination in such a patient may reveal a previously overlooked family history of relevance or a physical finding such as lymphadenopathy or an extrahepatic focus of infection. Cholestasis is a rare paraneoplastic manifestation of Hodgkin's disease or non-Hodgkin's lymphoma or an indirect consequence of systemic sepsis.

COMBINED AND COMPLEX CAUSES OF JAUNDICE

The case previously discussed under hepatocellular disease illustrates the problem of combined and complex causes of jaundice. There are two other situations in which many factors contribute to jaundice.

Jaundice in the Intensive Care Unit

The patient in the ICU who is observed to have suddenly developed jaundice produces an exciting challenge. Bilirubin overproduction, sepsis, drug toxicity, and ischemic injury may all contribute to "multifactorial jaundice." However, this label does not explain the jaundice, and in an individual patient it may, with experience, be possible to weigh all the contributing factors and search for others. Nowhere is medical detective snooping more rewarding.

Jaundice after Liver Transplantation

Jaundice after liver transplantation is more fully covered in the chapter on liver transplantation. However, besides all the causes of jaundice in anyone else, rejection of the allograft is added to the list of causes of jaundice in these persons. It should not be assumed, however, that jaundice after liver transplantation is attributable to rejection; indeed, sepsis and biliary obstruction are commoner causes than rejection in my experience.

SUMMARY

An approach to jaundice emphasizing the features that will help on history and physical examination to classify jaundice into one of four categories has been reviewed. The appropriate investigations common to all cases of jaundice are presented with an outline of the more specific detailed investigations for each category.

SUGGESTED READING

Balistreri WF: Neonatal cholestasis, Semin Liver Dis 7(2):Forward, 1987.

This is an overview of a special clinical problem and has enough detail for most clinicians.

Becker SD et al: Postoperative jaundice, Semin Liver Dis 8:183-190, 1988.

The "multifactorial" causes of this problem are placed in perspective in this article.

Blankaert N and Fevery J: Physiology and pathophysiology of bilirubin metabolism. In Zakim O and Boyer TD, editor: Hepatology, Philadelphia, 1990, WB Saunders Co.

A more detailed discussion of bilirubin chemistry with an excellent review of congenital syndromes, with 672 references is presented.

Frank BC et al: Clinical evaluation of jaundice: guideline of the patient care committee of the American Gastroenterologic Association, JAMA 262:3031-3034, 1989.

This is a very pragmatic, common-sense, and clinically oriented consensus.

Schorschmidt BF: Bile formation and cholestasis. In Zakim O and Boyer TD, editor: Hepatology, Philadelphia, 1990, WB Saunders Co.

Here is a research-oriented detailed account of cellular and molecular events in bile formation.

Zimmerman HZ and Deschner KW: Differential diagnosis of jaundice, Hosp Pract, pp 99-122, May 1987.

Here is practical advise with clinical gems from senior, experienced clinicians.

30 Diseases of the Biliary Tract

Frederick C. Johlin, Jr.

Gallstones are the most frequent cause of biliary tract disease, far outshadowing all other forms of biliary pathologic conditions. The emphasis of this chapter therefore is to promote a greater insight into the clinical presentation and the pathophysiology of gallstones. This chapter is also a discussion of some less frequent but no less clinically important entities that provide general insights into other clinical problems. Key points have been deliberately reiterated because one can never assume that the busy clinician will be able to read a chapter in its entirety. New options in the treatment of gallstones have recently become available. Some of these options have been introduced as a result of consumer pressure rather than as a result of careful scientific testing. Perhaps the most blatant example of this is laparoscopic cholecystectomy. The clinician must be furnished with new techniques in order to fulfill his or her role as patient advocate.

GALLSTONES

Seventy-five percent of gallstones are cholesterol stones (Figure 30-1). Calculated by percentage dry weight, "cholesterol" stones and "mixed" stones are 75% cholesterol anhydride. The remaining dry weight is made up of other lipids, amorphous material, and varying amounts of pigment. Cholesterol, the major sterol in bile, is a water-insoluble lipid that is secreted into the bile by the hepatocytes. The solubility of cholesterol is altered by other biliary lipids. The constituents of bile that solubilize cholesterol include the phospholipid lecithin and bile acids, products of cholesterol metabolism. Bile also contains glycoproteins, calcium carbonate, amorphous materials, and bilirubinate. Calcium bilirubinate is the main constituent of pigmented stones. Its concentration of calcium bilirubinate in bile varies significantly, depending on the rate of red blood cell turnover.

Gallbladder bile is made up of 0.7% cholesterol, 4% phospholipid, 12% bile salts, and 82% water. The aqueous phase of bile contains several electrolytes including bicarbonate. It takes 50 bile acid molecules to dissolve 1 cholesterol molecule, until lecithin is added. As lecithin is added, the ratio drops from 50:1 to 7:1. The maximum solubility of cholesterol in water is 20 μg/L. This can increase to 20 to 40 gm/L if the optimal concentrations of bile acids and lecithin are present.

The solubility of cholesterol in bile is also determined by a complex interaction of nucleation factors that either promote

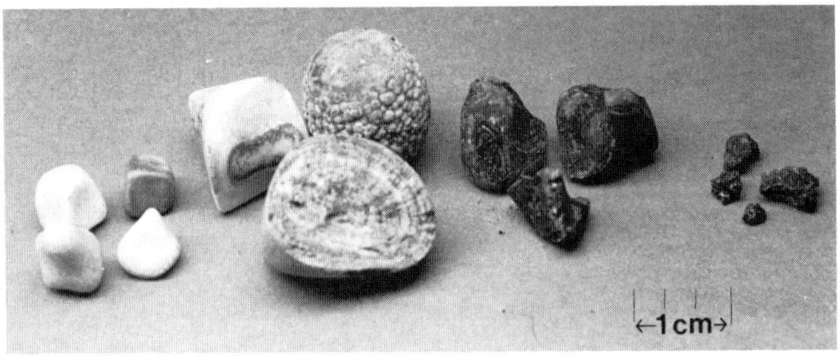

Figure 30-1
Choledochal cysts. Gallstones have varying degrees of cholesterol and bilirubinate. *Left,* "Pure" cholesterol stones; *right,* bilirubinate stones. The mixed stones in the middle have more pigment (bilirubinate) as one moves to the right. The stone that is fractured in two pieces has rings documenting the progressive growth of this stone.

or inhibit the formation of vesicles. Cholesterol crystals are the first physical stage in gallstone formation. The lithogenic index is a measure of the relative ratio of cholesterol to bile acids and phospholipids. Bile with a lithogenic index of less than 1 will dissolve cholesterol. Bile with a lithogenic index greater than 1 is saturated with cholesterol.

Colloidal interactions explain how cholesterol is solubilized in bile through the formation of micelles, mixed micelles, and unilaminar vesicles. Bile salts are amphiphiles. Their hydrophobic end can interact with the steroid nucleus of cholesterol while the hydrophobic end can interact with water (Figure 30-2, *A*). The hydrophilic end comprises a polar side chain, a conjugated carboxyl group (to glycine or taurine), and a polar hydroxyl group. This colloidal interaction forms a spherical micelle, with the hydrophobic cholesterol in the center (Figure 30-2, *B*). Phospholipids such as lecithin (which compromises 95.5% of the phospholipids in bile), lysolecithin, and phosphatidylethanolamine interact within the liquid crystal matrix between bile acids to improve the solubility of cholesterol. Biliary phospholipids are hydrolyzed by pancreatic enzymes and do not participate in the enterohepatic circulation.

Bile acids form the backbone of micelles and mixed micelles, and unilamellar vesicles are composed mostly of lecithin. The primary bile acid, cholic acid and chenodeoxycholic acid (Figure 30-3) are synthesized in the liver. Chenodeoxycholic acid is a dihydroxy bile acid, whereas cholic acid is a trihydroxy bile acid. The 7-hydroxy epimer of chenodeoxycholic acid is ursodeoxycholic acid. Despite their structural similarities, these bile acids differ in their clinical toxicity, because ursodeoxycholic is significantly less toxic and has fewer side effects. Bile acids that are not absorbed by the terminal ileum pass into the colon. Here, secondary bile acids, which are metabolites of primary bile acids, are formed by bacterial enzymes. Deoxycholic acid and lithocholic acid are the predominant secondary bile

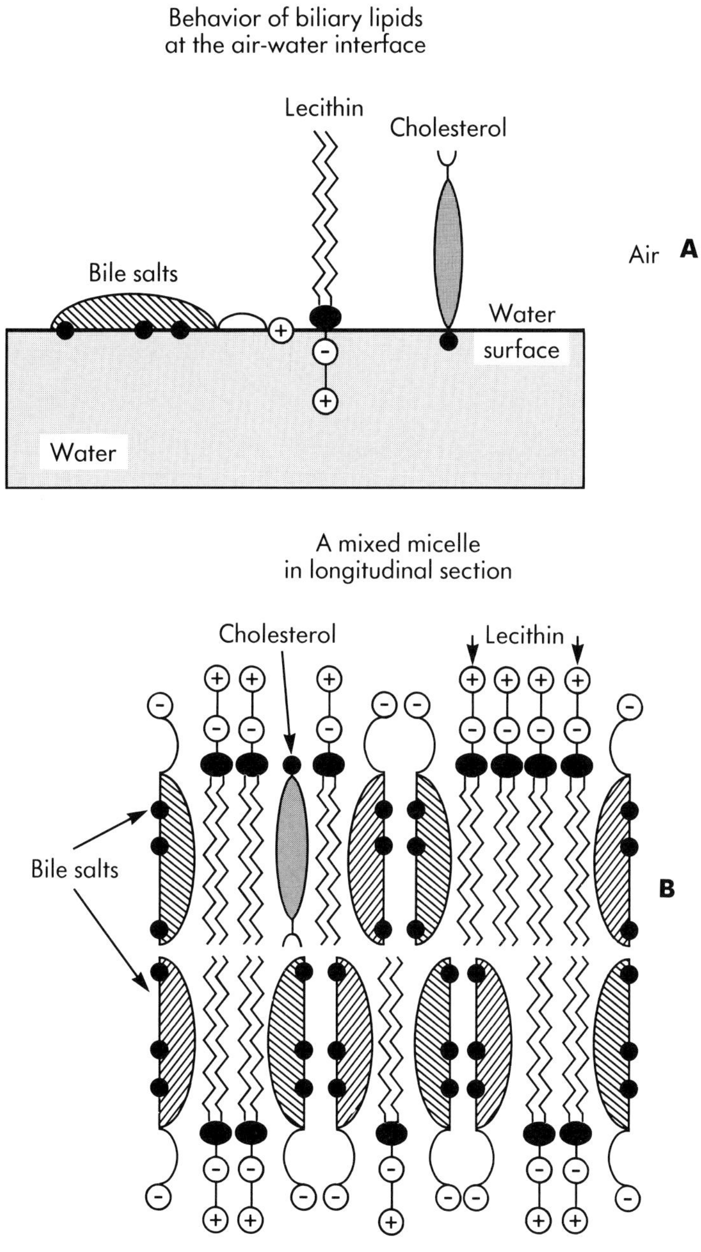

Figure 30-2
A, Behavior of biliary lipids. The interactions between bile salts, cholesterol, and lecithin with water are depicted. **B,** Mixed micelles. The way in which these biliary lipids interact with one another is also represented by the longitudinal section through a mixed micelle.

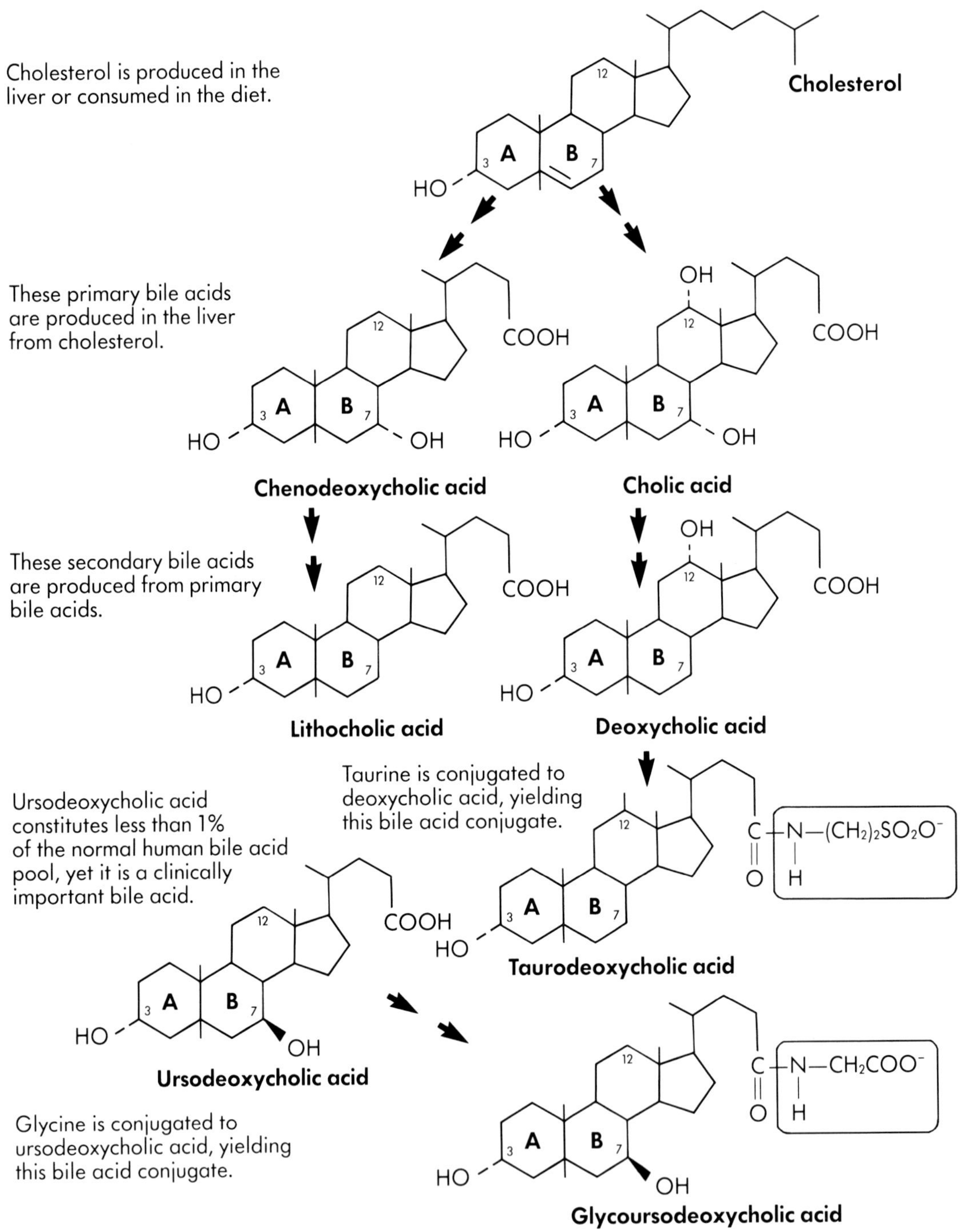

Figure 30-3
Human bile acid metabolism. The chemical structures of the three major groups of bile acids are shown. The primary bile acids are a metabolic product of cholesterol. In general, the solubility of bile acids in water is determined by the number of hydroxyl groups. Bile acid conjugates are also depicted: a taurine conjugate of deoxycholic acid, which is taurodeoxycholic acid, and the glycine conjugate of ursodeoxycholic acid, which is glycoursodeoxycholic acid.

acids. Lithocholic acid is only slightly absorbed, whereas deoxycholic acid undergoes enterohepatic circulation.

The total bile acid pool of a 70 kg male is estimated to be 5 gm, with 90% of the excreted bile acids being recovered by reabsorption into the enterohepatic circulation. Ten percent, or 500 mg of the bile acid pool, must be synthesized each day to replace stool losses. This consumes half of the body's cholesterol production per day. The loss of bile acids in the stool may be the only excretory route for endogenously produced cholesterol.

Genetic Factors

The serum cholesterol level correlates poorly with the risk of gallstone formation, except in patients with a type IV hyperlipidemia and, potentially, types I and IIb. Northern Europeans have a higher incidence of cholesterol gallstones than southern Europeans. American Indians, especially the Pima Indians, have one of the highest known incidences of gallstones, approaching 75% by the sixth decade. A familial history of gallstones also indicates an increased risk of developing gallstones. Persons on high caloric diets and those with obesity and frequent weight fluctuations are also at increased risk for gallstone formation.

Physical Factors

It is widely agreed that cholesterol gallstones require lithogenic bile for their formation. Although supersaturated bile is necessary, it is not always sufficient for stone formation. Many patients have supersaturated bile and yet do not develop gallstones. Fasting alone will elevate the cholesterol content of bile, but gallstones do not form. Cholesterol crystal growth appears to be facilitated by gallbladder mucus and inhibited by apolipoprotein and lecithin vesicles. Aspirin may reduce the risk of developing gallstones, presumably by reducing gallbladder mucus formation. A nucleation factor has long been proposed as an etiologic agent in the formation of gallstones. When bile is removed from persons who do not have stones and is mixed with bile from persons with cholesterol stones, cholesterol crystals can form without altering the cholesterol concentration. In addition to nucleation factors, the formation of gallstones is enhanced by the presence of a nidus. The nidus for gallstones can include such varied substances as mucus, bacteria, calcium bilirubinate, and foreign bodies such as suture material and metal clips. The role of biliary glycoproteins in the formation of gallstones continues to be an area of active investigation.

Bacteria

Bacteria are effective in producing deconjugated bile salts, which have a decreased ability to dissolve cholesterol. Colonies of bacteria can also form a nucleus for new stones. Bacterial contamination of gallbladder bile is more common in third-world countries than in the Sestern hemisphere. *Escherichia coli* and *Salmonella* are frequently found in the gallbladders of persons from Central America. *E. coli* is especially effective in the deconjugation of bile acids, thereby reducing cholesterol solubility. In Western countries, gallbladder bile is usually sterile at the time of cholecystectomy, and bacteria do not play a major role in the formation of most stones.

Drugs and Bowel Disease

Clofibrate and cholestyramine are therapies directed at lowering serum cholesterol and may increase the risk of gallstone formation by increasing the biliary excretion of cholesterol or by reducing the bile acid pool, respectively. Steatorrhea from either terminal ileal disease or pancreatic insufficiency will also increase the risk of forming gallstones. Terminal ileal disease and pancreatic insufficiency reduce the bile acid pool by reducing reabsorption of bile salts and thereby increase the lithogenic index of bile.

Gallbladder Statis

Gallbladder stasis increases the risk of stone and sludge formation. Several causes of gallbladder stasis exist. Those persons receiving parenteral nutrition without enteral feedings fail to empty their gallbladders and frequently develop biliary sludge and gallstones. Promoting gallbladder emptying by adding oral supplements or by using synthetic analogs of cholecystokinin may reduce gallbladder stasis. Vagotomy or visceral neuropathy reduces gallbladder emptying. Hormone excesses of somatostatin and glucagon prevent adequate gallbladder contraction.

Gender

Pregnancy is associated with reduced smooth muscle tone, impaired gallbladder contractility, and increased levels of estriol, especially during the third trimester. Estrogens reduce bile acid secretion. Prolonged estrogen use appears to increase the risk of developing gallstones twofold. Multiple pregnancies also increase the risk of gallstones by at least the same degree.

Age and Gallstone Disease

The incidence of concomitant choledocholithiasis, or bile duct stones, with cholelithiasis, or gallbladder stones, increases dramatically with age; on average it approaches 20% at the time of cholecystectomy. Between 50 and 60 years of age, 18% of those with gallstones will have symptoms. At the time of cholecystectomy, 14% of those patients will also have bile duct stones. In the 81- to 90-year-old age group, 57% of those people with gallstones will have symptoms and, if these patients have a cholecystectomy, over 90% will have bile duct stones. Therefore, with advancing age, the relative risk of symptomatic gallstones increases, as does the risk of bile duct stones.

Pigment Stones

Pigmented stones are small (see Figure 30-1) and are composed of 10% to 25% cholesterol (weight/weight). They are black or dark brown and derive their pigment from calcium bilirubinate. They also contain calcium phosphate, calcium carbonate, and cholesterol. Groups at risk to develop pigmented stones include those from the Orient and those persons with a chronic hemolytic process. Examples of the latter include hereditary spherocytosis, sickle cell anemia, and acquired hemolysis from prosthetic heart valves. The relative trace composition of calcium bilirubinate in cholesterol stones can increase with age and is higher in males than in females, thus adding some color to these stones.

Patients with cirrhosis have a high incidence of mixed or pigmented gallstones, despite having nonlithogenic bile. Normally, 80% of the body's cholesterol is formed in the liver. The remainder comes from diet and other tissues. However, in advanced liver disease, cholesterol production drops dramatically. Portal hypertension causing accelerated red blood cell destruction contributes to the formation of pigment stones or adds a pigment layer to the surface of previously formed cholesterol stones. A defect in the beta-glucuronidation of bilirubin is another source of bilirubinate stones.

Chronic inflammation of the bile ducts can result in primary bile duct pigmented-stone formation. These patients rarely have gallbladder stones. Oriental cholangiohepatitis (OCH) and sclerosing cholangitis are disorders in which this problem occurs (see discussion of choledocholithiasis, p.547). These patients rarely have gallbladder stones.

Chemical contact dissolution of pigment stones is not yet possible. Bile salts, methyl *tert*-butyl ether, and lithotripsy of the gallbladder will not free the patient of these stones. Therefore cholecystectomy is recommended for symptomatic patients with pigmented stones.

ACUTE CHOLECYSTITIS

In the United States, cholecystectomy is the most frequently performed elective surgery requiring hospital admission. It is estimated that 20 million Americans have gallstones. Over 500,000 gallbladder surgeries are performed each year for symptoms ranging from postprandial gas and bloating to acute cholecystitis (ACC). In 95% of cases, acute cholecystitis is caused by obstruction to bile flow through the cystic duct. This obstruction is caused by stones in 90% of the cases. Stone obstruction typically takes place in the neck or infundibulum (Hartmann's pouch) of the gallbladder. A closed-space infection may then develop in the gallbladder. Right upper quadrant abdominal pain, fever, nausea, and vomiting will bring these patients to medical attention. In 5% of episodes, ACC occurs in patients without stones. This condition is referred to as "acalculous acute cholecystitis."

Only 20% of the patients with cholelithiasis have symptoms. Of those with symptoms, 20% develop uncomplicated ACC whereas 10% have complications from ACC. The majority of those with symptoms, about 70%, will have chronic symptoms and chronic cholecystitis (CCC). A more appropriate term might be "intermittent gallbladder pain complex."

The combination of scintigraphy (see Figure 30-4, *C*) and ultrasonography in the management of patients with acute cholecystitis provides a diagnostic sensitivity and specificity of 95%.

Pathophysiology

Acute calculous cholecystitis. In Western societies, gallstones consist primarily of cholesterol. Gallstones are the source of 90% of ACC episodes. Gallstones grow slowly in ambulatory persons on a standard diet. Epidemiologic studies and radioisotope incorporation in the gallstones of people living near the Nevada nuclear test sites have demonstrated that stones grow slowly and may not produce symptoms for decades. Asymptomatic cholelithiasis is no doubt the precursor to symptomatic gallstones.

Acute acalculous cholecystitis. In an intensive care unit population the frequency of acalculous ACC may approach the frequency of calculous ACC. Acalculous ACC is often seen in situations that result in gallbladder stagnation. Clinical situations that place patients at risk for this condition are (1) multiple trauma, (2) extensive burns, (3) central venous nutrition, (4) mechanical ventilation, (5) prolonged general anesthesia, (6) heart failure, and (7) transfusion reaction. In the nonacute care setting, inflammation of the gallbladder without stones can be the result of a bacterial infection including (1) tuberculosis, (2) typhoid fever, (3) cholera, (4) syphilis, (5) leptospirosis, and (6) actinomycosis. Viral agents that cause acute acalculous ACC are typically confined to childhood illnesses, such as Kawasaki syndrome.

Clinical Manifestations

The essential findings suggestive of a diagnosis of acute cholecystitis are pain, nausea and vomiting, mild jaundice, and low-grade fever with leukocytosis. The pain is severe and steady but not colicky. The pain is typically in the hypochondrium or epigastrium, lasting 12 to 24 hours. Patients are sometimes admitted to the coronary care unit because of the severity of the pain and occasional substernal location of the discomfort. Voluntary guarding may obscure a focal point of palpable tenderness. If the edge of the gallbladder can be captured by direct palpation, inspiration may be arrested in midbreath, a finding known as Murphy's sign. Threefourths of patients vomit during the acute attack. It has been proposed that vomiting or other Valsalva maneuvers can dislodge the impacted stone resulting in pain relief in up to half of the patients. When the pain episode resolves, most patients will describe an area of residual tenderness. This corresponds to the contact point of the fundus of the gallbladder with the anterior abdominal wall. A palpable gallbladder should be expected in less than one fourth of patients, and one fourth will have clinical evidence of jaundice, i.e., a bilirubin greater than 3 mg/dl. Spiking temperatures, colicky intermittent pain, elevations of the amylase and lipase, and a bilirubin more than three times normal should be suggestive of a more complicated course or alternative diagnosis.

Patients that present with progressive jaundice, spiking fevers, colicky abdominal pain (Charcot's triad), and clinical deterioration have cholangitis attributable to bile duct stone or obstruction of the bile duct by the inflamed gallbladder (Figure 30-4, *A, B* and *C*). Liver-compression tenderness in these patients is not specific but is suggestive of a more diffuse hepatic inflammatory process than that seen with acute cholecystitis. Severe back pain, especially with an elevated serum lipase, should raise the question of gallstone pancreatitis.

Complications of Cholecystitis

Perforation, gangrene, and fistula of the gallbladder. The perforated or gangrenous gallbladder requires urgent surgery. Perforation should be suspected if there are diffuse peritoneal signs (bile peritonitis), crescendo pain, or rapid clinical deterioration. Rupture is most frequent in the fundus by erosion of the dilated Rokitansky-Aschoff sinuses. Gangrene may develop from vascular compromise of the cystic vessels by a cystic duct stone. Gangrene should be suspected if the pain and guarding is persistent or progresses after 12 hours of close observation. These findings may be difficult to detect in those patients who are diabetic, elderly, morbidly obese, or receiving steroids. Clinical deterioration may be manifested by fever spikes, persistent leukocytosis, hypotension, uncontrolled pain, and peritoneal signs. Rupture into surrounding structures is more frequent than into the free peritoneal cavity and may result in creation of a cholecystoenteric fistula (Figure 30-5).

Bacterial infections of the gallbladder. The organisms responsible for the infection complicating cystic duct obstruction are both anaerobic and aerobic. *Escherichia coli* or other coliforms and enterococci are the major aerobic bacteria. *Bacteroides fragilis* and *Clostridium perfringens* are the more common anaerobic organisms. *Clostridium welchii, E. coli,* and anaerobic and aerobic streptococci are implicated in acute emphysematous cholecystitis. Antibiotics alone are ineffective as long as the gallbladder is obstructed or gallstones are present.

Choledocholithiasis. Ninety percent of common bile duct stones originate in the gallbladder. The remaining 10% are primary bile duct stones. Complications from bile duct stones occur when they obstruct the bile duct or pancreatic duct. The type of symptoms depends on whether the bile is colonized with bacteria. The older patient with stones of the bile duct can present with painless jaundice, a finding typically assumed to be caused by malignant obstruction of the bile duct.

Cholangitis. Patients with cholangitis from bile duct stones must undergo an urgent biliary drainage procedure as soon as they have been hemodynamically stabilized with antibiotics and hydration. Medical therapy alone for cholangitis is universally ineffective. The gallbladder can be removed and the bile duct cleared by operative therapy. Bile duct obstruction can be treated by endoscopy and percutaneous drainage, but the gallbladder disorder will not be corrected if present. Sepsis, shock, abscess formation, and death will result if this process is not promptly recognized and treated with biliary drainage. Profound jaundice should be suggestive of coexistent common bile duct stones.

Gallstone pancreatitis. Gallstone pancreatitis occurs when a bile duct stone passes through the common channel of the bile duct and pancreas in the Ampulla of Vater. The triggering event may be common channel obstruction, obstruction with bile reflux into the pancreatic duct, or bile reflux with bacterial contamination. A randomized trial has demonstrated that patients with gallstone pancreatitis having greater than three Ranson criteria (see box) at presentation should be managed with urgent endoscopic clearance of the bile duct stones if a highly experienced endoscopist is available. Patients with fewer than three Ranson criteria fail to gain additional benefit from emergent therapeutic endoscopic retrograde cholangiopancreatography (ERCP). The majority of the less ill group pass their bile duct stones spontaneously and can be managed with a semielective cholecystectomy with operative cholangiography if they are a candidate for cholecystectomy, or with an elective ERCP if

RANSON CRITERIA FOR ACUTE PANCREATITIS *NOT* RELATED TO ALCOHOL

WBC >15,000 cells/μl
Blood glucose >180 mg/dl
Lactate dehydrogenase (LDH) >600 IU/L
Serum calcium <8.0 mg/dl
Serum albumin <3.2 gm/dl
AST >200 IU/L
P_{O_2} <60 mm Hg

A

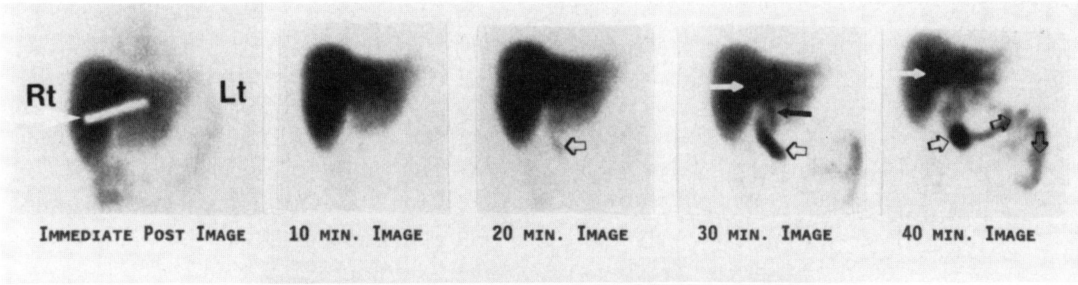
Rt
Lt
IMMEDIATE POST IMAGE
10 MIN. IMAGE
20 MIN. IMAGE
30 MIN. IMAGE
40 MIN. IMAGE

B

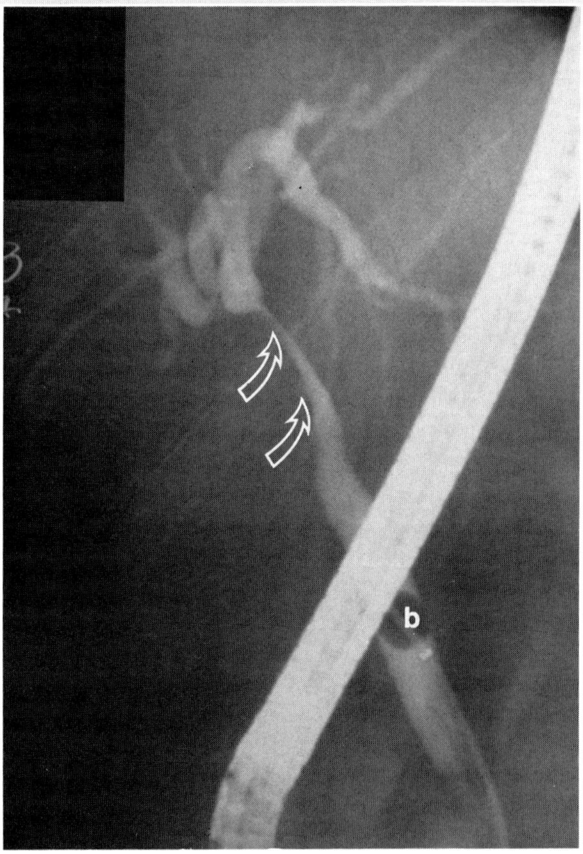
b

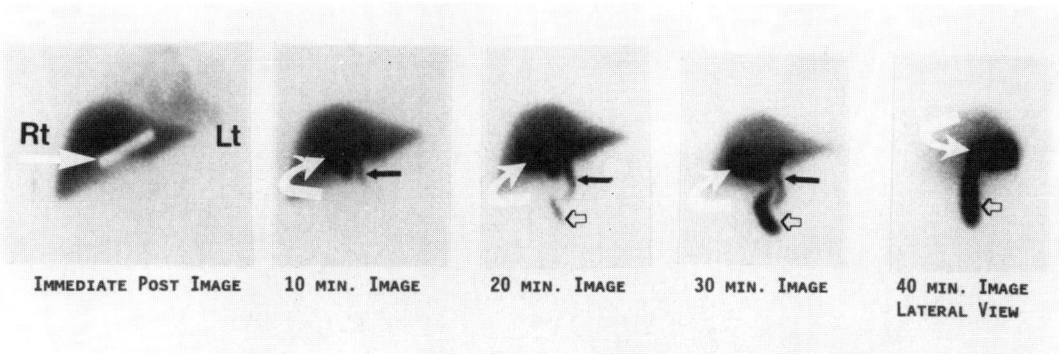

C

Figure 30-4

A, Abnormal ^{99m}Tc-DISIDA (diisopropyl iminodiacetic acid) as shown by scintigraphy from a 37-year-old woman was obtained when she presented with fevers, chills, abdominal pain, and jaundice. She had had a previous ultrasonogram that documented gallstones. These are anterior collimated images, except where otherwise indicated. The liver and blood pool are outlined in the image obtained immediately after injection of isotope. The 10-minute image does not demonstrate the duodenum, bile duct, or gallbladder. The 20-minute image demonstrates some duodenal activity, *open black arrow*. The 30-minute image demonstrates a greater hepatic duct isotope concentration, *white arrow,* than common bile duct activity, *black arrow,* and duodenal activity is also clearly evident, *open black arrow*. The 40-minute image indicates probable dilated hepatic ducts *(white arrow),* the absence of a gallbladder outline, and duodenal activity *(open black arrow)*. This study documents both cystic duct and partial hepatic bile duct obstruction. **B,** This corresponding retrograde cholangiogram is from a 37-year-old woman who presented with fevers, jaundice and abdominal pain. She had a ^{99m}Tc-DISIDA scan that documented a cystic duct obstruction in the face of known gallstones. Because she refused surgery, a retrograde cholangiogram was performed to relieve the bile duct obstruction. The bile duct obstruction was the result of a smooth inflammatory mass, *curved arrows,* caused by the acute cholecystitis. The injection catheter has an occlusion balloon, *b,* on it. **C,** This normal reference ^{99m}Tc-DISIDA scan is from a 42-year-old man who had recently undergone gallbladder lithotripsy. These are anterior collimated images, except where otherwise indicated. He sonogram documented the stone fragments, and this DISIDA scan documents prompt liver uptake of the isotope from the blood pool immediately after isotope injection.

The *straight white arrow* points to a 10 cm reference bar placed on the patient's anterior abdominal wall. The 10-minute image demonstrates the gallbladder, *curved white arrow,* and bile duct, *straight black arrow*. The duodenum, *open black arrow,* is faintly outlined on the 20-minute image. By 35 minutes, the blood pool and hepatocytes have greatly cleared the isotope, and the bile duct, *straight black arrow,* gallbladder, *curved white arrow,* and duodenum, *open black arrow,* are all outlined. This is a normal study.

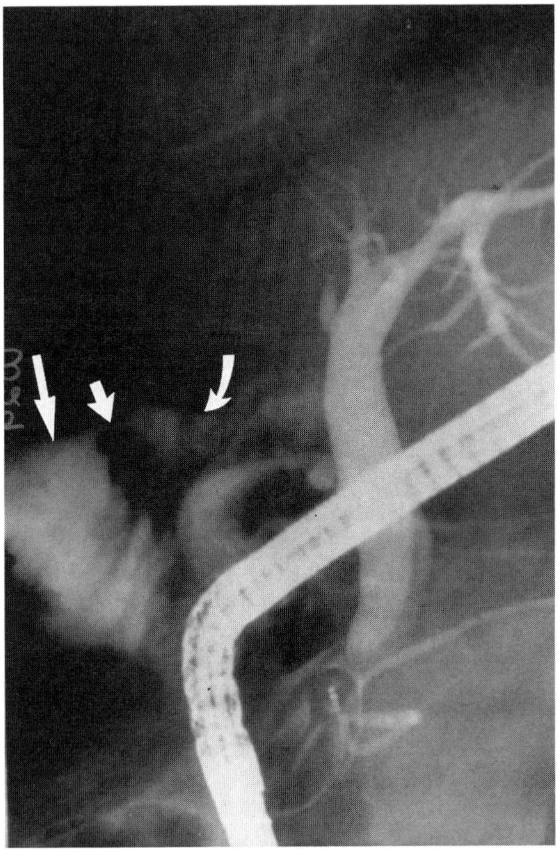

Figure 30-5
Fistula. This retrograde cholangiogram was obtained on a 77-year-old diabetic woman because she had an elevation of her γ-glutamyl transferase and alkaline phosphatase levels and an abnormal CT scan. The CT scan documented air in her biliary tree. A small contrast-filled gallbladder, *curved arrow,* is noted with two small stones. The gallbladder has a fistulous communication, *short arrow,* with the hepatic flexure, *straight arrow,* of the colon.

they are not a cholecystectomy candidate.

Hydrops of the gallbladder. The clear sterile mucus present in the gallbladder of these patients gives rise to the term "hydrops," though the fluid is rarely as clear as water. It develops in the face of prolonged cystic duct obstruction as the noninflamed gallbladder becomes distended with mucus, sometimes referred to as "white bile." It is frequently detected as a nontender palpable mass in the right upper quadrant. Cholecystectomy will determine the cause of the cystic duct obstruction and remove the risk of a future closed-space infection.

Lime bile syndrome. The hallmark of lime bile syndrome is an opacified gallbladder on plain abdominal films without prior contrast ingestion. In this condition, calcium carbonate (lime) is secreted by the gallbladder mucosa into the lumen. In sufficently high concentrations calcium carbonate is radiopaque. Lime bile may evolve from hydrops of the gallbladder. A gallbladder packed with radiopaque stones and a calcified gallbladder wall (porcelain gallbladder) can also present with the appearance of a radiopaque right upper quadrant mass.

Porcelain gallbladder. The name "porcelain gallbladder" is derived from the intramural calcification that is visible on plain films of the abdomen. The wall appears to be traced with a broken rather than solid line. The majority of these patients have a long history of intermittent gallbladder complaints, though at the time of obtaining the plain film the patient may have symptoms from another organ. The cancer risk in the porcelain gallbladder approaches 20%, and therefore cholecystectomy is strongly recommended in suitable candidates.

Cholesterolosis. The gallbladder with cholesterolosis is sometimes referred to as a "strawberry gallbladder." Yellow specks of mucosal cholesterol on a background of red mucosa is suggestive of the name. It is a completely benign condition. The diagnosis requires direct inspection of the gallbladder's inner surface. The ultrasonographic findings are nonspecific or, more typically, are normal. Histologically, fat-ladened macrophages are present in the gallbladder wall. The gallbladder wall is not significantly less pliable, even with the abundance of cholesterol in this mucosa. Some believe that patients with "strawberry gallbladders" can have symptoms similar to gallstone disease. Rarely, oral cholecystography and ultrasound examination of the gallbladder may cause confusion in the differentiation of cholesterolosis of the gallbladder wall from a fixed mass lesion. An elective cholecystectomy may be required, allowing exclusion of a gallbladder tumor. Polyps filled with cholesterol can also develop with cholesterolosis (see the discussion of gallbladder polyps).

Adenomyomatosi. Adenomyomatosis of the gallbladder results from a hyperplasia of the gallbladder wall. This disease, which is more common in women in their fourth decade, has three main forms: (1) segmental, (2) generalized, and (3) localized adenomyomatosis, on the basis of oral cholecystography. The clinical significance of this syndrome is uncertain, and it is not clear whether these patients benefit from cholecystectomy. This lesion is not premalignant.

Cystic duct syndrome. Some authors believe that patients with a long-retained cystic duct segment after cholecystectomy and who have persistent biliary-like symptoms may have the so-called cystic duct syndrome. It is difficult to imagine that patients develop pain syndromes from a cystic duct remnant in the absence

Table 30-1 Diagnostic testing for gallbladder disease

Factor	Ultrasonography	Cholescintigraphy	Oral cholecystography	Plain abdominal roentgenography
Preparation	6 hr (fasting)	2-4 hr (fasting)	1-2 days	None
Ionizing radiation	No	Yes	Yes	Yes
Risk	Very very low	Very low	Very low	Very low
Duration	10-15 min	60-240 min	10-30 min	2-6 min
Compromised by	Obesity, large wounds bones, dressings, air blocking	Liver disease, bile duct obstruction, alcoholic hepatitis, prolonged fasting, total parenteral nutrition, pancreatitis	Delayed gastric emptying, small bowel disease, liver disease, elevated bilirubin, tablets not taken, failure to follow preparation orders	Previously ingested contrast, air-filled bowel loops, excess colon stool
Cost	$150-$300	$200-$600	$135-$275	$35-$50
Sensitivity (%)				
Gallbladder disease	90-95		92-95	20-40
Acute cholecystitis		95-97	90-95	
Major criteria*	81-86			
Major and minor* criteria	90-98			
Acalculous cholecystitis	67	92		
Chronic cholecystitis	90-95	40-70	92-95	

Specificity (%)				
Gallbladder disease	94-98	90-97	95-100	60-70
Acute cholecystitis				
Major criteria*	94-98			
Major and minor† criteria	95-98			
Acalculous cholecystitis	70-90	70-86		
Chronic cholecystitis	94-98	90-97	95-100	
Determinates of a positive test	See footnote for major* and minor† criteria	ACUTE CHOLECYSTITIS None visualization by 1 hour yet isotope in the duodenum CHRONIC CHOLECYSTITIS Nonvisualization at 1 hr but visualization by 4 hours	Gallstones evident or gallbladder fails to be visualized	Calcifications or pneumobilia
Key advantages	Cost, speed availability	Cystic duct patency	Defines "stone load" Defines if the gallbladder can concentrate	Porcelain gallbladder, calcified stones, pneumobilia
Key disadvantages	Some user variability, especially if real time images are not analyzed	Cost	Diarrhea, long preparation time	Low yield

*Major criteria: (1) stones with shadowing, (2) nonvisualized gallbladder despite fasting.

†Minor criteria: (1) gallbladder wall thickening (>3.5 mm or >5.0 mm), (2) gallbladder enlargement (>5 cm), (3) gallbladder tenderness with directed ultrasound probe palpation, (4) round-shaped gallbladder.

of stones. In order to detect the retained stones, cholangiography is usually required. Retained cystic duct stones can be removed endoscopically. A retained nidus such as a metal clip or suture may require surgical removal if the stones reform and cause symptoms.

Diagnosis

Laboratory testing. Certain laboratory findings are useful in the diagnosis and management of patients with presumed cholecystitis. Typically, the white blood cell count is elevated in the range of 12,000 to 15,000/μl, with a predominance of neutrophils. The total bilirubin is usually less than 4 mg/dl. The asparate aminotransferase and other serum transaminases may be four times the normal range with a modest twofold elevation of the alkaline phosphatase. The serum amylase level may be twice normal with a normal serum lipase level. It should be emphasized that all the above tests are frequently within normal limits. Table 30-1 contains a tabulation of the key features of each of the major radiographic examinations used to evaluate the patient for gallbladder disease.

Plain films of the abdomen. A localized ileus may be noted in severe cases. Gallstone ileus refers to small bowel obstruction caused by a large stone migrating through the small bowel into the gut. Pneumobilia is suggestive of a biliary-enteric fistula contamination of the bile with gas-forming organisms (Figure 30-6). Intramural air in the gallbladder is suggestive of emphysematous cholecystitis. An abdominal plain film would likely demonstrate calcified gallstones in less than 15% of patients (Figure 30-7). One cannot accurately detect small amounts of calcium in stones at the time of an oral cholecystogram and therefore a plain film on or at a separate setting is recommended. A CT scan of the gallbladder is required to determine if the stones are calcified, but this is only important if one is considering chemolysis, with or without lithotripsy. In those patients at risk for chronic infections of the gallbladder and biliary tree or with hemolytic disorders, the presence of calcifications would be more likely. A calcified gallbladder wall is consistent with a porcelain gallbladder.

Oral cholecystography. The oral cholecystogram (OCG) is of very little utility in the setting of acute cholecystitis because of the failure of gallbladder visualization. OCG will document whether the gallbladder can concentrate bile. It can detect stones as small as 5 to 8 mm in diameter if the gallbladder functions, but the study is insensitive in detecting small amounts of calcium when compared to the plain film of the abdomen or the CT scan of the gallbladder. Ipodace (iopanoic acid), the contrast agent for this study, will obscure the calcification if present.

The reasons for nonvisualization of the gallbladder on an OCG study can include (1) patient noncompliance or emesis of the tablets, (2) small bowel mucosal disease, (3) lack of gastric or esophageal emptying, (4) cystic duct obstruction, (5) prolonged fasting, (6) fat intake just before the OCG, (7) chronic liver disease, (8) serum bilirubin greater than 3 mg/dl, and (9) extrahepatic biliary tree obstruction. The myriad of potential problems reduces the reliability of this tool.

Many centers use a 2-day protocol as the preparation for the OCG examination. Two days before the examination the patient consumes a normal evening meal. One hour later the patient takes six tablets of the Ipodace, one at a time, at

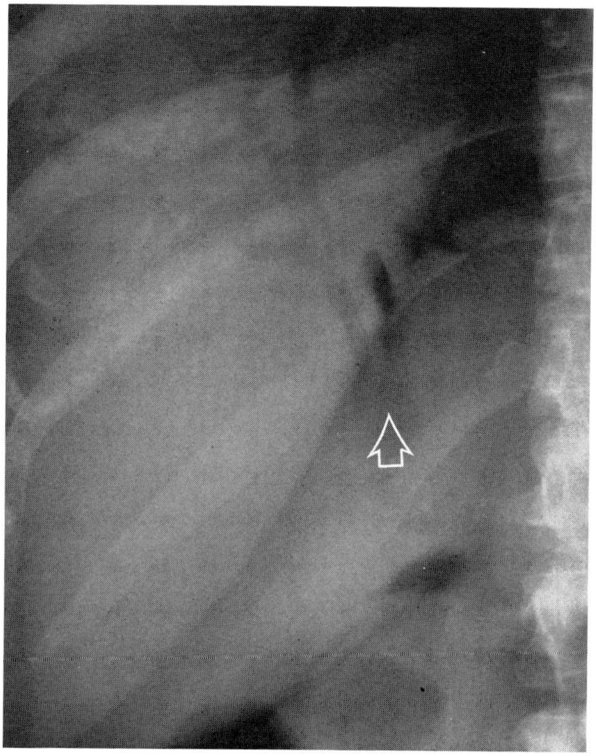

Figure 30-6
Pneumobilia. This upright film of the abdomen was obtained on a 43-year-old woman with a 2-week history of intermittent severe abdominal pain and progressive jaundice. The patient's stool was hemoccult positive. The retrograde cholangiogram documented pneumobilia from a biliary enteric fistula. Blood filled the distal bile duct, *below the open arrow,* and air filled the proximal bile duct, *open arrow and above.* The blood was swept from the bile duct and an elective cholecystectomy was performed for gallbladder stones.

10-minute intervals, with a small amount of water. All the following meals must be fat free. The evening before the examination the patient takes six more tablets. The patient is instructed not to eat or drink anything after midnight, until after the examination has been completed. Erect and supine oblique views are obtained (Figure 30-8). Small cholesterol stones may float; this is an important prognostic finding if bile salt therapy is anticipated.

Quantitative gallbladder emptying with a synthetic octapeptide of cholecystokinin (Sincalide) is difficult to reproducibly perform with OCG examinations, but reproducible quantitation is possible with scintigraphy. Bolus Sincalide stimu-

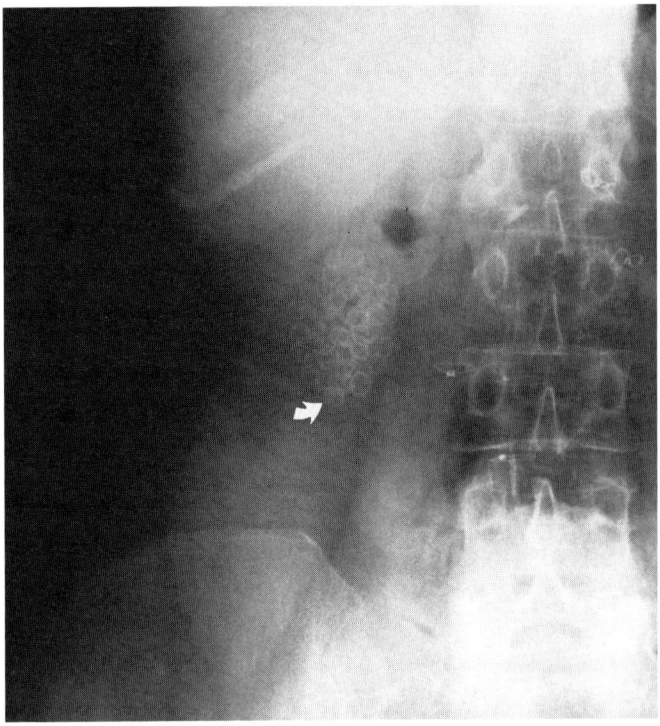

Figure 30-7
Calcified stones. This flat plate of the abdomen was obtained on a 61-year-old white woman as a screening test for a gallstone lithotripsy protocol. The stones, *curved arrow,* are more than 30 in number and contain calcium. As a result, the patient was not a candidate for either lithotripsy or dissolution therapy.

lation will result in poorer gallbladder emptying than an equal-sized dose given as a continuous infusion over 30 minutes. The nausea and cramping that develops with Sincalide stimulation, especially with the bolus dosing, is of no clinical value in defining the source of the patient's symptoms.

A serum direct bilirubin should be obtained before an OCG is ordered. If the direct bilirubin is greater than 3 mg/dl, it is unlikely that the gallbladder will be visualized. The bilirubin may also rise with the contrast ingestion because it competes with bilirubin for the excretory pathway.

Most centers use this study to determine whether (1) the gallbladder can concentrate, (2) the cystic duct is obstructed, (3) floating stones are present (greater cholesterol content), and (4) the gallbladder or gallstones have changed with lithotripsy or bile acid protocols. The study is also used to determine the type of adenomyomatosis.

Ultrasonography. Ultrasound is the first of two major tools used in the emer-

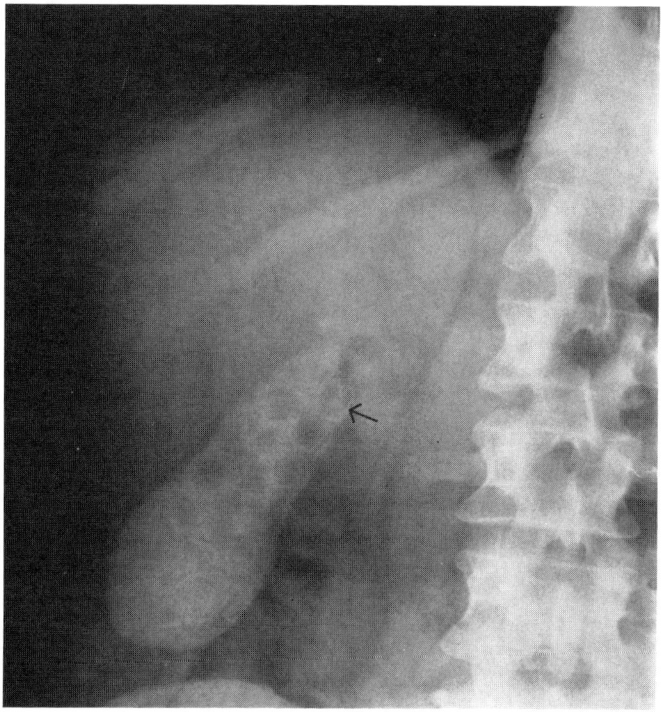

Figure 30-8
This oral cholecystogram documents that the gallbladder functions in a 53-year-old woman who was being evaluated for some vague gastrointestinal symptoms and a lung transplant. The stones indicate the presence of some rim calcification, *straight arrow*.

gency diagnosis of acute cholecystitis for the detection of gallstones. Ultrasound is a standard method used for stone detection and can detect gallstones 3 mm in diameter and larger. This instrument's sensitivity in detecting a pathologic condition can be user-dependent for complicated examinations. However, for a focused examination of the gallbladder, using real-time ultrasound, the sensitivity and specificity of detecting stones in a nonobese fasted patient approaches 95%. A significant advantage of ultrasound over other diagnostic imaging techniques used for the biliary tree is that it does not expose a patient to ionizing radiation. It is also less expensive than other forms of imaging. It had largely replaced oral cholecystography until information on gallbladder function was also required for lithotripsy and bile salt therapy (Figure 30-9).

A recent study suggests that an ultrasound examination of the gallbladder could predict a functioning gallbladder. A functioning gallbladder is one that will contract after a meal. This could replace

A

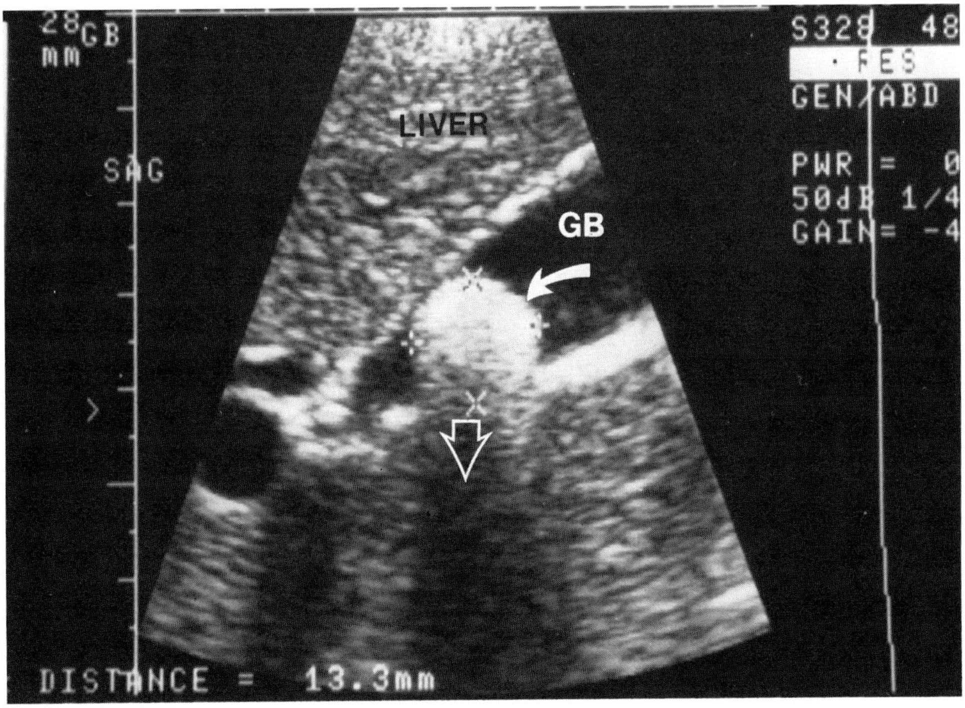

Figure 30-9
A, A pre–gallstone lithotripsy ultrasound examination of a 48-year-old woman with episodic, meal-related abdominal pain documents a solitary 13.3 mm gallstone, *curved arrow,* with echo shadowing, *open arrow*. **B,** A 12-hour post–gallstone lithotripsy ultrasound examination from the same patient in **A.** The gallstone was subjected to 1500 extracorporeal shock waves. The ×'s mark the margins of the largest fragment collection. Echo shadowing, *open arrow,* is still evident with other remaining fragments in the dependent portion of the gallbladder, *curved arrow*. **C,** A 6-week post–lithotripsy ultrasound examination from the same patient. The stone and stone fragments are no longer evident. The fragments disappeared while the patient was being treated with a bedtime dose of ursodeoxycholic acid (8 mg/kg). The dependent portion of the gallbladder wall is sharply outlined between the *open arrows*.

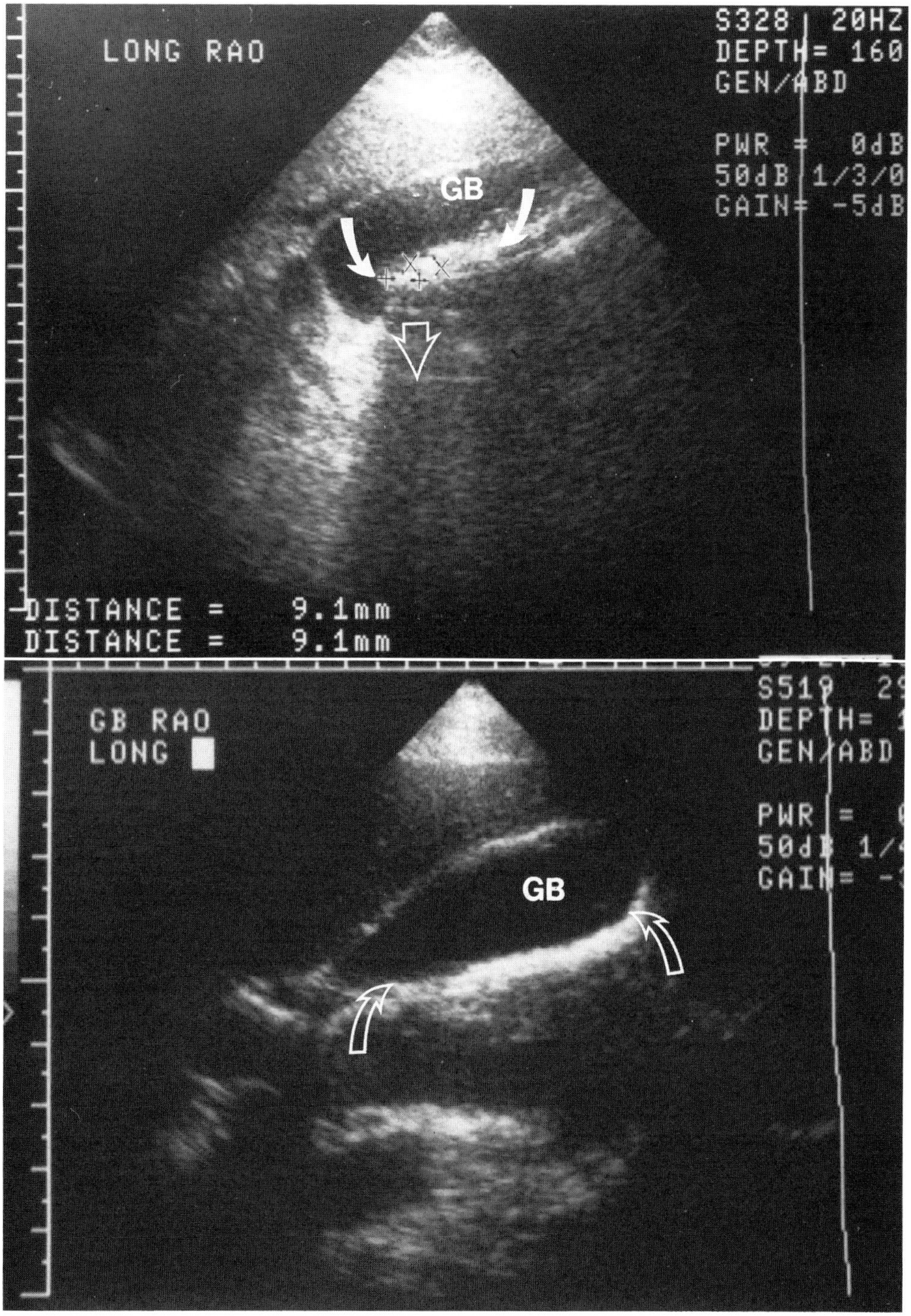

B

C

Figure 30-9, cont'd.

the combined OCG, ultrasound, and plain abdominal film with the latter two examinations. The advantage of this study technique would be the avoidance of radiation. The disadvantage is that the ultrasound is less accurate at determining stone density and total stone number than an OCG.

The ultrasonographic diagnostic criteria for cholelithiasis include demonstrating (1) mobility of the filling defect, (2) a defect casting an echogenic shadow, and (3) an echo dense defect (Figure 30-9, *A*). Internal echoes within the gallbladder indicate only gallbladder disease.

The specificity of ultrasound for acute cholecystitis can vary from 75% to 95% depending on which wall thickness is considered the upper limit of normal and whether the ultrasound probe is used to document Murphy's sign. Findings that are suggestive of acute cholecystitis are (1) a gallbladder wall thicker than 3.5 mm, (2) sonolucency of the gallbladder wall, (3) cystic echoes in the gallbladder wall, (4) a distended gallbladder, (5) Murphy's sign on probe presence, (6) fluid around the gallbladder wall, and (7) a pseudomembrane of the gallbladder wall.

Acute hepatitis can cause an inflammatory reaction in the wall of the gallbladder, as can heart failure, ascites, peritonitis, renal failure, and sepsis. Those patients with severe cholestatic hepatitis can have such a small contracted gallbladder that it may appear to be absent. Ultrasound examinations can be compromised by bowel gas, obesity, and the presence of a contracted gallbladder and are insensitive to common bile duct calculi (detecting less than 30%).

In acute acalculous cholecystitis the ultrasound administration may demonstrate only subtle findings. These findings may include an echo halo on the rim of a thickened gallbladder wall and a gallbladder filled with sludge. Coarse echoes in the gallbladder may reflect the presence of pus. Serial ultrasonograms, every 12 to 24 hours, will detect only two thirds of the patients with this disease. Criteria for the diagnosis include progressive enlargement of the gallbladder and progressive thickening of the gallbladder wall. It is important to note that a normal ultrasonogram does not rule out acute cholecystitis and that serial ultrasonograms are essential.

Hepatobiliary scintigraphy. Hepatobiliary scintigraphy (HS) is the second tool in making the diagnosis of acute cholecystitis (ACC). This method uses an isotope of the ^{99m}Tc-labeled IDA (iminodiacetic acid) most frequently marketed as PIPIDA or DISIDA. Metastable technetium 99 emits gamma radiation, which can be analyzed by surface counting. This provides an isotope outline of the liver and biliary tree (Figure 30-4, *A* and *C*).

This test has proved exceptionally accurate in the diagnosis of acute cholecystitis if the following diagnostic criteria are used: (1) biliary to bowel transit occurring within 1 hour and (2) nonvisualization of the gallbladder at 4 hours despite morphine administration. Using these criteria the accuracy is 95%, with a sensitivity of 97% and a specificity of 94%. The gallbladder can be visualized in 4% of patients with acute cholecystitis but typically only on the delayed images obtained at 4 hours.

False-positive results can occur in the face of alcoholic hepatitis, viral hepatitis, acute pancreatitis, chronic cholecystitis, parenteral nutrition and profound cholestasis. In cases of prolonged fasting, e.g., while one is receiving PN, consideration should be given to administration of Sincalide an hour before the scan to promote gallbladder emptying and reduce gallbladder stasis. If a false-positive result is still suspected, endoscopic retrograde cholangiopancreatography (ERCP) will determine cystic duct patency while also providing an opportunity for bile cultures, gram staining, and crystal examination. In selected cases, a transpapillary gallbladder drainage can also be performed. Morphine administration can reduce the number of false-negative HS examinations because morphine increases the tone of the sphincter of Oddi.

A very dilated proximal cystic duct can be confused with a small gallbladder, resulting in a false-negative scan. This dilemma may be resolved with ultrasonography. If the ultrasonogram is equivocal and an answer is essential, ERCP should be performed.

Acute acalculous cholecystitis is difficult to diagnose by ultrasound. Edema in or around the cystic duct may result in a functional obstruction. ^{99m}Tc-IDA scanning will have a true positive rate of 86% and a false-negative rate of 8% in this disorder.

Computerized tomography of the abdomen. CT scan is rarely indicated for the diagnosis of acute cholecystitis, but cholecytitis may be detected if the scan has been ordered in the evaluation of a febrile patient. The CT scan can accurately detect calcified stones. CT scans of the gallbladder may be useful in the obese patient, in those with marginal hepatic function, or in those with equivocal ultrasound findings.

Endoscopic retrograde cholangiopancreatography. Endoscopic retrograde cholangiopancreatography (ERCP) has a very limited role in uncomplicated cholecystitis. A recent prospective study from England addressed the role of ERCP in the preoperative management of patients with cholecystitis. The patients that had both a preoperative ERCP and a cholecystectomy had a higher morbidity and mortality than the control patients who were managed with cholecystectomy with operative cholangiography and common bile duct exploration when indicated. The morbidity of having both procedures was additive despite the theoretical advantage of having a common bile duct cleared of all stones before surgery. This should discourage the use of routine precholecystectomy ERCP in good-risk patients.

Percutaneous transhepatic cholangiography. Percutaneous transhepatic cholangiography (PTC) also has a very limited role in the diagnosis of acute cholecystitis. Ultrasound-guided percutaneous cholecystostomy catheters can be placed to drain the gallbladder in patients who are not surgical candidates or those who refuse surgery. This type of drainage is especially useful in the patient with acalculous cholecystitis.

Intravenous cholangiography. Intravenous cholangiography, using the contrast agent iodipamide, is a technique that was popular in the late 1970s. Iodipamide can be excreted by the liver into the bile without enzymatic conversion. This potentially dangerous technique caused severe systemic reactions to the contrast agent in 25% of patients. The biliary tree is poorly visualized under ideal circumstances and is often not seen at all if the serum bilirubin is above 3 mg/dl. This test is now considered obsolete and has largely been abandoned.

Management

The most established therapy for acute cholecystitis is cholecystectomy. The timing of the surgery may differ based on the clinical situation, the opinion of the surgeon, and the underlying general health of the patient. Surgery is usually undertaken after the first 24 hours of supportive therapy in patients who are a good operative risk. This may reduce the overall morbidity associated with this disease, in addition to being cost effective.

Supportive therapy focuses on maintaining adequate hydration, providing antibiotic coverage, and controlling pain. Food intake should be stopped until the patient recovers. If conservative care is elected, close observation is required to detect any signs that might indicate possible perforation, gangrene, or cholangitis. If operative therapy is not recommended for 2 to 3 months, a relapse should be resolved with an immediate cholecystectomy.

Mezlocillin and an aminoglycoside have recently been demonstrated to be as effective as the triple antibiotic regimen of ampicillin, gentamicin, and clindamycin for the stabilization of the ill patient with ACC. Antibiotics are indicated in all but the mildest episodes of ACC.

Diabetic patients have twice the frequency of gallstones when compared with age-matched controls. Diabetic patients with neuropathy may have minimal symptoms and signs despite having a perforation, gangrene, or peritonitis. Recent evidence has documented that the diabetic need not have a significantly greater hospital mortality than the nondiabetic patient. The diabetic with asymptomatic gallstones does not require prophylactic cholecystectomy, dissolution or fragmentation of their gallstones as previously suggested.

Summary

ACC is most frequently caused by cystic duct obstruction by gallstones. The emergency testing required includes biliary tract ultrasonography and hepatobiliary scintigraphy. Treatment is a timely cholecystectomy. One should manage complications by obtaining an accurate diagnosis of the complication or complications and then providing immediate intervention. Cholangitis must be managed with some form of urgent drainage after fluid resuscitation and antibiotics have been provided.

INTERMITTENT GALLBLADDER PAIN OR CHRONIC CALCULOUS CHOLECYSTITIS

Chronic cholecystitis (CCC) is a poorly defined clinical syndrome because of the wide spectrum of symptoms that some attribute to gallstones in these patients. It represents the most common clinical sequela of symptomatic cholelithiasis. Of those patients with symptomatic gallstones, 70% will fall into the CCC group. Within this group are two major subgroups: those who have classic biliary symptoms (50%) and those who have only vague, mild dyspeptic symptoms (20%). The unifying clinical characteristic of these patients is intermittent gallstone-related pain. The most reliable diagnostic criterion for this syndrome is based on histologic findings and cholecystectomy will verify the diagnosis. However, these patients can be successfully managed by a variety of therapies. The risk-to-benefit ratio of each of these procedures should be gauged against the severity of the symptoms (Table 30-2).

PATHOPHYSIOLOGY

The gallbladder in chronic cholecystitis is classically described as thick walled with varying degrees of calcification and cystic degeneration. This characterization may be overstated. Stagnant bile is frequently reported with characteristics of either

Table 30-2 Treatment strategies for gallbladder disease based on type of stone disease

Type of stone	Gallbladder disease treatment strategies: First option	Second option for poor surgical candidate	Second option for good surgical candidate
Asymptomatic stones	Observe	Observe	Observe
Symptomatic stones			
Functioning gallbladder			
Less than three radiolucent stones			
Small (<5 mm)	UDCA	MTBE*	LC†
Medium (6-20 mm)	ESWL*	MTBE*	LC†
Large (>20 mm)	MTBE*	ESWL*	
More than three radiolucent stones	MTBE*		LC†
Calcified stones	Cholecystectomy‡		
Nonfunctioning gallbladder	Cholecystectomy‡		
Inflamed gallbladder	Cholecystectomy‡		

ESWL, Extracorporeal shock-wave lithotripsy; *LC,* laparoscopic cholecystectomy; *MTBE,* methyl *tert*-butyl ether; *UDCA,* ursodeoxycholic acid.
*Investigational approach, not appropriate for acute cholecystitis.
†Unknown relative risk, not appropriate for acute cholecystitis.
‡The standard of care to judge all these therapies from is the time-honored open cholecystectomy.

sludge or mud. More severe involvement of the gallbladder may be revealed by ulcer formation and the deposition of collagen within the gallbladder wall. Special histologic stains can demonstrate the bands of collagen, whereas standard stains will demonstrate the lymphocytic infiltration with variable amounts of denuded gallbladder mucosa.

Clinical Manifestations

Meal-related pain is the symptom most ascribable to CCC. The discomfort tends to be located in the right upper quadrant and epigastrium. Either persistent or intermittent discomfort may be reported, and the pain may have a peak intensity 15 to 60 minutes after a large meal. Patients may alter their diet to avoid the pain. Rarely will pain last more than 1 hour. Gas and bloating are frequent complaints. Although nausea is common, vomiting is unusual. The physical examination may be remarkable for mild tenderness in the upper abdomen, especially the epigastrium and right upper quadrant. A palpable gallbladder should indicate an obstruction of the cystic duct with hydrops or tumor of the biliary tree.

Chronic dyspeptic symptoms may be

mislabeled as chronic cholecystitis. Empiric therapy with agents used to treat peptic ulcer disease will not reliably relieve symptoms in a patient with CCC.

Diagnosis

Nonbiliary studies, including complete blood counts, screening chemical profiles, and amylase and lipase determinations, are predictably normal in these patients. Nonvisualization of the gallbladder on the oral cholecystogram may document that the gallbladder is unable to concentrate bile, an indication of chronic cholecystitis or equally likely cystic duct obstruction.

The differential diagnosis for chronic cholecystitis is extensive. Acid peptic disease, "gas-bloat syndrome," aerophagia, functional bowel syndrome, chronic pancreatitis, lactose intolerance, and diseases of the hepatic flexure must be considered during the evaluation of these patients, especially if their symptoms are vague, meal-related discomforts. The diagnostic dilemma frequently provoked by these patients, if their chronic symptoms are disabling, may result in an evaluation that is costly and nondiagnostic.

A focused biliary tree evaluation with ultrasonography and scintigraphy would be appropriate in patients suspected of having chronic cholecystitis. The use of endoscopic evaluations of the colon and upper gastrointestinal track should be based on specific complaints registered by the patient and concerns raised on physical examination. CT scanning of the abdomen should be considered if a specific organ needs to be imaged based on the patient's presentation. No single test or combination of tests will always correctly identify patients with benign gallbladder disease.

Management

CCC can now be managed by several modalities. They include (1) cholecystectomy, (2) bile acid therapy, (3) gallbladder lithotripsy with bile acid therapy, (4) contact dissolution with methyl *tert*-butyl ether, and (5) laparoscopic cholecystectomy (see Table 30-2). Those patients with asymptomatic gallstones who do not have a calcified gallbladder wall do not require any therapy.

Cholecystectomy. Cholecystectomy is indicated in patients who have lime bile syndrome, calcification of the wall of the gallbladder, distinct ultrasonographic evidence of chronic inflammation, or scintigraphic evidence of cystic duct obstruction. Operative cholangiography is frequently indicated. Microscopic examination of the gallbladder after cholecystectomy should verify the preoperative diagnosis. Over 80% of those with classic gallbladder symptoms will respond to cholecystectomy, whereas the response to cholecystectomy in those 20% of CCC patients who have only dyspeptic symptoms has been disappointing.

Laparoscopic cholecystectomy. One of the first published series on laparoscopic cholecystectomy was from France. This procedure has now expanded precipitously throughout the United States. The safety and efficacy of this approach have not been tested in any controlled series. In the French study there were 36 patients, including 5 men and 31 women. None of the patients had acute cholecystitis, but did have symptoms of "biliary pain." Those authors excluded patients whom they suspected had common duct stones. All patients with evidence of acute cholecystitis were rejected from the endoscopic operation and then underwent minilaparotomy with conventional cholecystectomy. Complications of laparoscopic cholecystectomy included a cystic arterial bleed that occurred during one of the cases and required immediate laparotomy. Another patient required reoperation within 48 hours to evaluate persistent pain and fluid collection.

In theory this procedure should result in (1) a significant reduction in postoperative pain, (2) a reduction in the duration of hospitalization, (3) the ability to return to work after only a 1-week recovery period, and (4) the lack of a cosmetically unpleasant scar with preservation of an intact abdominal wall. The patient should also have a much lower risk of wound dehiscence. However the latter is primarily a problem in obese patients, and laparoscopic cholecystectomy is more difficult in the morbidly obese patient.

The safety and efficacy of this procedure remain to be proved. The profound proliferation of this procedure will, one would hope, not increase the risk of bile duct injuries and postoperative complications, as compared to patients with minilaparotomy cholecystectomies.

Bile acid therapy. Two bile salts, chenodeoxycholic acid (CDCA) and ursodeoxycholic acid (UDCA), are FDA approved for gallstone dissolution. The liver converts 500 mg of cholesterol to bile acids each day. Hydroxylation converts the hydrophobic cholesterol to the polar hydrophilic bile acids. The rate-limiting step in this process is the microsomal enzyme cholesterol 7-α-hydroxylase.

Chenodeoxycholic acid. The National Cooperative Gallstone Study, published in 1981, culminated in the approval of CDCA for cholesterol gallstone dissolution. When CDCA is taken orally 10 to 15 mg/kg/day, biliary lipids become less lithogenic and exogenous CDCA becomes the major biliary bile acid. Studies using this dose suggest that 14% to 30% of patients will become stone free within 2 years. Careful patient selection can result in a 60% stone dissolution rate, and partial dissolution may occur in an additional 30% of patients.

There are several side effects associated with CDCA use. Diarrhea is the most frequent side effect, occurring in 50% of the patients. Reducing the dose will end diarrhea in all but a few patients. CDCA also decreases the cholesterol saturation of bile through reduced hepatic secretion, but it increases the LDL level in serum. In addition, CDCA may reduce the intestinal absorption of cholesterol. About 33% of patients on CDCA will develop elevated serum aminotransferase levels. The mechanism of the hepatotoxicity is unknown, and the abnormalities noted in the chemical profiles are reversible when the drug is discontinued. Stone recurrence may develop in up to 50% of patients within 5 years.

Ursodeoxycholic acid. UDCA can desaturate bile at lower doses than CDCA. The usual dose is 600 to 900 mg per day as a bedtime dose, and this inhibits bile acid synthesis. In contrast to CDCA, UDCA can also solubilize cholesterol by the formation of liquid crystals, which is a major mechanism of stone dissolution with this agent, especially at the lower dosages. UDCA may reduce the biliary secretion of cholesterol by 50%. UDCA also appears to inhibit the intestinal absorption of cholesterol. UDCA has only rare side effects when compared with a placebo. The development of surface or rim calcification on the gallstones in patients on UDCA has been reported. Another equally effective therapy appears to be an equal dose mixture of CDCA and UDCA.

The ideal patient for bile acid therapy would be a thin female with a normal serum cholesterol and small stones (<1 cm) that float on a OCG examination. The success of stone dissolution in these patients may approach 60%.

Patients who respond poorly to this therapy include those with pigmented or calcified stones or multiple large stones. Solitary stones over 2 cm dissolve very slowly. Liver disease is associated with noncholesterol stones and is a relative contraindication for this therapy. These medicines have not been approved for pregnant women. CDCA therapy should not be used for patients with severe symptoms or in patients with asymptomatic cholelithiasis. Obese patients will have a very poor response to CDCA therapy and may require a higher dose if bile salt therapy is recommended. Antacids, cholestyramine, and charcoal bind bile acids and prevent their absorption.

Stones should become smaller by this therapy at a rate of about 1 mm per month. In theory, a smaller stone should be more likely to produce symptoms, but this has not been the case in any of the controlled trials. Patients had fewer symptoms on treatment, and the symptoms frequently resolved within 3 to 6 weeks after starting therapy. Those patients who will eventually respond to therapy will have evidence of stone-size reduction on imaging studies. If the stones have not responded by 6 months, another therapy should be considered.

Methyl* tert-*butyl ether. Methyl *tert*-butyl ether (MTBE) dissolution of gallstones has been popularized by Thistle and co-workers. Contact dissolution with this agent can be achieved by means of a small catheter passed by a percutaneous transhepatic approach into the gallbladder or by a transpapillary approach through the cystic duct. The catheter is wrapped around the stones, and the gallbladder and stones are then irrigated with MTBE.

MTBE has a boiling point of 52° C and therefore remains a liquid at body temperatures. This is distinctly different from ethyl ether, which vaporizes at body temperatures, making it unsuitable for in vivo stone dissolution. Gallstone dissolution can occur rapidly with MTBE if vigorous irrigation is used. Attempts to remove debris after the stones are dissolved is recommended. Any nondissolved particulate matter or material that remains after MTBE dissolution can serve as a nidus for stone recurrence. Patients who are selected should have cholesterol stones. Preprocedure CT scanning of the gallbladder is advocated because it can allow detection of small amounts of calcium in stones. Stones with a high content of calcium will not dissolve.

MTBE dissolution can be a low-risk procedure. If used properly, this chemical has a reasonable safety margin. Complications are frequently related to placement or removal of the catheter. Toxic side effects from this chemical occur when MTBE exits or leaks from the gallbladder. The reported complications include (1) hemorrhagic duodenitis, (2) ether anesthesia (MTBE absorbed after spillover), (3) hemolysis (MTBE absorbed into the bloodstream), (4) liver injury (with MTBE liver contact), and (5) stone recurrence (from remaining nidus). Hemorrhagic duodenitis from MTBE leakage into the duodenum through the biliary tree appears to respond to standard medical therapy without sequelae. The risk of general ether anesthesia requires that the patient be closely monitored during irrigation therapy. This is most easily accomplished by close attention to the return volume of MTBE with each irrigation in addition to careful observation of the patient's mental state. Catheter migration can result in contact destruction of liver and red blood cells if a side port migrates into the liver parenchyma. Repeated fluoroscopy with contrast infusion will allow detection of leaks while also allowing documentation of stone dissolution. Stone recurrence rates are similar to those seen with bile acid therapy. This treatment is not yet approved by the Food and Drug Administration.

Gallbladder lithotripsy. Fragmentation by extracorporeal shock-wave lithotripsy of gallbladder stones has gained significant attention since the initial reports were published by Paumgartner's group from Munich, Germany. The potential of a noninvasive method to fragment gallbladder stones with clearing of the residual fragments from the gallbladder was exciting because the risk of operative bile duct injury is avoided. Initial reports discussed the use of spark-gap lithotripsy. Since that time, there have become available several other forms of lithotripsy devices that are similar to the extent that they fragment stones by using shock waves. The available technologies are (1) spark gap, (2) piezoelectric, and (3) electromagnetic. The targeting mechanisms used by the lithotripsy units are primarily ultrasonography, on the machines designed to treat gallbladder stones, and fluoroscopy for those used to treat bile duct stones and kidney stones. It is estimated that between 80 to 100 lithotripsy units are presently in service in the United States. Up to now, none of them has received Food and Drug Administration approval.

The enthusiasm over gallbladder lithotripsy stems from the fact that this therapy can be performed on outpatients, requires only conscious sedation, produces minimal side effects, and minimizes lost work days because no real recovery period is required (see Figure 30-9).

Paumgartner's initial studies with carefully selected patients demonstrated that up to a 90% stone-clearance rate could be obtained. To achieve this high level of success, patients were selected who had a solitary noncalcified cholesterol gallbladder stone of 20 mm or less in diameter. After lithotripsy, the stone clearance at 1 and 2 years was 70% and 90% respectively. Patients with multiple stones or larger stones could be expected to have only a 40% to 50% stone-clearance rate after 1 year. Some of the smaller fragments pass through the cystic duct and eventually into the duodenum. However, the rate of stone clearance is greatly enhanced by the use of bile acids.

It is expected that less than 3% of patients will suffer serious side effects from lithotripsy. Mild hematuria or subcutaneous ecchymosis at the entrance site of the shock waves is not unusual and resolves promptly without sequelae. The most disconcerting side effect is gallstone pancreatitis or obstruction of the cystic duct. Theoretical risks of cavitation injury to the liver or kidney and interstitial hemorrhage in the lung have been largely avoided by the use of correct technique.

Summary

Chronic cholecystitis may be found in patients with vague or classic biliary symptoms. Those patients with distinct biliary symptoms or distinct abnormalities on ultrasonography, scintigraphy, oral cholecystogram, or plain films of the abdomen may benefit from cholecystectomy. Optional therapies are now available for those patients who wish to avoid surgery (Figure 30-3). These include bile acid dissolution therapy, lithotripsy with bile acid therapy, and contact dissolution with methyl *tert*-butyl ether, though the latter two therapies are still experimental. Stone recurrence will likely limit the use of these alternative methods until this drawback can be overcome. In younger patients, the use of extensive endoscopic and radiographic techniques to evaluate organs other than the gallbladder may not provide a cost-effective approach to evaluate patients with vague symptoms. Treating the gallstones in patients without clear-cut biliary symptoms will rarely reduce the severity of those presenting complaints.

CHOLEDOCHOLITHIASIS

The incidence of concomitant choledocholithiasis with cholelithiasis increases dramatically with age, approaching 20% at the time of cholecystectomy. Ninety percent of common bile duct stones have their origin as gallbladder stones. The remaining 10% are primary bile duct stones. Complications from bile duct stones occur when they obstruct the bile duct or pancreatic duct.

Pathophysiology

Nearly 20% of patients who are carefully studied at the time of cholecystectomy will have common bile duct stones. The incidence exceeds 50 by the seventh decade of life. Bile duct stones can form after cholecystectomy, and up to 5% of patients with bile duct stones may not have gallbladder stones (Figure 30-10). Primary bile duct stones tend to be softer and have a "mixed" composition. Bilirubinate-laden primary bile duct stones can be very hard and can be small in size and tend to develop only in patients with inflammatory diseases of the bile ducts such as sclerosing cholangitis (Figure 30-11) and oriental cholangiohepatitis (OCH) (Figure 30-12). Orientals who live in urban settings do not develop OCH. Bacteria or parasites play a central role in the formation of these stones. It has been suggested that OCH is a biliary expression of kwashiorkor. However, the presence of encrusted parasites in the nucleus of stones from patients with OCH would indicate a role for these parasites in stone formation. The responsible parasites are *Clonorchis sinensis* and *Ascaris lumbricoides*. Furthermore, waterborne bacteria can be cultured from the bile of patients with OCH. The lack of hepatic stones in persons from East Africa, where malnutrition is common, would further argue against a nutritional hypothesis for intrahepatic bilirubinate stones in OCH. Patients with sclerosing cholangitis can also develop primary intrahepatic pigmented stones, which can result in significant morbidity and mortality.

Clinical Manifestations

Patients with bile duct stones may present with a wide spectrum of symptoms and signs, ranging from vague pain to painless jaundice. The scenario is dependent on three major variables (1) where the stone obstructs, (2) whether the bile is sterile, and (3) the age of the patient. If a bile duct stone obstructs a biliary tract containing bile that is colonized with bacteria, the patient will present with fevers,

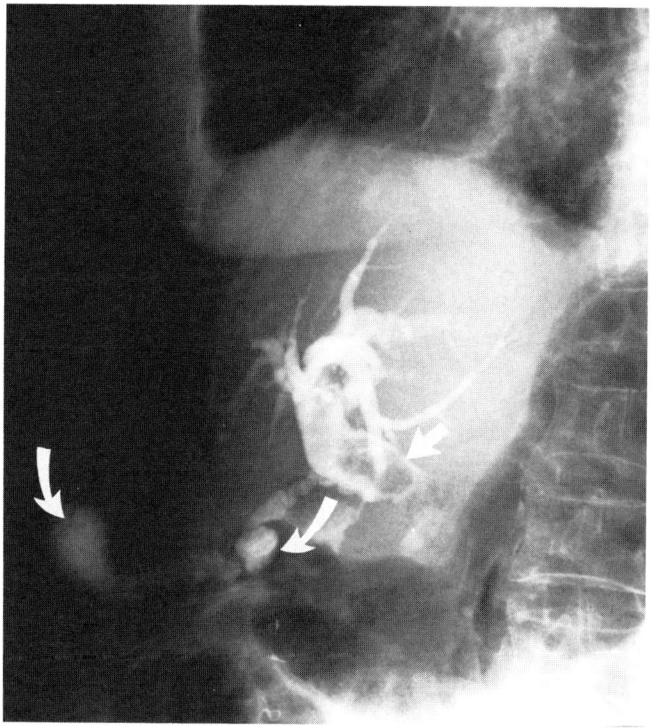

Figure 30-10
Bile duct with lithotripsy. This retrograde cholangiogram documents a 1.8 × 3.8 cm bile duct stone, *short arrow*, in a 75-year-old female who had jaundice without pain. She had positive blood cultures and a low peripheral white blood cell count. The stone was fractured with extracorporeal shock-wave lithotripsy. The gallbladder, *curved arrow*, was free of stones by both ultrasound examination and this retrograde study.

chills, jaundice, upper abdominal pain, nausea, vomiting, back pain, and septic complications. The bile may be frankly purulent at the time of emergent drainage. Medical therapy for cholangitis without concomitant drainage has a high mortality. Liver abscesses may complicate bacterial cholangitis. Frequently reported bacteria include *Klebsiella, Bacteroides,* anaerobic and aerobic streptococci, *Pseudomonas aeruginosa,* and *Clostridium* species. Elderly or diabetic patients with sterile bile may present with jaundice and vague symptoms. Their painless jaundice may be wrongly assumed to be attributable to a cancer. Bile duct stones that obstruct the pancreatic duct may produce acute pancreatitis. Bile duct stones may progress for years before they produce recognizable symptoms, especially in the elderly. It is believed that 30% or more of the patients with bile duct stones may

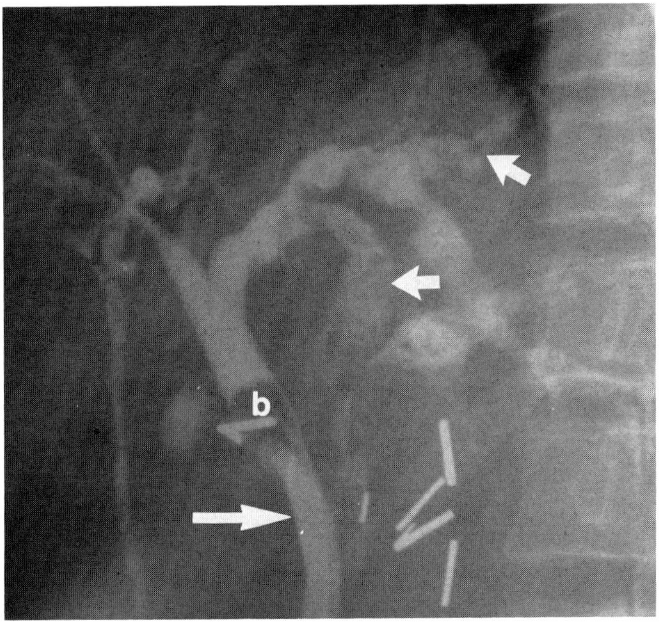

Figure 30-11
Primary sclerosing cholangitis with hepatic duct stones. This is a retrograde cholangiogram obtained in a 58-year-old man with a 10-year history of ulcerative colitis and a 4-year history of sclerosing cholangitis. He developed a rapidly rising alkaline phosphatase and bilirubin. The balloon catheter, *b,* allows the intrahepatic bile duct to fill, thereby outlining the innumerable stones, *short arrow*. The extrahepatic bile duct, *long arrow,* is remarkable for its lack of involvement. The patient required a liver transplant. Several metal clips are seen between the bile duct and the spine.

never have symptoms. However, when complications do occur, they may be life threatening.

Long-standing biliary obstruction from stones can clearly cause secondary biliary cirrhosis. Stones may act as a ball valve, resulting in only intermittent symptoms and a slightly elevated alkaline phosphatase. The level of jaundice will not always allow prediction of whether the obstruction is from stone or malignancy. It has been suggested that bilirubin levels rarely exceed 7 mg/dl from stone disease alone.

It remains unclear whether bile duct stones that pass through the distal bile duct result in clinically significant obstruction of the bile duct. The causes of ampullary stenosis are sufficiently unclear to only indicate bile duct stones as a possible cause.

Diagnosis

Serum chemistries are abnormal with biliary tract obstruction. The earliest change noted is an injury pattern seen in the serum transaminases, followed by a slower but progressive elevation of the alkaline

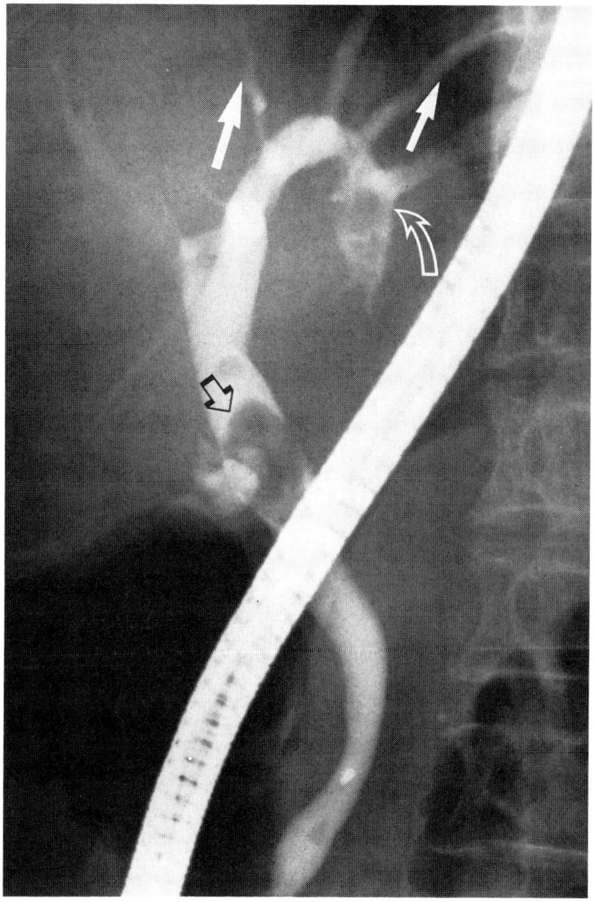

Figure 30-12
Oriental cholangiohepatitis. This cholangiogram was obtained on a 75-year-old woman who was born and raised in rural Thailand. She had suffered episodes of fevers, chills, and upper abdominal pain with associated nausea for decades. Shortly after arriving in the United States, she came to medical attention because of an episode of *Aeromonas* sepsis. The intrahepatic bile ducts, *long arrows,* have lost their arborization. The left lateral hepatic duct has an 11 mm bile duct stone, *curved arrow.* The common bile duct has a 25 mm stone, *open arrow,* and a small stone above it, *near open arrow.* The patient was made stone free after extracorporeal bile duct lithotripsy.

phosphatase and bilirubin. With uncomplicated acute obstruction of the biliary tract, the bilirubin will rise at a rate of 2 to 3 mg/dl/day. The white blood cell count may be only modestly elevated. The elderly or frail patient may demonstrate a low peripheral white blood cell count in the face of bacterial cholangitis. Blood cultures will typically be positive if the patient has bacterial cholangitis.

Plain abdominal films rarely demonstrate calculi, but air in the biliary tree may be evident (Figure 30-6). Ultrasound examination of the biliary tree may demonstrate intrahepatic and extrahepatic dilated bile ducts. Bile duct stones will rarely be demonstrated by ultrasound (<30%). Drainage of the infected bile and documentation of the cause typically requires an emergency endoscopic retrograde cholangiopancreatography (ERCP) or percutaneous transhepatic cholangiography (PTC). Only limited low-pressure cholangiograms should be obtained if the bile is infected. Both ERCP and PTC provide a method for immediate biliary drainage; ERCP also allows immediate stone clearance.

Endoscopic retrograde cholangiopancreatography. Endoscopic retrograde cholangiopancreatography (ERCP) permits the visualization of the pancreatic and biliary tracts by retrograde injection of contrast material using a transpapillary technique and natural orifices. ERCP has become the technique of choice to diagnose and treat a variety of pathologic processes of the bile ducts. Indications for diagnostic and therapeutic ERCP are as follows:

- Residual bile duct stones after cholecystectomy
- Bile duct stones in a poor operative candidate with gallbladder in situ
- Gallstone pancreatitis (highly selected patients)
- Evaluation of tumors of the ampulla of Vater
- Incision of a choledochocele
- Evaluation of drainage of the patient with obstructive jaundice
- Evaluation and stenting of a biliary fistula
- Biliary drainage of patients with cholangitis
- Diagnosis and potential therapy of patients with sclerosing cholangitis
- Biliary drainage of patients with obstructive jaundice
- Cytologic examination of bile duct strictures
- Performing biliary manometry
- Placement of transpapillary drainage tubes for stone dissolution.

Bile duct stones can be removed in 90% to 95% of patients. With only rare exceptions, patients with obstructive jaundice should have biliary drainage at the time of successful retrograde cholangiography. The role of ERCP in the face of acute cholecystitis should be limited to those patients who are poor operative candidates or those in whom the clinical course is highly atypical or complicated. ERCP may also have some utility in ruling out acute cholecystitis in the patient who shows clinical signs of alcoholic hepatitis but who also has signs suggestive of acute cholecystitis or cholangitis. Ill-conceived surgical exploration in the person with alcoholic hepatitis can result in a very high operative mortality.

Complications occur in 3% to 10% of ERCP diagnostic and therapeutic examinations. Pancreatitis is the most frequent complication. Bleeding is less frequent but can result in rapid exsanguination. Other complications including perforation, cholangitis, and instrument entrapment rarely occur. A skilled endoscopist should be able to successfully complete the procedure in more than 90% of patients.

Percutaneous transhepatic cholangiography. Percutaneous transhepatic cholangiography (PTC) also permits the direct visualization of the biliary tree. Contrast is injected through a thin-walled 22-gauge needle after a small peripheral bile duct is punctured. This procedure is successful in 75% of patients with nondilated ducts and 95% of patients with dilated ducts. The complication rate of a diagnostic PTC procedure is similar to that of retrograde cholangiography, whereas the complication rate for therapeutic drainage of the common bile duct may be higher with PTC, or PTC plus ERCP, than with ERCP alone. However, the types of complications for the two procedures are quite different. In a randomized trial comparing endoscopic and percutaneous drainage of malignant strictures, patients enrolled in the ERCP group had a 15% risk of stent- and manipulation-related complications, primarily cholangitis. Those in the percutaneous drainage group had a stent-related complication rate of over 25%, with infection problems occurring in 22%, bile leaks in 25%, and bleeding in 5% (Figure 30-13). The success at draining the patients was 61% for the percutaneous group and 81% for the endoscopic group.

Sifting. A widely neglected technique for detecting the passage of gallstones is the mechanical sifting of stool. A major disadvantage of this technique is that it involves the handling of excrement. Health care workers tend to strongly resist this examination, despite the fact that it can provide useful information on whether a patient has passed a bile duct stone.

Management

Antibiotic coverage in these patients is mandatory if any suggestion of infection is present. The duration of antibiotic coverage after clearing the bile duct of all stones remains controversial. Patients with frank cholangitis would normally be treated for a minimum of 10 days with parenteral therapy. Historically, ampicillin, gentamicin, and clindamycin have been the mainstays of therapy for this disorder. Mezlocillin with gentamicin appears to be an equally effective combination. The key step in the management of these patients is to relieve the obstruction and eventually remove all bile duct stones.

Good-risk patients with a gallbladder in situ should be managed with immediate cholecystectomy and common duct exploration. Patients who have a compromised status after cholecystectomy should be managed with endoscopic stone extraction if the expertise is available.

The morbidity from endoscopic stone extraction versus surgical stone extraction may be similar at some centers. Both ERCP and surgery require highly skilled technicians. The advantages of choosing endoscopic stone extraction center around the desire to minimize the number of hospital days and time of recovery. The success rate for both surgical and endoscopic stone extraction should approach 90%. A T-tube placed at surgery or a transpapillary drain placed endoscopically will assist in the management of any stones that could not be removed.

If retained stones are present, several options exist, including (1) stone extraction through a mature T-tube tract, (2) contact dissolution therapy with monooctanoin, and (3) extracorporeal bile duct lithotripsy.

T-tube extraction is a safe and effective therapy if a large-bore T-tube has been placed during the bile duct exploration. Once the tract matures, usually in 6

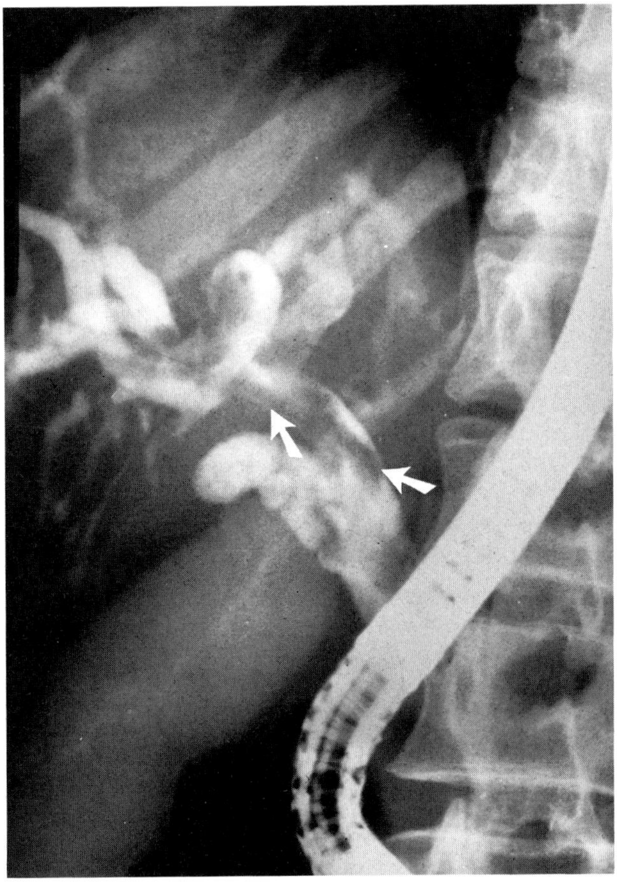

Figure 30-13
This retrograde cholangiogram demonstrates hemobilia in a 38-year-old woman 48 hours after having a combined endoscopic-percutaneous stent placed for a distal bile duct cholangiocarcinoma. *Arrows,* blood clots that partially fill the bile duct. The original bile duct stent and the biliary tree were plugged with clotted blood. The replaced endoprosthesis functioned well until the tumor could be successfully resected.

weeks, safe manipulations can be conducted through it. It has been shown that 60% to 90% of retained bile duct stones can be extracted through a T-tube tract manipulation such as basket fragmentation.

Monooctanoin (MON), a monoglyceride, can be used to dissolve bile duct stones. The solubility of cholesterol in MON and MTBE are similar. MON is a viscous, water insoluble cholesterol solvent. MON can dissolve 60% of the bile duct stones in the immediate postcholecystectomy period if the patient has known cholesterol gallbladder stones. In this instance, it is presumed that they

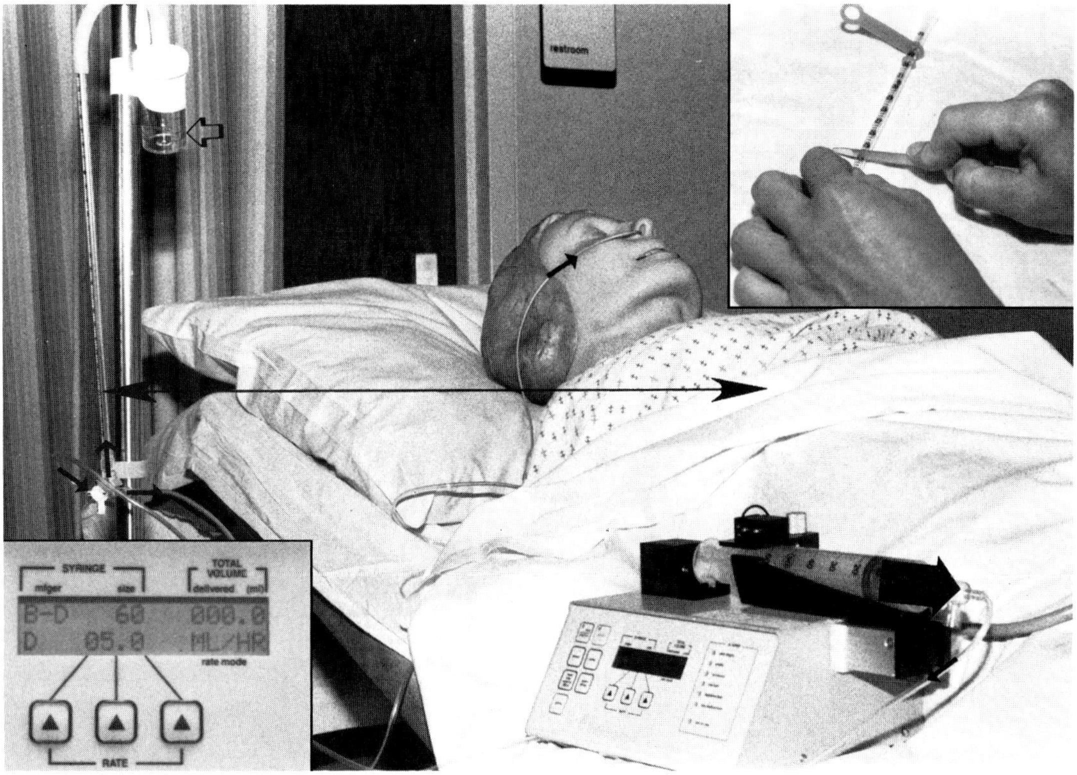

Figure 30-14
Infusion set monooctanoin. This mannequin is dressed with a perfusion setup to illustrate how a nasobiliary drainage catheter would be used for bile duct irrigation. The perfusion will flow in the direction of the arrows along the tubing. The manometer has been scored with a file and broken off at the 24 cm mark, *upper right inset.* The 0 cm park of the manometer is leveled with the anterior abdominal wall, as characterized by the *long thin arrow.* The top of the manometer is fitted with a trap, *open arrow,* to prevent any overflow from spilling onto the floor. The four-way valve on the manometer is kept open to all four directions so that the manometer can overflow if sufficient back pressure develops. The perfusion pump is a syringe pump that reproducibly delivers a prescribed volume and rate. The typical flow rate used is 3 to 10 ml/hr. The irrigation is stopped if pain, severe crampy abdominal distress, fever, chills, vomiting, or respiratory distress develops. If diarrhea develops, the irrigation rate should be reduced and the irrigation is stopped during meals and ambulation.

have cholesterol bile duct stones. Despite the fact that this solvent has been a food additive for years, it is a potent irritant to the small bowel mucosa. This agent should not be infused without use of an overflow manometer as a "safety valve" to prevent backdiffusion into the liver and thereby into the systemic circulation (Figure 30-14).

Bile duct lithotripsy has also proved efficacious. At the University of Iowa, 34 of 36 patients treated with extracorporeal lithotripsy for large nonextractable bile duct stones were discharged stone free. Twenty-two of the patients enrolled in the protocol were judged poor operative candidates because of chronic medical problems. None of the patients enrolled in this study required an operation to remove their bile duct stones, despite inclusion of patients with bile duct stones over 5 cm in diameter. The 30-day morbidity and mortality included three cases of reversible aminoglycoside nephrotoxicity and one death from endotoxic shock in a patient with a stone that was fragmented next to a liver abscess. The postmortem examination failed to document damage to the organs in the shock-wave path and the 3 cm stone was fragmented. Another patient with a retained intrahepatic bile duct stone above a post operative stricture had cirrhosis and alcoholism. He continued to abuse alcohol and died of variceal bleeding.

BILIARY DYSKINESIA

Approximately 20% of symptomatic patients undergoing cholecystectomy will not have relief from their complaints after the surgery. Three months postoperatively, nearly half will still have symptoms. This outcome has been labeled the postcholecystectomy syndrome, which is somewhat of a misnomer, because most of these patients have the same symptoms before and after cholecystectomy. The postcholecystectomy syndrome has evolved to include symptoms of bile reflux, gastritis, gas, and diarrhea. Pain is the chief complaint of the majority of these patients. The change in stool pattern and the bile reflux symptoms may respond to medical therapy.

The major cause for lack of improvement after cholecystectomy is that the patients' symptoms were not from the biliary tract. There is a smaller group of patients who have pain after cholecystectomy and have persistent biliary symptoms despite having their gallbladders removed. These patients may have worsening of symptoms after the gallbladder has been removed because they have lost a capacitance organ in the biliary flow circuit. Some of the patients classified as having postcholecystectomy syndrome have a dysfunction of the sphincter of Oddi. They may present with either biliary pain or pancreatitis. Persons with severe biliary pain should be directed toward studies that will define the structural and functional characteristics of the biliary system.

Geenen and Hogan have proposed a classification system that assists in the evaluation and classification of patients who may have dysfunction of the sphincter of Oddi. In the evaluation of these patients it is imperative to assess the size of the bile duct and to determine whether stones are present. A biliary ultrasonogram will accurately determine the common hepatic duct size yet may detect only 30% of the bile duct stones present. Serum chemistry values should be obtained during a typical episode in severe cases of biliary pain attacks. Patients who have twofold or more elevation of their AST, ALT, or alkaline phosphatase during pain episodes are a distinct group.

Patients with sphincter of Oddi dysfunction have been classified into three groups as follows: definite, presumptive and possible. These are sometimes called groups I, II, and III respectively. Sphincter of Oddi dysfunction can be caused by a multitude of problems. These disorders include structural or functional stenosis of the ampulla of Vater from congenital anomalies, neoplastic lesions, or inflammatory strictures. The dysfunctional sphincter can be characterized by (1) a hypertonic resting pressure greater than 40 mm Hg above duodenal reference pressure, (2) denervation (paradoxical response to cholecystokinin octapeptide), (3) tachyoddia (greater than eight contractions per minute), and (4) predominant retrograde peristalsis in the sphincter. The more typical pattern is one of reproducibly elevated basal pressure.

Several diagnostic tests have been advocated to evaluate the patient with biliary dyskinesia. Quantitative hepatobiliary scintigraphy may detect 60% of the patients who will have evidence on biliary manometry of sphincter of Oddi dysfunction. Along with a fatty-meal ultrasonograph examination, combined testing should produce the sensitivity of specificity that may detect 80% of those patients who would have an abnormal biliary manometry. For those patients who have severe symptoms, biliary manometry is essential, especially if the patients have failed to respond to conservative therapy with antispasmodics, a low-fat diet, and therapies directed at dyspepsia.

Criteria consistent with biliary dyskinesia on a standard ERCP include (1) a common bile duct greater than 15 mm in diameter and (2) a bile duct that requires more than 45 minutes to drain.

Biliary manometry is the "gold standard" with which to evaluate sphincter of Oddi dysfunction. Once anatomic lesions have been ruled out by the diagnostic portion of the ERCP, a standard 1.7 mm triple-lumen manometry catheter can be inserted into the common bile duct and its position documented by contrast injection or bile aspiration. The peristaltic and basal pressures within the sphincter are then measured. Optional provocative challenges can be performed by use of 2 to 5 μg of a cholecystokinin analog. Smooth muscle–relaxing agents such as nitroglycerin or amyl nitrate can be used for further evaluation of the sphincter's ability to relax. Therapy can be provided by an endoscopic sphincterotomy if the manometry is distinctly abnormal. Sphincterotomy is useful in treating those patients with basal pressures greater than 40 mm Hg, since up to 80% of the patients report a significant reduction in the severity and frequency of their pain.

Sphincterotomy without previous manometry in patients with presumptive or possible sphincter of Oddi dysfunction is not recommended. Patients with nondilated ducts have a higher risk of perforation and bleeding after sphincterotomy than patients with dilated bile ducts and stones. If the manometry is performed with a low-compliance transducer system, the accuracy afforded by this technique will assist in justifying the risk of a sphincterotomy in these patients.

BENIGN STRICTURES

In over 90% of cases, benign bile duct strictures are the result of surgical misadventures. Other causes of benign strictures include blunt trauma and inflammatory disease of the biliary tree. Primary bile duct stones may produce strictures of the bile duct, especially if chronic bacterial infection of the biliary tree is present.

Pathophysiology

Benign postoperative bile duct strictures represent the healing of an ischemic injury. The blood supply for the bile duct appears to flow hepatofugally. Transection of the bile duct will interrupt the blood and lymphatic supplies. Surprisingly, strictures may develop slowly, taking years to become clinically apparent.

Clinical Manifestations

Typically, patients with benign strictures of the biliary tree will not develop infectious complications of those strictures, unless there is a direct enteric anastomosis. Patients with enteric bile duct anastomoses present with cholangitis. More typically, these patients present with more indolent symptoms and signs. Mild laboratory abnormalities may be evident for years, until the patient eventually presents with jaundice and secondary biliary cirrhosis. Recovery of hepatic function in the presence of secondary biliary cirrhosis may be only temporary because these patients can develop complications associated with their portal hypertension and severe liver disease.

Diagnosis

Clinical investigation of these patients should include base-line laboratory tests and a physical examination with ultrasonographic visualization of the liver and biliary tree. The degree of ductal dilatation may be less impressive than the ductal dilatation seen with malignant distal bile duct obstruction. The presence of fibrous tissue in the liver may explain the lack of compensatory intrahepatic ductal dilatation. Isolated strictures at the site of the previous cholecystectomy or bile duct exploration is a consistent finding. Frequently there will be multiple metallic clips in the vicinity of the bile duct stricture. The term "surgical shrapnel" has been coined for this finding on a plain film of the abdomen.

The diagnosis of primary bile duct strictures is based on cholangiographic evidence (Figure 30-15). Differentiating these strictures from those of sclerosing cholangitis, malignancy, and encasement of the bile duct by tumor should be based on cytologic evaluation of the stricture, the clinical situation, and a close review from the operative report of any upper abdominal surgery.

Treatment

Surgical repair of the bile duct stricture is frequently advocated by biliary surgeons. Case series published in the surgical literature indicate that surgically treated patients may fare better than those patients treated with percutaneous bile duct stenting and drainage. Transhepatic catheter placement has significant disadvantages including the risk of fistula formation, bleeding, infection, and tube migration. However, surgery is not without risk. The list of complications associated with surgery are similar to those associated with percutaneous stenting and drainage. The frequency of complications has been lower in some surgical trials, but it is doubtful that the analysis of the data from these small series of cases has sufficient numbers to produce statistically significant power.

Endoscopic stent placement offers several attractive advantages over percutaneous drainage. Fistulas or drainage tracts

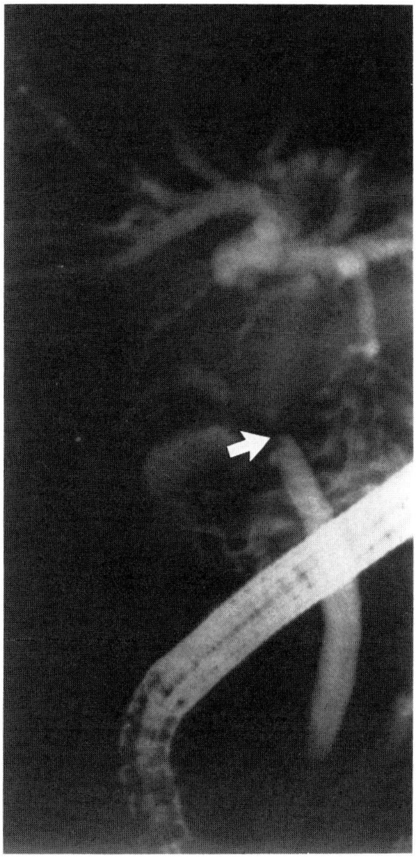

Figure 30-15
Benign stricture. This retrograde cholangiogram is from a 55-year-old man who had a bile duct injury at the time of cholecystectomy. He had two surgical repairs of the injured segment before this retrograde cholangiogram. A short narrow stricture, *short arrow,* is evident. The stricture was treated with dilatation and stenting and resulted in normalization of the serum transaminases bilirubin and alkaline phosphatase.

are not needed for endoscopic drainage. Stenting and dilatation can be performed on an outpatient basis with minimal risk of bleeding or cholangitis. Stent-induced pancreatitis is a risk, occurring in only 3% of patients. If decades of follow-up study are required to predict who has actually benefited from these therapies, further analysis is required. However, short-term endoscopic trials strongly indicate that endoscopic biliary dilatation affords adequate palliation of this problem.

Therapy for this problem should be based on the type of local expertise available. No matter which technique is used, long-term follow-up study with expectant management is dictated in all these patients. Liver transplantation in those patients with secondary biliary cirrhosis may be a more prudent course of action than extensive percutaneous, endoscopic, or surgical manipulations if significant impairments of hepatic synthetic function or coagulopathy are evident.

PRIMARY SCLEROSING CHOLANGITIS SYNDROME

Primary sclerosing cholangitis (PSC) is a chronic inflammatory disease of the liver and bile ducts of unknown cause. The dramatically increased frequency of this diagnosis over the past decade has been attributed to the proliferation of screening chemical profiles obtained on asymptomatic patients. Of patients with PSC, 50% to 75% have histologic evidence of chronic ulcerative colitis (CUC) or ulcerative proctitis. In contrast, only 2% to 5% of patients with chronic ulcerative colitis have PSC. Although exact prevalence data for primary sclerosing cholangitis are not available, extrapolation from statistics on patients with CUC would indicate that the prevalence of PSC may be between 1 to 5 per 100,000. This prevalence is similar to that seen for primary biliary cirrhosis. In contrast to primary biliary cirrhosis, PSC is a disease of young males. Seventy percent of the patients with PSC are males with a mean age of 43 years (range 15 to 70 years). The diagnosis of primary sclerosing cholangitis is based on clinical, biochemical, histologic, and radiographic criteria. The "gold standard" in making the diagnosis of sclerosing cholangitis is the retrograde cholangiogram.

Pathophysiology

Liver biopsy specimens in patients with inflammatory bowel disease may demonstrate a myriad of findings. PSC is characterized by progressive, onionskin-like fibrosis of the biliary tree. The mildest form of inflammatory bile duct disease appears to be portal triaditis. The liver histology in these patients demonstrates mild lymphocytic infiltration, eosinophil infiltration, portal edema, and very subtle bile duct changes.

Clinical Manifestations

Frequently, patients with inflammatory bowel disease are noted to have a twofold elevation of alkaline phosphatase for more than 6 months. Their medical regimen should be closely inspected for cholestatic drug usage. These patients are usually asymptomatic with respect to their biliary tree, and many patients with both PSC and CUC have only mild symptoms from their inflammatory bowel disease. There is no evidence, however, that their mild symptoms allow them to escape the risk of developing colon cancer.

Patients may present with more advanced disease, characterized by pruritus, jaundice, and right upper quadrant pain. They may also have signs and symptoms of frank cholangitis, including fever, leukocytosis, right upper quadrant pain, and even clinical sepsis. Those patients who present with clinical cholangitis will have had previous biliary tree surgery or will have primary strictures in the larger bile ducts.

Complications from sclerosing cholangitis almost always develop in the latter stages of the disease. Severe cholestasis will result in fat-soluble vitamin malabsorption disorders of coagulation and bone/calcium metabolism. Supplementation of these patients with fat-soluble vitamins is essential. Specific assays for vitamins A and D are available, and their levels should be monitored. Vitamin K deficiency will result in a prolonged prothrombin time that responds to vitamin K administration. The initial dose should be given by a subcutaneous injection to avoid confusion over vitamin absorption. Vitamin E supplementation in adults has no proved benefit.

Cholelithiasis and choledocholithiasis are frequent findings in sclerosing cholangitis. Up to 25% of patients have gallbladder stones, but most are asymptomatic. In contrast, intrahepatic bile duct stones may be exceptionally troublesome because these patients present with bacterial cholangitis (Figure 30-11). Retrograde cholangiography will allow one to make the diagnosis.

PSC may be a premalignant condition of the biliary tree just as CUC may be a premalignant condition of the colon. Cytology brushings of suspicious bile duct strictures will identify 75% of cancerous lesions. Cholangiocarcinoma is seen in 5% to 10% of the patients with advanced PSC.

Diagnosis

Endoscopic retrograde cholangiopancreatography. In PSC, cholangiography will demonstrate diffuse irregularities of the bile ducts. Stricturing followed by areas of sacculation and beading are classic findings. Strictures are most often diffuse, short, and annular. Although cholangiography is essential for making the diagnosis of PSC, it remains controversial whether patients who have minimal to no extrahepatic disease should be excluded from this diagnosis or included under the designation "intrahepatic sclerosing cholangitis."

When a diverticulum in the bile duct is long, or an irregular stricture is noted, a primary bile duct cancer may be present rather than PSC. Cytology tests are essential in this setting.

The presence of previous biliary surgery may obscure the diagnosis of PSC. Up to 7% of patients with PSC may have concomitant pancreatic ductal involvement. Congenital liver disease with strictures and cysts will not be confused with sclerosing cholangitis if adequate cholangiography is available.

Liver biopsy. The findings from liver histology are helpful in staging the severity of primary sclerosing cholangitis. Stage I (the portal stage) is defined as disease confined to the portal tracts. Stage II (the periportal stage) should demonstrate evidence of piecemeal necrosis, periportal fibrosis, and nonsuppurative cholangitis. Not all portal triads will be equally involved, and without adequate sampling, one may notice only portal tract enlargement. The ducts and ductules may be seen to proliferate during this stage. Stage III is defined as the septal stage. Intralobular bile ducts are lost in this stage as septal scar tissue forms. Areas of lymphocytic infiltration are noticed around the intralobular bile ducts. Histologic evidence of cholestasis will be noted, and special stains for copper deposition may be positive. The parenchymal changes, cholestasis and fibrosis, noted in stage III are presumed secondary to the loss of intralobular bile ducts. By stage IV, the patient is cirrhotic. Regenerative nodules are present. Some authors recommend grouping patients into a simpler classification of early (stages I and II) and late (stages III and IV) PSC. This grouping lends less risk of making an error in staging the patient because the severity of liver involvement may vary from one part of the liver to another.

Severely ill patients with inflammatory bowel disease frequently have severe fatty changes in the liver at the time of a bowel resection. It is presumed that this is a reversible lesion, possibly associated with their poor nutritional status. It is not clear whether these changes are related to steroid administration or parenteral nutrition in these patients. Similar histologic findings have been reported in patients with CUC who have not been on these treatments. Other reported histologic findings in patients with inflammatory bowel disease include postnecrotic cirrhosis and chronic active hepatitis.

A major advance in the care of the patient with bile duct strictures involving the extrahepatic bile duct has been dilatation of the primary large duct strictures. This therapy should be reserved for the patient who has recurrent cholangitis or progressive jaundice in the face of a dominant stricture, especially in the precirrhotic patient. Colectomy does not alter the natural history of PSC. Medical therapy for sclerosing cholangitis has not been shown to affect longevity or prevent the need for transplantation. Steroids are choleretics and may reduce the inflammation in the liver, but they accelerate bone wasting. Cyclosporin appears too toxic to become widely useful. Ursodeoxycholic acid may increase the flow of bile and may be beneficial, but the expense will dictate that further clinical studies be performed to document long-term benefit. The role of methotrexate remains uncertain.

Summary

PSC is a disease of unknown causes, though in the majority of patients PSC is associated with inflammatory bowel disease. There is no known treatment for this disorder except in the case of large duct strictures, in which dilatation may relieve the patient's jaundice. The disease will progress in the majority who present with jaundice, but the rate of progression in those who are detected because of minor abnormalities in their alkaline phosphatase is unclear. Liver transplantation should not be delayed unduly in those who have had clinical deterioration because transplantation offers an acceptable long-term outlook.

CHOLEDOCHAL CYST

Douglas described the clinical presentation and pathologic characteristics of choledochal cysts in 1852. Subsequently the greatest amount of literature has been from Japan where this lesion appears to be present with an increased frequency. The type I, II, and III cyst classification for choledochal cysts (Figure 30-16) is widely promoted. A type I cyst is simply a generalized enlargement of the extrahepatic bile duct, whereas a type II cyst represents a solitary diverticulum within the extrahepatic bile ducts. The type III cyst, or choledochocele, is described as a dilatation of the intraduodenal segment of the common bile duct. Type III choledochal cysts have been further subdivided into types IIIa, IIIb, and IIIc.

Pathophysiology

Choledochal cysts are "aneurysms" of the biliary tree. They are believed to represent an area of proliferated bile duct that became vacuolized during fetal development. The diverticula that develop with type I and type II cysts have no true mucosal lining and are therefore susceptible to neoplastic degeneration. Type III cysts can be demonstrated to have the mucosal linings of the duodenum and bile duct and are therefore considered to be more resistant to neoplastic degeneration. However, neoplasms have been noted within type III cysts.

Clinical Manifestations

Most patients with type I and type II choledochal cysts have either vague symptoms or none at all. The cyst may be detected in childhood as a cystic mass on physical examination or by a biliary imaging study obtained to evaluate an upper abdominal complaint. Intermittent jaundice or recurrent pancreatitis may be a presenting complaint in patients with a type III cyst. Evaluation of the liver in a child with congenital hepatic fibrosis may also reveal the presence of such a cyst. In adults, choledochal cysts can occasionally be found at the time of cholecystectomy. Rarely, the type II or III cysts may burst spontaneously or after blunt abdominal trauma.

Diagnosis

Laboratory analysis will be normal in patients with type I and II choledochal cysts. With type III cysts, mild elevations of the amylase and lipase levels between attacks of pancreatitis and persistent mild elevations of γ-glutamyl transferase and alkaline phosphatase levels may be noted.

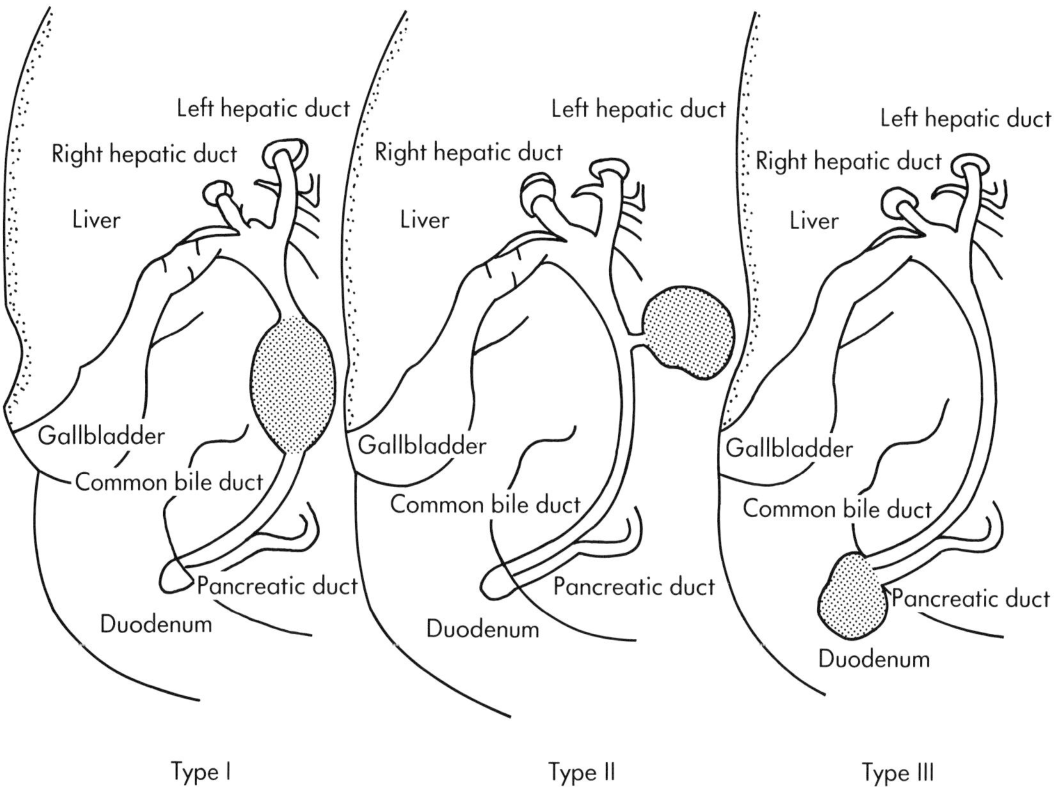

Figure 30-16
These drawings depict the three major types of choledochal cysts: type I, type II, and type III. The shaded areas document the anatomic level of the cysts' dilatation. Type III cysts are also referred to as "choledochoceles." The three further subdivisions of type III cysts are not depicted.

Biliary scintigraphy may demonstrate a dilated segment of the biliary tree. CT scans can demonstrate the cystic dilatation of the biliary tree. Cholangiography is essential to document the pathologic anatomy present in these patients (Figure 30-17).

Management

The mode of surgical management of the type I and type II choledochal cysts remains somewhat controversial. Most advocate cyst drainage in the symptomatic patient. The type I and type II choledochal cysts require a transabdominal laparotomy with cyst resection or Roux-en-Y choledochal cyst jejunostomy for drainage. Rarely, carcinoma has been demonstrated in cysts at the time of the operative procedure. The type III cysts can be treated endoscopically with a sphincterotomy and cyst incision. All

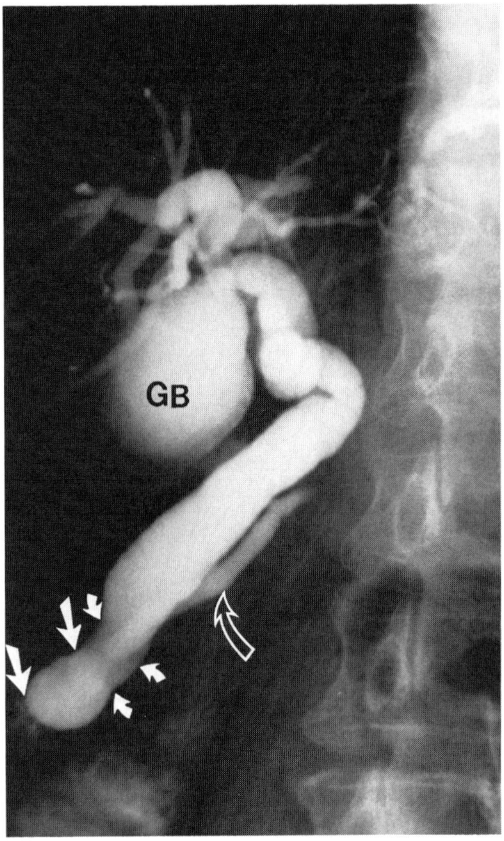

Figure 30-17
Choledochocele. This cholangiogram was obtained on a 63-year-old woman with severe chronic obstructive lung disease, a nonresolving pancreatitis, and elevated transaminases. Choledochocele is documented, *between straight arrows*. The intramural duodenal wall is shown between the *short curved arrows*. The pancreatic duct, *open arrow*, fills during bile duct filling. The choledochocele was incised by a retrograde sphincterotomy. The preprocedural pancreatic pain resolved immediately. A 5 mm sessile plaque in the base of the ampulla was biopsied and adenocarcinoma was evident on the histologic examination. The patient resumed eating within 24 hours, and a presumed curative resection was performed after a 6-week delay to allow the pancreatic edema to subside.

choledochal cysts should be considered to have a malignant potential. Patients with relapsing pancreatitis or abdominal pain can show dramatic improvement with drainage of a type III cyst.

Summary

All choledochal cysts may have a malignant potential with the greatest risk occurring in the type I and type II cysts. Choledochal cysts may be associated with biliary pain and pancreatitis, especially in type III cysts. Type I and type II cysts require surgical drainage with the use of a Roux-en-Y limb. Type III cysts can be treated endoscopically with a transpapillary approach.

CHOLANGIOCARCINOMA

Approximately 13,000 cases of cholangiocarcinoma (CLCA) are reported each year. CLCA may be found in 1 to 50 cases per 10,000 autopsies. Most believe the crude incidence is 2.0 to 2.8 per 100,000 for Western cultures, but it is much higher in the Far East, where biliary parasites are prevalent. The lowest incidence is found in West Africa. CLCA is associated with several types of liver and biliary tract diseases, which include (1) inflammatory bowel disease (even if PSC is absent), (2) primary sclerosing cholangitis, (3) choledochal cysts, (4) polycystic liver disease, (5) Caroli's disease, (6) Oriental cholangiohepatitis (*Clonorchis sinensis*), (7) biliary atresia, and (8) congenital hepatic fibrosis. Certain chemical exposures may increase the risk of developing CLCA. These higher risk exposures are (1) Thorotrast contrast, (2) benzidine (azo dye manufacturing and reagent for metal and blood detection), (3) 3,3′-dichlorobenzidine (azo dye manufacture), and (4) *m*-toluenediamide exposure. Thorotrast (thorium dioxide) was a radiographic contrast material that was widely used from 1930 to 1955. This agent has a biologic half-life of 400 years and emits alpha, beta, and gamma rays as it decays to lead. The CLCA that develop after Thorotrast exposure are almost all cholangiosarcomas, and the lag period between initial exposure and tumor development appears to be several decades.

Pathophysiology

CLCA may arise in any part of the biliary tree but is most frequently seen at the confluence of the right and left hepatic ducts (Klatskin tumor). When the relative frequency is divided by location, 50% are proximal, 21% are middle, and 21% are distal bile duct cancers. Five percent demonstrate diffuse involvement. The Klatskin type of CLCA is rarely resectable. Periductal invasion of liver, nerves, blood vessels, and lymphatics is frequently seen at the time of diagnosis. The majority of CLCA are adenocarcinomas arising from the biliary epithelium. Histologic elements include cuboidal and columnar cells, with abundant fibrous stroma beneath the surface epithelium. Based on cytologic features, CLCA can be difficult to distinguish from areas of dysplasia if significant acute and chronic inflammation are present.

Clinical Presentation

The clinical presentation is determined by the location of the cancer and therefore by the level of the biliary tree obstruction. The classic patient would be a 60- to 70-year-old male (with the male-to-female ratio being 3:1). He would have experienced weeks of epigastric distress. Jaundice would have developed insidiously but only if the cancer had obstructed both the right and left hepatic ducts. The patient with unilateral hepatic duct obstruction may not have jaundice and will relate only vague epigastric or upper abdominal complaints. The ipsilateral liver segments atrophy with prolonged obstruction. Weight loss, diarrhea, and acholic stool are noted in 60% to 75% of cases. The alkaline phosphatase and γ-glutamyl transferase enzyme levels would be abnormal, independent of the location of the obstruction. Anorexia and difficulty with fat absorption are common once the patient has jaundice. Bacterial cholangitis in patients who do not have an indwelling stent or a surgical anastomosis is uncommon at the time but may occur in the terminal stages of the disease. Peritoneal metastases are common late in the clinical course of these patients.

Diagnosis

An ultrasomogram of the liver and biliary tree may document the effects of the obstruction. Ultrasound examinations of patients with Klatskin lesions will frequently demonstrate dilated intrahepatic ducts and a contracted small gallbladder. Extrahepatic biliary tree dilatation occurs proximally to the level of obstruction. It is unlikely that a CT scan of the abdomen will demonstrate the mass lesion until late in the course of this disease, but it will certainly confirm the dilated ducts above the level of the obstruction.

Angiography is useful if surgery is contemplated. Those with vascular invasion are unresectable and therefore heroic surgical attempts should not be encouraged.

Cholangiography, either by ERCP or PTC, will demonstrate an obstructed bile duct at the level of the tumor (Figure 30-

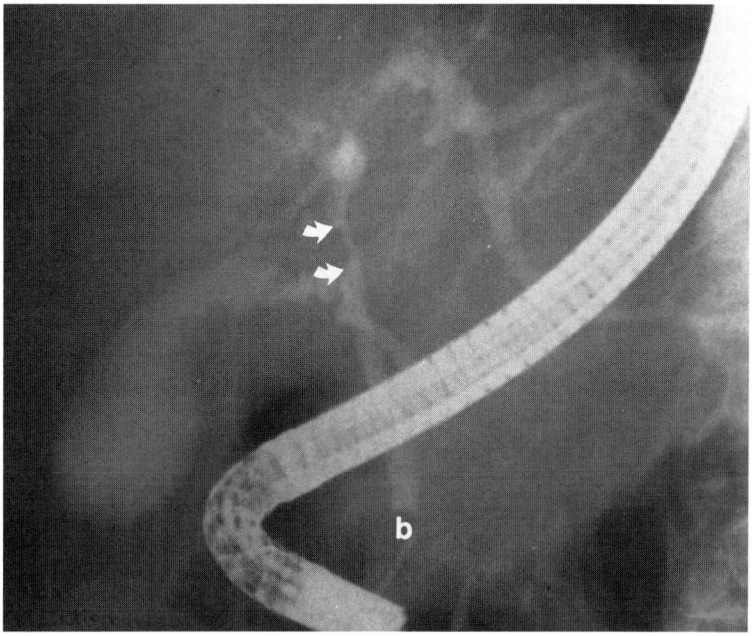

Figure 30-18
Cholangiocarcinoma. This retrograde cholangiogram was obtained on a jaundiced, pruritic 63-year-old man. Brushings and biopsies of the notched segment of bile duct documented a cholangiocarcinoma. Resection was not possible at the time of exploration, and the patient has been maintained with endoscopic stenting. The pruritus resolved promptly with stenting of the stricture.

18). Cytology brushing from the tumor surface will yield the diagnosis in 75% of cases.

Management

Death is more frequently related to hepatocellular failure from secondary biliary cirrhosis and chronic biliary tree obstruction than from metastatic destruction of the liver. Biliary drainage procedures may slow the progression to hepatic failure.

Palliative options that exist for these patients include resection of the tumor and, if possible, the establishment of biliary-enteric continuity. Lobectomy may be curative if unilateral disease is detected. Silicone rubber catheters, either straight or U-tube shaped, minimize the risk of recurrent cholestasis if they are exchanged on a regular basis. Biliary stents may be placed surgically, endoscopically, or percutaneously. Some surgeons believe that the drainage of a single side of a bilaterally obstructed liver will relieve the jaundice and pruritus while placing the patient at only a small risk for cholangitis in the contralateral lobe. As the jaundice resolves, the synthetic function of the liver will frequently recover and portal pressures may fall.

Percutaneous drainage using the right lateral approach between the ribs is an alternative. However, the patient may experience pain during breathing and motion of the torso. Percutaneous catheters may also migrate or damage the liver capsule. Drainage catheters that pass through the anterior abdominal wall by a left hepatic approach are preferred. If the tumor cannot be traversed on the first drainage attempt, internalization of the drainage is frequently possible after several days of external drainage. Failed drainage can lead to development of a fistula. A fistula can communicate with the peritoneal or pleural cavity or leak to the outside of the body.

Endoscopic drainage is an option that allows the resumption of biliary enteric continuity. The complications associated with endoscopic drainage in one controlled randomized trial were significantly lower than those noted with percutaneous drainage. Endoscopic drainage by a well-trained endoscopist should be possible in 85% of the cases. Failed endoscopic drainage will not result in a fistula tract forming, since no false tracts are created to perform the procedure. The optimal stent diameter is at least 3 to 4 mm. Newer metallic stents, which expand to 10 mm, are now available for both endoscopic and percutaneous placement and deserve further investigation. Smaller stents occlude earlier than the larger stents and have much poorer flow dynamics for bile. The rate of flow through a stent is proportional to the fourth power of the radius; i.e., a stent with twice the radius can transport 16 times as much fluid.

The 12-French stents (4 mm in diameter) may stay patent for 6 months. However, in an effort to avoid the morbidity, mortality, and hospital days associated with bacterial cholangitis after a stent occludes, many centers routinely exchange these devices every 4 to 6 months on an out-patient basis. Catheter-related sepsis is a frequent terminal event in these patients, and every effort should be focused on avoiding this problem.

Unresectable CLCA may be treated with radiation therapy. However, this tumor is relatively radiation resistant, and therefore some radiotherapists have advocated the addition of brachyradiotherapy with iridium implants (an investigational therapy). External beam radiotherapy of 5000 cGy is provided over 4 weeks at a divided dose. Brachyradiotherapy is then administered by use of an Iridium-192 wire that is threaded through the transpapillary nasobiliary stent or the percutaneous catheter. This provides an additional 4000 cGy of local radiation to the CLCA, with a limited tissue penetration of only 2 cm from the ^{192}Ir seed source. Only small numbers of patients have been treated with this modality, but a few patients may survive several years. Controlled trials have not been conducted because the number of patients with this disorder is so small. Presently available chemotherapy is ineffective against cholangiocarcinoma. Liver transplantation is rarely indicated because of the frequent recurrence of the tumor after transplant and the scarce nature of donor organs.

The 5-year survival rate for CLCA is a dismal 4% to 10%. Most patients die from liver failure or from infectious complications related to their lack of adequate biliary drainage. Inanition and anorexia are frequent in the terminal stages of the disease. Periductal spread of CLCA can result in invasion and occlusion of the portal vein and hepatic artery causing portal hypertension, ascites, and gastrointestinal bleeding. More effective forms of therapy are badly needed.

Summary

At the time of presentation of CLCA, it should be determined if there is a chance for curative resection. If the evaluation includes an ERCP, the patient can have a biliary drain placed at the time of the first diagnostic procedure. If the patient is discovered to be unresectable during the preoperative period or at the time of exploration, biliary enteric continuity will have already been established. Biliary decompression may improve the quality of life for these patients if their cancer is slowly growing. The endoprosthesis can then be used to assist in adjuvant radiotherapy, if indicated, by providing a radiopaque tube on which to focus. Brachyradiotherapy may be a useful addition, but greater experience with the technique is needed before it can be recommended as an acceptable treatment.

BENIGN AND MALIGNANT GALLBLADDER TUMORS

Polyps are surface protrusions into a lumen. Gallbladder polyps are typically less than 1 cm but may approach 1.5 cm. The three major types of polyps are (1) cholesterol polyps, (2) hyperplastic polyps, and (3) adenomas of the gallbladder. Polyps are seen incidentally in 5% of cholecystectomy specimens.

Pathophysiology

Polypoid lesions may be caused by simple hyperplasia or hypertrophy of the gallbladder mucosa. This is not a neoplastic process, and typically such lesions are found incidentally at the time of cholecystectomy.

Approximately 90% of the benign polyps of the gallbladder are cholesterol polyps. These polyps represent a more focal example of cholesterolosis of the gallbladder wall and are composed of fat-laden cells. They have no known malignant potential.

Hyperplastic polyps of the gallbladder represent about 5% of gallbladder polyps and are associated with cholesterolosis of the gallbladder and chronic cholecystitis. Histologically they contain epithelial elements without muscular stroma and are classified as being of either villous type or spongy type. The villous polyps are characterized as having tall, delicate papillary projections that protrude into the lumen of the gallbladder. The spongy type of hyperplastic polyps are typically flat and contain dilated cystic glands. Rare case reports of dysplasia in these polyps have been noted.

Adenomatous polyps of the gallbladder are small with a smooth surface. They are more typically sessile than stalked. A smooth surface covers a structure interlaced with stroma and proliferative glands that contain dilated cystic structures. The sessile adenomas may be difficult to differentiate from gallbladder cancers on the basis of an ultrasound examination. The risk of cancer in adenomatous polyps less than 1.2 cm is very low. There is a risk of carcinoma in gallbladder polyps larger than 1.2 cm in diameter, even though it is only a small risk. The histologic characteristics of adenomas of the gallbladder are similar to those of villous hyperplasia of the gallbladder. These small polyps have delicate branched villous projections that protrude into the lumen. Their epithelium is either columnar or cuboidal. They rarely exceed 2 cm in size and are frequently laden with cholesterol. In approximately 30% of patients they will occur in more than one location in the gallbladder. Adenomatous polyps of the gallbladder may occur as an isolated finding, or they may be associated with several diseases. These disease processes include (1) ulcerative colitis with or without primary sclerosing cholangitis, (2) Gardner's syndrome, (3) Peutz-Jeghers syndrome, and (4) cholesterolosis of the gallbladder. Some physicians believe that small adenomas of the gallbladder are not premalignant. Larger polyps may harbor carcinoma in situ. The polyp-to-malignancy concept proposed for colon polyps presumably holds for gallbladder polyps as well.

Clinical Manifestations

The detection of a gallbladder polyp typically occurs at the time of a gallbladder-imaging study. Small polyps should produce no symptoms, since they are associated with chronic cholecystitis and symptoms associated with chronic cholecystitis. Contrast or ultrasonic studies of the gallbladder will demonstrate a small fixed lesion. Except for size, there are no distinguishing characteristics that will accurately allow one to be certain that the polyp present in the gallbladder, if sessile, is not in fact a gallbladder cancer. The most common lesion is obviously the cholesterol polyp.

Management

Cholecystectomies directed at gallbladder polyps are best reserved for lesions larger than 12 mm. The reported malignant potential for polyps less than 12 mm is very low.

CARCINOMA OF THE GALLBLADDER

Gallbladder cancer (GBC) is unusual but is the most common cancer of the biliary tree. GBC in the United States is detected in about 0.6% to 1% of autopsy cases and in almost 2% of biliary surgeries. Females are affected three times as often as males. The crude incidence of GBC in England is about 11.6 per million. GBC in Mexico is found in 3.5% of the gallbladders removed. Additional ethnic groups at risk for GBC are the American Indians and Japanese immigrants.

Pathophysiology

Gallstones are present in 95% of patients who have GBC, and chronic inflammation in the gallbladder is also classically noted. It is believed that the inflammation in the gallbladder predisposes the patient to develop cancer. In the hamster animal model, elevated biliary levels of the carcinogen dimethylnitrosamines can be produced if the gallbladder has been contaminated with bacteria. One study suggested that persons who are chronic carriers of typhoid may have a sixfold greater risk of developing cancer of the gallbladder and biliary tree than patients with uncomplicated gallstones.

Papillary cancers may progress from a polyp to a cancer, starting as an adenoma. Nearly 85% of gallbladder cancers are adenocarcinomas. The other cancers noted in the gallbladder include (1) anaplastic carcinoma, (2) squamous cell carcinoma, (3) adenosquamous carcinoma, (4) carcinoid tumors, (5) melanomas, and (6) sarcomas of the gallbladder.

Certain occupations increase the risk of developing cancer of the gallbladder and biliary tree. These occupations include (1) textile workers, (2) metal fabrication workers, (3) workers in the rubber industry, and (4) employees exposed to wood-finishing products. The common denominator in these occupations is aromatic chemical exposure.

Clinical Manifestations

The classic clinical presentation of gallbladder cancer would be that of a 60- to 80-year-old woman who presents with symptoms similar to those seen with chronic cholecystitis. If the patient presents in the latter stages of the disease, 75% of patients will have pain, jaundice, and weight loss. Hepatomegaly would be noted in about 66%.

Gallbladder cancers spread by six primary pathways. These include (1) direct extension, (2) lymph node metastasis, (3) direct extension in the blood vessels, (4) peritoneal metastasis, (5) invasion into nerves, and (6) extension into the surrounding bile ducts. Metastatic spread of these cancers is usually related to direct extension or lymphatic metastasis. Those patients with jaundice may have widely metastatic disease at the time of presentation. Direct invasion into the liver occurs early. Direct extension into the colon, stomach, or duodenum may be detected as a biliary enteric fistula.

Management

The only hope for cure in patients with GBC is surgery. However, surgical cures occur in only about 10% even though the majority are discovered incidentally at the time of surgery.

The Beltz and Condon classification, based on the stage of the disease, correlates well with survival and helps one to review the surgical options. Group A patients have cancers that are seen in the cholecystectomy specimen but not detected at surgery. These patients have an excellent prognosis. Surgery is curative in most patients, though reports of deaths from metastatic disease have been published. In group B patients, the tumor is discovered during the cholecystectomy, and an extended cholecystectomy may be indicated with lymph node dissection. If the cancer is confined to the gallbladder and the tumor margins are free of cancer, surgery may be curative. The benefits of a liver wedge resection added to cholecystectomy have not been clearly documented, especially for the patients of groups A and B. Group C patients have an extensive tumor load and are able to be palliated during the surgery with a biliary bypass and enteric bypass. Group D patients are those who undergo an exploration and biopsy only, because their disease is too extensive for palliation. The group C and D patients typically have evidence of metastatic involvement of the liver, bile duct, or lymph nodes at the time of their staging laparotomy.

Adjuvant chemotherapy with radiation therapy has been advocated. The improvement in survival of patients who received 5-fluorouracil and radiation therapy was measured in added months of life. This survival increase with adjuvant therapy is slight but statistically significant. Patients who are not resectable may have palliation of their jaundice and pruritic symptoms by endoscopic or percutaneous biliary drainage.

Summary

Gallbladder cancer that is discovered incidentally may have an excellent prognosis. Surgery offers those patients a hope for cure. The patient who presents with larger GBC will have palliative procedures directed at improving the quality of life. Local metastatic disease causes most of the morbidity and mortality in patients with GBC. For the group C and D patients, less than 4% will survive 5 years. The patient experiences limited benefit from chemotherapy.

SUGGESTED READINGS

Beckman I, Dash N, Sefczek RJ, et al: Ultrasonographic findings in acute acalculous cholecystitis, Gastrointest Radiol 10:387-389, 1985.

This short paper provides some insight into how a noninvasive study using ultrasound might assist in the evaluation of the patients that are at risk for acalculous cholecystitis. The findings of a thickening (a change noted on serial examinations) gallbladder wall, a subserosal "halo" of edema, pericholecystic abscess formation, and noticeable gallbladder distention were all consistent findings that should assist in making the diagnosis of acute acalculous cholecystitis.

Christensen AH and Ishak KG: Benign tumors and pseudotumors of the gallbladder, Arch Pathol 90:423-432, 1970.

This is a hallmark publication that includes 180 cases of benign tumors and pseudotumors of the gallbladder. The gross findings and microscopic findings are presented and discussed.

Dubois F, Icard P, Berthelot G, and Levard H: Coelioscopic cholecystectomy, Ann Surg 211(1):60-63, 1989.

The authors in this article describe the technique involved in intra-abdominal endoscopic (laparoscopic) cholecystectomy. They discuss 36 patients who were treated by this technique, after perfection of the technique on an animal model, the pig. This was one of the articles that resulted in the widespread proliferation of this technique throughout the United States.

Fromm H: Gallstone dissolution therapy with urodiol: patient selection, Dig Dis Sci 34(12):36S-38S, 1989.

This is one of the articles published from a sponsored symposium on advances in bile and acid therapy. This article discusses the ideal patient selection and rational use of screening techniques to evaluate patients who might benefit from bile acid therapy.

Geenen DJ, Geehen JE, Hogan WJ, et al: Endoscopic therapy for benign bile duct strictures, Gastrointest Endosc 35:367-371, 1989.

This report discusses an endoscopic approach to benign bile duct strictures and presents data from a prospective study. This study suggests that the combination of progressive hydrostatic balloon dilatation and stent placement provides a safe and effective therapy for benign bile duct strictures.

Health and Policy Committee, American College of Physicians: How to study the gallbladder: position paper, Ann Intern Med 109:752-754, Nov 1988.

This paper provides an authoritative review of the current understanding of the diagnostic testing needed to evaluate patients with gallbladder disease.

Helzberg JH, Petersen JM, and Boyer JL: Improved survival with primary sclerosing cholangitis: a review of clinicopathologic features and comparison of symptomatic and asymptomatic patients, Gastroenterology 92:1869-1875, 1987.

This paper describes the clinicopathologic features and long term follow-up study (over a 30-year span) of patients with primary sclerosing cholangitis. This paper brings to focus that when PSC is detected before the onset of signs and symptoms this disease does not have the dismal outlook the earlier literature suggested was the case.

Jutras JA and Levesque HP: Adenomyoma and adenomyomatosis of the gallbladder: radiologic and pathologic correlations, Radiol Clin North Am 4:483-500, 1966.

This is an excellent review of the anatomic and histologic findings of adenomyomatosis of the gallbladder with radiologic correlates. The paper includes a discussion of the literature.

Leese T, Neoptolemos JP, Baker AR, and Carr-Locke DL: Management of acute cholangitis and the impact of endoscopic sphincterotomy, Br J Surg 73:988-992, 1986.

The paper outlines the need for decompression of an infected biliary tract.

Lokich JJ, Kane RA, Harrison DA, and McDermott WV: Biliary tract obstruction secondary to cancer: management guidelines and selected literature review, J Clin Oncol 5:969-981, 1987.

The authors present an authoritative review of the literature and recommendations for management. The evidence presented suggests that prophylactic biliary stenting to prevent cholangitis is not supported by the literature, despite the fact that it has become the standard of care at many centers.

Marton KI and Doubilet P: How to image the gallbladder in suspected cholecystitis, Ann Intern Med 109:722-729, Nov 1988.

The authors review the more commonly used gallbladder-imaging techniques used in the evaluation of patients with cholecystitis. They also outline some diagnostic strategies in the cost-effective use of these techniques. The review avoids discussion of testing required to evaluate patients for bile duct stones even though one would expect an overlap of the two processes.

Mueller PR, van Sonnenberg E, and Simeone JF: Fine-needle transhepatic cholangiograph, Ann Intern Med 97:567-572, 1982.

The authors review the technical aspects, safety, and problems associated with skinny-needle cholangiography.

Neoptolemos JP, Carr-Locke DL, and Fossard DP: Prospective randomized study of preoperative endoscopic sphincterotomy versus surgery alone for common bile duct stones, Br Med J 294:470-474, 1987.

The role of preoperative endoscopic sphincterotomy vs. surgery alone is addressed in this study.

Neoptolemos JP, Hofman AF, and Moossa AR: Chemical treatment of stones in the biliary tree, Br J Surg 73:515-524, 1986.

This review article provides an excellent discussion of the current understanding of the contact dissolution agents. The discussion is designed as a practical outline for the practicing physician.

Neoptolemos JP, London NJ, James D, et al: Controlled trial of urgent endoscopic retrograde cholangiopancreatography and endoscopic sphincterotomy versus conservative treatment for acute pancreatitis due to gallstones, Lancet 2(8618):979-983, Oct 29, 1988.

This report discusses the results of a prospective trial that involved examination of whether urgent endoscopic retrograde cholangiopancreatography with sphincterotomy offered an advantage over conservative supportive therapy alone.

Pitt HA, Kaufman SL, Coleman J, et al: Benign postoperative biliary strictures, Ann Surg 210:417-425, 1989.

This article is a retrospective chart review that is an attempt to provide some insights into the complications and response to treatment of benign bile duct strictures. The study compares the results of patients treated with percutaneous transhepatic balloon dilatation to surgery.

Ransohoff DF, Miller GL, Forsythe SB, and Hermann RE: Outcome of acute cholecystitis in patients with diabetes mellitus, Ann Intern Med 106:829-832, 1987.

This paper presents data that no longer allow one to support the practice of prophylactic cholecystectomy for diabetic patients with silent gallstones. They found that surgery does not increase life expectancy or the quality of life.

Speer AG, Russell RCG, Hatfield ARW, et al: Randomized trail of endoscopic versus percutaneous stent insertion in malignant obstructive jaundice, Lancet 2(8550):57-62, July 11, 1987.

This prospective randomized study compares percutaneous biliary drainage with endoscopic drainage in terms of success and safety in patients with malignant obstruction who were judged unfit for surgery.

Summers RW and Johlin FC: The pathophysiology, evaluation and management of motility disorders of the biliary tract, Gastroenterol Clin North Am 18(2):425-435, 1989.

This review provides a discussion of the management and evaluation of patients with presumed motor disorders of the biliary tract.

31 Hepatobiliary Trauma

Kenneth L. Mattox and *Robert Richardson*

The following diagnostic and therapeutic considerations of hepatobiliary injury have one common theme: the prime directive in the treatment of liver trauma is hemostasis. Throughout history, authors have noted the propensity of the injured liver for hemorrhage. Diverse maneuvers attempting to achieve hemostasis have been employed in the past. Some, such as the Pringle maneuver, have had success. Others, such as perihepatic packing, have fallen into disrepute, only to be revived in recent years.

ANATOMIC CORRELATIONS

The liver is suspended in the right upper quadrant of the peritoneal cavity by the falciform, triangular, and coronary ligaments, from which the liver may avulse during rapid deceleration. For practical purposes in dealing with trauma patients, the peritoneal cavity lies between the nipples (fourth or fifth intercostal space) and the pubis. It should be understood that the upper extent of diaphragm travel is this intercostal level; therefore entry wounds near the fourth or fifth interspace may have traversed the peritoneal cavity. In the right upper quadrant, the dome of the liver may rise to the level of the nipple during expiration (Figure 31-1).

The liver is composed of soft parenchyma penetrated with a ductular and vascular framework. It is a dense organ, easily fractured or penetrated if force is directly applied to its surface. Glisson's capsule is a thin layer of visceral peritoneum surrounding the liver. A fracture of the underlying hepatic parenchyma without injury to Glisson's capsule leads to the development of a subcapsular or intrahepatic hematoma. There is a bare area devoid of this covering posteriorly where the hepatic veins join the vena cava. Injuries in this area are highly lethal and difficult to approach.

The hepatic pedicle is composed of the portal vein, common bile duct, and hepatic artery. These structures lie in the lateral aspect of the hepatoduodenal ligament. Placing a clamp across these structures to occlude inflow to the liver is known as a "Pringle maneuver." Posteriorly to the hepatic pedicle lies the vena cava. Overlying and parallel to each other, the vena cava and hepatic pedicle are a fingerbreadth apart. Injuries common to both structures must be suspected and excluded during exploration.

Anatomically the liver is divided into right and left lobes, which are further subdivided for purposes of formal resection. Rarely do the effects of blunt force

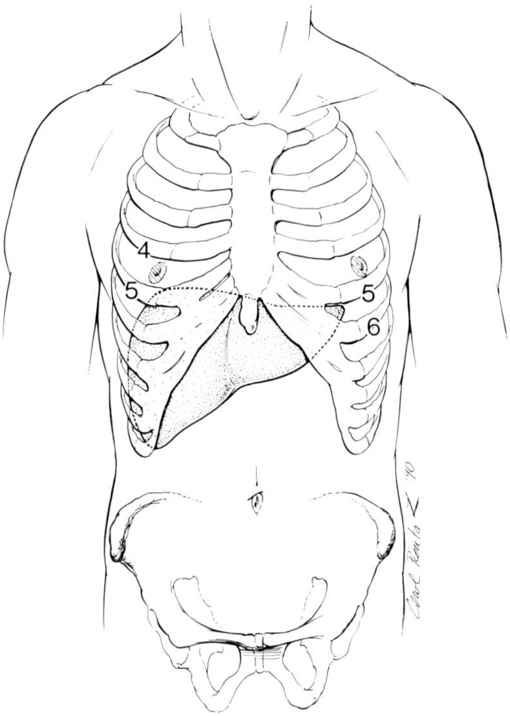

Figure 31-1
Anatomic relationship of liver within the rib cage. The dome of the liver may rise to the level of the fourth intercostal space. Penetrating trauma entering the right side of the chest commonly involves the diaphragm and liver.

and penetrating trauma correspond to lines of anatomic resection. On rare occasions of extensive lobar destruction, one may consider lobectomy.

Several organs share proximity to the liver and may be concurrently injured. The left lobe of the liver overlies part of the esophagus, stomach, and duodenum. Common to both lobes is the gallbladder. In proximity to the right lobe is the duodenum, hepatic flexure of the colon, right kidney, and vena cava. Located superiorly is the diaphragm on the right and pericardium on the left.

MECHANISMS OF INJURY

Liver injury is discovered in 30% of laparotomies for blunt trauma and 20% of laparotomies for penetrating trauma. It is the largest and heaviest solid intra-abdominal organ. It is suspended superiorly and posteriorly by ligamentous attachments, which the extent of its support. Protection is provided by the bony thorax, and force great enough to fracture ribs certainly may injure the liver. The liver may be injured during rapid deceleration, such as that experienced in falls and motor vehicle accidents. Avulsion of the liver from the vena cava may occur, leading to massive hemorrhage. Crush injuries or the localized application of force over the liver may be sustained in fights or assaults with blunt objects. Rib fractures may be associated with this mechanism, and they are suggestive of the presence of hepatic injury. Fragments of fractured ribs may be driven into the hepatic parenchyma compounding the degree of injury. Livery injury has also occurred secondary to cardiopulmonary resuscitation.

Penetrating trauma accounts for 80% of abdominal trauma seen in large urban trauma centers such as the Ben Taub General Hospital in Houston, Texas. Gunshot wounds, stab wounds, and shotgun wounds involving the liver occur in 20% of the cases. Iatrogenic liver injury does occur and may result from percutaneous liver biopsy, laparoscopy, and transhepatic cholangiogram.

Gradation of liver injury has been proposed in similar forms by Pachter,

Moore, and Flint and is useful for description of injury severity.

Grade 1 Simple laceration or tear.
Grade 2 Simple laceration or tear. Requires hepatorrhaphy.
Grade 3 Parenchymal disruption from blunt or penetrating force resulting in the development of a subcapsular hematoma, intrahepatic hematoma, or hemoperitoneum. Hepatorrhaphy or tractotomy is usually sufficient.
Grade 4 Major parenchymal disruption of one or both lobes. Requires adjunctive maneuvers for hemostasis such as packing.
Grade 5 Hepatic venous injury or retrohepatic vena cava injury.

INITIAL CONSIDERATIONS

The initial evaluation and resuscitation of the injured patient should proceed in a rational fashion, such as that described in the American College of Surgeons Advanced Trauma Life Support course. Presentation of the patient with liver injury depends on the extent of hepatic injury, extent of associated injuries, and the resulting degree of hemorrhage. Hemodynamic presentation can range from the asymptomatic to profound shock. Liver trauma, apart from other injuries, is difficult to diagnose without the assistance of imaging studies or direct visualization at surgery.

Any history of a forceful deceleration or trauma localized to the right upper quadrant or right flank may indicate the presence of liver injury. This is in addition to the obvious presence of entry wounds from a stabbing or gunshot wound.

To the physician caring for the hypotensive patient with a distended abdomen either from blunt or penetrating trauma, the main concern should be getting the patient to the operating room as rapidly as possible. If, on the other hand, the patient is not rapidly deteriorating and is in a relatively stable condition, signs and symptoms of liver injury may be systemic or localized. Systemic signs and symptoms of significant liver injury are those of hemorrhage such as hypotension, tachycardia, decreased urine output and altered mental status. Localized signs and symptoms may include abdominal distention, decreased bowel sounds, and abdominal pain and tenderness in the right upper quadrant. The tenderness encountered on examination is variable and may include pain from rib fractures, an overlying soft tissue injury, or blood in the peritoneal cavity, which causes a diffuse tenderness without rigidity.

The intensity of the above findings can range from the barely perceptible to a state in extremis. Frequently these findings are encountered in the management of patients with additional injuries to other organs. In the presence of suggestive signs and the history of significant blunt or penetrating trauma to the right upper quadrant, liver injury is highly likely. The state of shock does not correspond to the degree of liver trauma. With the tamponade effect of the closed peritoneum, a patient may appear deceptively stable, only to become very hypotensive when the peritoneum is opened in the operating room.

In the multiply injured patient, liver injury may occur in a cluster of injuries to multiple systems with varied signs and symptoms. Whatever the presentation, strict adherence to the principles of initial resuscitation cannot be overemphasized.

The orderly and rational application of resuscitation algorithms favorably affects outcome. Initially, all patients must have the assurance of a secure airway. Efforts must be taken to address any problem, such as a pneumothorax, that may prevent the adequate exchange of oxygen. Hemorrhage should be arrested concurrently with the treatment of hypovolemia. If this cannot be achieved in the emergency center, preparations are made to expeditiously take the patient to the operating room. A rapid, thorough physical examination is of paramount importance to elucidate those "hidden" entry wounds.

The unstable patient with intraabdominal hemorrhage from hepatic injury is best treated in the operating room. Mattox in 1978 reported that laparotomy with packing of the liver in the emergency center does not increase survival. Patients with this type of injury should not be kept in the emergency center to be "stabilized" before exploration. However, the initiation of intravenous fluids for resuscitation is acceptable. Multiple large bore intravenous lines or a Swan-Ganz introducer sheath with a side port are placed. Because of their small caliber, standard central lines should not be used for volume resuscitation. They may, however, be used to measure central venous pressure in cases of suspected cardiac tamponade. Blood samples should be sent for type and cross matching. In the acutely hypotensive patient, the use of uncrossmatched, type-specific packed red blood cells that can be obtained in 3 to 5 minutes is recommended, rather than the use of O-negative blood.

DIAGNOSTIC STUDIES

The diagnosis of liver injury may be supported by laboratory values. Although not specific for liver injury, decreased hemoglobin and hematocrit values are suggestive of hemorrhage. These values may be monitored serially to determine the presence of ongoing hemorrhage in the stable patient. The white blood cell count may be elevated from associated injuries or a demargination effect.

Liver enzymes and bilirubin levels may be elevated; however, this is usually not seen in the acute setting. Patients that present in delayed fashion can have jaundice, especially from injuries to the biliary tract. Bilirubin levels that double in a 24-hour period can be seen from the intraperitoneal absorption of bile. Amylase values are not helpful with the diagnosis of liver injury. Elevations are usually seen with pancreatic, salivary gland, or small bowel injury.

Abdominal radiographs are generally not helpful in diagnosing hepatic trauma because they are rather nonspecific. Retrospectively, an elevated right hemidiaphragm has been observed in some cases of significant injury.

After disruption of hepatic parenchyma, nuclear scintigraphy such as the HIDA (dimethyliminodiacetic acid) or PIPIDA (paraisopropyl IDA) scan may be abnormal. This study is also helpful in diagnosing injuries to the biliary tract and gallbladder. Nuclear scans can also be used in follow-up studies to document the resolution of an intrahepatic hematoma. Logistical limitations usually restrict this study to patients presenting in a delayed fashion or in the stable patient when CT scan is not available in the acute setting.

The CT scan is an extremely useful tool in the diagnosis of blunt hepatic injury in hemodynamically stable patients. It can demonstrate hepatic parenchymal injury, intraperitoneal fluid, and associated injuries to other solid organs, such as the pancreas and spleen. The CT scan is the study of choice in the patient injured from a blunt assault with a suspected hepatic injury in whom a negative study or demonstration of a minimal injury would result in nonoperative management.

For the CT scan to be a useful tool in the management of patients with hepatic injury, it must be available 24 hours a day in a timely fashion. The accuracy of the CT scan for solid organ injury is 85% to 90%, whereas that for hollow organ injury is significantly less even with the use of contrast agents.

In some clinical settings, the CT scan may not be appropriate. For example, a hypotensive patient with a right hemothorax, rib fractures, a slightly distended abdomen and a fractured femur will not benefit from CT scan of the abdomen. In this case, diagnostic peritoneal lavage is the study of choice to rule out significant intraabdominal hemorrhage. Peritoneal lavage, though not specific for hepatic injury, can be performed in a rapid manner, and if grossly positive, results are immediate.

NONOPERATIVE MANAGEMENT

Approximately 15% of isolated liver injuries occurring in adults may be considered for nonoperative management. The percentage is somewhat higher in the pediatric population. Nonoperative management should be considered only by those experienced in the care of trauma patients and treatment of hepatic injuries. Although nonoperative treatment has been employed successfully in pediatric and some adult populations, one must clearly understand that this modality can be contemplated only in patients whose hemodynamic stability is beyond question. Vital signs should be stable over time with blood pressure and pulse rate in acceptable ranges. Abdominal pain and tenderness associated with rib fractures, soft-tissue injury, or intraperitoneal blood do not obviate the need for serial examination of the abdomen, since increasing pain or the development of peritonitis may signal the presence of an associated injury.

Blunt trauma is the etiology of injury in almost all cases of nonoperative management. A CT scan best demonstrates the injury, which may be a subcapsular hematoma (Figure 31-2), intrahepatic hematoma (Figure 31-3), or lobar fracture. Ultrasound has been used to diagnose solid organ injury in an emergency setting but is not widely used at present.

Proponents of nonoperative management advocate observation in the intensive care unit until hemodynamic stability is assured. Initial resuscitation should be the same as for any trauma patient with significant hemorrhage. Initial laboratory studies should include blood for type and cross matching and clotting parameters. Liver enzymes and bilirubin may become slightly elevated in the days after injury. Pronounced and rapid elevation of bilirubin may indicate biliary tract injury, and additional studies should be obtained in preparation for possible exploration.

The diet should be withheld and patients kept at bed rest for 2 to 3 days after the injury to decrease the chances of rebleeding in the acute setting. Hemoglobin values may drift downward to the point where transfusion is considered. Advocated by some, transfusion of blood products is a key element in the supportive therapy of these patients. However, requirements exceeding one half the patient's blood volume are administered with extreme caution. When this limit is approached, continued hemorrhage is occurring. Transfusion therapy should not

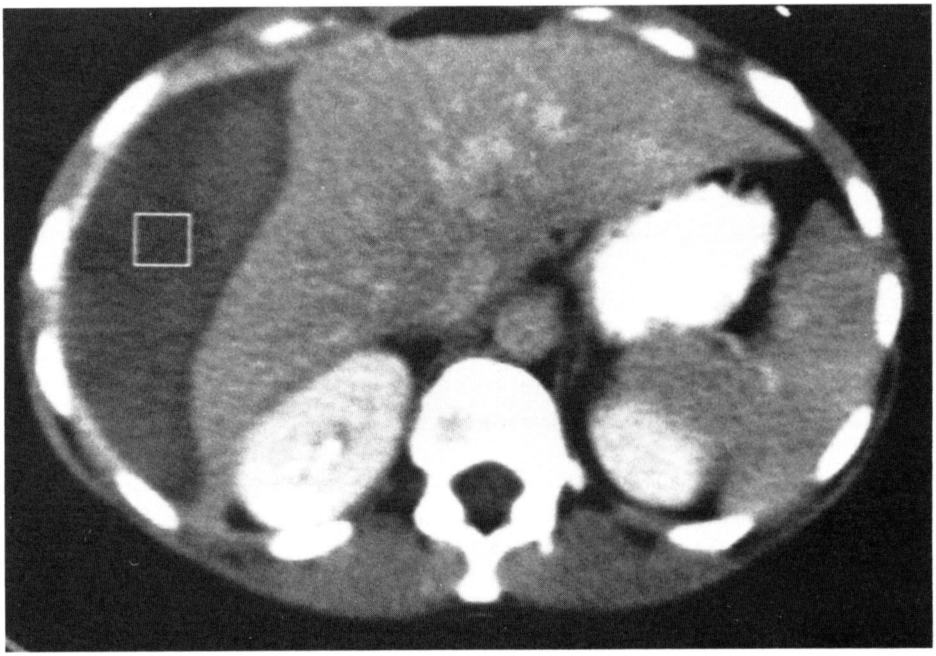

Figure 31-2
CT scan demonstrating a large subcapsular hematoma of the right lobe of the liver.

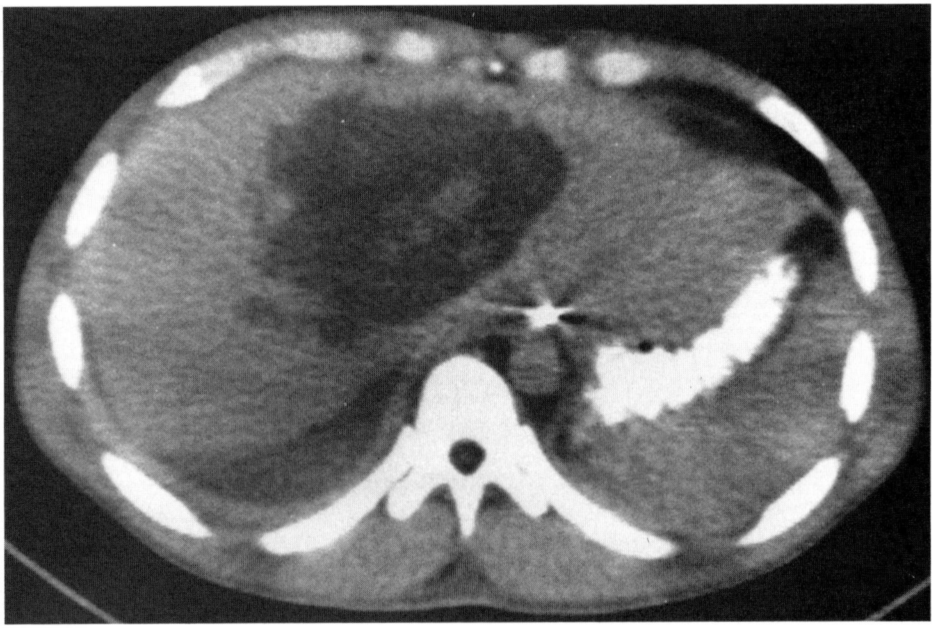

Figure 31-3
CT scan demonstrating a large intrahepatic hematoma.

be employed to treat persistent hypotension in the posttraumatic patient with liver injury, and exploration is warranted to address ongoing hemorrhage.

A follow-up scan should be obtained before discharge to document the absence of hematoma enlargement. Patient activity is restricted for 4 to 6 weeks. Morbidity is to be expected in up to 20% of patients after major injuries. Potential complications include postinjury fever, intraabdominal abscess, other septic complications, and hematobilia. Hospital stays may also be prolonged up to 3 weeks in some cases. Despite this, nonoperative management is successful in 90% of pediatric cases with failed attempts at nonoperative therapy requiring surgery because of continued hemorrhage, bile peritonitis, or associated injuries.

The rationale for nonoperative management is to avoid exploration of patients with isolated liver injuries that will stop bleeding and resolve spontaneously. When this can be achieved without the use of blood products, it is beneficial to the patient. Even though the risk of transfusion therapy is minimal, it is constantly present, and the liberal use of blood products to avoid surgery may not be ultimately beneficial to the patient.

OPERATIVE TREATMENT

The nature of significant hepatic injury is difficult to characterize without direct visualization. Frequently all that can be determined preoperatively about the nature of intraabdominal injuries is whether the patient requires an operation. Indications for laparotomy in abdominal trauma are based on the presence of any one of the following: peritonitis, hemodynamic instability, positive peritoneal lavage, gunshot wounds involving the peritoneal cavity, and selected stab wounds of the abdomen.

Once the decision is made to take the patient with intra-abdominal hemorrhage to the operating room, some initial considerations are worthy of mention. Before one makes the incision in an unstable patient who is rushed to the operating room with a hemoperitoneum, it is often prudent to wait the few extra minutes needed to obtain packed red blood cells. The tense hemoperitoneum will act to tamponade the injury. Opening the abdomen before anesthesia personnel are ready to keep up with ongoing blood loss will only further increase volume deficits as clots are dislodged and bleeding starts again. The brief waiting time is not wasted as additional intravenous access is obtained, initiated transfusions are completed, and equipment such as the BRAT (Baylor Rapid Autotransfusion) device is set up.

Once the abdomen is opened, the nature of the bleeding is assessed by a rapid evacuation of blood in the peritoneal cavity. This is best achieved by use of dry laparotomy pads in rapid succession to absorb the blood, which can later be suctioned by the autotransfusion device. Using only suction devices to aspirate blood in this setting is slow and inadequate. If massive bleeding is encountered, pressure is applied with laparotomy pads and the anesthesia personnel are appropriately cautioned that significant blood loss is imminent. Almost all liver bleeding can be temporarily stopped by pressure from laparotomy pads or pressure from the first assistant (Figure 31-4). By doing this, the anesthesiologist is therefore able to stabilize the patient as much as possible before continued exploration and further

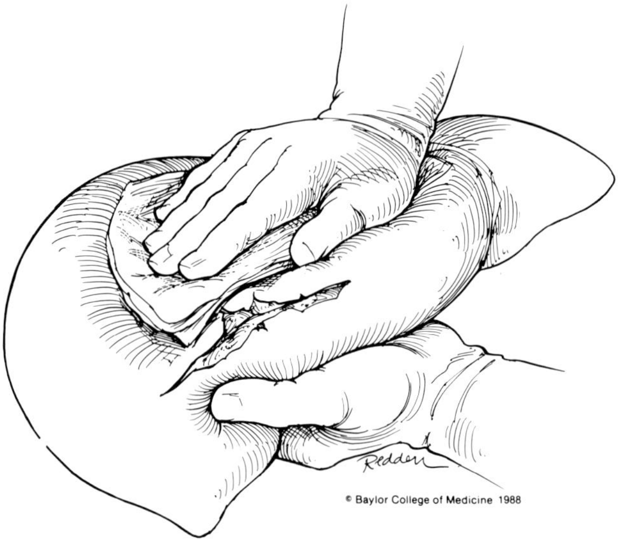

Figure 31-4
Bimanual compression of the liver effectively arrests hemorrhage in the massively bleeding liver.

blood loss. The concept of teamwork and communication cannot be overemphasized in this particular setting.

Initial exploration of the abdomen includes rapid assessment of all injuries with decisive efforts directed at control of active bleeding. In the profoundly hypotensive patient with multiple injuries, temporary aortic occlusion to aid in the control of hemorrhage and the augmentation of cerebral blood flow may be considered. This step may be achieved by descending thoracic aortic occlusion, aortic occlusion at the diaphragmatic hiatus, or balloon catheter occlusion of the aorta via the femoral artery.

A key concept in the exposure of liver injuries is mobilization. Incomplete exposure will impede efforts to repair or ligate bleeding vessels. Exposure is achieved by division of the falciform and right or left triangular ligaments as indicated. The liver can then be rotated medially into the wound, thereby providing adequate exposure.

If continued hemorrhage is massive, placement of a clamp across the hepatic pedicle to occlude the portal vein and hepatic artery may decrease bleeding (Figure 31-5). This Pringle maneuver may allow the surgeon to adequately visualize injured vessels so that repair can be accomplished. Clamp times in excess of 1 hour have been reported without any sequelae. If massive bleeding continues, retrohepatic venous injury must be suspected.

SPECIFIC INJURY TYPES

Simple Lacerations

Simple lacerations and capsular tears occur frequently (50% to 60% of all liver injures) and a significant number of these injuries are not actively bleeding when they are exposed during exploration despite a moderate amount of blood encountered in the peritoneal cavity. In the absence of active bleeding, nothing need be done to the injury. If bleeding is seen at exploration, hemostasis might be ob-

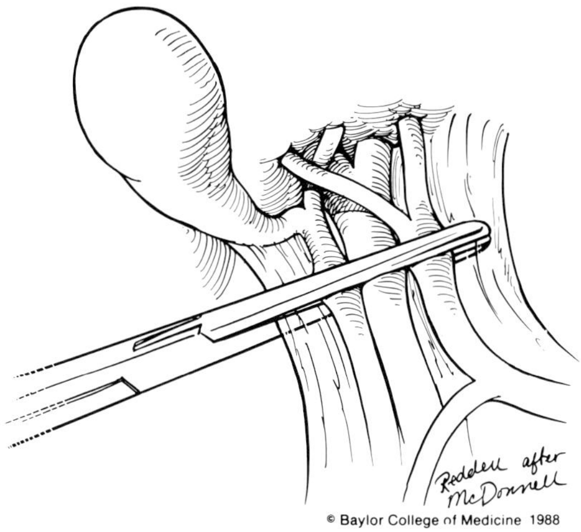

Figure 31-5
The placement of a clamp across the hepatic pedicle is known as a "Pringle maneuver." Controlling hemorrhage in this manner facilitates visualization and repair of the injury. Continued hemorrhage after placement of the clamp may indicate the presence of a retrohepatic venous injury.

tained by simple measures such as application of local hemostatic agents. If these maneuvers are not successful, suture hepatorrhaphy in a figure-of-eight fashion should suffice. A sheet of hemostatic agent may be placed over the injury which is then sutured, though this procedure is not usually necessary. Suture material should be number 0 or 1 chromic on a large, blunt-tipped needle. Gentle pressure should be applied when one is tying the suture, to avoid tearing the liver capsule or necrosing portions of liver tissue.

The decision to place a drain is based on the probability of developing a bile leak. Traditionally, extensive injuries require drainage, whereas very minimal injuries do not. On rare occasions, transient bile leaks have developed after minimal injuries, and some surgeons have adopted a routine drainage policy of all injuries. On the other hand, surgeons do not routinely drain wedge biopsy sites of the liver. Therefore, drainage of selected grade 2 injuries when bile staining is observed is recommended.

Shallow Fractures of One or Both Lobes

Shallow fractures of the lobes result from a direct blunt assault causing the capsule to rupture and the parenchyma to fracture. The injury configuration may be stellate or linear with little devitalized tissue. The injury is not deep but may bleed profusely. The bleeding is easily controlled by direct pressure, but the continued application of pressure is usually not successful in permanently arresting the hemorrhage.

Bleeding vessels in the injury should be ligated or repaired when they can be easily identified without increasing the area of injury. For the shallow fracture, suture hepatorrhaphy is appropriate if dead space will not be created within the parenchyma. Drainage is recommended for this type of injury.

Bleeding Missile Tracts

Missile tracts may be caused by gunshot wounds, other projectiles, and stab wounds. The amount of bleeding encountered is variable, and involvement of ma-

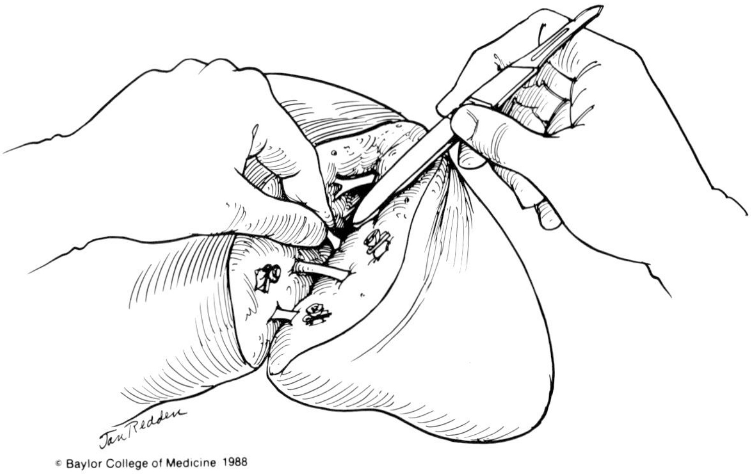

Figure 31-6
Tractotomy through the substance of the liver to the level of vascular injury is a useful technique. Upon exposure, the injury may be repaired under direct visualization.

jor vascular structures is not always readily apparent. Location of the wound may help determine major vessel involvement, and profuse bleeding, if present, is an ominous sign. Suture hepatorrhaphy of the entry and exit wound is associated with the creation of an intrahepatic collection, which has the potential for infection and subsequent abscess development. Hemobilia can also result from this technique.

A more direct approach is tractotomy to the level of the injury (Figure 31-6). This technique involves unroofing of the tract through the substance of the liver to the level of the injury. The finger fracture technique is utilized to directly approach the bleeding vessel for repair or ligation (Figure 31-7). It is important to ligate all lacerated biliary radicles when encountered to aid in the prevention of postoperative bile leaks. After hemostasis is attained, the parenchyma may be loosely approximated and drained. As an alternative, a tongue of greater omentum is placed into the crevice created by the tractotomy to function as a viable drain (Figure 31-8).

Subcapsular Hematoma

Fracture of the liver parenchyma without rupture of the liver capsule leads to the development of a subcapsular hematoma. This occurs in 7% of patients with liver injury but is identified with increasing frequency because of the availability of CT scanning. Patients may present in an acute or delayed fashion. If no other injuries that may cause shock are present, these patients are hemodynamically stable. The diagnosis is suspected by the history of blunt abdominal trauma and right upper quadrant pain without signs of peritonitis. Liver tests may be mildly elevated. In those patients whose only injury is a subcapsular hematoma, diagnostic

A

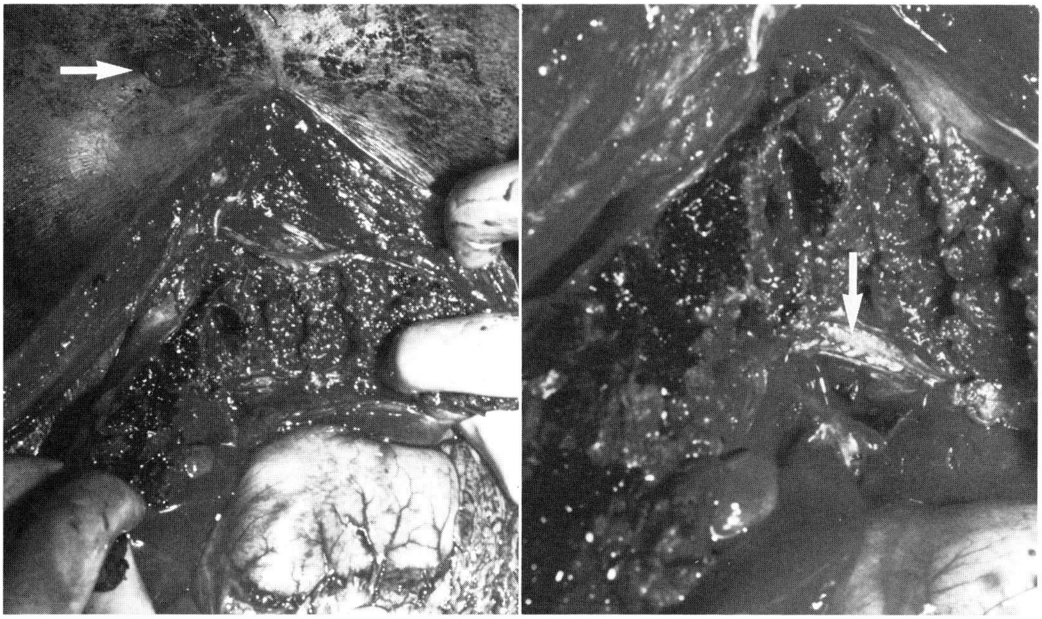

B

Figure 31-7
A, Gunshot wound entering the right lower chest, *white arrow,* and tractotomy performed to the level of the injury. **B,** Lateral venorrhaphy of the left portal vein near the bifurcation, *black arrow.*

A

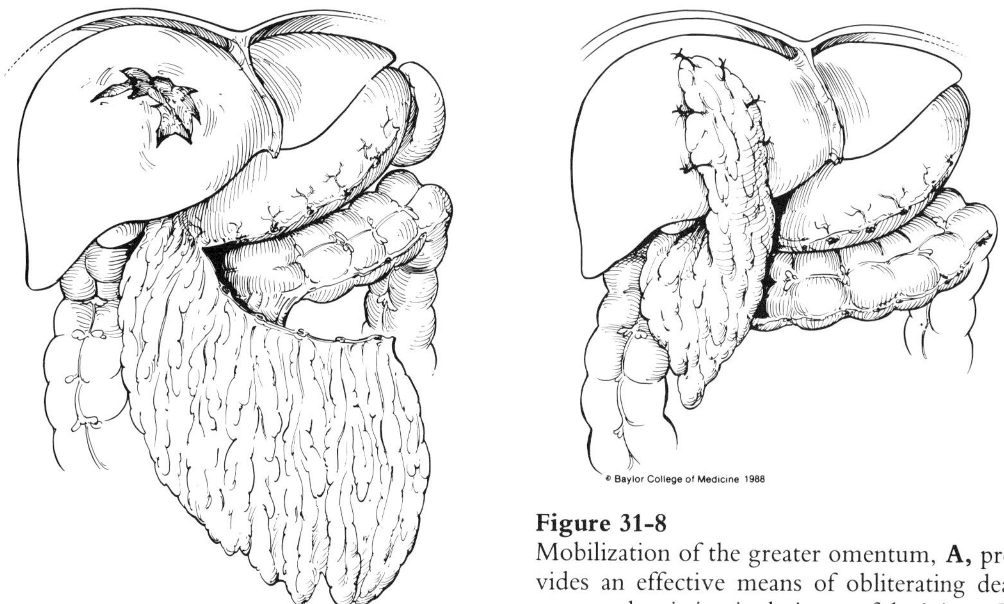

B

Figure 31-8
Mobilization of the greater omentum, **A,** provides an effective means of obliterating dead space and assisting in drainage of the injury, **B.**

peritoneal lavage is negative because of the absence of intraperitoneal blood. Hemoglobin and hematocrit may be slightly decreased but should remain stable over time. CT scan reveals a perihepatic hematoma without free fluid in the peritoneal cavity. The value of repeated clinical examination cannot be overemphasized should the patient develop signs of peritonitis during the in-hospital observation period. Transfusion for hemodynamic support should be given cautiously, if at all. If the patient becomes hemodynamically unstable with signs of hemorrhage, laparotomy is indicated.

Patients should undergo intensive observation for 2 to 3 days, and the duration of hospitalization may extend beyond several days. Hemoglobin levels are monitored serially, and meals are withheld until hemodynamic stability is assured. Blood is kept on hold in the blood bank, and coagulation parameters are measured. The use of prophylactic antibiotics is controversial, but those, who support their use, such as Tunnell and Elkins et al., cite the desire to prevent infection of the hematoma as the rationale. A CT scan before discharge from the hospital is recommended to ensure that the hematoma is not enlarging. Physical activity should be restricted for 4 to 6 weeks or until near resolution can be documented.

Traditional teaching has held that subcapsular hematomas should be opened to achieve hemostasis because of the risk of delayed rupture and hemorrhage. If the CT scan reveals a large fracture of hepatic parenchyma associated with a subcapsular hematoma, it should be opened; however, if the subcapsular hematoma is small, nonexpanding, and not associated with major parenchymal injury, it can be observed and followed.

Major Lobar Disruption

Lobar disruption of one or both lobes is associated with high velocity bullet wounds and blunt trauma from high energy impact. Bleeding is profuse, and patients are usually hypotensive in the field. The abdomen is distended, and patients manifest signs of circulatory collapse. A chest radiograph may reveal right-sided rib fractures. A right-sided pleural effusion may be seen from a diaphragmatic tear that allows blood to egress into the pleural cavity from the liver injury. With these injuries, CT scan and peritoneal lavage would only confirm strong suspicions of intraabdominal hemorrhage; therefore one is not indicated.

At exploration, initial considerations are to rapidly visualize and characterize the injury. Of primary concern, is achieving hemostasis. It may be necessary to control active bleeding by pressure tamponade of the liver while further evaluation and stabilization is accomplished. The percentage of cases with associated injuries requiring treatment is approximately 80%.

As it becomes evident that major lobar injury is present, adjunctive maneuvers to achieve hemostasis are considered. Mobilization of the liver is helpful in this situation. When visualization is poor because of ongoing blood loss, it is important to remember when dividing the triangular ligaments not to proceed too far medially because the hepatic veins may be inadvertently encountered.

Bleeding vessels should be ligated or repaired whenever possible, but these procedures are almost impossible to perform from within the injury. Bleeding seldom is exclusively arterial in nature. In general, hepatic arterial ligation is rarely successful in completely arresting the hemorrhage but can be performed without major sequelae if portal venous perfusion is maintained.

After control of major hemorrhage, débridement of devitalized tissue is performed. A considerable amount of necrotic tissue may be present; however, formal lobectomy is not routinely indicated in this setting. In fact, this procedure may be hazardous in the emergent situation because of the associated blood loss.

For larger fractures of the hepatic parenchyma, approximation of liver tissue after control of major vessels may not achieve complete hemostasis. In this situation, an alternative to hepatorrhaphy of deep lacerations is packing with a viable segment of mobilized greater omentum (see Figure 31-8). Placing omentum against the injured surface functions to obliterate closed space and to provide a vascularized surface to aid in the absorption of a serous or bilious effluent from the liver.

POSTOPERATIVE CARE

Postoperatively, hemoglobin and hematocrit are monitored serially for 24 to 48 hours. After liver injury, most drains are placed prophylactically to function as a conduit should a bile leak occur. If drains are used, they should be left in place for 48 hours. If a bile leak is not observed, removal of the drain is considered. A nasogastric tube may be required initially, but usually can be removed in 24 hours. Meals are withheld for 36 to 48 hours. Antibiotics, if employed as a prophylaxis against septic complications, should be continued for no more than 24 to 48 hours. Patients are seen in follow-up sessions 1 week and 1 month after injury.

SPECIAL CONSIDERATIONS

On occasion, it may be totally impossible to arrest bleeding from liver parenchyma by use of the methods described above. Up to 5% of patients with liver injuries may experience a bilobar burst or crush, the development of a coagulopathy, or a retrohepatic venous injury.

The temporary placement of laparotomy pads around the liver to tamponade bleeding has been a very useful tool (Figure 31-9). Indications for packing include the development of a coagulopathy or uncontrollable parenchymal bleeding. The goal of packing is to rapidly arrest hemorrhage with laparotomy pads, which compress the liver and tamponade the bleeding. When using this procedure, care must be taken not to occlude the vena cava. Depending on the size of the patient, 10 to 20 laparotomy pads are used. A folded plastic Steri-drape is placed on the surface of the liver to prevent undue adherence of the pads to the liver and to facilitate removal. Drains are not placed at this time.

The patient should be kept intubated because of the increased intraperitoneal volume and elevation of the right hemidiaphragm, which makes continued normal excursion impossible. Packs are left in place approximately 48 hours. During this time, coagulation factors are replaced, and the patient is warmed and stabilized. Upon reexploration, the bleeding has stopped or is controllable in 90% of patients. At the time of reexploration, the abdomen should be irrigated with warm normal saline and a careful search carried out for additional injuries. The liver should also be drained and an abdominal radiograph obtained in the operating room to document the recovery of all laparotomy pads. On rare occasion, it may

A

B

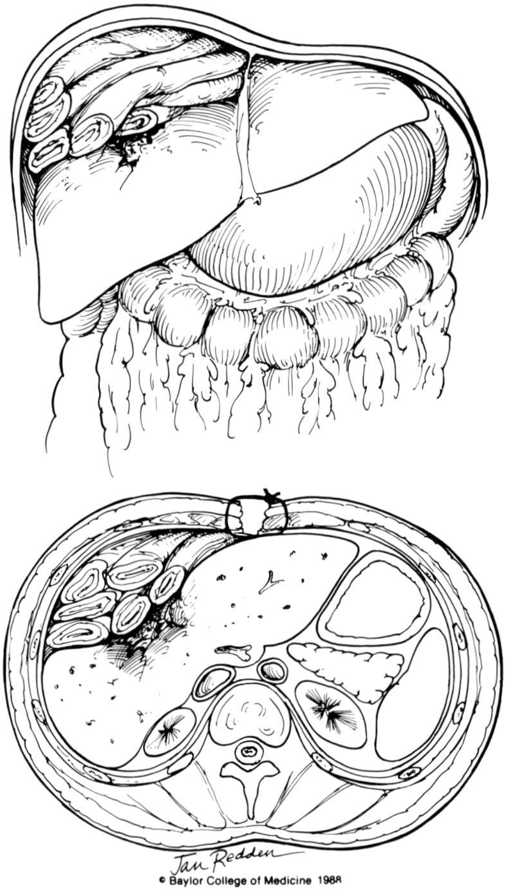

Figure 31-9
A, Temporary placement of laparotomy pads around the liver to arrest hemorrhage. **B,** Care should be taken to avoid occlusion and compression of the vena cava.

be necessary to repack the patient because of continued bleeding and wait another 48 hours before reexploration.

The development of a coagulopathy during the treatment of massive liver trauma is dependent on several factors. Some of the reasons include clotting factor consumption, hemodilution, and hypothermia. During exploration in a seriously injured patient with considerable blood loss, a subtle transition becomes apparent. Despite the ongoing administration of blood, fresh-frozen plasma, and platelets, the patient is no longer able to form a clot. Previously dry areas begin to bleed and hypothermia becomes pronounced from the administration of cold fluids and exposure of the peritoneal cavity to room air temperatures. As bleeding worsens, fluids are given at an even higher rate increasing hemodilution and straining the ability of anesthesia personnel to keep up with the losses. Blood warmers and rapid transfusion devices may delay the onset of a coagulopathy; however, the effect is only temporary if bleeding remains uncontrolled.

In the unstable, coagulopathic patient, further attempts at hepatic repair will actually worsen hypothermia and increase blood loss to the point that chances for survival begin to disappear. Maneuvers to rapidly stop bleeding and close the abdomen would be advantageous. Packing of the liver injury will assist in hemostasis, but abdominal fascial approximation may be an insurmountable task because of the packing and edematous small bowel, which may be massive from the administration of considerable amounts of crystalloid. When expeditious abdominal closure is necessary, application of towel clips to temporarily close the abdomen is advised. In less than 1 minute, 30 to 40 sequentially placed towel clips (1.5 cm apart) can approximate the skin of the abdominal wall. A sterile towel placed on the clips is then covered with an adhesive, plastic, sterile drape. The patient is rapidly taken to the ICU for supportive care and warming. The patient is returned to the operating room for formal abdominal closure when the edema, hypothermia, and coagulopathy have been reversed. Usually this requires 36 to 48 hours. This technique is especially useful for planned reoperations of any kind. There have not been any wound problems specifically related to the application of towel clips. The mortality of patients requiring towel clip closure is 60% to 70%, which reflects the severe degree of injury.

RETROHEPATIC VENOUS INJURIES

The mortality of retrohepatic venous injuries exceeds 90%. Exploration may reveal massive hemorrhage that is not affected by clamping the hepatic pedicle, or some patients may demonstrate a contained hematoma. Repair of the hepatic veins or retrohepatic vena cava may be attempted by medial rotation of the liver after extensive mobilization (Figure 31-10). If this is not feasible, the injury may be directly approached through the substance of the liver by finger fracture technique. Control of the hemorrhage may necessitate placement of a bypass intracaval shunt (Figure 31-11). Simply clamping the vena cava and hepatic pedicle to control hemorrhage during repair would obstruct venous return to the heart, predisposing the patient to cardiac arrest from hypovolemia. Once vascular isolation of the liver is achieved, repair may then be carried out. Use of autotransfusion devices are extremely helpful in this situation. Successful use of the shunt depends on the presence of experienced and knowledgeable personnel.

COMPLICATIONS OF HEPATIC INJURY

Biliary Fistula

Bile leakage after liver trauma is caused by ductular disruption of varying degrees. This complication is seen in approximately 5% to 10% of patients after grade 3 injuries and above. In general, if a fistula is to occur, it is seen within 48 hours. Fistulas are usually self-limited and resolve within 1 to 2 weeks if no associated distal obstruction or biliary tract injury is present.

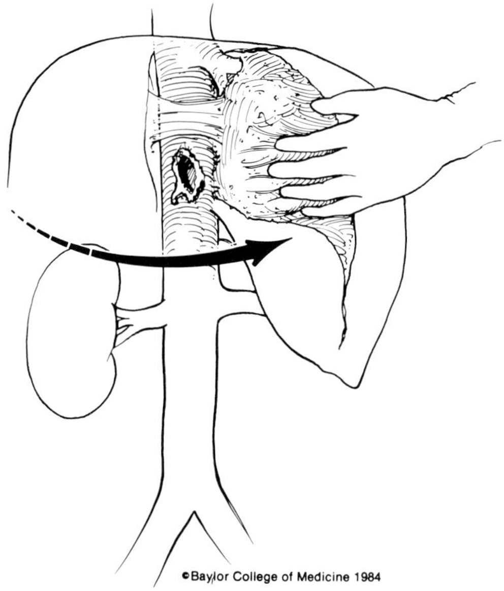

Figure 31-10
Division of the triangular ligaments will permit the medial rotation and elevation of the right lobe of the liver so that retrohepatic vena cava and hepatic venous injuries may be exposed.

Placement of a Penrose or closed-suction drain does not always guarantee complete evacuation of the bile should a fistula occur. Intraperitoneal bile may not cause peritonitis unless it is infected or inspissated. In the presence of an unrecognized diaphragmatic injury, biliary fistula patients may develop a thoracobiliary fistula. Intraabdominal bile collections may be drained by CT-guided catheter placement. If this does not achieve permanent resolution of the collection, investigative

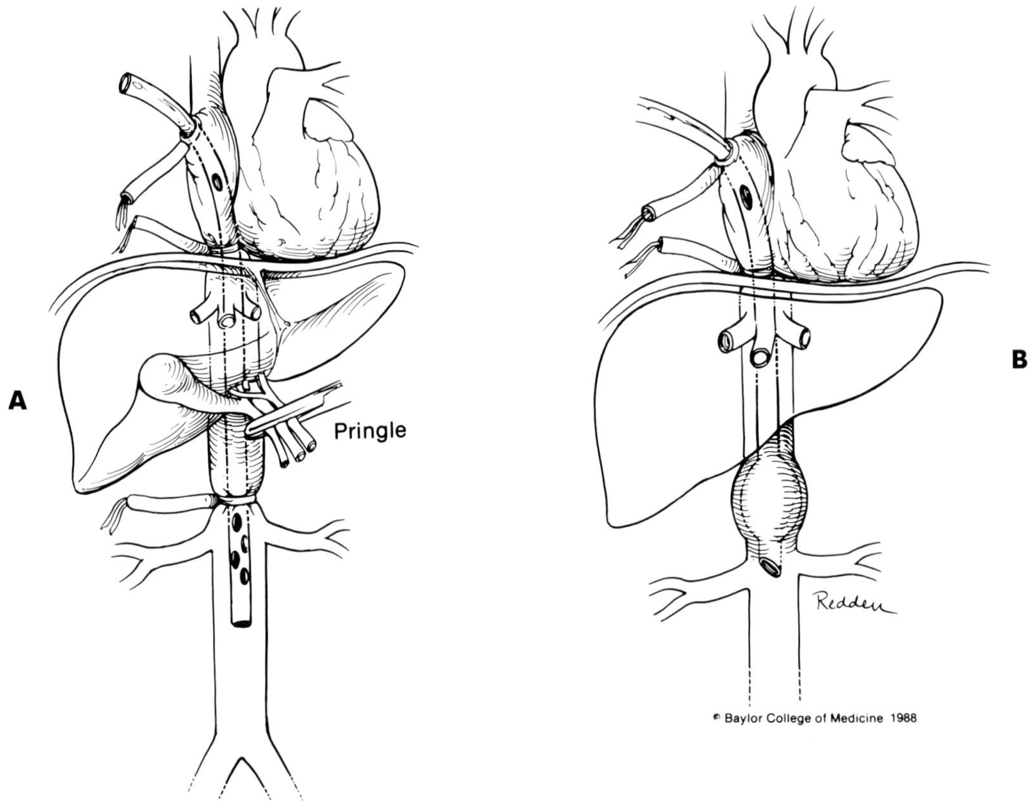

Figure 31-11
With use of a chest tube, **A,** or endotracheal tube, **B,** the atriocaval shunt is inserted through the right atrium. Use of the endotracheal tube obviates the need to control the suprarenal inferior vena cava below the liver because of the inflatable cuff. However, if it is performed, it must be done above the renal veins to prevent bleeding during the repair. The supradiaphragmatic inferior vena cava must be exposed and isolated to prevent retrograde bleeding in all cases. Care must be taken to create a port in the shunt between the atriotomy and proximal inferior vena cava to permit venous return to the heart. The application of a Pringle maneuver and insertion of the shunt will achieve vascular isolation of the liver. Further mobilization will reveal the injury so that direct repair can be performed.

studies should be obtained if the patient is asymptomatic and stable. An endoscopic retrograde cholangiopancreatoscopy (ERCP) may demonstrate the level of the fistula. If the injury is minor, endoscopic sphincterotomy will decrease the duration of drainage if spontaneous resolution is expected. If this is not successful, operative drainage should be performed.

Hematobilia

Hematobilia may occur from days to weeks after hepatic injury and is seen in less than 1% of patients. It results from a traumatic communication of the biliary tract and hepatic vascular system. The patient demonstrates signs of hemorrhage, episodic right upper quadrant pain and jaundice. Lower gastrointestinal bleeding is present in some form in all patients, and 80% develop melena. Fewer than 20% of patients will develop hematemesis. Endoscopy reveals a normal stomach proximal to the pylorus; however, visualization of the papilla may reveal a bloody effluent or clot. Bleeding can be intermittent or massive in nature.

A CT scan, ultrasonogram, or HIDA scan may reveal an intrahepatic hematoma. An angiogram will reveal the arterial source of bleeding in most cases, and the biliary tree may even be visualized in some patients.

Preferred treatment is embolization of involved arterial branches. If unsuccessful, hepatic resection or selective arterial ligation may be considered. Portal venous bleeding into the biliary tree is usually self-limited but may become a problem if the patient has portal hypertension.

Peri-hepatic Abscess

Incomplete hemostasis and drainage of liver injuries contribute to development of perihepatic fluid accumulation. Inadequate débridement of devitalized tissue leads to development of necrotic tissue. In certain patients, the above circumstances may be instrumental in the development of a perihepatic abscess. Intrahepatic abscess may develop from contamination of an intrahepatic hematoma.

Diagnosis is best confirmed by CT scan on a postoperative patient manifesting signs of infection on postoperative days 7 to 10. Liver tests of alkaline phosphatase and bilirubin may show elevated levels. Antibiotics to cover gastrointestinal flora are started, and CT-guided aspiration of the collection is successful in 70% of cases. If the patient does not demonstrate clinical improvement in 24 to 48 hours, operative drainage is indicated.

Liver Fever

"Liver fever" is a phenomenon often described by residents. A typical patient has suffered a moderate fracture of one lobe of the liver and, on postoperative days 4 to 7, is beginning to manifest modest elevations in temperature (99° to 101° F). The fever is attributed to resolution of devitalized hepatic parenchyma. No signs of systemic sepsis are present, and the condition remains self-limited.

ADDITIONAL CONSIDERATIONS

Injuries to the extrahepatic biliary tree are seldom isolated, but they do occur. Penetrating trauma accounts for the majority (90%), whereas blunt trauma accounts for the remainder. Peritoneal lavage may be positive for bile but can be from associated enteric injuries.

If patients present in a delayed fashion, symptoms may include jaundice and right upper quadrant pain. Liver tests may show elevation of bilirubin and alkaline phosphatase values. Endoscopic retrograde pancreatography, transhepatic cholangiography, or liver scanning may be helpful in defining the level of injury. To avoid missing injuries, one should investigate any bile staining seen at initial exploration, and one should explore hematomas in the vicinity of the biliary tree.

Injuries to the gallbladder and cystic duct should be managed by cholecystectomy. If the extent of injury is not fully apparent, a cholangiogram is recommended to exclude injury to the common or hepatic duct. If the patient is unstable or the liver cirrhotic, alternatives to cholecystectomy include simple repair and cholecystostomy. Routine drainage is recommended in cases of cholecystectomy for trauma.

Eighty percent of injuries to the extrahepatic biliary tree involve the common bile duct or common hepatic duct. Simple lacerations involving less than one half the circumference should be primarily repaired and drained by a T-tube. Preferably, the T-tube exits the duct by a separate incision rather than through the repair.

Complete divisions and near transection should be repaired in a tension free manner and with minimal dissection to preserve the blood supply. Injuries to the biliary tree are repaired when discovered, preferably at the initial operation if the patient is assumed to be stable enough to undergo repair. Tension and ischemia of the repair will lead to the development of a stricture of the duct. Transection injuries to the right or left hepatic duct, common hepatic duct, or common bile duct are repaired by drainage into a defunctionalized jejunal limb. An acceptable alternative is creation of a choledochoduodenostomy when applicable. Repairs should be stented and drained. Stents are left in place for 3 to 4 weeks. Whether to include cholecystectomy is controversial; however, removal of the gallbladder is recommended if the patient is stable. The gallbladder ceases to function after a choledochoenteric anastomosis because it is unable to fill adequately. The most likely reason for malfunction is absence of backpressure from the excluded sphincter.

The portal vein should be repaired when injured. It is almost never a solitary injury, and the mortality of patients with portal vein injury is 40%. The most preferable repair technique is lateral venorrhaphy; however, ligation has been reported by one author to be feasible if repair seems impossible or unsafe. Interposition grafting using synthetic or autogenous material has been performed with success. On occasion, division of the neck of the pancreas is safe and may afford better visibility of the junction of the superior mesenteric vein and splenic vein to form the portal vein. In general, portacaval shunting for injuries to the portal vein should be a last resort if no other technique is available or signs of portal hypertension are evident.

During exploration of the abdomen for blunt trauma, hematomas of the suprarenal retrohepatic area are occasionally discovered. By virtue of its presence, exploration of the area may seem warranted. Interestingly, routine exploration of nonexpanding, retrohepatic hematomas often reveals only venous injuries at the cost of increasing blood loss, time of operation, and, on occasion, necessitating the placement of the atriocaval shunt for vascular control. In a small number of patients, nonexploration of this area has been successful in these circumstances. The success of this technique is attributed to the low pressure of the venous system.

SUMMARY

The propensity of the injured liver for major hemorrhage must be recognized. CT scanning adequately demonstrates the extent of hepatic injury and allows identification of those patients with minimal injury. Isolated minor injuries in stable patients may be safely observed; however, one must be ever vigilant for signs of associated injuries and clinical deterioration. Suture hepatorrhaphy, though appropriate for the less extensive injuries, is not recommended for large, actively bleeding fractures. In this circumstance, tractotomy (if necessary) and selective vascular ligation is preferred. Massive bleeding from hepatic injury may be complicated by hypothermia and a dilutional coagulopathy. In this circumstance the operation should be rapidly terminated. Perihepatic packing and towel-clip closure of the abdomen are helpful in this situation. Complications after liver injury include hemobilia, perihepatic fluid collection, abscess, and biliary fistula. Management of injuries to the biliary tract include primary repair if less than half the circumference is involved. More serious injuries require defunctionalized jejunal limb drainage. Portal vein injuries should be repaired, however, when necessary ligation is well tolerated.

SUGGESTED READINGS

Burch JM, Feliciano DV, and Mattox KL: The atriocaval shunt: facts and fiction, Ann Surg 207:555-568, 1988.

This paper is an excellent review of 31 patients with retrohepatic venous injuries requiring placement of the shunt. Emphasis is on decision making, technique, and pitfalls.

Defore WW et al: Management of 1,590 consecutive cases of liver trauma, Arch Surg 111:493-497, 1976.

The summary of 1590 patients with liver injuries seen in a major urban trauma center is presented. Management techniques, mortality, and morbidity are emphasized.

Franklin RH, Bloom WF, and Schoffstall RO: Angiographic embolization as the definitive treatment of posttraumatic hemobilia, J Trauma 20:702-705, 1980.

Embolization is the preferred therapy for hemobilia. Infarction of the liver, distal to the embolized vessel, does occasionally occur but does not seem to be a problem.

Geis PW et al: The fate of unruptured intrahepatic hematomas, Surgery 90:689-696, 1981.

Nonoperative treatment is recommended initially. Late complications may occur up to 28 days later.

Ivatury RR, Rohman M, and Stahl WM: Liver packing for uncontrolled hemorrhage: a reappraisal, J Trauma 26:744-753, 1986.

Used only for severe injuries, the mortality was 60%, and 80% of patients developed an intraabdominal abscess.

Mays ET: The hazards of suturing certain wounds of the liver, Surg Gynec Obstet 143:201-203, 1976.

This is a review of the consequences of suturing deep fractures of the liver. Complications include hemobilia, secondary hemorrhage, sepsis, and liver failure. Emphasis is on selective vessel control and drainage.

Moore EE: Critical decisions in the management of hepatic trauma, Am J Surgery 148:712-716, 1984.

This is a concise and well-written review by an experienced trauma surgeon from a major metropolitan trauma center.

Oldham KT et al: Blunt liver injury in childhood: evolution of therapy and current perspective, Surgery 100:542-549, 1986.

A combination of CT scanning and good clinical judgment will lead to successful nonoperative management of hepatic trauma in children. Major complications occurred in 8% of patients; 21% of patients required a transfusion; the incidence of hollow-viscus injury was 1.1%.

Pachter HL et al: Experience with the finger fracture technique to achieve intrahepatic hemostasis in 75 patients with severe injuries of the liver, Ann Surg 197:771-778, 1983.

37% of 200 patients had extensive injuries. With this technique the mortality was about 5%.

Pachter HL et al: The management of juxtahepatic venous injuries without an atriocaval shunt: preliminary clinical observations, Surgery 99:659-575, 1986.

Using extensive finger fracture, 5 consecutive patients survived. The mortality of hepatic venous injuries repaired by use of the atriocaval shunt is 60% to 100%.

Sheldon GF et al: Management of injuries to the porta hepatis, Ann Surg 202:539-545, 1985.

Vascular injuries are repaired primarily, and repair of ductal injuries may be delayed. Hepaticojejunostomy is recommended for hepatic duct injury.

32 Fulminant Hepatic Failure

S.C. Pappas

Fulminant hepatic failure (FHF) is the term used to refer to the syndrome that arises as a result of major hepatic dysfunction in a person in whom there is no identified antecedent hepatic dysfunction. The definition has incorporated the development of hepatic encephalopathy (HE) occurring within a defined period of time after initial symptoms (usually jaundice), with the most commonly proposed time period being 8 weeks. However, a syndrome of FHF with late-onset HE is well recognized, and this syndrome has been variously referred to as subacute hepatic failure or, preferably, subfulminant hepatic failure. Despite their overlapping pathophysiologic and clinical features, the distinction between fulminant and subfulminant hepatic failure may be important, since certain causes of liver failure may be associated more commonly with a subfulminant course and the prognoses of the two disorders may differ. For the purposes of discussion, the term "fulminant hepatic failure" will be used in this chapter to include both fulminant and subfulminant hepatic failure except where practical differences may be important. It is proposed that fulminant hepatic failure refer to the syndrome of liver failure with hepatic encephalopathy occurring within 2 weeks after the onset of symptoms and that the term "subfulminant liver failure" allude to the occurrence of HE 2 to 24 weeks after the initial symptoms. These definitions are certainly not perfect because a syndrome of FHF can be the initial manifestation of chronic liver disease as is seen occasionally in patients with Wilson's disease or delta superinfection in a patient with chronic hepatitis B. Fortunately, from the practical point of view the clinical features and management of these types of patients closely resemble those of patients with more clearly defined FHF.

ETIOLOGY

The most important causes of FHF are listed in Table 32-1. The various causes of FHF can be grouped into the four types indicated: infection with acute viral hepatitis, toxic liver injury, vascular or ischemic insults to the liver and a group of miscellaneous disorders. Viral hepatitis is the commonest cause of FHF in North America, generally accounting for 50% to 75% of all cases. Toxic liver injury is the second commonest cause of FHF, accounting for 15% to 40% of cases in most series. Acetaminophen is uniformly the

Table 32-1 Causes of fulminant hepatic failure

Group		Examples
I	Infection	Viral hepatitis A, B, C, D, E, cytomegalovirus, herpes simplex
II	Toxins	Acetaminophen, halothane, valproic acid, mushroom poisoning
III	Vascular or ischemic	Budd-Chiari syndrome, systemic hypotension, hypoxemia
IV	Miscellaneous	Metabolic (Wilson's disease, tyrosinemia), neoplastic (metastatic liver disease), autoimmune liver disease, microvesicular steatosis syndromes (fatty liver of pregnancy, tetracycline), others

commonest drug implicated in most series though this varies from country to country. Mushroom poisoning is a well-recognized cause of FHF in Continental Europe. Vascular or ischemic injury of the liver is actually believed to occur quite commonly but is not usually identified as a patient's primary diagnosis, since the injury occurs in patients with multiple medical problems, which overshadow the presence of FHF (such as massive myocardial infarction with cardiogenic shock). Budd-Chiari syndrome, or acute veno-occlusive disease of the liver, account for less than 2% to 5% of cases of FHF in most series. Although in part the etiology of FHF is not relevant to the subsequent complications, prognosis, and supportive management, there are several important cause-specific considerations. For example, the prognosis of the 0.05% to 0.1% of patients with hepatitis A who develop FHF appears to be better relative to other causes of FHF, with survival rates of up to 40% having been reported. On the other hand, the mortality of patients with FHF caused by sporadic hepatitis C has been higher than that with either hepatitis A or B. This may in part reflect a higher percentage of such cases presenting as subfulminant hepatic failure with a longer interval between the onset of jaundice and the occurrence of HE. Acetaminophen has uniformly been reported as the cause of FHF associated with the most favorable prognosis, with an overall survival rate of approximately 50%. In addition to the relationship between cause and prognosis, certain causes of FHF merit special consideration in regard to treatment. For example, orthotopic liver transplantation is probably the most appropriate therapy in a young person with Wilson's disease or acute Budd-Chiari syndrome presenting as FHF. Intravenously administered acyclovir may be of value in the rare patient with FHF caused by herpes simplex infection, and in contrast to other causes of FHF, antithrombin 3 infusion may be useful in the management of accompanying coagulopathy in patients with acute fatty liver of pregnancy. It also seems reasonable to employ corticosteroids in drug-induced FHF accompanied by a hypersensitivity syndrome as may occur with halothane or phenytoin hepatotoxicity. In children with inborn errors of metabolism and FHF (i.e., with galactosemia, tyrosinemia) specific dietary therapy should be started. The cause is certainly an important consideration when one is contemplating orthotopic liver transplantation for FHF with considerable controversy remaining regarding the appropriateness of this procedure in patients with fulminant viral hepatitis. For example, there is a high 40% to 80% 1- and 2-year posttransplantation mortality in patients undergoing transplantation for liver disease related to delta virus. This represents a much poorer outcome compared to patients undergoing transplantation for acute hepatitis C or hepatitis B infection alone. Finally, the recognition of neoplastic liver disease as the cause of FHF will considerably alter the therapeutic approach.

PATHOLOGY

The pathologic appearance of FHF is usually that of extensive hepatocellular necrosis involving adjacent acini and leaving residual islands of surviving hepatocytes, many of which show features indicative of hepatic regeneration. Liver injury however may not always be overt, and a more focal hepatocyte necrosis may be the only histologic abnormality demonstrated. In acute fatty liver of pregnancy or tetracycline-related FHF, the liver injury is characterized by microvesicular fat with the liver dysfunction occurring as a result of impaired organelle function. This is reflected in the accompanying observation that patients with these disorders tend to have modest increases in serum transaminases and lesser degrees of hyperbilirubinemia; patients with Wilson's disease and FHF may have similar features.

The precise pathophysiologic condition of the various complications that ensue when the liver fails remains unclear. The pathophysiologic mechanisms operative are best discussed within the context of the various clinical features of FHF.

CLINICAL MANIFESTATIONS

Hepatic Encephalopathy (HE)

As suggested by its inclusion in the definition of FHF, hepatic encephalopathy (HE) is one of the cardinal features of the syndrome. In general the clinical features of HE in FHF are very similar to those of HE complicating chronic liver disease, and the same clinical grading system may be employed. Patients with stage IV HE (coma) should be further described in terms of a coma-grading scale such as the Glasgow coma scale or equivalent. Increasing neurologic depression is the general clinical course with progressive FHF though in children and young adults agitation or hypomania may occur with the earliest stages of HE. Seizures and myoclonus, uncommon features of HE with chronic liver disease, may occur in up to 5% to 10% of patients with FHF. Electroencephalographic (EEG) changes include a progressive reduction of the usually dominant alpha-wave rhythm and the occurrence of increased theta-wave activity with paroxysmal slow waves. This results in the pattern of so-called triphasic waves. It has been proposed that the occurrence of triphasic waves is associated with a poor prognosis, but there are little data to substantiate this. If triphasic waves are seen and found to demonstrate decreasing amplitude without a return to normal EEG frequencies with stage IV HE, this usually indicates the development of increased intracranial pressure, and this pattern is a particularly ominous sign.

Surprisingly, despite intensive studies, the precise neural mechanisms leading to HE remain unclear, with several theories in existence. As with studies of HE in chronic liver disease, interest has recently focused on the potential role of the γ-aminobutyric acid (GABA)–benzodiazepine receptor in HE complicating FHF.

Cerebral Edema

Although clearly the occurrence of cerebral edema in FHF may be of relevance to HE, this particular complication of FHF is probably best discussed as a separate entity. Cerebral edema is a frequent postmortem finding in FHF because 60% to 80% of patients dying with FHF demonstrate histologic cerebral edema; Cerebral edema has been implicated as the cause of death in approximately 50% of such patients through the mechanism of brainstem coning. Intracranial pressure (ICP) measurements in patients with FHF and stage IV HE have demonstrated that over three fourths of patients with FHF and hepatic coma have raised ICP, probably as a result of cerebral edema. One must keep in mind that raised ICP does not necessarily equate with the presence of cerebral edema since ICP may also be increased as a result of increased vascular volume within the intracranial space. For example, cerebral blood flow is increased in FHF, and this appears to result from a relative cerebral vasodilatation; this may be associated with an increased vascular volume leading to elevated ICP. However, from a practical point of view, in patients with FHF it is probably safe to assume that the finding of raised ICP in large part reflects the presence of cerebral edema. The clinical manifestations of raised ICP in patients with FHF are those that are typical of most patients with raised ICP of other causes. The main neurologic signs that may indicate a raised ICP are listed in the box below. The clinical assessment of possible cerebral edema is difficult however because some of the typical signs such as papilledema, vomiting, and bradycardia may be absent in patients with FHF or occur so late as to be little more than manifestations of a terminal agonal state. The placement of extradural pressure transducers to monitor ICP certainly allows the diagnosis to be made in the absence of typical clinical findings, but the value of the routine use of such monitoring has not been rigorously assessed (see p. 624-625). The availability of an ICP measurement does allow the precise calculation of cerebral perfusion pressure, which one can calculate by subtracting ICP from mean arterial pressure. Optimal cerebral function requires a cerebral perfusion pressure greater than 60 mm Hg, and lower values may occur as a result of raised ICP acting in concert with a lower than normal mean arterial pressure.

The pathophysiologic features of cerebral edema of FHF remains controversial. It is unclear whether this cerebral edema is a vasogenic type occurring as a result of damage to the blood-brain barrier or

FINDINGS THAT MAY BE PRESENT IN PATIENTS WITH FULMINANT HEPATIC FAILURE AND RAISED ICP

- Decreased level of consciousness (usually stage IV hepatic encephalopathy)
- Absent or abnormal pupillary light reflexes
- Absent or abnormal oculovestibular reflexes
- Seizure activity, myoclonus
- Hypertension, bradycardia
- EEG asymmetry

whether it occurs as a result of a cytotoxic mechanism that might occur as the result of an entry of toxins through an intact blood-brain barrier causing the cellular accumulation of water; it is quite conceivable that both mechanisms are operative. The autoregulation of cerebral blood flow appears to be intact in FHF, despite some increase in total cerebral blood flow, until the very terminal stages when there may be a loss of normal autoregulatory mechanisms.

Coagulopathy

Bleeding is a potentially severe problem in FHF and a significant coagulopathy occurs in virtually all patients. Clinical evidence of bleeding occurs in 50% to 80% of patients, with the major site of blood loss being from the upper gastrointestinal tract. Other common sites include skin puncture sites, the nasopharynx, lungs (particularly in intubated patients), and retroperitoneal areas; bleeding from the last site may be difficult to diagnose without a high index of suspicion and the appropriate imaging studies, which may include ultrasonography or abdominal CT scanning. Since the liver is capable of synthesizing almost all coagulation factors except for factor VIII and some of the inhibitors of coagulation and fibrinolysis, the coagulopathy of FHF is a result of factor deficiency. A low-grade disseminated intravascular coagulation (DIC) may be demonstrated in most patients with FHF though the role of this, if any, in causing a bleeding diathesis is unclear. Abnormal platelet production and function are well documented to occur with FHF and certainly contribute to the bleeding diathesis.

Hypotension

Approximately 50% of patients with FHF demonstrate systemic hypotension with a systolic blood pressure less than 90 mm Hg. This hypotension may be the result of gastrointestinal bleeding or cardiopulmonary dysfunction in some cases, but in about 60% of cases the cause of hypotension is not apparent. The decrease in mean arterial pressure is associated with a decreased total peripheral resistance and a relative bradycardia and an increased cardiac output, the pattern resembling the hemodynamic picture of sepsis. Indeed, a factor that may be responsible for the hemodynamic picture may be spontaneous endotoxemia with a consequent reduction in peripheral resistance and increased capillary permeability. Raised ICP and pulmonary dysfunction with hypoxemia may also contribute to causing the hemodynamic derangements.

Lactic acidosis with a raised mixed venous lactate greater than 2.5 mmol/L occurs in 60% to 70% of patients with FHF and was initially attributed to disordered lactate metabolism resulting from decreased liver function. However, more recent studies have indicated that the lactic acidosis is more likely related to a "covert" tissue hypoxia occurring at the microcirculatory level and involving splanchnic and extrasplanchnic vascular beds. Accordingly, this type of lactic acidosis is not directly correlated with the occurrence of systemic hypotension and may not improve with maneuvers to correct any obvious hemodynamic derangements. Hyperlactatemia with refractory metabolic acidosis is a particularly ominous sign in patients with FHF.

Cardiopulmonary Complications

Respiratory failure is reported to occur in 30% to 60% of patients with FHF, with the adult respiratory distress syndrome occurring in about one third of patients. The latter is correlated with the severity of the accompanying coagulopathy and most commonly occurs in patients with raised intracranial pressure and presumably cerebral edema. The pulmonary wedge pressure is low and an increased lung vascular permeability is believed to be an important pathophysiologic mechanism for the occurrence of noncardiogenic pulmonary edema. Intrapulmonary arteriovenous shunting of blood contributes to the occurrence of hypoxemia and may occur in the absence of pulmonary edema. A variety of arrhythmias occur in patients with FHF and include sinus tachycardia and bradycardia, supraventricular tachyarrhythmias, atrial fibrillation, ectopic beats, and heart block. These arrhythmias generally reflect inadequate myocardial oxygenation.

Acid-Base and Electrolyte Disturbances

Respiratory alkalosis is the most common derangement of acid-base balance occurring in FHF with 80% to 100% of patients demonstrating a mild respiratory alkalosis. This probably results from a direct stimulation of the respiratory center by some as yet unidentified substance that accumulates because of liver failure. A metabolic alkalosis may supervene when severe vomiting or hypokalemia occurs. Hypokalemia is a most important electrolyte abnormality occurring with FHF because it may be severe and exacerbate the predisposition to hepatic encephalopathy. Interestingly, the mechanisms responsible for the occasionally severe hypokalemia that occurs with FHF are unclear but may be related to a relative hyperinsulinism that drives serum potassium into the intracellular compartment of tissues. This may be compounded by a fundamental disturbance of intracellular electrolyte handling favoring the trapping of potassium within cells. Urine potassium excretion may also be increased, with the mechanism by which this occurs being unclear. Serum sodium tends to be low in patients with FHF though hypernatremia may also occur. Hyponatremia may result from actual loss of total body sodium in the urine or as a result of the administration of hypotonic fluids, commonly glucose solutions.

Renal Dysfunction

Some form of renal dysfunction occurs in approximately 50% to 80% of patients with FHF. Prerenal azotemia as a result of overvigorous diuresis or hemorrhage may occur. Acute tubular necrosis (ATN) may also occur as a result of prolonged volume contraction, or ATN may supervene after a period of so-called "functional renal failure" of FHF. The latter is part of a spectrum of renal dysfunction typified by established hepatorenal syndrome. This progressive renal failure is associated with avid sodium retention and hyperosmolar urine. This functional renal failure probably occurs as a result of intense renal vasoconstriction related to a disturbed prostaglandin mechanism in conjunction with putative circulating vasoactive substances that result in reduced renal cortical perfusion. From the clinical point of view, a typical scenario is of a patient with FHF presenting with prerenal azotemia, which initially can be corrected with volume replacement but with the subsequent development of an increasing serum creatinine and a urine sodium less than 10 mEq/L despite euvolemia. After a variable period with this functional renal failure, the patient develops further increasing serum creatinine associated with high urinary sodium greater than 40 mEq/L and an active urine sediment indicative of ATN.

Hypoglycemia

Hypoglycemia with a blood glucose of less than 2.8 mmol/L (50 mg/dl) occurs in upwards of 40% of patients with FHF though this is not clinically apparent. Severe hypoglycemia is actually not common with FHF and probably occurs in less than 10% of patients. Hypoglycemia arises as a result of depleted liver glycogen stores and impaired gluconeogenesis with relative hyperinsulinemia. The clinical features of hypoglycemia are the usual findings of increasing obtundation, and frank hypoglycemia can mimic or aggravate the manifestations of HE. Hypoglycemia can develop rapidly, particularly in children, and may be relatively refractory to correction even when relatively large volumes of glucose are administered. Its presence is easily determined using bedside Dextrostix estimations.

Pancreatitis

Clinical acute pancreatitis occurs in less than 10% of patients with FHF and is associated with the usual clinical features of epigastric pain, nausea, and vomiting. The serum amylase is elevated in 25% to 30% of patients with FHF, with postmortem examination of the pancreas demonstrating hemorrhage and fat necrosis in approximately 40% of patients dying with FHF. The precise pathophysiologic features involved are unclear, but it is likely that the acute pancreatitis arises as a result of multiple factors including impaired pancreatic microcirculation, concomitant sepsis, hypoxemia, and associated coagulopathy.

Infection

In most series of patients with FHF, bacterial infection has occurred in 25% to 50% of patients. Common sites of infection include the respiratory and urinary tracts in addition to spontaneous gram-negative bacteremia and spontaneous bacterial peritonitis. The clinical manifestations of infection are usually not present or are attributed to other specific complications of FHF. Septicemia is often clinically inapparent, and a high index of suspicion must be maintained; the surveillance for infection must include the routine bacteriologic examination of blood, urine, sputum, and stool samples even in the absence of clinical features suggestive of infection. Systemic candidiasis complicating FHF has been described, particularly in patients receiving H_2-receptor antagonist drugs for the prophylaxis of gastrointestinal tract bleeding. The reduction in gastric acid production predisposes to gastric overgrowth with *Candida* organisms, and systemic candidiasis appears to result from impaired defense mechanisms. Diminished opsonization resulting from a decreased level of serum complement and defective leukocyte chemotactic function contribute to the propensity to infection.

DIAGNOSIS

The diagnosis of the syndrome of FHF is not difficult as suggested by the clinical definition of the disorder. Severe failure of normal hepatic function is associated with hyperbilirubinemia, and the presence of jaundice immediately draws attention to the diagnostic consideration of FHF. It has been suggested in the literature that established FHF with HE may occur without obvious jaundice though precise figures indicating the incidence of this are not available. In the experience of most clinicians the sequence of HE preceding jaundice is extremely rare if it occurs at all. The diagnostic efforts in patients with

FHF should be directed toward establishing the specific cause, and a battery of diagnostic tests to assist in this regard may be performed. The remaining investigations that should be conducted can be grouped within two categories consisting of (1) tests to evaluate the degree of hepatic function and injury as well as complications of FHF (assessment tests) and (2) tests that need to be performed as part of an appraisal for subsequent orthotopic liver transplantation (pretransplant tests). These tests are listed in the box at right. Remember that it is not necessary that all tests be carried out in every patient. It is also important to note that some of these tests must be requested on an urgent basis and this will include tests that are not normally ordered as such (e.g., hepatitis serology, urine copper excretion). Finally, regular monitoring with serial investigations, including frequent neurologic assessment, is extremely important and particularly relevant for the assessment of blood glucose. It is recommended that Dextrostix estimations or their equivalent be performed hourly in patients with a progressive clinical course because the treatable complication of hypoglycemia may develop rapidly and may go unrecognized in patients with stage IV He as described previously.

MANAGEMENT

A checklist for the management of patients with FHF is presented in the box on p. 623. The treatment of FHF can be divided into supportive care and specific therapy. The overall managements of patients with FHF involves the application of aggressive intensive-care surveillance and nursing with the general principle that such treatments should take place in

THE INVESTIGATION OF PATIENTS WITH FULMINANT HEPATIC FAILURE (FHF)

Diagnostic tests

Viral hepatitis serology
Acetaminophen levels, drug screen
12- or 24-hour urinary copper excretion, serum ceruloplasmin
Peripheral blood film examination for evidence of hemolysis
Autoimmune serology
Abdominal ultrasonography
(Transjugular liver biopsy)

Assessment tests of hepatic function and injury or complications of FHF

Blood glucose, electrolytes, urea nitrogen, creatinine
Arterial blood gases, electrocardiogram, chest radiograph
Bilirubin, AST, ALT, alkaline phosphatase, albumin
Prothrombin time, partial thromboplastin time (with or without coagulation screen including thrombin time, fibrin degradation products
Factor VII levels
Serum amylase
Urine electrolytes
Blood, urine, sputum, and stool cultures
Electroencephalogram, CT scan (head)
(Transjugular liver biopsy)

Pretransplant tests

Blood group typing and reserve
Echocardiogram
HIV serology
CT scan (head)

> **CHECKLIST FOR THE MANAGEMENT OF PATIENTS WITH FULMINANT HEPATIC FAILURE**
>
> 1. Admit to intensive care unit
> 2. Notify laboratory, blood bank, liver transplantation team
> 3. Perform detailed base-line neurologic assessment
> 4. Obtain appropriate diagnostic, assessment, and pretransplant tests (see box on p. 622).
> 5. Order serial testing of prothrombin time, blood glucose, liver biochemistry, and renal function
> 6. Institute indicated supportive management (Table 32-2)
> 7. Consider specific therapy (if available)

specialized intensive care units preferably associated with a liver transplantation service. There are data available supporting the contention that the application of standard intensive care is the major factor responsible for the increased survival of patients with FHF over the past 10 to 20 years.

Supportive Care

The major complications of FHF and their treatment are summarized in Table 32-2. As can be seen, the treatment of the individual complications of FHF are not intricate or exotic; the tendency for multiple problems to occur simultaneously or within short periods of time leads to the complexity of management. For example, patients with pronounced hypokalemia may require large volumes of fluid to correct this important electrolyte imbalance resulting in fluid overload as a consequence of associated renal failure. This may further exacerbate pulmonary edema, and the resulting hypoxemia may impair cardiac function. Systemic hypotension may ensue, further compounding the problem of renal failure. Complications that in other patients might be regarded as minor and easily treatable may well be the first step in a cascade culminating in multisystem organ failure in the patient with FHF. A few specific comments should be made with regard to certain aspects of supportive therapy. Hypokalemia may be particularly severe, and although the majority of patients require 150 to 200 mEq of potassium per day, up to 600 mEq of potassium per day is necessary in some patients. In general, treatment of hyponatremia is not indicated and should be reserved for those patients with profound hyponatremia (serum sodium levels less than 110 mEq/L) and in whom worsening neurologic deterioration may be attributed to this electrolyte abnormality. Dialysis is useful in the management of fluid overload, hyperkalemia, and metabolic acidosis of FHF with the usual indications for dialysis prevailing. Peritoneal dialysis may be performed in patients with FHF and indeed may be preferable because of the avoidance of the need for anticoagulation. However, experience with this supportive therapeutic measure in FHF is limited. Prophylactic antibiotic therapy for the prevention of systemic infections is not recommended in patients with FHF, and, similarly, prophylactic treatment of the coagulopathy of FHF is not indicated. Fresh frozen plasma and platelets may be administered at the time of any invasive procedures, and vitamin K should be given by slow intravenous infusion on admission and weekly thereafter, since a liver recovering

Table 32-2 Complications of fulminant hepatic failure and their management

Complication	Treatment
Hypoglycemia	IV glucose (300 gm of glucose/day, minimum)
Hypokalemia	IV potassium chloride (150 to 200 mEq/day)
Hyponatremia	Hypertonic saline not usually required
Renal failure	
Metabolic acidosis	Dialysis
Fluid overload	
Hypoxemia	Assisted ventilation
Pulmonary edema	
Infection	Antibiotics for identified infection
Increased intracranial pressure	Mannitol (1 gm/kg of body weight)
Hypotension	IV fluids, vasopressors if indicated
Gastrointestinal bleeding	Sulcralfate suspension, 1 gm q6h by nasogastric tube or H_2-receptor antagonist IV 3 times daily or equivalent
Coagulopathy with bleeding	Vitamin K Fresh-frozen plasma, platelets, blood
Disseminated intravascular coagulation	Heparin not usually indicated
Pancreatitis	Nasogastric suction, IV fluids, nothing by mouth
Hepatic encephalopathy	Zero protein intake initially Lactulose (if gastrointestinal bleeding present)
Seizures	Diazepam 2 to 5 mg IV as required Pentobarbital for status epilepticus

from massive hepatic necrosis may be responsive to vitamin K at a later point in time even when previous administration was not effective. Active bleeding must clearly be treated, with the general principle being that of attempting to ameliorate the coagulopathy and stop bleeding as opposed to attempting to correct coagulation tests. For example, it may be possible to correct coagulation test abnormalities by the administration of large volumes of activated clotting factors, but this often results in volume overload and potentially the exacerbation of the low-grade disseminated intravascular coagulation that may occur with FHF. Prophylaxis for gastrointestinal tract bleeding should clearly be employed, since this now represents the second commonest cause of death in most series; the administration of cytoprotective sulcralfate suspensions via nasogastric tube (1 gm qid) would appear to be the optimal prophylactic treatment, since this obviates the need to adjust systemic drug doses to account for impaired hepatic metabolism and may be associated with a lower incidence of nosocomial pneumonia particularly in the intubated ICU patient. Analogous to the treatment of coagulopathy and hyponatremia, the systemic hypotension accompanying FHF should be treated only if the systemic blood pressure is sustained below a level of 80 to 90 mm Hg in concert with deteriorating renal function or obvious neurologic deterioration. Again, treatment aimed to arbitrarily increase the blood pressure to within the normal range may involve the administration of large volumes of fluid, which may exacerbate the tendency to pulmonary edema and left ventricular failure. When indicated, short courses of vasopressor drugs may be administered, particularly when cerebral perfusion pressures demonstrate a sustained fall below 60 mm Hg.

The most difficult complication of FHF to treat is the problem of raised intracranial pressure (ICP), and this currently represents the commonest cause of death in these patients. It has been demonstrated that steroids and controlled hyperventilation are of no value in the treatment of raised ICP in FHF. Mannitol administered as a bolus of a 20% solution at a dose of 1 gm/kg of body weight to a maximum of 100 gm is effective for treatment of sustained increases in ICP above a range of 20 to 30 mm Hg for more than 5 minutes. This therapy can be repeated as indicated but should not be continued if a favorable clinical response is not present, direct ICP monitoring demonstrates a lack of response, or there is renal failure with oliguria. Thiopental-induced coma and pancuronium bromide (Pavulon)–induced paralysis have been employed in patients with FHF as adjunctive measures for the control of raised ICP and appear to be of some benefit in patients with high ICP measurements (generally over 30 mm Hg) not responsive to mannitol or in patients with renal failure in whom mannitol cannot be given. Experience with this type of therapy is limited. A major problem with the management of raised ICP is that it may escape detection even with meticulous surveillance by repeated neurologic examination. Although intuitively it would seem that the placement of extradural pressure transducers is quite reasonable, there are no data to support their routine use at present and their placement is not without risk.

The treatment of HE complicating FHF is not significantly different from that for treating HE in chronic liver disease, with the most important principle of therapy being that of the identification and treatment of exacerbating factors. Although lactulose or neomycin therapy is commonly employed in the setting of FHF, there are no good data demonstrating the value of these agents in FHF. Lactulose should probably be reserved for those patients with an associated gastrointestinal tract hemorrhage where a cathartic effect may be of benefit. The temptation to use sedative or hypnotic drugs should be avoided as much as possible, despite the common occurrence of hypomania or aggressive combative behavior particularly in children or young adults with stage II-III HE. Seizures must be treated, however, if they are repetitive, and conventional treatment can be undertaken with the general principle that the drugs employed should be used in doses adjusted for the presence of hepatic failure. Diazepam appears to be the safest drug to employ in this setting, with doses of 2 to 10 mg administered intravenously generally being all that is required. Recurrent refractory seizures usually indicate pronounced ICP increases though alternative causes for the seizure activity should be sought (e.g., intracranial hemorrhage or infection, hypoglycemia). Anecdotal reports have recently described the benefit of a benzodiazepine receptor antagonist drug in ameliorating HE in FHF and offer some prospects for future therapies.

Specific Therapy

Unfortunately, clinicians have little choice with regard to specific therapy, if any, that can be employed in the management of patients with FHF. Evidence is available demonstrating the lack of efficacy of corticosteroids (perhaps with the exception of halothane or phenytoin-induced FHF) and regular exchange transfusions, and these therapeutic measures should not be employed. Postdilution hemofiltration and newer plasma exchange procedures using techniques of on-line plasma separation and replacement have been performed in patients in FHF with favorable results, and these approaches would appear to require further study. Charcoal hemoperfusion has not been demonstrated to be effective when studied within the context of a properly controlled clinical trial, and although attempts at developing an effective artificial hepatic support system continue, the use of these techniques cannot currently be routinely advocated. Prostaglandin administration (e.g., PGE_1) has been reported to be of benefit in patients with fulminant viral hepatitis, but the precise role of this therapy in patients with FHF remains unclear.

Orthotopic liver transplantation can be carried out in patients with FHF, and indeed accumulated data have indicated that this procedure may be successful in improving survival rates in FHF to approximately 55% to 60%. Accordingly, in general, most patients with FHF should be considered for liver transplantation as soon as the diagnosis is made and stage IV HE supervenes. Exceptions of course would include patients with acetaminophen ingestion in a suicide attempt where this type of aggressive specific therapy might be difficult to justify on ethical grounds though clearly cases must be considered on an individual basis. Furthermore, higher survival figures for patients with FHF related to acetaminophen, even with stage IV HE, argue against liver transplantation in this group of patients. Delta hepatitis–related FHF appears to have a favorable short-term outcome when treated by liver transplantation, but the poor long-term posttransplant survival statistics noted above probably do not justify the routine transplantation of such patients. Patients with Wilson's disease or Budd-Chiari syndrome and FHF appear to be the best patients to treat by use of liver transplantation. In addition, the high mortality for patients with subfulminant hepatic failure, particularly related to viral hepatitis C, and the frequent occurrence of decompensated chronic liver disease in those patients that do survive, indicates that these patients would benefit most from liver transplantation. The major problems with this form of specific therapy at the current time include organ availability, determining the precise timing of the operation, and the identification of factors predictive of fatality in patients with FHF to facilitate patient selection (see below). Of patients with FHF awaiting transplantation, 25% to 40% die before an organ becomes available. Equally as important, 15% to 20% of patients with FHF in whom a decision has been made to perform a liver transplantation improve while awaiting a donor organ and subsequently survive, underscoring the need to more effectively select patients who would most benefit from this procedure.

Prognostic Factors Outcome and Sequelae

The management of patients with FHF would be considerably facilitated by the identification of clinical or laboratory features identifying those patients who are unlikely to survive and thus be considered for a specific therapy such as artificial hepatic support or liver transplantation. It is not surprising that mortality tends to be greater the deeper the stage of HE or with the presence of one or more of the complications cerebral edema, renal failure, and noncompensated or refractory metabolic acidosis. Children with FHF appear to have a better survival in comparison to adults. The type of cause appears to affect outcome as noted earlier. Several laboratory tests have been examined for their prognostic value. The prothrombin time is probably the single best test; although as an independent variable that can be applied as a clinically useful measurement in individual patients, even this test is limited. Unfortunately, serial measurements of α-fetoprotein and factor VII levels have not proved to be widely applicable clinically useful prognostic indicators though factor VII estimation may be of some value. Factor VII levels greater than 9% were associated with 100% survival in one study (with 95% confidence limits for a predictive value being 54% to 100%). The increasing use of the transjugular route to obtain hepatic tissue in patients with FHF despite a pronounced coagulopathy has provided some prognostic information in FHF. In a normal liver, hepatocytes average 80% to 85% of the total volume of tissue. It appears that when this volume falls to below 35% to 40%, the survival rate is greatly reduced compared to patients with a higher percentage of hepatocytes. It has been suggested that this information may be helpful in determining the need for and the timing of liver transplantation. For this reason, if available, transjugular liver biopsy should probably be attempted in most patients with FHF. The diagnostic value of a transjugular liver biopsy in patients with FHF remains unclear though presumably the tissue obtained could be used to establish a specific cause (e.g., the findings of nuclear inclusion bodies and herpes simplex antigen–positive immunoperoxidase staining in a case of herpes hepatitis–related FHF).

The outcome of patients with FHF remains poor, with the survival rate for patients with stage IV HE treated with supportive care alone being approximately 20% to 35% in most recent series. The inclusion of liver transplantation as part of therapy has resulted in some additional improvement, with survival rates of 60% to 70% being reported in patients who ultimately undergo liver transplantation. If one considers patients dying while awaiting a donor organ, overall survival rates are in the neighborhood of 45% to 55% in terms of short-term survival. It is interesting that 30% to 40% of patients dying from FHF have evidence of hepatic regeneration at postmortem examinations, an indication that the potential for survival was present. The antemortem identification of such patients would identify them as the optimal patients whom artificial liver support would benefit.

In general, survivors of FHF demonstrate a complete return of liver function to normal without the development of chronic active hepatitis or cirrhosis. The latter two entities appear to develop in over 50% of patients with subfulminant hepatic failure, however, an indication that these patients are the ones most likely to require additional subsequent specific therapy if available (e.g., immunosuppressive therapy for autoimmune chronic active hepatitis). In addition, this type of patient may well be best managed with orthotopic liver transplantation as noted above. With the spontaneous recovery of liver function, overt neurologic sequelae appear to be quite rare. The precise incidence of minor degrees of neurologic impairment after FHF is unknown though it appears to be less than the reported 30% incidence of persistent neurologic problems (mental retardation, spasticity, seizure disorder) reported to occur in survivors of Reye's syndrome with deep coma, a somewhat analogous clinical syndrome.

SUMMARY

Fulminant hepatic failure remains among the most challenging syndromes encountered in clinical medicine. The majority of cases are related to acute viral hepatitis or toxic liver injury with the remainder attributable to a large number of miscellaneous disorders. Regardless of cause, the pathologic condition observed is usually that of extensive hepatocellular necrosis with microvesicular steatosis characterizing the liver injury in some settings. The clinical manifestations that arise as a result of FHF involve multiple organ systems, and the complications that ensue often lead to multiorgan failure. Chief among these complications is the problem of raised intracranial pressure, which is associated with the development of cerebral edema such that, currently, this remains the most difficult problem to treat and the one most commonly responsible for death. The management of patients with FHF involves the aggressive application of supportive care aimed at correcting the multiple complications that occur. Specific therapy most commonly involves orthotopic liver transplantation, a therapy that has resulted in the best survival statistics up to now. In view of the fact that many patients dying with FHF have postmortem evidence of hepatic regeneration, efforts to develop artificial hepatic assist devices are continuing. In contrast to patients with subfulminant hepatic failure in whom there is a high incidence for the subsequent development of decompensated chronic liver disease in survivors, patients with FHF who recover do very well without residual sequelae. It is hoped that with a better understanding of the pathophysiology of FHF, particularly with reference to the problem of raised intracranial pressure, newer approaches to the therapy of this serious clinical problem will develop.

SUGGESTED READINGS

Bernuau J, Rueff B, and Benhamou JP: Fulminant and subfulminant liver failure definitions and causes, Semin Liver Dis 6:97, 1986

The authors give a detailed description of the reported causes of FHF with a complete reference list.

Ede RJ and Williams R: Hepatic encephalopathy and cerebral edema, Semin Liver Dis 6:107, 1986

This is a very well-referenced discussion of the problem of cerebral edema in FHF with the presentation of important clinical observations.

Martin P and Pappas SC: Fulminant hepatic failure, Dig Dis, 8(3):138, 1990.

This is a well-referenced review article on the clinical aspects of FHF.

O'Grady JG, Gimson AES, O'Brien CJ, et al: Controlled trials of charcoal hemoperfusion and prognostic factors in fulminant hepatic failure, Gastroenterology 94:1186, 1988.

Two controlled trials with a large number of patients studied and a concise analysis and discussion regarding prognosis related to causes and complications are presented. The accompanying editorial by Berk and Goldberg in the same issue provides an important perspective from which studies in FHF may be interpreted.

Pappas SC: Fulminant hepatic failure. In Bayless TM, editor: Current therapy in gastroenterology and liver disease—2, Philadelphia, 1986, BC Decker Inc.

This is an overview of the practical management of patients with FHF.

Schafer DF and Shaw BW: Fulminant hepatic failure and orthotopic liver transplantation, Semin Liver Dis 9:189, 1989.

This is a concise review of the authors' experience with this treatment modality with some practical clinical recommendations and discussion; key references are provided.

33 Transplantation of the Liver

Byers W. Shaw, Jr.

You have come to the final chapter of this book. If you have arrived here not after a thorough reading of the preceding chapters (all excellent works by recognized authorities) but rather after a brief peek at their contents, you should be forgiven. You are obviously a scholar of the 1990s, and you recognize where the solutions lie. You know that all that has preceded this chapter is mostly anguish over the singular incapacity of Medicine (as a science) to either prevent or adequately treat most of the more common forms of end stage liver disease. This is the only reason that this chapter remains relevant.

Lest you mistake chagrin for arrogance, let me add perspective. We all know the old saw about the value of prevention over cure. In heeding this maxim, Medicine has become a war of biochemistry. The greatest battles are won by learning to control the interactions of molecules. The public health worker who daily adds fluoride to the city water supply of the Bronx does more for the health of the public tooth than do all the dentists in Manhattan. Closer to home, a few good scientists have already shown us how mere micromoles of the right antigen can confer immunity against type B hepatitis and thus do more to eliminate liver disease than can all the liver transplant surgeons in Pittsburgh. We should never lose sight of the real goal of Medicine. In essence, after the final victory over molecules, we should no longer have a need for transplant surgeons . . . or dentists.

In the meantime, I must support my claim that all treatment featured in the preceding chapters is just procrastination. In the following pages, I discuss the status of liver transplantation in the treatment of liver disease, including indications and contraindications, techniques and regimens, new developments and future concerns. Permeating much of this discussion is a certain foreboding imparted by the specter of increasing demand in the face of limited supply.

INDICATIONS FOR LIVER TRANSPLANTATION

A graphic breakdown of the diseases for which liver transplantation is an effective treatment is presented in Figure 33-1. These data are taken from a report of the Pittsburgh-United Network for Organ Sharing (PITT-UNOS) Liver Transplant Registry summarizing the experience

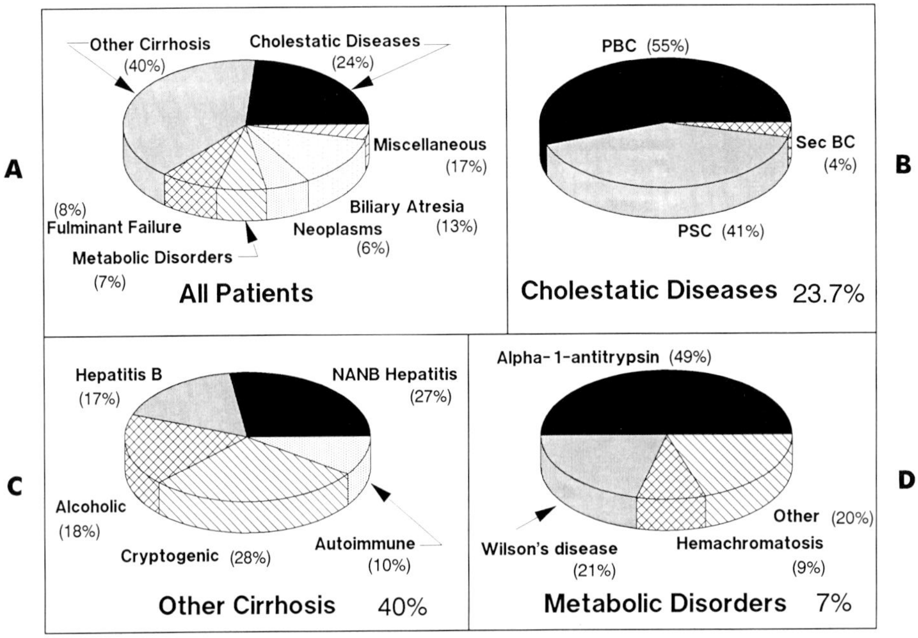

Figure 33-1
A, Primary disease categories for liver transplantation in 1377 recipients reported to the PITT-UNOS Liver Transplant Registry, October 1, 1987 through September 30, 1989. Percentages represent fraction of the total number of patients for each diagnosis category. **B** to **D,** Breakdown of cholestatic diseases, other cirrhosis, and metabolic disorders into specific diagnoses. Percentages are for the fraction of the patients in each category.

with 1377 liver transplants performed between October 1, 1987, and September 30, 1988. The most common diagnosis among adult patients was the "other cirrhosis" category (39.8%), with cirrhosis secondary to non-A, non-B hepatitis (some of which will be proved by retrospective testing to be type C hepatitis) representing 10.9% of all patients who underwent transplantation. The most common single diagnosis among all patients was primary biliary cirrhosis (13.1%), with biliary atresia second (12.7%). Biliary atresia was the most common diagnosis among children receiving liver transplantation, representing 84% of the patients 5 years of age or younger reported to UNOS. Primary sclerosing cholangitis was also an important disease entity among adults. Among metabolic disorders, α_1-antitrypsin deficiency is the most common followed by Wilson's disease with all other metabolic disorders combined representing fewer than 2% of all cases. Of those patients who received transplantation primarily for treatment of neoplasms, hepatocellular carcinoma represented the most common tumor type, with cholangiocarcinoma being second.

Fulminant hepatic failure represents an indication for emergency transplantation. The causes of fulminant failure include viral infection, drugs and toxins, and metabolic disorders (e.g., Wilson's disease and hereditary tyrosinemia).

Any disorder that can cause liver failure should be considered a possible indication for transplantation. However, controversy exists regarding the role of liver transplantation in the treatment of hepatic malignancies. For the most part, this controversy arises because of the relative ineffectiveness of any other treatment modality. Thus, even though the 2-year survival rates in this group of patients average only 20% to 30% in most series, remarkable long-term survival has been obtained in cases believed hopeless without transplantation.

Because of the high rate of recurrence in the hepatic allograft, type B hepatitis was at one time believed to represent a contraindication to liver transplantation. However, long-term survival rates after transplantation for this disease range from 50% to more than 80% in different series. A review of several series, including my own, reveals that conversion to a negative serologic result occurs very rarely. Seroconversion has not been reported after transplantation in recipients who are hepatitis B e antigen positive. Among those who remain surface antigen (HBsAg) positive, approximately 2 in 7 will develop significant liver dysfunction and either require retransplantation or die, 3 in 7 will experience recurrent acute hepatitis and go on to develop chronic hepatitis with minimal to mild symptoms, and the remaining 2 in 7 will become so-called healthy carriers with no apparent clinical activity. The coexistence of recurrent rejection episodes with recurrent hepatitis presents a difficult challenge. Deaths occur from hepatic failure or from sepsis associated with both overimmunosuppression and hepatic failure. The role of passive immunoprophylaxis with specific hepatitis B immune globulin has not been defined. Likewise, the use of α-interferon has not yet proved efficacious in transplant recipients with recurrent chronic hepatitis.

CONTRAINDICATIONS TO LIVER TRANSPLANTATION

Patients with acquired immunodeficiency syndrome (AIDS) or AIDS-related complex (ARC) and patients with failure of another vital organ system that is deemed not treatable by any medical or surgical measures should not undergo liver transplantation. The latter group would include patients with advanced cardiac or pulmonary failure who are not candidates for transplantation of the heart or lungs. It would also include patients with documented cerebral death. The latter might seem an obvious contraindication, but the necessity of documenting that cerebral death has **not** occurred **before** transplantation is sometimes overlooked in emergency situations such as in the treatment of fulminant hepatic failure.

In the past, authors mentioned advanced age, portal vein thrombosis, a history of multiple procedures in or around the liver, sepsis, and the presence of extrahepatic malignancy as contraindications to liver transplantation. By the late 1980s none of these factors should independently exclude a patient from transplantation. Nevertheless, each of these complicating variables can contribute to increased morbidity and mortality, and each must be considered important modifiers in any decision regarding candidacy for transplantation.

By 1990, several centers had reported a positive experience with liver transplantation in older patients. At our own center, we have performed liver transplantation in 21 patients over 60 years of age, 4 of whom were 65 or older. Overall, 17 of 21 have survived (81%). However, when one looks at those patients who were not hospitalized in the intensive care unit at the time of transplantation, survival is 17 of 19 or 89%. Although the numbers of patients are small, the observation that only three of these patients have developed a rejection episode after transplantation indicates that advanced age may have a desirable effect on the immune response to an allograft. However, the potential disadvantage of this apparent blunted immune response is a lower tolerance for infectious complications. Older patients must also go through a thorough search for prohibitive risk factors resulting from age-related diseases of other organ systems.

Experience providing transplantation for patients with documented portal vein thrombosis also removed this problem from the list of contraindications. In virtually every case, portal vein inflow to the allograft can be obtained from mesenteric venous collaterals or from the superior mesenteric vein (SMV) itself. In a recent 48 year old patient with complete thrombosis of the portal vein, SMV, and splenic vein, the donor portal vein was anastomosed end to side with a huge gastroepiploic vein running along the inferior border of the gastric antrum. Because one can almost always find a vein that will provide adequate long-term mesenteric inflow to the liver allograft, I do not consider portal vein thrombosis a contraindication to transplantation.

Liver transplantation also has provided dramatic recovery from multiorgan failure and sepsis in patients with advanced liver failure. In these cases, rapid treatment (transplantation) is mandatory. A protracted pretransplant course is associated with death from superinfection, antibiotic-resistant organisms, or invasive fungal infection. Careful judgment is required in assessing the suitability of these patients for transplantation.

The recent literature contains three reports of palliation of metastatic neuroendocrine tumors with liver transplantation. In Pittsburgh, 3 of 5 such patients survived the procedure with a median survival of 12 months. On the other hand, the known experience with liver transplantation for treatment of metastatic pancreatic, colonic, or other adenocarcinomas reveals no cases of long-term cure and death from recurrence within 2 years in 90% of patients.

DONOR-RECIPIENT MATCHING

Except for an occasional case report, all 5000+ liver transplants performed in the United States during the past 4 years were orthotopic. For those who cannot remember their Greek, that means that the native liver was removed and the new graft was put in the same location.

In matching donors and recipients, the current policy at most centers is to follow the general rules of blood group compatibility. No one has attempted, on a large scale or as a matter of principle, to achieve the best tissue match. In addition, a compatible lymphocyte crossmatch, though an absolute requirement in kidney transplantation, is not regarded as necessary in liver transplantation. However, a recent report from Iwaki in Pittsburgh suggests that preformed antibodies may affect graft survival in liver transplantation, a phenomenon not observed in any previous study.

The penalty for crossing a blood group barrier is not well documented. The Pittsburgh group has reported a higher incidence of hepatic arterial thrombosis in small children who received blood group–incompatible allografts. On the other hand, several centers cross blood-group barriers in situations of critical need. Our own policy is to consider blood-group A2 donors compatible with all blood groups, the same as with O blood type but different from the A1 subgroup. Blood group–compatible but nonidentical donor-recipient combinations carry the risk of graft vs. host (GVH) phenomena, including major hemolytic reactions. However, GVH disease is usually self-limited and responds to increased immunosuppression.

In orthotopic transplantation, one also needs to be wary of donor-recipient size discrepancies. A general rule-of-thumb is to match donor and recipient weight within 20% of one another. However, body weight is a very imprecise reflection of liver size. Tall thin donors will yield much larger allografts than short obese donors with the same weight. I have also learned that obese recipients have a great deal less intraabdominal space than their thinner counterparts. Massive abdominal ascites or hepatomegaly often provide enough extra space to allow such recipients to accept a much larger donor liver than one would normally accept on the basis of body weight.

THE OPERATIVE PROCEDURE

Some surgeons will claim that taking out the old liver is the hardest part and the rest of the operation is easy. This is, in a word, nonsense. The worst cases usually develop after an ill-advised comment from an errant assistant who, wanting to reassure the wistful anesthesiologist, blurts out an overly optimistic estimate of a finish time. I remain deeply superstitious. The best cases are the ones I approach with utmost trepidation and then find surprisingly straightforward. Humility seems to exact a lesser punishment than does pride.

The Initial Dissection

Previous surgery on or around the liver leads to adhesions of bowel, omentum, and the abdominal wall to the liver. In the face of portal hypertension, these adhesions become the site of extensive collateralization between the mesenteric venous system and the systemic venous system. I often encounter veins 1 to 2 cm in diameter running between the liver and the abdominal wall or coursing from the omentum to the liver surface and up to the site of the previous incision. With appropriate patience, this phase of the operation will take more time but not significantly more transfused blood than in patients without previous surgery. Several publications have not shown a relationship between previous abdominal surgery and either operative blood loss or mortality after transplantation.

The more common recipient factors affecting both operative blood loss and mortality are indicators of the severity of liver failure before transplantation. This was well documented in a study of preoperative risk factors published in 1985. Massive ascites, severe encephalopathy, and very high serum bilirubin (>35 mg/dl) were independent and covariant variables associated with both greater blood losses and higher 6-month mortality after transplantation in adults.

In effect, the goal of the initial phase of the recipient operation is to isolate the native liver so that it can be removed by the simple expediency of clamping and dividing the bile duct and three blood vessels (the inferior vena cava above and below the liver, the portal vein, and the hepatic artery). In most cases, I remove a small segment of the intrahepatic vena cava with the native liver. I cut the septa between each hepatic vein and the inferior vena cava to create a single, large opening for anastomosis with the upper vena cava of the donor liver. For preparation of the native hepatic artery, I usually dissect as far proximal as the origin of the splenic artery. Many times, the take-off of the gastroduodenal artery is a widened area of the common hepatic artery that I can open and fashion into a trumpeted end that serves as a good size match for the celiac axis of the allograft. Many times I will leave a rim of native aortic wall around the celiac origin (a Carrel patch) to match the fluted end of the native artery. This allows the creation of an anastomosis that is at least as wide if not wider in diameter than the proximal and distal vessels. I believe this is important in reducing the incidence of arterial thrombosis.

What about bypass?

In adults, I routinely use a venous bypass during the anhepatic phase. Several publications have described the technique and hemodynamic advantages of this adjunct. I do not believe that selective use of a bypass is either practical or warranted. Routine use has eliminated any time penalties and is not associated with any increased risk to the recipient. Venous bypass is not necessary to successful transplantation as several years of excellent results preceding its introduction had already shown. However, it maintains normal hemodynamics during the anhepatic phase. This allows the opportunity to extend the anhepatic time for upwards of several hours, if necessary, to allow accomplishment of certain technical tasks (such as obtaining complete hemostasis in the hepatic bed). Bypass provides an important advantage in patients with cardiac dysfunction, particularly those with high-output cardiac failure related to long-standing severe portal hypertension or those with severe pulmonary hypertension associated with cholestatic liver disease. Venous bypass has also aided in the extension of the upper age limit for liver transplant candidacy.

Insertion of the bypass tubing is a simple task. I expose the greater saphenous vein and the axillary vein through small cutdowns in the groin and axilla respectively. The cannula that carries blood from the infrahepatic vena cava is inserted through the greater saphenous vein and positioned in the ipsilateral common iliac vein. A second, larger cannula is placed into the portomesenteric venous system either through the cut end of the portal vein or through the inferior mesenteric vein. Two groups have reported using the latter technique and claim that it has advantages in allowing the surgeon to perform the portal vein anastomosis without having to discontinue portal venous bypass and remove the cannula. Although it carries theoretical advantages, this extra step has not appeared to be necessary in our practice.

Venous bypass is not indicated in children undergoing liver transplantation. This applies to most patients under 11 to 13 years of age and to all patients less than 40 kg in weight. Unlike adults, children exhibit almost no perceptible hemodynamic changes during the anhepatic phase and, even without venous bypass, do not require vigorous volume expansion to maintain adequate systemic blood pressure. I have speculated that this may be related to the greater capacity in children of both normal and abnormal (associated with portal hypertension) collateral channels to accommodate the need for increased flow during the anhepatic phase. We also recognize that children simply might have a more efficient compensatory response than adults to the hypovolemia associated with sudden interruption of venous return from the inferior vena cava.

Rapture and judgement

If a liver transplant surgeon's *raison d'être* is doing liver transplants, then his apotheosis is performing the vascular anastomoses. For many (and no less so for the patient!) it may also be the moment of truth. If all that precedes the vascular anastomoses has gone well, if the surgical field has remained under the surgeon's control, and if the surgical team is properly organized, any surgeon with vascular experience can sew in the new liver. I will describe briefly our preferred technique. This is probably similar to the steps taken by most liver transplant surgeons.

The suprahepatic vena cava anastomosis is performed first followed by the lower or infrahepatic vena cava anastomosis in a similar end-to-end fashion. While the surgeon is sewing the latter anastomosis, the donor liver is flushed with cold 5% albumin solution (500 ml in patients over 40 kg of body weight, 250 ml for those under 40 kg) through a cannula in the donor portal vein. This serves two purposes: (1) it flushes out the preservation solution, and (2) it displaces air in the donor vena cava segment with fluid. Both the high potassium content and the adenosine in the UW solution have been implicated as causes of cardiac arrests occurring at the time of revascularization of the liver in the recipient.

The portal vein anastomosis is completed next. The portal vein bypass cannula is clamped and removed from the cut end of the recipient portal vein, and the vein is clamped as far proximal as possible in the recipient. The donor portal vein is cut to proper length and sewn end to end to the native vein. Finding the correct portal vein length is critical in preventing thrombosis.

In most cases, I prefer to restore flow to the liver immediately after completing the portal vein anastomosis. Release of the three clamps is coordinated with the anesthesiologists. In an effort to prevent cardiac arrest, they usually premedicate the recipient with a calcium compound, sodium bicarbonate, and, when hyperkalemia is severe, glucose and insulin. They also ready their batch of resuscitation drugs in case of arrest. We routinely have defibrillation paddles immediately available beside the operating table at the time of revascularization.

The portal vein clamp is released first and then the lower vena cava clamp, followed by the suprahepatic clamp. This order is not critical, and surgeons vary somewhat in their beliefs about the proper order. My own thought has simply been to release the most accessible vessels first so that if massive bleeding occurs from an unrecognized open vessel in the liver, the inflow can be reclamped immediately. Others have argued in favor of unclamping the outflow vessel first in order to avoid venous congestion in the donor liver. We have done it both ways, can see no difference in early graft function, and so do what seems easiest.

Once all vessels are unclamped, a quick search is made for important bleeding sites. Those are the ones that, provided that the anesthesiologist is not engaged in a cacophonous display of displeasure, the surgeon can hear. Venous bypass should be discontinued as soon as it is clear that reclamping of the vena cava is not necessary. The next step is the arterial anastomosis.

Much has been written about the causes of arterial thrombosis in the hepatic allograft. The anastomosis involves two small vessels and is a bit more challenging than joining big, forgiving veins. If the anastomosis clots off, it causes two problems, only one of which is important. The first problem involves the unwitting recipient. Because the newly transplanted liver does not have any source for collateral flow, early arterial thrombosis usually leads to necrosis of the liver. Retransplantation is often the only recourse. The other problem is the surgeon's and probably accounts for the reason so much has been written by surgeons about arterial thrombosis: a clot in a vessel anastomosis implies something about the skill of the anastomoser.

Some events that are not directly related to the anastomosis and that increase the likelihood of arterial thrombosis include polycythemia (e.g., overtransfusion, hemochromatosis, polycythemia rubra vera), a hypercoagulable state (e.g., malignancy, antithrombin III deficiency, thrombocytosis, protein C deficiency), or recipient vascular disease (e.g., atherosclerosis, intimal dissection, celiac axis stenosis, anatomic anomalies). However, most of these conditions should not appear as surprises during the evaluation of an episode of arterial thrombosis, since they are all either preventable or treatable conditions. Other factors implicated as causes of arterial thrombosis include endothelial injury during reperfusion or from immunologic attack.

In any event, arterial thrombosis is a potentially lethal complication. It is almost always preventable, usually has a technical cause, and should occur in fewer than 5% to 10% of a center's experience. The impact of arterial thrombosis has been lessened by recent experience with early detection and operative thrombectomy. For example, we have salvaged seven grafts using this approach, reducing the retransplantation rate for arterial thrombosis from 6% to less than 2% in our series.

After the arterial clamps are released, the artery should have an easily palpable thrill. In adults, especially older patients or any patient with autoimmune disease, the recipient vessel should be carefully inspected for any sign of intimal dissection. Ultimately, the surgeon must be absolutely certain of the quality of arterial inflow before completion of the operation. He can use other measures, such as intraoperative Doppler ultrasonography or arteriography to evaluate more fully suspected problems.

Penance and atonement

A question frequently asked by patients is, "How long does a liver transplant take?" The answer is or should be, "It depends." And although it depends on multiple factors, it usually depends most on what happens after revascularization.

If the anesthesiologist has been adept at doing everything necessary to maintain normal coagulation, if the new liver begins working immediately, and if the surgeon has kept the operative field dry up to the point of revascularization, the operation can be completed within an hour (or less than 2 hours) after revascularization. A thorough search for anastomotic bleeding or for bleeding from open vessel branches should take very little time provided that the rest of the operative field does not begin to bleed profusely. The most common causes of the latter disappointment are thrombocytopenia, fibrinolysis, or consumptive coagulopathy. The distinction between the various forms and causes of coagulopathy that appear at this stage is sometimes subtle and blurs even further when one realizes that the problem is usually a combination of events. The operative personnel, working together as a closely knit team, usually solve the problem the same way that the crew of the starship *Enterprise* always seemed to get out of a particularly hopeless fix: the surgeon's call for "more clot, Scotty . . . give me more clot!" is followed by the anesthesiologist's plaintive "Aye, Captain, but I've given it all she'll take!" Somehow, the surgeon puts enough suture in the right places, the anesthesiologist gives just a little more of the right factor, good triumphs over evil, Klingons are vanquished, and the bleeding suddenly stops. Although much has been written about the causes and treatment of the coagulopathies associated with liver transplantation, experience indicates that most of those authors know somewhat less about their subject than Mr. Roddenberry does about warp drive and Klingons.

The keys to successful passage through the revascularization phase include (1) anticipation of bleeding disorders, leading to early (if occasionally unnecessary) treatment; (2) frequent use of methods for assessing the status of coagulation, including the thromboelastograph or the Sonoclot device; (3) proper timing of both diagnostic tests and therapeutic maneuvers; and (4) specific treatment. The experienced anesthesiologist recognizes that within a few minutes of revascularization, none of the tests of coagulation performed only 20 minutes earlier are valid. An experienced surgeon can also provide useful information by noting whether clots are forming and whether lysis of previously formed clots has taken place and by ensuring that all "surgical bleeding" (the kind that requires sutures) has been eliminated.

Who Was Achilles?

Several years ago, I was performing the biliary reconstruction during a liver transplant procedure when the medical student playing third hook on my left, who was until then quiet and perhaps ruing her offer to help out, suggested that I probably could leave and let the surgery resident and her finish this relatively trivial part of the operation. In answer, I quoted the recently (at the time) knighted Sir Roy Calne of Cambridge by stating that the biliary reconstruction was the "Achilles heel of liver transplantation." I took the brief silence that followed as arising from contemplation of this Hellenic metaphor. That we had uncovered a problem that night that ran deeper than knowledge of things surgical became evident when the student's barely audible "*Whose* heel?"

was pushed aside on my personal scale of alarm by the senior surgery resident's attempt to fake an answer having something to do with a Renaissance anatomist who first knew about tendons in the heel and a former center for the Boston Celtics who always had trouble with his. Although we learned very little about biliary anastomoses, we did review how a lapse in attention to details, either in baptisms or biliary tract procedures, might eventually prove lethal.

Comments on the content if not the quality of modern education aside, Sir Roy was referring to an incidence of biliary tract problems that at the time exceeded 50% in the Cambridge series. This included major leaks and obstructions and carried a 25% to 30% mortality in both the Cambridge and Denver series. Calne in fact adopted for transplantation a technique first described by Waddell that made use of the gallbladder to form a conduit between donor and recipient ducts. Perhaps because the lower doses of steroids used after the introduction of cyclosporin A promoted better tissue healing and perhaps because of greater experience, both the incidence and the impact of biliary tract complications have fallen dramatically in the last decade. Recent studies that include all postoperative problems involving the bile duct report an incidence of 12% to 18% and mortality rates (independent of biliary necrosis associated with arterial thrombosis) at less than 1 in 50.

The problems that present within 1 to 14 days of transplantation include biliary leaks (around the T-tube insertion site in 7 of our 23 cases of biliary tract complications) and migration or dislodgment of the T-tube. Biliary obstruction at this stage is extremely rare but can occur in association with an expanding mucocele of a cystic duct stump (donor or recipient) or because of an injury to the donor bile duct either at the time of the donor operation or during implantation. These surgical errors, and others involving initial placement of stents or tubes, should be discovered by use of routine cholangiography after completion of the biliary reconstruction. If neither a T-tube nor a cystic duct stump is available for injection of radiographic contrast material, a 25-gauge needle can be inserted into the donor duct and a cholangiogram obtained with as little as a few milliliters of contrast.

A simple duct-to-duct anastomosis can be used in patients who have a normal native bile duct of sufficient length and caliber. In patients with diseased or absent extrahepatic biliary ducts (e.g., sclerosing cholangitis or biliary atresia), a 25 to 35 cm Roux-en-Y limb of jejunum is constructed and brought up to the duct either in front of or behind the transverse colon. The end of the duct is then sewn to the antimesenteric side of the jejunum near its terminus. In constructing the choledochocholedochostomy, a T-tube is positioned in the native duct with the long vertical base of the T leaving the side of the native duct. One end of the horizontal limb is positioned across the anastomosis with its open end located just shy of the donor biliary confluence. The other horizontal limb is placed into the distal native duct but not through the sphincter of Oddi.

I use a small-caliber (8, 10, or 12 French) plastic tube several centimeters in length as a stent for performing the choledochojejunostomy. Although I used to leave this tube in place in the belief that it reduced the incidence of early strictures, I now routinely remove them (by transmural manipulation) from the duct after completion of the anastomosis. The incidence of early or late strictures associated with choldedochojejunostomy is 3.4%, about the same as the 4.6% rate seen with duct-to-duct connections, and it is not influenced by immediate removal of the stent. The stimulus for prompt removal was experience with three patients in a 4-year period who required removal of retained stents because of concretions and sludging. The stents now serve only as aids for sizing and completing a patent anastomosis, and they play no role in long-term success.

I routinely remove the gallbladder from the donor liver. Some surgeons report a lack of problems leaving it in place. The traditional teaching that the thing should come out is based on two principles: the theoretical risk of a high rate of cholecystitis in the denervated gall bladder and anecdotal experience with that very problem in the early days at Denver. Our own philosophy is that leaving it in place does not solve any problems that any of our patients have encountered and may lead to new problems that we have never encountered.

I have seen two cases of biliary obstruction arising from expanding mucoceles of a cystic duct stump. One involved a duct-to-duct anastomosis in an adult and the other a choledochojejunostomy in a child. In both cases, in the donor liver, the cystic duct had not yet joined with the common hepatic duct at the point of severance and appeared as a separate opening behind the distal terminus of the common duct. In performing the anastomosis, I purposely closed off the distal end of the cystic duct by the anastomotic sutures. Since the more proximal, gallbladder end of the cystic duct had also been ligated, this created a closed pocket of mucus epithelium. The resulting mucocele expanded and became large enough to occlude the common hepatic duct just proximal to the anastomosis with the recipient. Both cases were successfully treated by excision of the mucocele. Since then, I routinely avoid ligating the cystic duct when I see a separate lumen at the level of the biliary anastomosis.

The final puzzle about the biliary reconstruction involves the T-tube: When is the best time to remove it? We were taught that the tube should stay in a minimum of 3 months. This gave the best chance for avoiding biliary strictures, we were told, and lessened the risk of a bile leak (from the tube exit site) severe enough to cause bile peritonitis. Two years ago I increased this interval to 6 months because about 60% of patients had symptomatic bile leaks and two required operative intervention to close the small hole in the side of the native duct. This has lessened the incidence to just over 50%, but the difference is not statistically important. In the meantime, several surgeons raised on another philosophy say that they remove T-tubes at 2 or 3 weeks, never have leaks, and never have late strictures. I would like to believe they are right, but none has published confirmatory reports. In short, no good science yet dictates the art of T-tube removal. Since I have not seen any problems related to leaving the tubes in too long, I suspect the right time lies somewhere between 2 weeks and greater than 6 months.

IMMUNOSUPPRESSION

Perhaps a bit overbuoyed by his recent success in describing the triangulation technique for vascular anastomoses, Alexis Carrel in 1906 wrote an article in *Science* describing the "successful transplantation" of kidneys from one dog to another. That the single animal on which he had operated died on the ninth day was omitted from this report that described the animal on the *eighth* day as "jumping up and running around." Having later met with repeated failures in performing allotransplants in cats, he proved himself the consummate surgeon when he clarified his earlier optimism by offering the following:

> Should an organ, extirpated from an animal and replanted into its owner by a certain technique, continue to functionate normally, and should it cease to function when transplanted into another animal by the same technique, the physiological disturbance could not be considered as brought about by surgical factors. The changes undergone by the organ would be due to the influence of the host, that is, the biological factors.

Now, 78 years after Alexis Carrel became the first scientist in America to receive a Nobel Prize, we surgeons still seek solace from our failures among biologic factors. In truth, we cannot completely prevent, treat, or even reliably diagnose rejection. It remains the single most important source of failure in organ transplantation.

The battle against immunologic destruction of engrafted tissue has been fought for more than 35 years on two major fronts: suppression of the immune response and modification of the immune response to achieve tolerance. We have had success in achieving the former but would like to make immunosuppression obsolete by accomplishing the latter.

Starting in 1963, the first immunosuppressive protocol used for liver transplantation by Starzl and his group at the University of Colorado was combination azathioprine and prednisone. Although azathioprine was unacceptably hepatotoxic in dog models of liver transplantation, the Denver group already had proved the efficacy and safety of the drug in human kidney recipients. In the mid-1970s, antilymphocyte serum was used as was thoracic duct drainage. Cyclosporin A was first used in liver recipients in 1979 and became available for general use after Food and Drug Administration approval in September 1983. A mouse monoclonal antilymphocyte antibody with specific activity against CD3-positive T-lymphocytes (OKT3) has been used in liver transplantation since 1984. It can be used either during the so-called induction phase (meaning the interval of initial presentation of donor antigens to the host) or for treatment of rejection episodes. In 1988, Starzl and colleagues at Pittsburgh began using a novel compound called "FK506." This drug, a macrolide discovered in soil samples collected from Tsukuba, Japan, and produced by Fujisawa Pharmaceutical Co., Ltd., has activity similar but not identical to cyclosporin A. The Pittsburgh group has used the drug in over 500 patients, either as baseline immunosuppression or for treatment of established rejection resistant to conventional immunosuppression. In many patients, the Pittsburgh group has found that concomitant use of steroids with FK506 is not necessary. Although the new drug is nephrotoxic (one of the major disadvantages of cyclosporin), FK506 may have a wider therapeutic index than cyclosporin A does.

The same can be said of many other approaches to both prevention and treatment of rejection. Another macrolide attracting interest is rapamycin. This drug was named after the South Pacific island, Rapa Nui, from whose soil the compound was first isolated. It was originally produced as an antifungal agent but abandoned when it proved too immunosuppressive. Kahan and colleagues in Houston have shown that rapamycin is synergistic with cyclosporin in a rat transplant model. Other groups are reporting initial successes combining cyclosporin at lower than usual doses with bromocriptine or thalidomide. These investigators hope that one of these drugs will provide the extra margin of safety that azathioprine never did when combined with cyclosporin.

An increasing number of monoclonal antibodies are being made available. Clinical transplant trials are already underway involving an anti-CD4 (helper cell) antibody and an anti-Tac (a murine anti–interleukin-2 receptor antibody). Future human use of antibodies to CD2 (anti-T11 in humans, the T-cell erythrocyte receptor), to anti-TNF (tumor necrosis factor), and to CD45R and T-cell integrin may prove useful as clinical immunosuppressants.

My own thoughts are that monoclonal antibodies will be most useful as the means of manipulating an immune response once we understand that response better. We need to know more about the intricacies of the cascade of events that occur so that we will know when and where to intervene in very discrete ways. Monoclonal antibodies that target effector cells alone do not address the true complexity of the human immune response. In some instances, this is the immunosuppressive equivalent of targeting infantrymen when what we should be trying to do is negotiate a cease-fire further up the chain of command.

Recent attempts at achieving immunologic tolerance in clinical transplantation have been interesting if not conclusive. Several groups, including Barber and colleagues from Alabama, have obtained improved survival in kidney recipients who received intravenous infusion of donor bone marrow 7 days after completion of an induction course of antilymphocyte globulin. Kidney-graft survival in the treatment group (90%) was significantly better ($p < .02$) than that in the control group (71%). They did not report results of testing for donor-specific responsiveness in these recipients.

Strober at Stanford has demonstrated true donor-specific tolerance in three kidney transplant recipients treated with total lymphoid irradiation (TLI). Myburgh and colleagues in South Africa have had some success in achieving tolerance in baboons who received solid organ transplants after TLI.

Many years before cyclosporin became available, TLI was abandoned by the transplant community, largely because of its extremely narrow therapeutic window. However, our group has been encouraged by some initial experience with TLI in combination with cyclosporin and have initiated several protocols. The results of this experience are too preliminary to allow comment other than to say that the treatment has proved to be relatively nontoxic.

This decade shows promise of being the most interesting period in transplantation immunosuppression. Never since the days more than 35 years ago, when the need for immunosuppression was first recognized, have more approaches and more agents been under investigation in human trials. In his American Society of Transplant Surgeons presidential speech, Barry Kahan demanded that rigor be the guiding principle of scientific investigations during the coming years, warning that testimonial, regardless of its sincerity, not be accepted as a substitute. With so much at stake, with interest in the surgical pursuit of transplantation becoming widespread, and with the availability of donor organs falling increasingly short of new demands, his words should not be taken for granted.

TIMING IS EVERYTHING (ALMOST)

"No one cares about those details," Dr. Starzl once told me. "They only want to know the bottom line: how many survived and how many died." It was May of 1983, and we were preparing for the National Institutes of Health Consensus Development Conference on liver transplantation to be held less than 1 month later in Bethesda. He was looking over the latest summary of our survival statistics at Pittsburgh and they were not as good as he had expected and not as good as previous reports. We were searching for reasons, and he proffered this gentle admonition after I had opined that we were tackling much higher risk patients than represented in the previous analyses. Although no one could argue with the accuracy of this contention, we were able to show a distinct difference in patient survival depending on the level of care required before transplantation. Patients called in from home had a 6-week survival rate of 68% compared to only 42% for those in the intensive care unit before surgery. Another large group of patients comprised those who were in the hospital but not requiring intensive care before surgery. For reasons yet unexplained, they had an even better survival rate than the outpatient group with 86% surviving the first 6 weeks after surgery.

The second opportunity for discovering the profound effect of preoperative morbidity on outcome after transplantation occurred when we compared the survival of the first 56 consecutive adults who underwent liver transplantation with the use of venous bypass with a historical control group of 63 consecutive adult patients. Although the bypass group had a survival advantage 30 and 60 days after transplantation, by 6 months the difference in survival was not significant.

Suspecting that the advantages of bypass might be obtained mostly in the first month after surgery and that deaths after 1 month might be related to factors other than intraoperative events, I divided the two patient groups into the same three risk groups that we had defined for the NIH conference. We found that both the outpatient and the non-ICU inpatient group who underwent transplantation under bypass showed better survival at all intervals than the nonbypass group. The most disappointing finding was that the ICU-bound bypass group, though obtaining a 61% to 30% advantage over their nonbypass counterparts at 30 days (an advantage we hypothesized but could not prove was attributable to the use of bypass), experienced an alarming mortality rate during the next 60 days.

The first attempt at developing a scoring system that used patient variables (rather than location of care) was ours at

Table 33-1 The risk score developed in 1985 from a multivariant analysis of patient variables affecting survival after liver transplantation

	Risk score		
Grade or step	**Coma**	**Malnutrition**	**Ascites**
None	0	0	0
Mild/moderate	+1	+1	+1
Severe	+2*	+2	+2
Serum bilirubin >30 mg/dl			+2
Serum bilirubin <10 mg/dl			−1
Prothombin <15 seconds			−1
Patient age >40 years			−1
SUBTOTAL SCORE			—
If subtotal > 5 and age <25 years			−2
TOTAL PREOPERATIVE SCORE			—
Transfusion requirement >39 units of PRBC			+1
Preoperative score >5 and transfusion <10 units			−1
FINAL POSTOPERATIVE SCORE			—

Low risk	= 0-3 points
Medium risk	= 4-6 points
High risk	= >6 points

*For stage IV coma, score 6 points

Pittsburgh in 1985. Multivariant analyses revealed that, in adult patients, survival was highly related to severity of illness as reflected by a patient's level of encephalopathy, severity of malnutrition, ascites volume, serum bilirubin level, and prothrombin time. We also found that the amount of blood lost during the operation correlated very closely with both severity of illness and survival. In fact, the scoring system that we developed allows for a preoperative score to be modified if blood loss is either higher or lower than expected for the corresponding risk category. See Table 33-1 for an outline of the specific scoring system.

This risk score was applied to a group of patients who underwent transplantation during a 3-year period at Nebraska between 1985 and 1988. We again found the method useful in segregating high-, medium-, and low-risk patients based on preoperative variables. More importantly, we were able to show that only 45% of patients who were considered high risk before transplantation survived the first year after transplantation. The causes of death in this group were usually directly

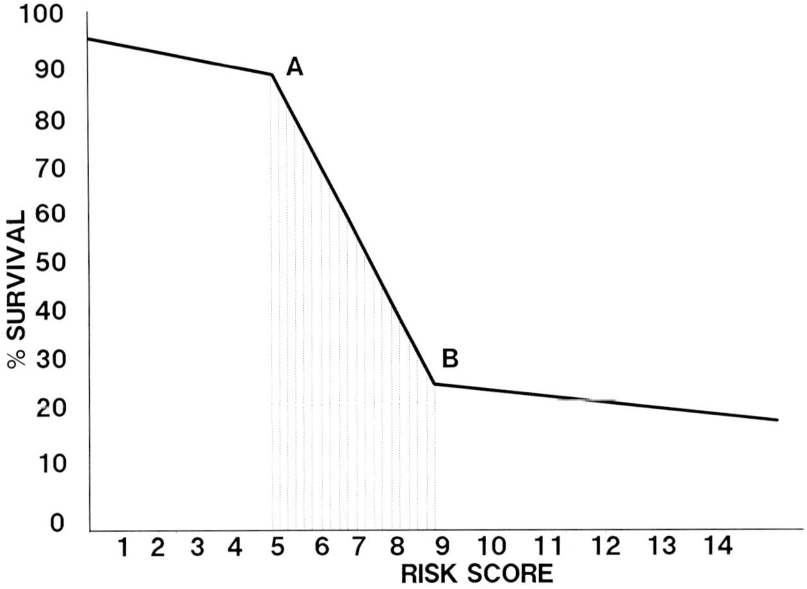

Figure 33-2
Nonlinear relationship between preoperative risk score and posttransplant mortality.

attributable to pretransplant morbidity. Low- and medium-risk patients, on the other hand, had a 85% to 91% survival rate. We could attribute almost all the deaths in this group either to unusual events or to technical errors. We also found that although the average hospital costs associated with providing liver transplantation for the greater than 90% of the low-risk patients who survived was less than \$80,000 the mean hospital costs for all high-risk patients, whether they lived or died, was greater than \$200,000

The relationship between any measure of preoperative morbidity and survival after transplantation is not linear but sigmoid in shape (Figure 33-2). This is a curve described by a third-order equation and is typical of the relationship between continuous biologic variables and their relevance as measures of risk. The two inflection points on the curve represent values of the variable associated with a sudden change in the increment of risk associated with a change in the value of the variable. In other words, at point *A* the value of variable x has reached a point where any further increase in its value is associated with a much greater decrease in the value of y than for any value of x less than that at *A*.

All that this means is that because of this particularly nonlinear relationship any scoring system that uses biologic variables to assign points will effectively separate patients (or whatever possesses the biologic variable) into two distinct groups, with a third group riding on the steep part of the curve. If the overall risk score is on the x axis and the probability of survival on the *y*, one can separate low- and high-risk patients distinctly and will have a medium-risk group somewhere in between. The relevance of this discussion is twofold. First, patients should be referred for transplantation before they get to the bottom of the steep part of the curve. Second, to the extent that small changes in the value of the risk score are associated with large changes in survival probability, the scoring system is likely to be least accurate where one would find it most useful for distinguishing risk, i.e., between the inflection points. The overall message is that early referral is better than late. I always use additional variables to make decisions about the timing of transplantation.

This relationship between survival probability and preoperative morbidity has important implications for the future. A clear understanding of this relationship must be part of any evaluation of a specific center's results in any discussion of patient selection criteria, in assessments of the costs of treatment, and in the distribution of the limited supply of donor organs. Clearly, we have not reached a point in the evolution of liver transplantation where we can categorically exclude patients on the basis of risk. However, we are reaching the point where we must begin to make difficult decisions about how we are going to ration an increasing shortfall of donor organs.

OF FISHES, LOAVES, AND LIVERS

"Look, you don't understand." A mother with a 3-year-old girl who needed a liver transplant was being interviewed by a reporter from the local newspaper. The reporter had suggested to the mother that maybe she was bitter that another child who had received extensive attention in the national news was in the operating room undergoing transplantation while her child was still waiting. Although her child had required hospitalization for several months, the mother had endured the transplantation of several other children who had either been waiting longer or were more desperately ill.

"Any attention focused on the need for donor organs will benefit all of the children waiting, including my baby. The public needs to know that from one terrible tragedy several lives can be saved. The attention this other child has gotten will increase the number of organs available for the next week or so and hopefully my little girl will be the next lucky one."

In the early 1980s when liver transplantation was a little known treatment performed at only a few centers in the world, liver allografts were procured from only a fraction of the cadaver donors that provided kidneys. The concept of multiple-organ procurement was neither understood nor widely accepted by the larger transplant community. Reports in the literature, such as ours from Pittsburgh, showing that multiple organ procurement did not jeopardize the quality of the kidneys, were important in allaying some of the fears of kidney transplant groups. But for all of the negative connotations attached to news media stories by the professional community, those very stories arguably did the most to bring the new and growing need for extrarenal donor organs into both the public and professional conscience.

In 1984, the National Transplant Act was enacted. Among other things, it called for the establishment of a national organ procurement and transplantation

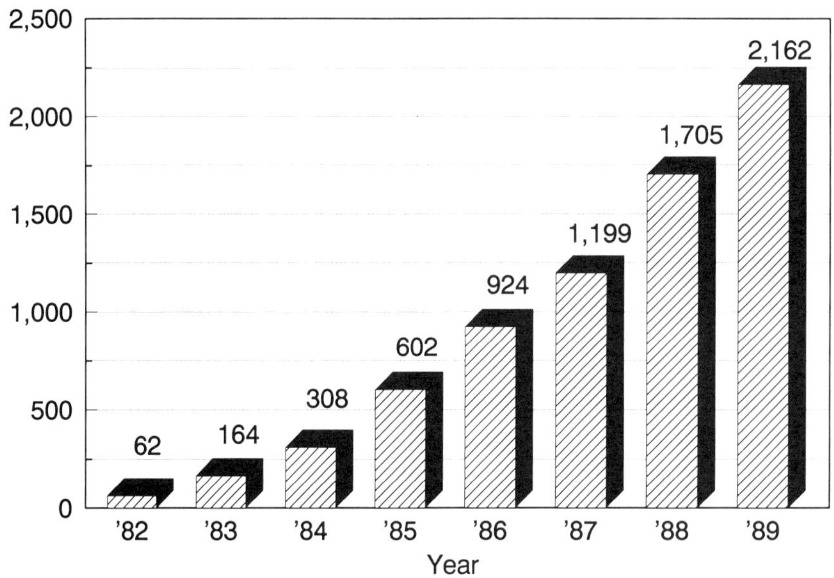

Figure 33-3
The growth of liver transplantation in the United States from 1982 to 1989.

network (OPTN) that would govern the distribution of donor organs. In addition to ensuring the fair and equitable distribution of organs, the OPTN would be required to establish criteria for transplant centers, surgeons, and physicians in all organ systems, maintain a registry of all organ donors and recipients, and establish a scientific registry in organ transplantation. In October 1987, the United Network for Organ Sharing (UNOS) began operations as the contracting agency for both the OPTN and the scientific registry.

To appreciate the growth that has occurred in liver transplantation, one only need look back over the past 9 years. In 1981, the total number of liver transplantations performed in the United States was less than 50. Figure 33-3 shows the exponential growth that has taken place since, fueled in large part by Food and Drug Administration approval of cyclosporin in September 1983. As recently as 1982, fewer than five liver transplant centers were active in this country. Early in the summer of 1990, the number had swollen to over 85, distributed across the country as shown in Figure 33-4.

The actual national need for liver transplantation is difficult to estimate. Past conjectures have yielded several figures, including (1) 20 liver recipients per year per million population and (2) 5000 patients annually nationwide who have liver disease caused by an accepted indication for transplantation and who have about a 50% 1-year survival without transplantation (suggesting that at least 2500 per year should receive transplantation).

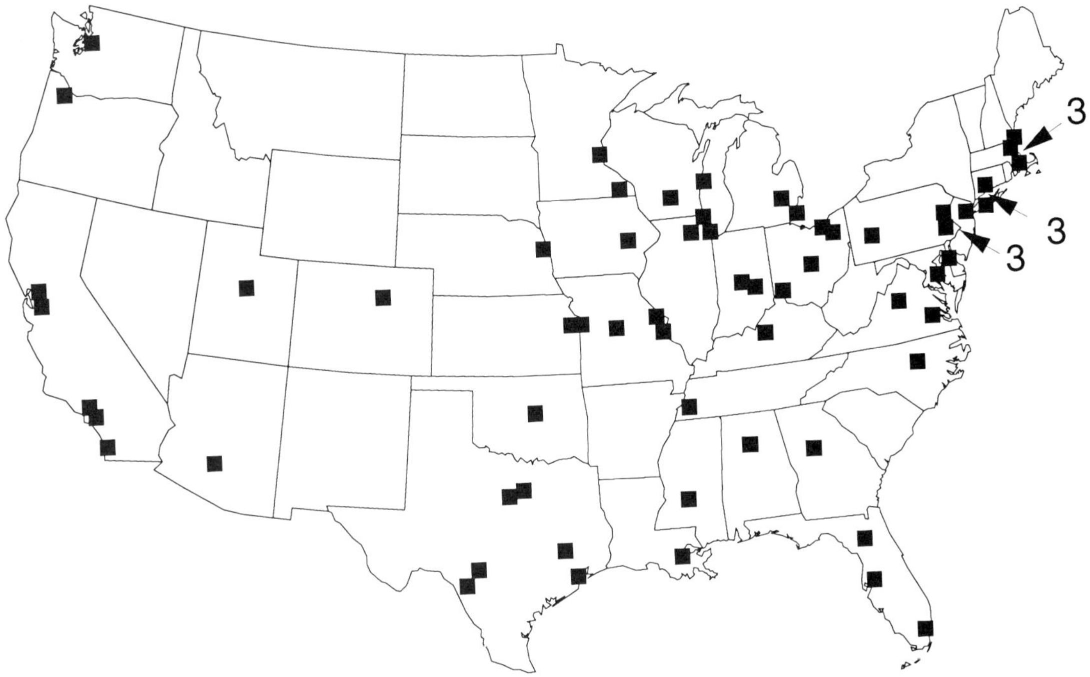

Figure 33-4
Geographical locations of liver transplant centers registered with the United Network for Organ Sharing (UNOS) as of May 1990.

Although both of these estimates have appeared in the literature, I am unaware of any recent scientific surveys that would corroborate them. In fact, since these figures have been circulating since the early 1980s, their relevance today is questionable. As I discussed earlier in this chapter, the accepted indications for liver transplantation have increased in recent years, particularly with the addition of Laennec's cirrhosis and acute hepatic failure. The conquest of such technical barriers as a thrombosed portal vein or previous biliary surgery also has resulted in an increase in the pool of potential recipients. The improved survival probabilities anticipated with the availability of better immunosuppression undoubtedly will lead to more liberalization of patient-selection criteria and even earlier referral of patients for transplantation. With the continued proliferation of transplant centers, the demand for donor livers will swell well beyond all previous estimates.

In the meantime, what of the supply? In 1989, a total of 3797 cadaver donors yielded kidneys for transplantation compared to 2365 that provided livers. At any time during 1989, between 700 and 850 patients were on the waiting list for donor livers. At a recent ASTS meeting, Gordon and colleagues reported that among the 1340 patients entered on the transplant waiting list for the University of Pittsburgh during 25 months from October 1987 to November 1989, 120, or 9.2%, died without receiving a new liver, including 12% of infants, 4% of children, and 11% of adults. Although UNOS has not released corresponding data for the national waiting list, we can only conclude that the mortality among waiting patients is alarmingly high.

We also have been dismayed by recent surveys that show a decrease in the rate of consent for organ donation. Thus far, the reasons for this apparent trend are not known. Speculation includes an increased rate of request (claiming that a greater percentage of a less willing population are being approached), an increase in the number of requests made by inexpert personnel (previous studies have shown a correlation between the success of requests and the skill of the requester), and an increasing public apathy toward organ donation and transplantation (believed to be part of a proposed new distrust of high technology medicine).

Surveys from several state organ procurement networks have suggested that legislative attempts to address the donor organ shortage may have backfired to some degree. Required request or routine inquiry legislation has been blamed for more inexpert (and often insensitive) requests having been made. A few months after the first few West Coast states enacted required request legislation, I saw a television interview of a California physician who, though once an enthusiastic recruiter of organ donors at his hospital, had become disenchanted by all of the new bureaucracy. It seems he and his colleagues were being told they were legally required to do what for many years they already had been accomplishing out of altruism. It was part of his answer to why organ donation had fallen dramatically in his community since the new legislation had gone into effect. Unfortunately, little more than theory based on such anecdotes has been proffered thus far on a national level. The transplant community must strive to foster new and continuing public support of organ donation.

The past 5 years have also witnessed several technical breakthroughs that have increased the availability of donor livers. The concept of using a portion of a liver graft to provide transplantation for children has served in small part to address the most critical shortage. Likewise, several groups, including our own, have used a single liver to provide transplantation for two recipients.

The most recent evolvement of this technology is living-donor liver transplantation. Broelsch and his group at the University of Chicago perform left hepatic lobectomy on the living parent donor and transplant the left lateral segment into the child. This technique has captured the imagination of parents terrorized by fears their child with liver disease will die before a donor organ becomes available. It also appeals to the technical instincts of the surgeon who seeks new challenges in the operating room. The capacity of this option to provide a safe and ready source of new donor organs for the teeming pool of waiting candidates remains uncertain.

One of the most important advances in the history of liver transplantation was the extension of preservation times from the 4 to 6 hours afforded by Collins' solution and its derivatives to the 24 hours possible with University of Wisconsin (UW) solution. Introduced for clinical use in 1987, UW solution affords a luxury of time that, in my opinion, has been the most important factor in extending selection criteria for cadaver liver donors. Previously the time constraints imposed by the inadequacies of preservation obviated any risk taking in the selection of organ donors. For all trips more than an hour or two drive from the transplant center, a charter aircraft was required to transport a surgical team from the transplant center to the donor hospital and back. The recipient operation was always timed so that the native liver could be removed and the donor organ implanted soon after the donor team returned. This prevented the development of any methods for assessing allograft quality before implantation, since in most cases the recipient team had crossed the proverbial Rubicon by the time the donor liver arrived at the transplant center. With the addition of a few (16 to 20) hours to the limits of safe preservation and with dissemination of skills in multiple-organ procurement, an on-site team can remove a liver allograft and send it by commercial airline (even when en route connections are necessary). The recipient team can then inspect the liver, perform a histologic examination (by either frozen or rapid-process permanent section) of a biopsy specimen, and make a decision about suitability for transplantation before ever committing the recipient to an operation. This added safety combined with a transportation price of as little as $39.95 (compared to over $10,000 for charter jet aircraft) has encouraged us to accept donor organs from donors that would have been excluded previously. This includes elderly donors (60 to 80 years of age), donors with marginal clinical histories or laboratory studies, and donors with a history of alcohol abuse. Although we are still learning the value of pretransplant histologic examination of donor livers, we feel confident we can diagnose preexisting chronic liver disease as well as extensive ischemic necrosis and macrovesicular steatosis. More sophisticated and accurate means of assessing liver graft viability before implantation will undoubtedly be forthcoming.

Several years ago, I picked up the local paper and found a picture of a bearded man in a checked shirt and blue jeans carrying a liver by the vena cava in each hand as he crossed a section of interstate highway. In the background a police cruiser diverted traffic. Scattered like giant slugs across the pavement were about three-score livers, which the caption explained had spilled out of a truck the pictured man had wrecked. The picture served as an odd reminder that we live in a time of scarcity in the face of plenty. If immunology were not such a barrier, the solution to our most irreconcilable problem might be found in mundane sources all around us.

Between 1963 and 1964, Starzl and his group in Denver performed xenotransplantation of the liver in three children. Chimpanzees served as donors. Although all three recipients died, the deaths apparently were not caused by rejection. Survival times were 26 hours and 9 and 14 days. These trials took place at a time when only a few recipients had obtained long-term survival after allograft liver transplantation.

Recent laboratory research in xenotransplantation seeks to define the role of both preformed antibodies and cell-mediated events in xenorejection. In reality, the immunologic success of concordant primate-to-human xenotransplantation would present a potentially more formidable barrier: public acceptance of the sacrifice of nonhuman primates as organ donors. Even with public approval, we likely would need 8 to 10 years to develop a renewable source of chimpanzee organs to meet the current need for donor livers. Baboons might provide a more ready source, but they represent a more discordant match for humans than do chimps. Although the most likely species combinations to yield successful results are those with the least discordance, no one has shown this in a liver model of primate transplantation.

In the absence of a clear solution to the dilemma of increasing shortage of donor organs, we are faced with a problem of rationing. If not everyone can be treated, whom should we choose to treat? The complete discussion of all the ramifications of this issue requires more space than the editors of this text would allow me, even if I did know what I was talking about. The ethics of distributive justice, as far as I can tell, would allow us to do whatever we choose as long as we follow one of the major guiding principles. We can choose to be purely egalitarian and base distribution on a first-come, first served scheme. Alternatively and somewhat at the other end of the spectrum, we can be purely utilitarian and do whatever will ostensibly provide for the greatest good. The latter approach gets a little sticky when we get into the details of just how much good we want to provide versus how much bad we want to avoid. It gets even more nasty when the ethicists start talking about assessing the social value of the persons we are talking about choosing or ignoring.

Overriding all of this drivel about distributive justice is the natural abhorrence of most physicians to accept the need for or engage in rationing. We all seek to treat the patients who desperately need our help. With liver disease, these are sometimes the poorest risk patients imaginable. We see them as having no chance without our specific treatment and find *that* stark reality to be more compelling than any more global arguments about utilitarianism. Perhaps in times of war, natural disaster, epidemics, or famine we become indoctrinated by a sense of community need that is simply inconceivable when faced with individual patients awaiting our specialized care.

These issues do not have easy solutions. On the one hand, we must have policies for organ distribution that are both equitable and logical. On the other, we have yet to devise a method that we can all agree accurately estimates survival probabilities after transplantation. Even assuming we develop such a method, what level of estimated survival should we decide is too low to warrant rationing a piece of the dwindling pie? Perhaps we make such judgments on an informal basis even now. Even so, my guess is that we have different ideas about what is hopeless. Nevertheless, equitable treatment demands that we ration on the basis of formal policies that can tolerate the most severe public scrutiny.

SUGGESTED READINGS

Broelsch CE et al: Liver transplantation, including the concept of reduced-size liver transplants in children, Ann Surg 208:410, 1988.

This is the first report of an American experience downsizing large livers for transplantation into small recipients.

Colonna JO et al: A prospective study on the use of monoclonal anti–T3-cell antibody (OKT3) to treat steroid-resistant liver transplant rejection, Arch Surg 122:1120, 1987.

A trial showing utility of OKT3 in liver transplantation is reported.

Kalayoglu M et al: Extended preservation of the liver for clinical transplantation, Lancet 1:617, 1988.

This is the early clinical report that led to a new era in liver allograft preservation.

Markin RS: Hepatic allograft pathology: evaluation of post-transplant biopsies. In Balistreri WF and Stocker JT, editors: Pediatric hepatology, New York, 1990, Hemisphere Publishing Corporation.

This is a comprehensive review of liver transplant histopathology.

Shaw BW Jr et al: Venous bypass in clinical liver transplantation, Ann Surg 200:524, 1984.

The initial documentation of the advantages of venous bypass in liver transplantation is reported.

Shaw BW Jr et al: Stratifying the causes of death in liver transplant recipients: an approach to improving survival, Arch Surg 124:895, 1989.

This is a study that categorizes deaths in a large series of adult liver recipients and then correlates causes of death, mortalities, and costs of therapy with preoperative risk score.

Sorrel MF and Shaw BW Jr, guest editors: A primer of liver transplantation for the referring physician, Semin Liver Dis 9:159, 1989.

This is a guide for the practitioner on the preoperative and postoperative care of liver transplant recipients.

Starzl TE, guest editor: Hepatic transplantation, Semin Liver Dis 5:309, 1985.

An entire volume of the journal was devoted to a series of state-of-the-art articles, still relevant years later.

Starzl TE et al: Liver transplantation with the use of cyclosporin A and prednisone, N Engl J Med 305:266, 1981.

This is the original study from Denver and Pittsburgh demonstrating a >70% 1-year survival rate in liver recipients under cyclosporin immunosuppression.

Starzl TE et al: Evolution of liver transplantation, Hepatology 2:614, 1982.

This is a landmark paper heralding the proliferation of liver transplantation therapy throughout the world.

Starzl TE et al: Orthotopic liver transplantation for alcoholic cirrhosis, JAMA 260:2542, 1988.

Data suggesting that alcoholics should not be categorically refused liver transplantation are presented.

Starzl TE et al: A flexible procedure for multiple cadaveric organ procurement, Surg Gynecol Obstet 158:223, 1984.

Complete with excellent color drawings, this article outlines the technical details of procuring multiple donor organs from the same donor.

Todo S et al: Liver, kidney and thoracic organ transplantation under FK 506, Ann Surg 212(3):295, 1990.

This is the initial experience with a new immunosuppressant in different organ systems, presented at the American Surgical Association meeting in 1990.

Hepatology 4(Suppl 1):1S, 1984.

These papers were presented at the June 1983 National Institutes of Health Consensus Development Conference documenting the efficacy of liver transplantation for the treatment of many liver disorders.

Gastroenterol Clin North Am 17:1,1988.

These are a series of papers on liver transplantation from the University of Pittsburgh.

Index

Page numbers in *italics* indicate boxed material and illustrations. Page numbers followed by *t* indicate tables.

F

N

O

P

T

U

V